D0781046

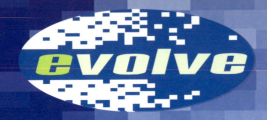

The Latest *Evolution* in Learning.

Evolve provides online access to free learning resources and activities designed specifically for the textbook you are using in your class. The resources will provide you with information that enhances the material covered in the book and much more.

Visit the Web address listed below to start your learning evolution today!

▶▶ **LOGIN:** *http://evolve.elsevier.com/phtls/*

Evolve Student Learning Resources for PHTLS: *Basic and Advanced Prehospital Trauma Life Support* offers the following great features:

- **Weblinks**
  Active websites and journal articles relevant to prehospital trauma care.

- **PHTLS Course Information**

- **PHTLS Course Materials Information**

Think outside the book... *evolve.*

PHTLS

Basic and Advanced Prehospital Trauma Life Support

"*The fate of the wounded rest in the hands of the one who applies the first dressing.*"

Nicholas Senn, Surgeon

Fifth Edition

PHTLS

Basic and Advanced Prehospital Trauma Life Support

Prehospital Trauma Life Support Committee of The National
Association of Emergency Medical Technicians in Cooperation with
The Committee on Trauma of The American College of Surgeons

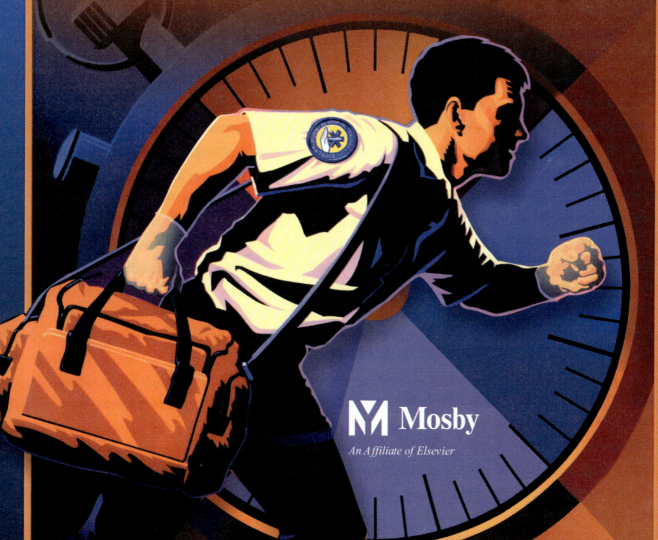

M Mosby

An Affiliate of Elsevier

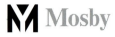 Mosby

An Affiliate of Elsevier

11830 Westline Industrial Drive
St. Louis, Missouri 63146

NOTICE

Pharmacology is an ever-changing field. Standard safety precautions must be followed, but as new research and clinical experience broaden our knowledge, changes in treatment and drug therapy may become necessary or appropriate. Readers are advised to check the most current product information provided by the manufacturer of each drug to be administered to verify the recommended dose, the method and duration of administration, and contraindications. It is the responsibility of the licensed prescriber, relying on experience and knowledge of the patient, to determine dosages and the best treatment for each individual patient. Neither the publisher nor the editor assumes any liability for any injury and/or damage to persons or property arising from this publication.

Previous editions copyrighted 1986, 1990 by Educational Direction, Inc., Akron, Ohio; 1994, 1999 by Mosby, Inc.

International Standard Book Number 0-323-02744-X

Executive Editor: Claire Merrick
Senior Developmental Editor: Kelly Trakalo
Publishing Services Manager: Catherine Jackson
Project Manager: Jeff Patterson
Design Coordinator: Amy Buxton

GW/KPT

Printed in the United States of America

Last digit is the print number: 9 8 7 6 5 4 3 2

Scott B. Frame, MD, FACS, FCCM
January 31, 1952 - March 14, 2001

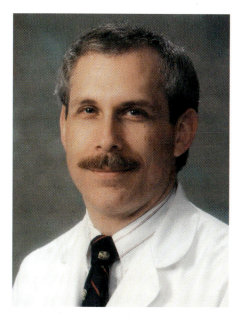

Scott Frame grew up in Albuquerque, New Mexico, where he learned the value of competition both in academics and athletics. For the last 2 years of high school he had the fastest time in the state in both the high and low hurdles. He went to college at the University of New Mexico and stayed there for medical school. He completed his residency training at Portsmouth Naval Hospital as a member of the United States Navy Medical Corps. After completing his residency and a tour of duty he realized that more education in Trauma/Critical Care was important. At Tulane University School of Medicine he completed the USN Trauma/Critical Care Fellowship. While at Tulane he became an avid prehospital care supporter. On the faculty at the University of Tennessee, Knoxville, he continued his work in trauma and was actively involved in the flight medical service. He took over as Director of the Division of Trauma/Critical Care

at the University of Cincinnati where he continued his prehospital care interest in Cincinnati, nationally and internationally, through PHTLS.

He was the Associate Medical Director for the PHTLS program. His major emphasis was in the development of the audio-visuals for PHTLS and its promulgation internationally. At the time of his untimely death, he had assumed the responsibility of putting together the Fifth Edition of the PHTLS course. This included not only the revision of the textbook, but also of the instructor manual and all of the associated teaching materials, such as the slides and CD. He accepted the appointment to become Medical Director of the PHTLS course as soon as the Fifth Edition was published. He published chapters and articles on EMS and trauma in major textbooks and scientific journals.

Scott was liaison for the American College of Surgeons Committee on Trauma for the PHTLS program and for the National Association of EMTs. Additionally, Scott was active in the Eastern Association for the Surgery of Trauma, the American Association for the Surgery of Trauma, the National Association of EMS Physicians, and the Pan American Trauma Society. In the midst of all of this, as an avid scuba diver, Scott was the Director of Continuing Medical Education for the International Society of Aquatic Medicine.

Joyce was his mainstay in life. She was his constant companion whether working on PHTLS, traveling to meetings, or just staying at home relaxing. Joyce was with Scott throughout his terminal illness, providing him with love, companionship, long days in the hospital, and assistance in all the decisions necessary for the planning of his medical care. She was Scott's love and life and he, hers.

The PHTLS program grew immeasurably under Scott's leadership. Its continuation into the future will be because of what Scott did and the part of his life that he lent to PHTLS and to his patients.

Contributors

EDITORS

Norman E. McSwain, Jr., MD, FACS, NREMT-P
PHTLS Editor-in-Chief
Professor of Surgery
Tulane University School of Medicine
New Orleans, Louisiana

Scott Frame, MD, FACS, FCCM
Associate Professor of Surgery
Director, Division of Trauma/Critical Care
University of Cincinnati Medical Center
Cincinnati, Ohio

Jeffrey P. Salomone, MD, FACS, NREMT-P
PHTLS Scientific Editor
Associate Professor of Surgery
Emory University, School of Medicine
Atlanta, Georgia

ASSOCIATE EDITORS

Peter Pons, MD, FACEP
Associate Medical Director, PHTLS
Denver Health Medical Center
Denver, Colorado

Chief Will Chapleau, EMT-P, RN, TNS, CEN
Chairperson, PHTLS
Fire Chief
Chicago Heights Fire Dept.
Chicago Heights, Illinois

Gregory Chapman, EMT-P, RRT
Vicechair, PHTLS
Program Director
Hudson Valley Community College
Troy, New York

Steve Mercer, EMT-P, MEd
Education Coordinator, PHTLS
Iowa Department of Public Health
Bureau of EMS
Des Moines, Iowa

CONTRIBUTING REVIEWER/ EDUCATION CONSULTANT TO PHTLS

Melissa Alexander, MS, NREMT-P
Asssistant Professor of Emergency Medicine
The George Washington University
Washington, DC

CONTRIBUTORS

Augie Bamonti, BA, NREMT-P
Chicago Heights, Illinois

Gregory Chapman, RRT, EMT-P
Program Director
Hudson Valley Community College
Troy, New York

Blaine L. Endersen, MD, FACS, FCCM
Chief, Division of Trauma/Critical Care
University of Tennessee Medical Center
Knoxville, Tennessee

Larry Hatfield, MEd, EMT-P
Omaha, Nebraska

Craig Jacobus, DC, CPM
Orland Park, Illinois

Jon A. King, MS, NREMT-P
Director of EMS Education
Emory University
Atlanta, Georgia

Merry McSwain, RN, NREMT-P, BSN
Masters Candidate in Trauma/Critical Care
University of Alabama in Birmingham
School of Nursing
Birmingham, Alabama

Norman E. McSwain, Jr., MD, FACS, NREMT-P
Medical Director, PHTLS
Tulane University Department of Surgery
New Orleans, Louisiana

Eric Ossman, MD, FAAEM
Assistant Professor of Emergency Medicine
Emory University
Atlanta, Georgia

Peter Pons, MD, FACEP
Associate Medical Director, PHTLS
Denver Health Medical Center
Denver, Colorado

Valerie J. Phillips, MD
Director, Department of Emergency Medicine
EMS Medical Director
Good Samaritan Hospital
Downers Grove, Illinois

Brian Reiselbara, BA, NREMT-P
Melbourne, Florida

Jeffrey P. Salomone, MD, FACS, NREMT-P
Associate Medical Director, PHTLS
Emory University, Department of Surgery
Atlanta, Georgia

David M. Tauber, NREMT-P-IC
Director Advanced Life Support Institute
Conway, New Hampshire

Robert K. (Bob) Waddell II
EMS Systems Specialist
Emergency Medical Services for Children
National Resource Center
Washington, DC

Keith Wesley, MD, FACEP
Director EMS Education
Sacred Heart Hospital
Eau Claire, Wisconsin

Doug York, EMT-P
University of Iowa Hospitals and Clinics
Iowa City, Iowa

Alida Zamboni, RN, BA, ECRN
Warrenville, Illinois

MILITARY CONTRIBUTIONS

Gregory H. Adkisson, Capt., MC, USN
Commanding Officer
Defense Medical Readiness Training Command (DMRTC)
San Antonio, Texas

Morris L. Beard, SFC, USA, NREMT-P
Special Operations Forces Liaison
Joint Medical Readiness Training Center (JMRTC)
San Antonio, Texas

Frank K. Butler, Jr., Capt., MC, USN
Biomedical Research Director
Defense Medical Readiness Training Command (DMRTC)
San Antonio, Texas

Milton R. Fields III, Tsgt., USAF NREMT-P
Military PHTLS Coordinator
Joint Medical Readiness Training Center (JMRTC)
San Antonio, Texas

John Mechtel, Capt., USAF, NC
Assistant Chief, Professional Programs
Joint Medical Readiness Training Center (JMRTC)
San Antonio, Texas

Dale C. Smith, PhD
Chairperson, Department of Military History
Uniformed Services University Health Sciences
Bethesda, Maryland

Kenneth G. Swan, MD
Professor of Surgery
Chief, Section of General Surgery
UMDNJ/New Jersey Medical School;
Chief, Division of Thoracic Surgery
University Hospital
Newark, New Jersey

K.G. Swan, Jr., BS
First Year Medical Student
Cornell University Medical College
New York, New York

Steven J. Yevich, LTC, USA, MC
Chief of Staff
Joint Medical Readiness Training Center (JMRTC)
San Antonio, Texas
Clinton, Mississippi

REVIEWERS

Rosemary Adam, RN, EMT-P
EMS Learning Resources Center
The University of Iowa Hospital
Iowa City, Iowa

Jameel Ali, MD, M.Med Ed, FRCSC, FACS
Division of General Surgery, Trauma, and Critical Care,
St. Michael's Hospital
Professor of Surgery, University of Toronto
Toronto, Ontario, Canada

Mary-Ann Clarkes, EMT-A
Canadian College of Emergency Medical Services
Edmonton General Hospital
Edmonton, Alberta, Canada

Greg Clarkes, EMT-P MICP, NREMT-P
President & Education Coordinator
Canadian College of Emergency Medical Services
Edmonton General Hospital
Edmonton, Alberta, Canada

Neil Coker, BS, EMT-P
Department of EMS Professions
Temple College
Temple, Texas

John Czajkowski
Transportation Rescue Consultants, Inc.
Apopka, Florida

Heather Davis, MS, NREMT-P
UCLA Center for Prehospital Care
Inglewood, California

Nita Ham, EMT-P
Department of EMS Training
Georgia Public Safety Training Center
Forsyth, Georgia

J. Steven Kidd
Transportation Rescue Consultants, Inc.
Apopka, Florida

William Metcalf
Division Chief
North Lake Tahoe Fire Protection District
Incline Village, Nevada

James B. Miller, EMT-P
U.S. Army EMT Program Manager
U.S. Army Academy of Health Sciences
Fort Sam Houston, Texas

Keith A. Monosky, MPM, BS, EMT-P
Department of Emergency Medicine
The George Washington University
Fairfax, Virginia

Jeanne O'Brien, BSN, REMT-P
Department of Fire and EMS
Tacoma Fire Department Paramedic Training
Tacoma, Washington

David S. Pecora, PA-C, NREMT-P, RN
Department of Emergency Medicine
West Virginia University
Morgantown, West Virginia

INTERNATIONAL ACKNOWLEDGMENTS

Dr. Jameel Ali
Toronto, Canada

Dr. Nikki Blackwell
Mt. Isa Base Hospital
Mt. Isa, Australia

Dr. Chris Carney
Royal College of Surgeons
London, England

Dr. Ricardo Ferrada
Emergency Department and Trauma Unit
Bogota, Columbia

Dr. Fernando Magallenes-Negrete
Hospital Centrar Militar
Lomas de Sotelo, Mexico

Dr. Anna Notander
Stockholm, Sweden

Professor Sergio Olivero
Cattedra di Cirurgia D'urgenza
Turin, Italy

Dr. Renato Poggetti
Brazilian American College of Surgeons
Sao Paulo, Brazil

Dr. Oswaldo Rois
Fundacion EMME
Buenos Aires, Argentina

Dr. Mario Uribe
American College of Surgeons-Chile
Santiago, Chile

PHTLS EXECUTIVE COUNCIL

Chief Will Chapleau, EMT-P, RN, TNS, CEN
Chairperson, PHTLS
Fire Chief
Chicago Heights Fire Dept.
Chicago Heights, Illinois

Gregory Chapman, EMT-P, RRT
Vicechair, PHTLS
Program Director
Hudson Valley Community College
Troy, New York

Steve Mercer, EMT-P, MEd
Education Coordinator, PHTLS
Iowa Department of Public Health
Bureau of EMS
Des Moines, Iowa

Derek Hanson, BS, NREMT-I
Communications Coordinator, PHTLS
EMS Coordinator
St. Alexius Medical Center
Bismarck, North Dakota

Dennis Rowe
Knoxville, Tennessee

NATIONAL ASSOCIATION OF EMTs

Nathan Williams, EMT
President

John Roquemore, EMT
Vice President

Pat Moore, EMT
Secretary

Ken Bouvier, EMT-P
Treasurer

Deborah Knight-Smith, EMT
Immediate Past President

Brian Reiselbara
Melbourne, Florida

Mark Stevens, EMS Chief
Aloha, Oregon

Corine Curd
PHTLS International Office Director
NAEMT Headquarters
Clinton, Mississippi

Norman E. McSwain, Jr., MD, FACS, NREMT-P
Medical Director, PHTLS
Tulane University Department of Surgery
New Orleans, Louisiana

Jeffrey P. Salomone, MD, FACS, NREMT-P
Associate Medical Director, PHTLS
Emory University, Department of Surgery
Atlanta, Georgia

Peter Pons, MD, FACEP
Associate Medical Director, PHTLS
Denver Health Medical Center
Denver, Colorado

PHTLS Honor Roll

PHTLS continues to prosper and promote high standards of trauma care all over the world. It would not be able to do this without the contributions of many dedicated and inspired individuals over the past two and a half decades. Some of the names below were instrumental in the development of our first textbook. Others were constantly "on the road" spreading the word. Still others "put out fires" and otherwise problem solved to keep us growing. The PHTLS Executive Council, along with the editors and contributors of this, our fifth edition, would like to express our thanks to all of those listed below. PHTLS lives, breathes, and grows because of the efforts of those who volunteer their time to what they believe in.

Jameel Ali, MD

J.M. Barnes

Ann Bellows

Chip Boehm

Don E. Boyle, MD

Susan Brown

Alexander Butman

H. Jeannie Butman

Steve Carden

Edward A. Casker

Bud Caukin

Philip Coco

Michael D'Auito, MD

Alice "Twink" Dalton

Judith Demarest

Joseph P. Dineen, MD

Leon Dontigney, MD

Betsy Ewing

Sheryl G.A. Gabram, MD

Capt. Bret Gilliam

Vincent A. Greco

Walter Idol

Len Jacobs

Lou Jordan

Richard Judd

Dawn Loehn

Mark Lockhart

Robert Loftus

William McConnell, DO

Fernando Magallenes-Negrete, MD

Scott W. Martin

Don Mauger

Claire Merrick

Bill Metcalf

George Moerkirk, MD

Stephen Murphy

Lawrence D. Newell

Jeanne O'Brien

Joan Drake-Olsen

Dawn Orgeron

James Paturas

Thomas Petrich

James Pierce

Brian Plaisier, MD

Mark Reading

John Sigafoos

Paul Silverston, MD

David Skinner, FRCS

Richard Sobieray

Sheila Spaid

Michael Spain

Don Stamper

J.J. Tepas III, MD

Richard Vomacka

Michael Werdmann, MD

Elizabeth Wertz

Roger White, MD

David Wuertz

Kenneth J. Wright, MD

Al Yellin, MD

Again, thanks to all of you, and thanks to everyone all over the world for making PHTLS work.

PHTLS Executive Council
Editors and Contributors of PHTLS

Acknowledgments

In 1624 John Donne wrote that "No man is an island, entire of itself." This describes in many ways the process of the publication of a book. Certainly, no editor is an island. Textbooks such as the PHTLS book and especially courses that involve audiovisual material, instructor manuals, and the textbook cannot be published by editors in isolation. As a matter of fact, much, if not most, of the work in the publishing of a textbook is done not by the editors and the authors whose names appear on the cover and on the inside of the book, but by the editorial staff. The fifth edition of PHTLS is certainly no exception.

Alex Butman and Rick Vomacka worked diligently and frequently using money out of their own pockets to bring the first two editions of the PHTLS program to fruition. Without their help and work, PHTLS would never have begun.

From the American College of Surgeons Committee on Trauma, James E. Wilberger, MD, FACS, Chairman of the Emergency Services Committee–Prehospital; Steve Parks, MD, FACS, Chairman of the Advanced Trauma Life Support Committee; and, of course, Irvene Hughes, RN, the National/International Coordinator of ATLS, have provided major support of PHTLS generally and the fifth edition specifically. The Committee on Trauma, Executive Secretary, Carol Williams and the current Chairman of the Committee on Trauma, David Hoyt, MD, FACS, have provided outstanding support for this edition as well as PHTLS.

Within Mosby, Claire Merrick has been an outstanding supporter of PHTLS and has continued through this edition as our executive editor. Derril Trakalo has done an outstanding job with the public relations of this book. Jeff Patterson, with the support of his production team, has been outstanding. In addition, thanks to Rick Brady for the new photographs, Jeanne Robertson for the new illustrations, and Studio Montage for the wonderful new design and look of the fifth edition.

A special thanks is given to the Chicago Heights Fire Department for the use of their facilities and to the crews who participated in the photo shoot for this book.

One person within Elsevier Science stands out far above the rest: Kelly Trakalo. Never in my life of writing articles, book chapters, and books over the past 35 years have I run into anybody with the knowledge, aggressiveness, and dedication to a project that Kelly Trakalo has had. There is no question in my mind, or in the minds of any of the other members of the Editorial Board, that without Kelly Trakalo this book would never have met its deadlines. Kelly is the *be all and end all* to this edition. Kelly, from the bottom of our hearts . . . **THANKS.**

The family of the editors and authors whose wives, children, and significant others have put up with the long hours in the preparation of the material are obviously the backbone of any publication.

And finally, in my own life, thank you to Vanessa Angelety-Lee, my assistant, confidante, friend, and supporter, without whom I could not function on this or any other project.

Norman E. McSwain, Jr, MD, FACS, NREMT-P

Preface

When becoming a prehospital care provider, one should accept the responsibility to provide patient care as close to absolutely perfect as possible. This cannot be achieved with insufficient knowledge of the subject. We must remember that the patient did not choose to be involved in a traumatic situation. The provider, on the other hand, has chosen to be there to take care of the patient. The prehospital care provider is obligated to give 100% of his or her effort during contact with every patient. The patient has had a bad day; the provider cannot also have a bad day. The prehospital care provider must be sharp and capable in the competition between the patient and death and disease.

The patient is the most important person at the scene of an emergency. There is no time to think about the order in which the patient assessment is performed or what treatments should take priority over others. There is no time to practice a skill before using it on a particular patient. There is no time to think about where equipment or supplies are housed within the jump kit. There is no time to think about where to transport the injured patient. All of this information and more must be stored in the mind and all supplies and equipment must be present in the jump kit when arriving on the scene. Without the proper knowledge or equipment, the provider may neglect to do things that could potentially increase the patient's chance of survival. The responsibilities of a provider are too great to make such mistakes.

Those who deliver care in the prehospital setting are integral members of the trauma patient care team, as are the nurses or physicians in the emergency department, operating room, intensive care unit, ward, and rehabilitation unit. Prehospital care providers must be practiced in their skills so that they can move the patient quickly and efficiently out of the environment of the emergency and transport the patient quickly to the closest appropriate hospital.

WHY PHTLS?

Course Education Philosophy

Prehospital Trauma Life Support (PHTLS) focuses on **principles**, not preferences. By focusing on principles of good trauma care, PHTLS promotes critical thinking.

The Executive Committee of the PHTLS Division of the National Association of Emergency Medical Technicians (NAEMT) believes that, given a good fund of knowledge, prehospital care providers are capable of making reasoned decisions regarding patient care. Rote memorization of mnemonics is discouraged. Furthermore, there is no one "PHTLS way" of performing a specific skill. The principle of the skill is taught, then one acceptable method of performing the skill that meets the principle is presented. The authors realize that no one method can apply to the myriad of unique situations encountered in the prehospital setting.

Up-to-Date Information

Development of the PHTLS program began in 1981, immediately on the heels of the inception of the Advanced Trauma Life Support (ATLS) program for physicians. As the ATLS course is revised every 4 to 5 years, pertinent changes are incorporated into the next edition of PHTLS. This fifth edition of the PHTLS program has been significantly revised based on the 2002 ATLS course. While still following the ATLS principles, PHTLS is specifically designed for the unique requirements of caring for trauma patients in the prehospital setting. Two new skills (face-to-face intubation and two-person rapid extrication) have been added. Many chapters now include algorithms to better illustrate the flow of patient care. We have also included a CD-ROM with video clips of skills and practice questions. Note that throughout the book, the 💿 symbol references where more information can be found on the CD-ROM.

Scientific Base

The authors and editors have adopted an "evidence-based" approach that includes references from the medical literature supporting the key principles. Additionally, several of the position papers published by the National Association of EMS Physicians (NAEMSP) have been included, where applicable.

Support for NAEMT

The NAEMT provides the administrative structure for the PHTLS program. No proceeds from the PHTLS program (surcharges or royalties from the text and audiovisuals) have ever gone to the American College of Surgeons

Committee on Trauma nor any other physician-oriented organization. All profits from the PHTLS program are channeled back into NAEMT in order to provide funding for issues and programs that are of prime importance to EMS professionals, such as educational conferences and lobbying of legislators on the behalf of prehospital care providers.

PHTLS Is a World Leader

Because of the unprecedented success of the fourth edition of PHTLS, the program has continued to grow by leaps and bounds. PHTLS courses continue to proliferate across the United States, and the U.S. military has adopted it, teaching the program to armed forces personnel at over 100 training sites worldwide. PHTLS has been exported to over 25 nations, and many others are expressing interest in bringing PHTLS to their country in efforts to improve the level of prehospital trauma care.

Prehospital care providers have the responsibility to assimilate this knowledge and skills in order to use them for the benefit of the patients for whom they are responsible. The editors and authors of this material and the Executive Committee of the PHTLS Division of the NAEMT hope that you will incorporate this information into your practice and daily rededicate yourself to the care of those persons who cannot care for themselves—the trauma patients.

Jeffrey P. Salomone, MD, FACS, NREMT-P
Editor
Norman E. McSwain, Jr., MD, FACS, NREMT-P
Editor in Chief, PHTLS

Contents

PHTLS—EXTENDING THE HANDS OF EDUCATION ACROSS THE GLOBE

Past, Present and Future

In 1979, care of trauma patients took a giant step forward with the inauguration of the Advanced Trauma Life Support (ATLS) course. The first chairman of the ATLS ad hoc committee for the American College of Surgeons and Chairman of the Prehospital Care Subcommittee on Trauma for the American College of Surgeons, Dr. Norman E. McSwain, Jr., FACS, knew that what they had begun would have a profound effect on the outcome of trauma patients. Moreover, he had a strong sense that an even greater effect could come from bringing this type of critical training to prehospital care providers.

Dr. McSwain, a founding member of the board of directors of the National Association of Emergency Medical Technicians (NAEMT), gained support of the Association's president, Gary Labeau, and began to lay plans for a prehospital version of ATLS. President Labeau directed Dr. McSwain and Robert Nelson, NREMT-P, to determine the feasibility of an ATLS-type program for prehospital care providers.

As a professor of surgery at Tulane University School of Medicine in New Orleans, Louisiana, Dr. McSwain gained the University's support in putting together the draft curriculum of what was to become Prehospital Trauma Life Support (PHTLS). With this draft in place, in 1983, a PHTLS committee was established. This committee continued to refine the curriculum, and later that same year, pilot courses were conducted at Tulane; Marian Health Center in Sioux City, Iowa; Yale University School of Medicine in New Haven, Connecticut; and Norwalk Hospital in Norwalk, Connecticut.

Tulane also hosted the first National Faculty course in early 1984. This was followed in the summer of 1984 by a course in Denver, Colorado. The graduates of these early courses formed what would be the "Barnstormers," PHTLS national and regional faculty members who traveled the country training more faculty members, spreading the word that PHTLS had arrived.

Early courses focused on advanced life support (ALS). In 1986, a course that encompassed basic life support (BLS) was developed. The course grew exponentially. Beginning with those first few enthusiastic faculty members, first dozens, then hundreds, and now thousands of providers annually participate in PHTLS courses all over the world.

As the course grew, the PHTLS committee became a division of the NAEMT. Course demand and the need to maintain course continuity and quality necessitated the building of networks of affiliate, state, regional, and na-

tional faculty members. There are national coordinators for every country, and in each country there are regional and state coordinators along with affiliate faculty members to make sure that information is disseminated and courses are consistent whether you participate in a program in Chicago Heights, Illinois, or Buenos Aires, Argentina.

Throughout the growth process, medical direction has been provided by the American College of Surgeons Committee on Trauma. For nearly 20 years the partnership between the American College of Surgeons and the NAEMT has ensured that course participants are given the opportunity to give trauma patients everywhere their best chance at survival.

PHTLS in the Military

Beginning in 1988, the U.S. military aggressively set out to train its medics in PHTLS. Coordinated by DMRT, the Defense Medical Readiness Training Institute at Fort Sam Houston in Texas, PHTLS is taught all over the United States, Europe, and Asia and anywhere the flags of the U.S. military fly. In 2001, the Army's 91WB program standardized the training of over 58,000 Army medics to include PHTLS.

The participation of the U.S. military in the program includes providing a chapter to cover the particular needs of the military and provide information on tactical medicine that is of interest to any population in the modern world.

International PHTLS

The sound principles of prehospital trauma management emphasized in the PHTLS course have led to prehospital care providers and physicians outside of the United States to request the importation of the program to their various countries. This had been assisted by ATLS faculty members presenting ATLS courses worldwide. This network provides medical direction and course continuity.

As PHTLS has moved across the United States and around the globe, we have been struck by the differences in our cultures and climates and also by the similarities of the people who devote their lives to caring for the sick and injured. All of us who have been blessed with the opportunity to teach overseas have experienced the fellowship with our international partners and know that we are all one people in pursuit of caring for those who need care the most.

The nations in the growing PHTLS family include the following: Australia, Argentina, Barbados, Bolivia, Brazil, Canada, Chile, China, Colombia, England, Greece, Holland, Ireland, Israel, Italy, Mexico, New Zealand, Norway, Panama, Saudi Arabia, Sweden, Switzerland, Trinidad, the

United States, and Venezuela. Demonstration courses have been run in Bulgaria, Macedonia, and soon Croatia, with hopes to establish faculty members there in the near future. Peru, Portugal, Denmark, Japan, Korea, South Africa, and Nigeria all hope to join the family in the near future.

Vision for the Future

The vision for the future of PHTLS is family. The father of PHTLS, Dr. McSwain, is the root of the growing family that provides vital training and contributes knowledge and experience to the world. The inaugural international PHTLS Trauma Symposium was held near Chicago, Illinois, in the year 2000. This first program pitted the controversies facing trauma care against the will and energy of prehospital trauma providers. These programs will bring the work of practitioners and researchers around the globe together to determine the standards of trauma care for the new millenium.

The support of the PHTLS family worldwide, all volunteering countless hours of their lives, allows the PHTLS leadership to keep PHTLS growing. This leadership consists of the following:

The PHTLS Executive Council

Medical Director of PHTLS International:

Norman E. McSwain, Jr., MD, FACS, NREMT-P	1983-Present

Associate PHTLS Medical Directors:

Scott B. Frame, MD, FACS, FCCM	1994-2001
Jeffrey Salomone, MD, FACS, NREMT-P	1996-present
Peter Pons, MD, FACEP	2000-present

International PHTLS Chairs:

Richard Vomacka, REMT-P	1983-1985
James L. Paturas	1985-1988
David Wuertz, EMT-P	1988-1990
John Sinclair, EMT-P	1990-1991
James L. Paturas	1991-1992
Elizabeth M. Wertz, RN, BSN, MPM	1992-1996
Will Chapleau, EMT-P, RN, TNS	1996-present

As we continue to pursue the potential of the PHTLS course and the worldwide community of prehospital care providers, we must remember our commitment to the following:

- Rapid and accurate assessment
- Identification of shock and hypoxemia
- Initiation of the right interventions at the right time
- Timely transport to the right place

It is also fitting to reprise our mission statement written in a marathon session at the NAEMT conference in 1997. The PHTLS mission continues to provide the highest quality prehospital trauma education to all who wish to avail themselves of this opportunity. The PHTLS mission also enhances the achievement of the NAEMT mission. The PHTLS program is committed to quality and performance improvement. As such, PHTLS is always attentive to changes in technology and methods of delivering prehospital trauma care that may be used to enhance the clinical and service quality of this program.

National Association of Emergency Medical Technicians

The NAEMT represents the interests of prehospital care providers all over the world.

NAEMT was founded with the help of the National Registry of EMTs (NREMT) in 1975. Since its inception, the association has worked to promote professional status for prehospital care providers from the first responder to the administrator. Its educational programs began as a way of providing meaningful continuing education to providers at every level and have become the standard of prehospital continuing education all over the world.

NAEMT has reciprocal relationships with dozens of U.S. and international federal and private agencies that influence every aspect of prehospital care. The NAEMT's participation ensures that the voice of prehospital care is heard in determining the future of our practice.

NAEMT MISSION

The mission of the National Association of Emergency Medical Technicians, Inc., is to be a professional representative organization that will receive and represent the views and opinions of prehospital care personnel and to influence the future advancement of EMS as an allied health profession. NAEMT will serve its professional membership through educational programs, liaison activity, development of national standards and reciprocity, and the development of programs to benefit prehospital care personnel.

With this mission clearly defined and passionately pursued, NAEMT will continue to provide leadership in this developing specialty of prehospital care into the new millenium.

PHTLS

Basic and Advanced Prehospital Trauma Life Support

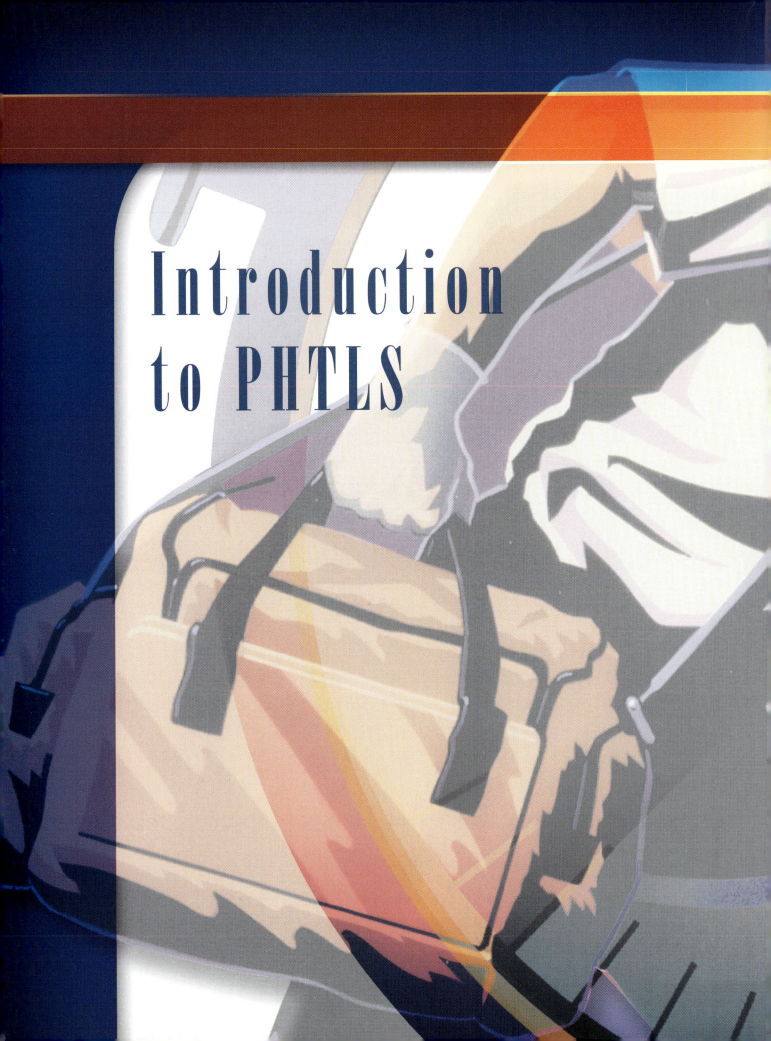

Introduction to PHTLS

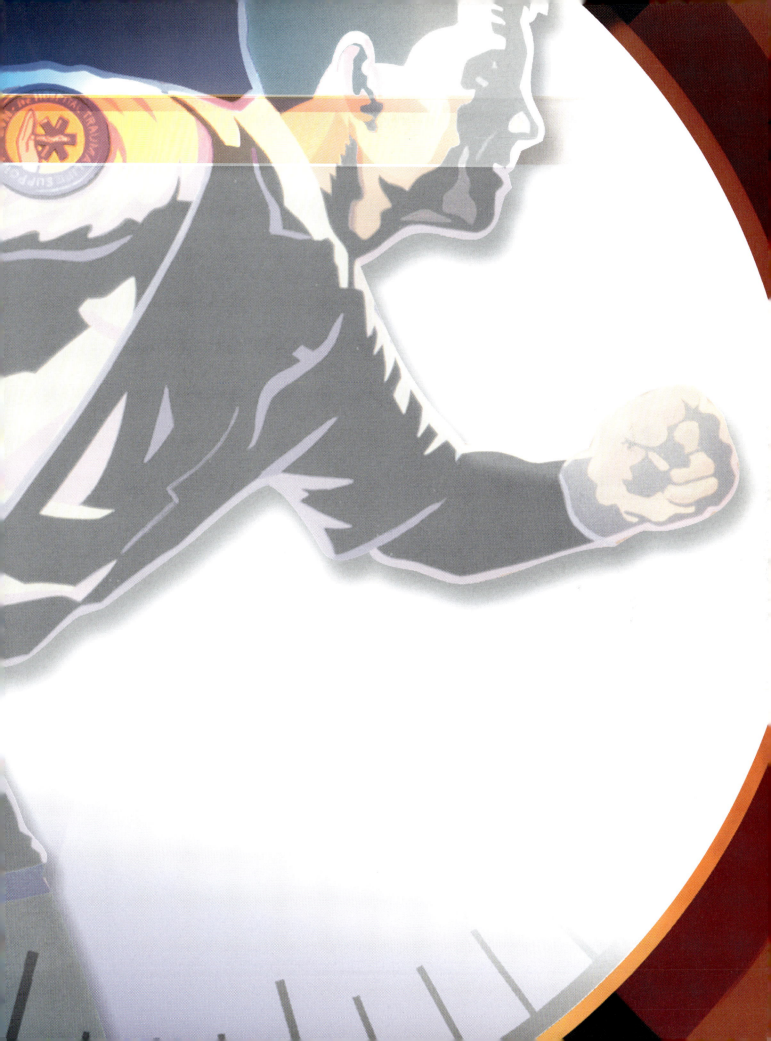

Our patients did not choose us. We have chosen to treat them. We could have chosen another profession, but we did not. We have accepted the responsibility for patient care in some of the worst situations: when we are tired or cold, when it is rainy and dark, and often when conditions are unpredictable. We must either accept this responsibility or surrender it. We must give our patients the very best care that we can—not with unchecked equipment, not with incomplete supplies, not with yesterday's knowledge, and not with indifference. We cannot know what medical information is current, and we cannot claim to be ready to care for our patients without reading and learning each day. The Prehospital Trauma Life Support (PHTLS) course contributes to the knowledge of a prehospital care provider and, more importantly, ultimately benefits the patient. At the end of each run, we should feel that the patient received nothing short of our very best.

Trauma Care in the Twenty-First Century

The opportunity for a prehospital care provider to help another person is greater in the management of trauma patients than in any other patient encounter. The number of trauma patients is higher than most other patient populations, and the chance of survival of the trauma patient who receives good hospital care is probably greater than that of any other patient. The prehospital care provider can lengthen the life span of the trauma patient and benefit society because of the number of productive years saved. Therefore the prehospital care provider, through effective management of the trauma patient, has a significant influence on society.

Understanding, learning, and practicing the principles of PHTLS is more beneficial to patients than any other educational program. The following facts have led to the inclusion of a chapter on injury prevention in this edition of *Prehospital Trauma Life Support*.

Trauma is the leading cause of death in persons between 1 and 44 years of age. About 80% of teenage deaths and 60% of childhood deaths are secondary to trauma. Trauma continues to be the seventh leading cause of death in the elderly. Three times more Americans die of trauma each year than died in the Vietnam War. Every 10 years more Americans die of trauma than have died in all U.S. military conflicts combined. Only in the fifth decade of life do cancer and heart disease compete with trauma as a leading cause of death.

Prehospital care can do little to increase the survival of a cancer patient. However, for the trauma patient, prehospital care can often make the difference between life and death; between temporary, serious, or permanent disability; or between a life of productivity and a life of destitution and welfare. In the United States, about 60 million injuries occur each year, 30 million will require medical care, and 9 million of these are disabling. About 8.7 million will be temporarily disabled, and 300,000 will be permanently disabled.

The cost for care of trauma patients is staggering. Billions of dollars are spent on the management of trauma patients, not including the dollars lost in wages, insurance administration costs, property damage, and employer costs.

Lost productivity from disabled trauma patients is the equivalent of 5.1 million years at a cost of over $65 billion. For patients who die, 5.3 million years of life are lost (34 years per person) at a cost of over $50 billion. Comparatively, the costs (measured in dollars and in years lost) for cancer and heart disease

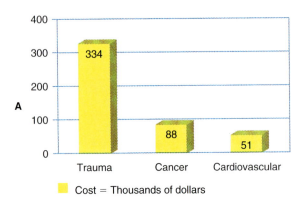

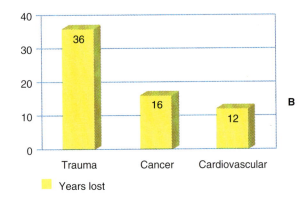

Figure I-1 **A,** Comparative costs in thousands of dollars to United States victims of trauma, cancer, and cardiovascular disease each year. **B,** Comparative number of years lost as a result of trauma, cancer, and cardiovascular disease.

are much less, as illustrated in Figure I-1. For example, proper protection of the fractured cervical spine by a prehospital care provider may make the difference between lifelong quadriplegia and a productive healthy life of unrestricted activity. Prehospital care providers encounter many more examples almost every day.

Trauma care is divided into three phases: preevent, event, and postevent. The prehospital care provider has responsibilities in each phase.

Preevent Phase

Trauma is no accident. An *accident* is defined as either "an event occurring by chance or arising from unknown causes" or "an unfortunate occurrence resulting from carelessness, unawareness, ignorance." Most trauma deaths and injuries fit the second definition and are preventable. Traumatic incidents fall into two categories—intentional and unintentional. In working toward prevention in both of these areas, prehospital care providers must educate the public to increase the use of vehicle occupant restraint systems, promote methods to reduce the use of weapons in criminal activities, and promote nonviolent conflict resolution. In addition to caring for the trauma patient, all members of the health care delivery team have a responsibility to reduce the number of victims. Currently, violence and unintentional trauma cause more deaths annually in the United States than all diseases combined. Violence accounts for over one third of these deaths (Figure I-2). Motor vehicles and firearms are involved in more than one half of all trauma deaths, most of which are preventable (Figure I-3).

Motorcycle helmet usage laws are one example of legislation that has had an effect on injury prevention. In 1966 Congress gave the Department of Transportation the authority to mandate that states pass legislation requiring the use of motorcycle helmets. The use of hel-

mets subsequently increased to almost 100%, and the fatality rate decreased dramatically. In 1975 Congress rescinded this authority. More than half of the states repealed or modified the existing legislation, leading to an increase in related fatalities. As some states reinstate or repeal these laws, the rates have changed. Recently more states have repealed rather than instituted such laws, resulting in increased death rates in 1998 and 1999. Figure I-4 shows the recent change.

Another example of preventable trauma deaths involves drunk driving. As a result of pressure to change state laws for the level of intoxication while driving and through the educational activities of such organizations as Mothers Against Drunk Drivers (MADD), the number of drunk drivers involved in fatal crashes has been consistently decreasing since 1989.

Another way to prevent trauma is through the use of child safety seats. Many trauma centers, law enforcement organizations, and emergency medical services (EMS) conduct programs to educate parents in the correct installation and use of child safety seats.

Event Phase

Whether driving a personal vehicle or an emergency vehicle, prehospital care providers must protect themselves and teach by example. They should always drive safely, follow traffic laws, and use the protective devices available, such as vehicle restraints, in the driving compartment and in the passenger or patient care compartment.

Postevent Phase

Donald Trunkey, MD, has described a trimodal categorization of trauma deaths. The first phase of deaths occurs within the first few minutes of and up to an hour after an incident. These deaths would likely occur even with prompt medical attention. The best way to combat

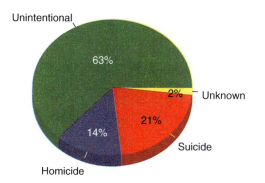

Figure I-2 Unintentional trauma and violence account for more deaths than all other causes of death combined.

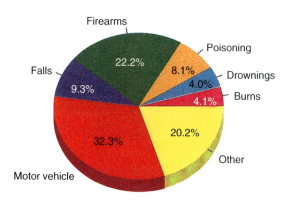

Figure I-3 Motor vehicle trauma and firearms account for more than half of the deaths that occur as a result of trauma and violence.

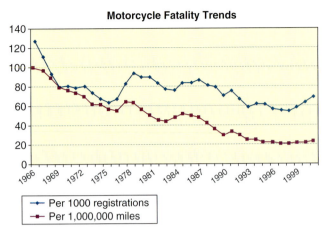

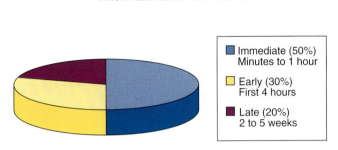

Figure I-4 Motorcycle helmet legislation and therefore the mandated use of helmets significantly reduce the motorcycle fatality rate. Repeal of this law in 1975 produced a marked increase in the number of fatalities. Many states have reinstated their own laws, reducing the number of fatalities for registered motorcyclists to as low as it was before the repeal of this law.

Figure I-5 When patients die from trauma. Immediate deaths can be prevented only by injury prevention education because the only chance some patients have is for the incident to not have occurred. Early deaths can be prevented through timely appropriate prehospital care to reduce mortality and morbidity rates. Late deaths can be prevented only through prompt transport to a hospital appropriately staffed for trauma care.

these deaths is through injury prevention and safety strategies. The second phase of deaths occurs within the first few hours of an incident. These deaths can be prevented by good prehospital care and good hospital care. The third phase of deaths occurs several days to several weeks after the incident. These deaths are generally due to multiple organ failure. Much more needs to be learned about managing and preventing multiple organ failure; however, early and aggressive shock management in the prehospital setting can prevent some of these deaths (Figure I-5).

R Adams Cowley, MD, founder of the Maryland Institute of Emergency Medical Services (MIEMS), one of the first trauma centers in the United States, described and defined what he called the "Golden Hour." Based on his research, Cowley believed that patients who received definitive care soon after an injury had a much higher survival rate than those whose care was delayed. One reason for this improvement in survival is preservation of the body's ability to produce energy to maintain organ function. For the prehospital care provider this translates into maintaining oxygenation and perfusion and providing rapid transportation to a facility set up to continue that process.

An average urban EMS system has a response time (from the time the incident occurs until arrival on the scene) of 6 to 8 minutes. A typical transport time to the receiving facility is another 8 to 10 minutes. Between 15 and 20 minutes of the magic "Golden Hour" are used just to get to the scene and transport the patient. If prehospital care at the scene is not efficient and well organ-ized, an additional 30 to 40 minutes can be spent on the scene. With this time on the scene added to the transport time, the "Golden Hour" has already passed before a physician has an opportunity to treat the patient. Research data are starting to support this notion. One study showed that critically injured patients had a significantly lower mortality rate (17.9% vs. 28.2%) when transported by a private vehicle rather than an ambulance. This unexpected finding was most likely the result of prehospital care providers spending too much time on the scene. One trauma center in the locale where the study was conducted documented that EMS scene times averaged 23 minutes for patients injured in motor vehicle crashes (MVCs) and 22 minutes for victims of penetrating trauma. This begs the questions that all prehospital providers should ask: "Is what I'm doing going to benefit the patient? Does that benefit outweigh the risk of delaying transport?" One of the most important responsibilities of a prehospital care provider is to spend as little time on the scene as possible. In the first precious minutes a prehospital care provider must rapidly assess the patient, perform lifesaving maneuvers, and prepare the patient for transportation.

A second responsibility is actually transporting the patient to an appropriate facility. The factor most critical to any patient's survival is the length of time that elapses between the incident and definitive care. For a cardiac arrest patient, definitive care is the restoration of normal heart rhythm and adequate perfusion. Cardiopulmonary resuscitation (CPR) is merely a holding pattern. For a patient whose airway is compromised, definitive care is

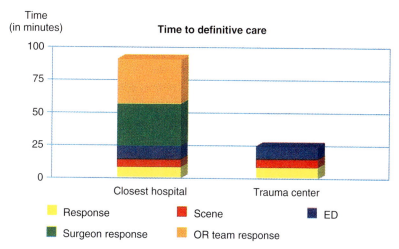

Figure I-6   In locations where trauma centers are available, bypassing hospitals not committed to the care of the trauma patient can significantly improve patient care. In severely injured trauma patients, definitive patient care must occur in the operating room. An extra 5 to 10 minutes spent en route to a hospital with an in-house surgeon and in-house operating room staff will significantly reduce the time to definitive care. The *green* indicates surgical response from out of hospital. The *yellow* indicates operating team response from out of hospital. In hospitals with in-house surgical and operating room staff, these delays do not exist.

the management of the airway and restoration of adequate ventilation. The reestablishment of either ventilation or normal cardiac rhythm by defibrillation is usually easily achieved in the field; therefore transportation time is not as critical for the cardiac patient.

The management of trauma patients is different. Definitive care is usually hemorrhage control and restoration of adequate perfusion. Hemostasis (hemorrhage control) cannot always be achieved in the field or in the emergency department; it must often be achieved in the operating room. Therefore in determining an appropriate facility, the prehospital care provider must consider the transport time to a given facility and the capabilities of that facility.

A trauma center that has an in-house surgeon and an operating room team can often have a trauma patient with life-threatening hemorrhage in the operating room within 10 to 15 minutes of the patient's arrival. On the other hand, a hospital without in-house surgical capabilities must await the arrival of the surgeon and the surgical team before transporting the patient from the emergency department to the operating room. Additional time may then elapse before the hemorrhage can be controlled, resulting in an associated increase in mortality rate (Figure I-6).

History of EMS

This text, the PHTLS course, and care of the trauma patient are based on the objectives developed and taught by the early pioneers of prehospital care. The list of these innovators is long; however, a few especially deserve our recognition.

As early as the late 1700s, Baron Dominick Jean Larrey, Napoleon's chief military physician, recognized the need for prompt prehospital care. He developed the horse-drawn "flying ambulance" for timely retrieval of men injured on the battlefield and introduced the premise that individuals working in these "flying ambulances" should be trained in medical care to provide on-scene and en route care for patients.

J.D. "Deke" Farrington, MD, the father of modern EMS, stimulated the development of improved prehospital care with his landmark article "Death in a Ditch." His work as chairman on three of the initial documents establishing the basis of EMS (the essential equipment list for ambulances of the American College of Surgeons, the KKK standards of the Department of Transportation, and the first EMT basic training program) also propelled the idea and development of prehospital care. Robert Kennedy, MD, was the author of "Early Care of the Sick and Injured Patient." Sam Banks, MD, who with Dr. Farrington taught the first prehospital training course to the Chicago Fire Department in 1957, initiated proper care of the trauma patient. Minimal change occurred between the 1700s and the time that Farrington and the early leaders, such as Oscar Hampton, MD, and Curtis Arts, MD, brought the United States into the modern era of EMS and prehospital care.

A 1965 text edited and compiled by George J. Curry, MD, a leader of the American College of Surgeons and its Committee on Trauma, states the following:

Injuries sustained in accidents affect every part of the human body. They range from simple abrasions and contusions to multiple complex injuries involving many body tissues. This demands efficient and intelligent primary appraisal and care, on an individual basis, before transport. It is obvious that the services of trained ambulance attendants are essential. If we are to expect maximum efficiency from ambulance attendants, a special training program must be arranged.

Although prehospital care was rudimentary when Curry wrote this passage, the words still hold true as prehospital care providers address the specific area of prehospital trauma care rather than the broad field of general EMS.

Curry's call for specialized training of "ambulance attendants" has been answered during the past 25 years by this text and by the landmark "white paper" *Accidental Death and Disability: The Neglected Disease of Modern Society.* The National Academy of Science's National Research Council issued this paper just 1 year after Curry's call. The first efforts to answer Curry's call were primitive and have come a long way in a brief time. However, despite the continual rush of new developments, procedures, equipment, provider levels, and standards, a need exists to go back and rethink issues to fill in the spaces left by the march of progress through the field of EMS.

All of these innovators have taught several basic principles that have been expanded upon and refined over time. These principles are as follows:

- Rapidly respond to the patient.
- Provide efficient but prompt care to reestablish adequate ventilation, provide sufficient oxygenation, and preserve adequate perfusion to maintain the needed energy production for organ preservation.
- Rapidly transport the patient to the most appropriate facility.

Rapid access to the patient depends on a prehospital care system that offers easy access to the system. This access can be aided by a single emergency phone number (e.g., 9-1-1 in the United States, other numbers in other countries), a good communication system to dispatch the unit, and well prepared and trained prehospital care providers. Many people have heard that early access and early CPR save the lives of those experiencing cardiac arrest. Trauma can be approached the same way. The three principles listed previously can save lives.

Efficient on-scene medical care requires prehospital care providers who are well trained in rapid identification of the patient's condition and skilled in airway management, shock management, and proper immobilization procedures. The prehospital care provider must exercise good judgment to decide what action to

take on the scene, how to perform it efficiently, and which steps to carry out en route to the receiving facility.

The prehospital care provider must ensure that the patient is transported to an appropriate facility. This facility is the one that can most promptly and most appropriately provide definitive care to the patient. The prehospital care provider often has no choice in a rural area with only one hospital available in the community. The next hospital may be miles away, and the trauma center could be even farther. In this instance, the prehospital provider must decide whether helicopter transport from the scene is warranted. This is a fairly simple calculation. The approximate time of ground transportation is on one side of the equation. On the other side is the time necessary for helicopter alert and lift off, travel to the scene, management on the scene, and travel back to the hospital. The prehospital care provider determines the means of transportation based on which of the two times is shorter.

PHTLS is designed to rapidly assess patients and begin life-saving therapy early and appropriately. Two studies conducted by Dr. Jameel Ali in Trinidad and Tobago demonstrated an improved process in patient care resulting in a decrease in the mortality rate from trauma after teaching PHTLS to all prehospital care providers (Figure I-7). This text and the PHTLS course provide the necessary tools to save lives. Prehospital care works.

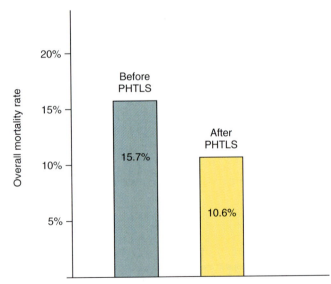

Figure I-7 Trauma deaths decreased by about one third after the introduction of PHTLS to the nations of Trinidad and Tobago. (*Adapted from Ali J, Adam RU, Gana TJ et al: Trauma patient outcome after the prehospital trauma life support program,* J Trauma 42:1018, 1997.)

REFERENCES

Ali J, Adam RU, Gana TJ et al: Effect of the prehospital trauma life support program (PHTLS) on prehospital trauma care, *J Trauma* 42:786, 1997.

Ali J, Adam RU, Gana TJ et al: Trauma patient outcome after the prehospital trauma life support program, *J Trauma* 42:1018, 1997.

Cornwell EE, Belzberg H, Hennigan K et al: Emergency medical services (EMS) vs. Non–EMS transport of critically injured patients: a prospective evaluation, *Arch Surg* 135(3):315, 2000.

Demetriades D, Chan L, Cornwell EE et al: Paramedic vs. private transportation of trauma patients: effect on outcome, *Arch Surg* 131:133, 1996.

Farrington JD: *Death in a ditch*, Chicago, 1967, American College of Surgeons.

Kennedy R: *Early care of the sick and injured patient*, Chicago, 1964, American College of Surgeons.

National Academy of Sciences/National Research Council: *Accidental death and disability: the neglected disease of modern society*, Washington, DC, 1966, NAS/NRC.

Rockwood CA, Mann CM, Farrington JD et al: History of Emergency Medical Services in the United States, *J Trauma* 16:299, 1976.

Trunkey DD: Trauma, *Scientific American* 249:28, 1983.

Chapter 1

Injury Prevention

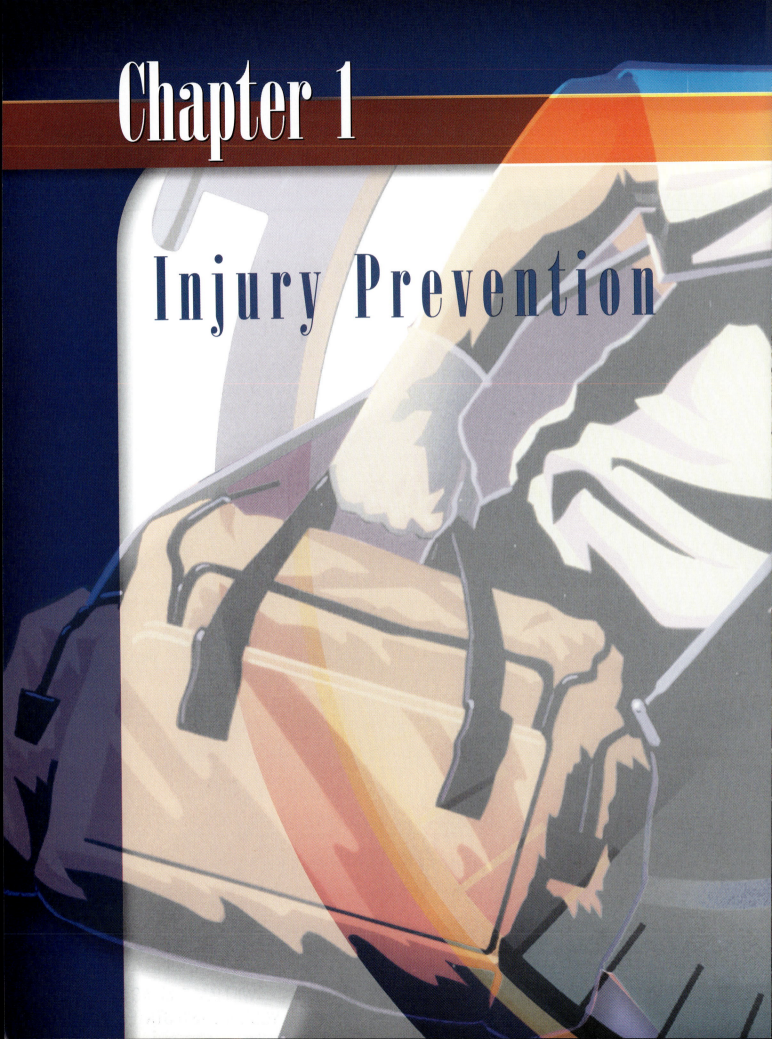

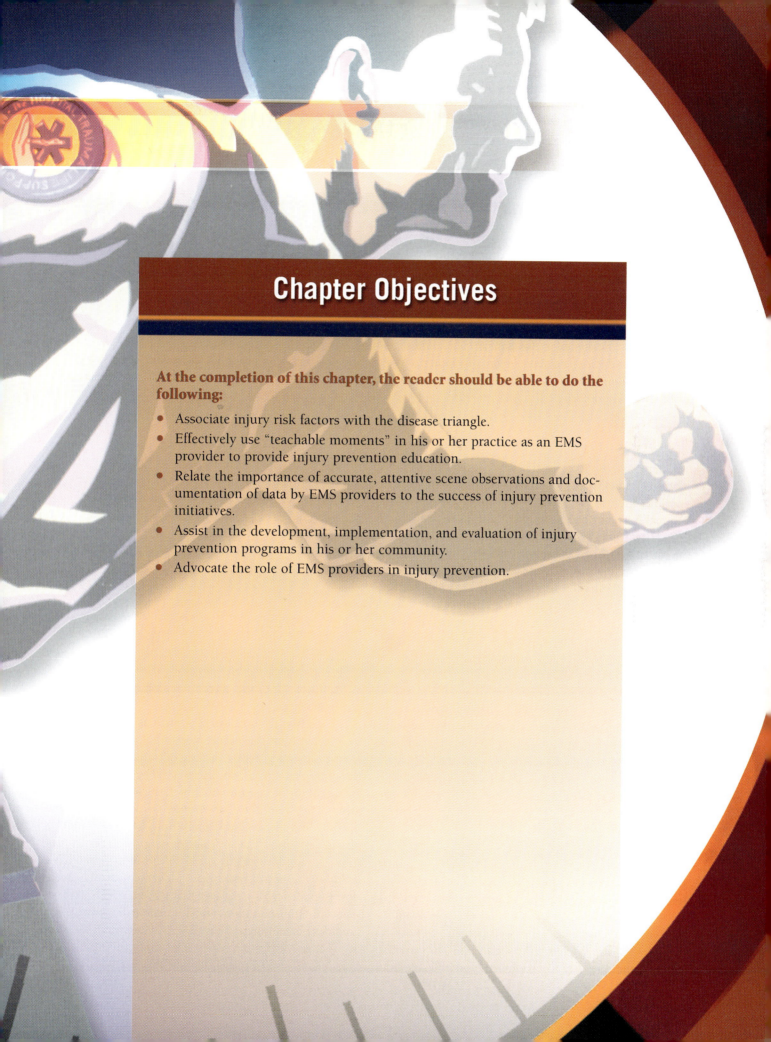

Chapter Objectives

At the completion of this chapter, the reader should be able to do the following:

- Associate injury risk factors with the disease triangle.
- Effectively use "teachable moments" in his or her practice as an EMS provider to provide injury prevention education.
- Relate the importance of accurate, attentive scene observations and documentation of data by EMS providers to the success of injury prevention initiatives.
- Assist in the development, implementation, and evaluation of injury prevention programs in his or her community.
- Advocate the role of EMS providers in injury prevention.

Scenario

Mark and Pam have been partners as EMS providers in a large, urban EMS system for 5 years. They are stationed in a district where nearly 100% of the residents are indigent and in which they have a high call volume. Mark and Pam have become increasingly frustrated by calls that involve tragic intentional and unintentional injuries. Shortly after beginning their shift today, they received a call for a child struck by a vehicle. On arrival, they find an 8-year-old male who was struck by a vehicle while riding his bike in the street. The child was not wearing a helmet and received devastating head trauma. The patient is apneic and bradycardic on the scene. Despite their 3-minute response time, 7-minute scene time, excellent prehospital management, and rapid transport to a level-one trauma center, the patient dies within 40 minutes.

What factors contributed to this injury? How could this injury and countless others have been prevented? What could Mark and Pam have done before this injury to reduce the incidence of injury in the community they serve? How do you think EMS providers' perceptions about their jobs are affected by exposure to such a high number of calls that involve injuries?

The major impetus in the development of modern emergency medical services (EMS) systems was the publication of the 1966 "white paper" by the National Academy of Science/National Research Council (NAS/NRC) entitled, *Accidental Death and Disability: The Neglected Disease of Modern Society*. The paper spotlighted voids in injury management in the United States, which helped launch a formal system of on-scene care and rapid transport for patients injured as a result of "accidents." This educational initiative was instrumental in the creation of a more efficient system to deliver prehospital care to the sick and injured.

Death and disability from injury in the United States have fallen since publication of the white paper. Despite this progress, injury remains a major public health problem. Over 146,000 Americans die from injuries annually, and millions more are adversely affected to some degree. Injury is a global problem as well. Approximately 5.8 million people worldwide died from injuries in 1998. Injuries remain a leading cause of death for all age groups. For some age groups, particularly children, teenagers, and young adults, injury is *the* leading cause of death.

The desire to care for patients stricken by injury draws many into the field of EMS. The Prehospital Trauma Life Support (PHTLS) course teaches prehospital providers to be *more* efficient and effective in injury management. The need for well-trained prehospital providers to care for injured patients will always exist; however, the best way to be efficient and effective is to prevent injury from happening in the first place. Prehospital care providers at all levels must play an active role in injury prevention to achieve the best results.

Even in 1966, the authors of the NAS/NRC white paper recognized the importance of injury prevention when they wrote the following:

> The long-term solution to the injury problem is prevention . . . . Prevention of accidents involves training in the home, in the school, and at work, augmented by frequent pleas for safety in the news media; first aid courses and public meetings; and inspection and surveillance by regulatory agencies.

Prehospital personnel can easily play an active role in most, if not all, of the current recommendations for injury prevention.

Prevention of some diseases, such as rabies, has been so effective that the occurrence of a single case makes front-page news. Public health officials now recognize that prevention results in the greatest reward toward the amelioration of disease. To spur EMS systems to take a more active role, the *EMS Agenda for the Future*, developed by and for the EMS community, lists prevention as one of 14 attributes to further develop in order to "improve community health and result in more appropriate use of acute health resources." Movement in that direction is evidenced by the fact that the latest U.S. Department of Transportation (DOT) paramedic curriculum includes prevention training. EMS systems are transforming themselves from a solely reactionary discipline to a broader, more effective discipline that includes prevention. This chapter is designed to introduce key concepts of injury prevention to the prehospital care provider.

Scope of the Problem

Death from injuries is a major health problem worldwide resulting in almost 16,000 deaths *daily* (Box 1-1). In few countries, regardless of their level of development, do injuries not appear among the five leading causes of death. Although types of injury deaths vary little between countries, wide variability exists between which types influence specific age groups. Because of economic, social, and developmental issues, the cause of injury-related death varies from country to country and even region to region within the same country.

In low- and middle-income countries of the Western Pacific the leading injury-related causes of death are road traffic injuries, drowning, and suicide. In Africa the leading causes are war, interpersonal violence, and road traffic injuries. In high-income countries of the Americas the leading cause of death among people between 15 and 44 years of age is road traffic injuries. In low- and middle-income countries of the Americas the leading cause is interpersonal violence. Figure 1-1 demonstrates that injury plays a role in at least 1 of the top 15 leading causes of death in every age group, particularly the young, worldwide.

In the United States injuries are the third leading cause of death behind cardiovascular disease and cancer, accounting for over 146,000 deaths annually (Figure 1-2). Injury is an especially serious problem for the youth of America and of most industrialized nations of the world. In the United States, injury kills more children and young adults than all diseases combined (nearly 19,000 in 1997).

Unfortunately, deaths from injury are only the tip of the iceberg. The "injury triangle" provides a more complete picture of the public health impact of injury (Figure 1-3, p. 15). In the United States in 1997, just over 146,000 people died from injury, but another 2.5 million were hospitalized because of nonfatal injuries. Injury also resulted in 37 million emergency department visits.

The impact on a nation can best be understood by examining the number of years of potential life lost (YPLL) as a result of injury. YPLL is calculated by subtracting the age at death from a fixed age, usually 65 or 70 years or the life expectancy of the group in question. This measure shows how injury compares with other causes of death in terms of years of life lost. Injury unnecessarily kills or maligns people of all ages, but it disproportion-

ately affects children, youth, and young adults, especially in industrialized nations. Because injury is the leading killer of Americans between 1 and 44 years of age, it is responsible for more YPLL than any other cause. In 1995, injury stole an estimated 3.5 million years from its victims compared with 2 million years for cancer even though cancer claims more lives than injury.

Another measure of injury severity can be demonstrated in dollars spent. Economic costs of injury are felt far beyond the patient and/or his immediate family. All members of society feel the effect because the costs of injury are borne by federal and other agencies, private insurance programs, and employers as well as the patient. As a result, everyone pays when an individual is seriously injured. Cost estimates for injury run as high as $325 billion dollars annually, which includes the direct cost of medical care and indirect cost such as lost earnings.

The toll of injury in terms of morbidity, mortality, and economic stress is excessive.

> Injuries have always been a threat to the public's well-being, but until the mid-twentieth century, infectious diseases overshadowed the terrible contribution injury made to human morbidity and mortality. Public health's success in other areas has left injury as a major public health concern, one that has been termed "the neglected epidemic." (Christoffel and Gallagher, 1999)

Society is calling upon all segments of the medical community to increase their prevention activities. With more than 600,000 prehospital providers in the United States alone, EMS systems stand to make a tremendous contribution to community-based injury prevention efforts.

Concepts of Injury

Definition of Injury

A discussion of injury prevention should begin with a definition of the term *injury*. The wide variability of the causes of injury initially represented a major hurdle in the study and prevention of injury. For example, what does a fractured hip resulting from a fall by an elderly person have in common with a self-inflicted gunshot wound to the head of a young adult? All possible causes of injury, from vehicle crashes, to stabbings, to suicides, to drownings, have one thing in common—energy transfer. *Injury* is now commonly defined as a harmful event that arises from the release of specific forms of physical energy or barriers to normal flow of energy.

Typically, energy exists in five physical forms—mechanical, chemical, thermal, radiation, or electrical. Mechanical energy, the most common cause of injury,

Box 1-1

Injury-Related Statistics

INJURY OVERALL

- Road traffic and self-inflicted injuries are the leading causes of injury-related deaths worldwide.*
- Five of the top ten causes of death in the world for persons 15 to 44 years of age are the result of injuries.*
- In high-income countries, road traffic injuries, self-inflicted injuries, and interpersonal violence are the three leading causes of death among people 15 to 44 years of age.*

MOTOR-VEHICLE–RELATED INJURIES

- Motor vehicle crashes are the leading cause of injury death in the United States for people 1 to 34 years of age.[†]
- In the United States in 1997, nearly 42,000 people died as a result of motor vehicle crashes and another 3.5 million sustained nonfatal injuries.[†]
- Motor vehicle crashes took the lives of 5606 teenagers and 2027 children in 1998.[†]
- In the United States in 1998, 5220 pedestrians died from traffic-related injuries and another 69,000 pedestrians sustained nonfatal injuries.[†]
- The United States has witnessed a 90% decrease in the annual death rate involving motor vehicle crashes despite a steep increase in the number of drivers, vehicles, and vehicle miles traveled.[‡]
- Worldwide, road traffic injuries are the leading injury-related cause of death and burden of disease in males.*

BICYCLE INJURIES

- In the United States in 1997, 813 bicyclists were killed in crashes with motor vehicles. Of these, 31% were younger than 16 years of age and 97% were not wearing helmets.[‡]
- An estimated 140,000 children in the United States are treated each year in emergency departments for head injuries sustained while bicycling.[‡]
- Almost 600,000 people in the United States are treated in emergency departments for bicycle-related injuries annually. In 1998, 758 bicyclists died from this type of injury.[†]

HOME AND RECREATION INJURIES

- Drowning is the second leading cause of injury death among children (1 to 14 years of age).[†]
- In the United States in 1996, nearly 4000 people drowned, including 1000 children younger than 15 years of age.[‡]
- In the United States in 1997, residential fires accounted for 3360 deaths and caused an estimated $4.6 billion in residential property damage.[†]
- Working smoke alarms reduce the risk of death from residential fires by 40% to 50%.[‡]
- Every 40 seconds someone in the United States seeks medical care because of a dog bite.[†]
- In the United States, falls are the leading cause of injury deaths among people 65 years of age or older. One out of three Americans 65 years of age or older falls each year.[†]
- Falls are the leading cause of nonfatal unintentional injuries and emergency department visits for children between birth and 14 years of age.[†]
- Each year in the United States, 200,000 preschool and elementary school children visit emergency departments for injuries sustained on playground equipment (about one injury every 2½ minutes). About 35% of these injuries are severe (e.g., fractures, internal injuries, concussions, dislocations, amputations, crushes).[‡]

*As gathered from multiple sources and reported by the World Health Organization.
[†]As gathered from multiple sources and reported by the National Center for Injury Prevention and Control.
[‡]As gathered from multiple sources and reported by the Society for Public Health Education.

Rank	0—4 years	5—14 years	15—44 years	45—59 years	>60 years	All ages
1	Perinatal conditions 2,155,000	Acute lower respiratory infections 213,429	HIV/AIDS 1,629,726	Ischemic heart disease 887,146	Ischemic heart disease 6,239,562	Ischemic heart disease 7,375,408
2	Acute lower respiratory infections 1,850,412	Malaria 209,109	Road traffic injuries 600,312	Cerebrovascular disease 600,854	Cerebrovascular disease 4,247,080	Cerebrovascular disease 5,106,125
3	Diarrheal diseases 1,814,158	Road traffic injuries 161,956	Interpersonal violence 509,844	Tuberculosis 407,737	Chronic obstructive pulmonary disease 1,974,652	Acute lower respiratory infections 3,452,178
4	Measles 887,671	Drowning 157,573	Self-inflicted injuries 508,621	Trachea/bronchus /lung cancers 305,982	Acute lower respiratory infections 1,184,698	HIV/AIDS 2,285,229
5	Malaria 793,368	Diarrheal diseases 133,883	Tuberculosis 427,314	Cirrhosis of the liver 264,117	Trachea/bronchus /lung cancers 889,873	Chronic obstructive pulmonary disease 2,249,252
6	Congenital abnormalities 404,849	War injuries 57,285	War injuries 372,935	HIV/AIDS 214,571	Tuberculosis 570,513	Diarrheal diseases 2,219,032
7	HIV/AIDS 349,885	Nephritis/nephrosis 44,640	Ischemic heart disease 244,556	Liver cancers 205,394	Stomach cancers 561,527	Perinatal conditions 2,155,000
8	Pertussis 345,771	Congenital abnormalities 43,056	Cerebrovascular disease 195,983	Stomach cancers 205,212	Diabetes mellitus 426,964	Tuberculosis 1,496,061
9	Tetanus 302,668	Inflammatory cardiac disease 40,802	Cirrhosis of the liver 142,445	Chronic obstructive pulmonary disease 203,192	Colon/rectum cancer 424,463	Tracheal/bronchus/ lung cancers 1,244,407
10	Protein–energy malnutrition 214,717	HIV/AIDS 39,042	Drowning 141,922	Self-inflicted injuries 178,478	Cirrhosis of the liver 355,615	Road traffic injuries 1,170,694
11	Drowning 125,301	Fires 38,968	Fires 122,666	Road traffic injuries 172,312	Nephritis/nephrosis 307,832	Malaria 1,110,293
12	STDs excluding HIV 118,178	Cerebrovascular disease 38,349	Maternal hemorrhage 116,771	Breast cancers 132,238	Esophagus cancers 296,550	Self-inflicted injuries 947,697
13	War injuries 103,323	Tuberculosis 38,093	Acute lower respiratory infections 115,100	Esophagus cancers 117,352	Liver cancers 295,756	Measles 887,671
14	Road traffic injuries 82,429	Interpersonal violence 34,938	Rheumatic heart disease 104,635	Diabetes mellitus 104,855	Inflammatory cardiac disease 268,545	Stomach cancers 822,069
15	Meningitis 60,198	Leukemia 34,503	Liver cancers 103,131	Inflammatory cardiac disease 97,511	Self-inflicted injuries 227,724	Cirrhosis of the liver 774,563

Source: World Health Report 1999 Database

Figure 1-1   Worldwide leading causes of death, both sexes, 1998. *Blue,* death from unintentional injury; *Red,* death from intentional injury committed by others; *Green,* death from intentional injury committed by self.

is expended when an unrestrained driver collides with the windshield during a vehicle crash. Injury from chemical energy occurs when a curious child drinks ammonia found in an unlocked cabinet in the kitchen. Thermal energy causes injury when a cook sprays lighter fluid on actively burning charcoal in an outdoor grill. Radiation energy produces sunburn to the teenager searching for a golden tan for the summer. Electrical energy damages the skin, nerves, and blood vessels of a prehospital care provider who fails to do a proper scene assessment before touching a vehicle that hit a power pole.

The body requires basic elements such as oxygen and heat to produce the internal energy needed to function properly. If conditions arise that prevent the body from using these necessary elements, injury can result. Suffocation and hypothermia are physical injuries that result from an interruption of the body's normal energy flow.

Any form of physical energy in sufficient quantity can cause tissue damage. The body can tolerate energy transfer within certain limits. If this threshold is breached, an injury results. A bullet fired from a pistol

	Age Groups										
Rank	**<1**	**1-4**	**5-9**	**10-14**	**15-24**	**25-34**	**35-44**	**45-54**	**55-64**	**65+**	**Total**
1	Congenital anomalies 6,178	Unintentional injury and adv. effects 2,005	Unintentional injury and adv. effects 1,534	Unintentional injury and adv. effects 1,837	Unintentional injury and adv. effects 13,367	Unintentional injury and adv. effects 12,598	Malignant neoplasms 17,099	Malignant neoplasms 45,429	Malignant neoplasms 86,314	Heart disease 606,913	Heart disease 726,974
2	Short gestation 3,925	Congenital anomalies 589	Malignant neoplasms 547	Malignant neoplasms 483	Homicide & legal intervention 6,146	Suicide 5,672	Unintentional injury and adv. effects 14,531	Heart disease 35,277	Heart disease 65,958	Malignant neoplasms 382,913	Malignant neoplasms 539,577
3	SIDS 2,991	Malignant neoplasms 438	Congenital anomalies 223	Suicide 303	Suicide 4,186	Homicide & legal intervention 5,075	Heart disease 13,227	Unintentional injury and adv. effects 10,416	Bronchitis Emphysema Asthma 10,109	Cerebro-vascular 140,366	Cerebro-vascular 159,791
4	Respiratory distress syndrome 1,301	Homicide & legal intervention 375	Homicide & legal intervention 174	Homicide & legal intervention 283	Malignant neoplasms 1,645	Malignant neoplasms 4,607	HIV 7,073	Cerebro-vascular 5,695	Cerebro-vascular 9,676	Bronchitis Emphysema Asthma 94,411	Bronchitis Emphysema Asthma 109,029
5	Maternal complications 1,244	Heart disease 212	Heart disease 128	Congenital anomalies 224	Heart disease 1,098	HIV 3,993	Suicide 6,730	Liver disease 5,622	Diabetes 8,370	Pneumonia & influenza 77,561	Unintentional injury and adv. effects 95,644
6	Placenta cord membranes 960	Pneumonia & influenza 180	Pneumonia & influenza 76	Heart disease 185	Congenital anomalies 420	Heart disease 3,286	Homicide & legal intervention 3,677	Suicide 4,948	Unintentional injury and adv. effects 7,105	Diabetes 47,289	Pneumonia & influenza 86,449
7	Perinatal infections 777	Perinatal period 75	HIV 62	Bronchitis Emphysema Asthma 79	HIV 276	Cerebro-vascular 678	Liver disease 3,508	Diabetes 4,335	Liver disease 5,253	Unintentional injury and adv. effects 31,386	Diabetes 62,636
8	Unintentional injury and adv. effects 765	Septicemia 73	Bronchitis Emphysema Asthma 50	Pneumonia & influenza 65	Pneumonia & influenza 220	Diabetes 620	Cerebro-vascular 2,787	HIV 3,513	Pneumonia & influenza 3,759	Alzheimer disease 22,154	Suicide 30,535
9	Intrauterine hypoxia 452	Benign neoplasms 65	Anemias 38	Cerebro-vascular 51	Bronchitis Emphysema Asthma 201	Pneumonia & influenza 534	Diabetes 1,858	Bronchitis Emphysema Asthma 2,838	Suicide 2,946	Nephritis 21,787	Nephritis 25,331
10	Pneumonia & influenza 421	Cerebro-vascular 56	Benign neoplasms 35	Benign neoplasms 41	Cerebro-vascular 188	Liver disease 516	Pneumonia & influenza 1,394	Pneumonia & influenza 2,233	Septicemia 1,852	Septicemia 18,079	Liver disease 25,175
11	Neonatal hemorrhage 339	HIV 54	Septicemia 34	HIV 40	Diabetes 129	Congenital anomalies 454	Bronchitis Emphysema Asthma 886	Homicide & legal intervention 1,869	Nephritis 1,832	Athero-sclerosis 15,273	Alzheimer disease 22,475
12	Homicide & legal intervention 317	Meningo-coccal 45	Perinatal period 27	Anemias 25	Benign neoplasms 115	Bronchitis Emphysema Asthma 357	Viral hepatitis 734	Septicemia 1,188	HIV 1,065	Hypertension 11,627	Septicemia 22,396
13	Remainder respiratory 274	Meningitis 44	Cerebro-vascular 25	Meningitis 18	Complicated pregnancy 87	Septicemia 235	Septicemia 634	Viral hepatitis 952	Hypertension 1,003	Liver disease 10,226	Homicide & legal intervention 19,846
14	Intestinal infections 200	Bronchitis Emphysema Asthma 41	Meningo-coccal 19	Septicemia 18	Septicemia 86	Benign neoplasms 187	Congenital anomalies 534	Nephritis 867	Homicide & legal intervention 853	Suicide 5,728	HIV 16,516
15	Septicemia 196	Anemias 40	Meningitis 15	Two tied 15	Anemias 85	Nephritis 179	Nephritis 448	Hypertension 586	Benign neoplasms 726	Hernia 5,725	Athero-sclerosis 16,057

Produced by: Office of Statistics and Programming, National Center for Injury Prevention and Control, CDC
Data source: National Center for Health Statistics (NCHS) Vital Statistics System.

Figure 1-2   Leading causes of death in the United States by age group, 1997. *Blue,* death from unintentional injury; *Red,* death from intentional injury committed by others; *Green,* death from intentional injury committed by self.

at point-blank range easily passes through skin and soft tissue, causing massive injury. If the intended victim is far enough away, theoretically the victim can simply stick out a hand and the bullet would hit the palm and fall harmlessly to the ground. The bullet's energy dissipates in the air on its flight. Therefore it does not have enough energy on impact to exceed the body's tolerance level.

Energy Out of Control

People harness and use all five forms of energy in many productive endeavors every day. In these instances en-

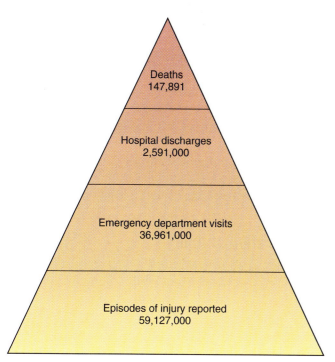

Figure 1-3   Injury triangle.

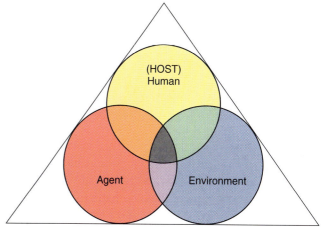

Figure 1-4   Disease triangle.

in concentration at the very moment when additional skill is required may lead to a crash. Injury occurs during the crash because of amounts of uncontrolled, sudden energy release in excess of the body's tolerance level.

Injury as a Disease

The following must interact simultaneously for an illness to occur: (1) an agent that causes the illness, (2) a host in which the agent can reside, and (3) a suitable environment in which the agent and host can come together. Once public health professionals recognized this "disease triangle," it discovered how to combat the disease (Figure 1-4). Eradication of certain diseases has been possible by vaccinating the host, destroying the agent with antibiotics, reducing environmental transmission through improved sanitation, or a combination of all three. Illness can be attacked by modifying the host and environment as well as by destroying the agent.

Only since the late 1940s has significant exploration of the injury process occurred. Pioneers in the study of injury demonstrated that in spite of the obviously different results, illness and injury behave similarly. Both require the presence of the three elements of the disease triangle, and therefore both are treated as a disease:

1. For an injury to occur, a host (i.e., the human being) must exist. As with illness, susceptibility of the host does not remain constant from individual to individual; it varies as a result of internal and external factors. Internal factors include intelligence, sex, and reaction time. External factors include intoxication, anger, and beliefs. Susceptibility also varies over time within the same person.

ergy is under control and is not allowed to adversely affect the body. A person's ability to maintain control of energy depends on two factors—task performance and task demand. As long as a person's ability to perform a task exceeds the demands of a task, energy is released in a controlled, useable manner.

However, in three instances demand may exceed performance, leading to an uncontrolled release of energy:

1. *When the difficulty of the task suddenly exceeds the individual's performance ability.* For example, a prehospital care provider may operate an ambulance safely during normal driving conditions but loses control if the vehicle hits a sheet of black ice. The sudden increase in the demands of the task exceeds the prehospital care provider's performance capabilities, leading to a crash.
2. *When the individual's performance level falls below the demands of the task.* Falling asleep at the wheel of a vehicle while driving down a country road causes a sudden drop in performance with no change in task demand, leading to a crash.
3. *When both factors change simultaneously.* Talking on a cellular phone while driving may reduce a driver's concentration on the road. If an animal darts in front of the vehicle, task demand suddenly rises. Under normal circumstances, the driver may be able to handle the increased demands of the task. A drop

2. As described previously, the agent of injury is energy. Velocity, shape, material, and time of exposure to the object that releases the energy all play a role in whether the host's tolerance level is overwhelmed.
3. The host and agent must come together in an environment that allows the two to interact. Commonly, the environment is divided into physical and social components. Physical environmental factors can be seen and touched. Social environmental factors include attitudes, beliefs, and judgments. For example, teenagers are more likely to participate in risk-taking behavior because they have more of a sense of invincibility than other age groups.

In the case of injury, the host might be a curious, mobile 2 year old; the agent of injury might be a swimming pool filled with water with a beach ball floating just beyond the edge; the environment might be a pool gate left open while the baby-sitter runs inside to answer the telephone. With the host, agent, and environment all coming together at the same time, an unintentional injury—in this case, drowning—can occur.

Haddon Matrix

Dr. William J. Haddon, Jr., is considered the father of the science of injury prevention. Working within the concept of the disease triangle, in the mid-1960s he recognized that an injury can be broken down into three temporal phases:

1. *Preevent*. Before the injury.
2. *Event*. The point when harmful energy is released.
3. *Postevent*. The aftermath of the injury.

By examining the three factors of the disease triangle during each temporal phase, Haddon created a nine-cell "phase-factor" matrix (Figure 1-5). This grid has become known as the *Haddon Matrix*. It provides a means to graphically depict the events or actions that increase or decrease the odds that an injury will occur. It can also be used to identify prevention strategies. The Haddon Matrix demonstrates that *multiple* factors can lead to an injury and therefore multiple opportunities exist to prevent or reduce its severity. The matrix played a major role in dispelling the myth that injury is the result of a single cause, bad luck, or fate.

Figure 1-5 depicts a Haddon Matrix for a vehicle crash. The components in each cell of the matrix are different depending on the injury being examined. The preevent phase includes factors that can contribute to the likelihood of a crash. However, during this time, energy is still under control. This phase may last from a few seconds to several years. The event phase depicts the factors that influence the severity of the injury. During this time, uncontrolled energy is released and injury occurs if energy transfer exceeds the body's tolerance. The event phase is typically very brief. It may last only a fraction of a second but rarely lasts more than a few minutes. Factors in the postevent phase affect the outcome once an injury has occurred. Depending on the type of event, it may last from a few seconds to the remaining life span of the host.

Classification of Injury

A common method to subclassify injuries is based on intent. Injury may result from either intentional or unintentional causes. While this is a logical way to view injuries, it underscores the difficulty of injury prevention efforts.

Intentional injury is typically associated with an act of interpersonal or self-directed violence. Problems such as homicide, suicide, spousal abuse, and war fall into this category. Previously, prevention of intentional injury was thought to be the sole responsibility of the criminal justice and mental health systems. Although these agencies are integral to reducing violent deaths, intentional injuries can best be prevented through a broad multidisciplinary approach, which includes the medical profession.

In years past, unintentional injuries were called *accidents*. The authors of the NAS/NRC white paper appropriately referred to them as accidental death and disability because that was the vocabulary of the time. Health care providers now understand that the term *accidental* does not describe unintentional injury resulting from vehicle crashes, drownings, falls, and electrocutions. EMS systems have embraced this concept by using the term *motor vehicle crashes* (MVC) rather than *motor vehicle accidents* (MVA). However, public perception has changed much more slowly. News reporters still describe persons injured in "automobile accidents" or "accidental shootings." The term *accident* suggests that a person was injured as a result of fate, divine intervention, or bad luck. It implies that the injury was random and therefore unavoidable. As long as this misperception exists, implementation of corrective measures will be difficult.

Prevention as the Solution

Preventing injury is even more important than treating injury. When injury is prevented it spares the patient

Time Phases \ Disease Triangle Factors	HOST	AGENT	ENVIRONMENT
PREEVENT	• Driver vision • Alcohol consumption • Experience and judgment • Amount of travel • Level of fatigue • Adherence to driving laws	• Maintenance of brakes, tires, etc. • Defective equipment • Center of gravity • Speed of travel • Ease of control • Vehicle inspection programs	• Visibility hazards • Road curvature and gradient • Surface coefficient of friction • Narrow road shoulder • Traffic signals • Speed limits • Weather conditions • Attitudes about alcohol • Laws related to impaired driving • Support for injury prevention efforts • Roads used as primary playgrounds
EVENT	• Safety belt use • Osteoporosis • Injury threshold • Ejection	• Speed capability • Vehicle size • Automatic restraints • Hardness and sharpness of contact surfaces • Steering column	• Lack of guard rails • Median barriers • Distance between roadway and immovable objects • Speed limits • Oncoming traffic • Attitudes about safety belt use • Laws about safety belt use • Enforcement of child safety seat laws • Motorcycle helmet use laws
POSTEVENT	• Age • Physical condition • Type or extent of injury • Knowledge of first aid	• Fuel system integrity • Entrapment	• **Emergency communication system** • **Distance to and quality of EMS** • **Training of EMS personnel** • Availability of extrication equipment • Support for trauma care systems • Rehabilitation programs

Figure 1-5   Haddon Matrix for a vehicle crash.

and family from suffering and economic hardship. The National Center for Injury Prevention and Control (NCIPC) of the Centers for Disease Control and Prevention (CDC) estimates the following:

- $1 spent on smoke detectors saves $69.
- $1 spent on bicycle helmets saves $29.
- $1 spent on child safety seats saves $32.

- $1 spent on center and edge lines on roads saves $3 in medical costs alone.
- $1 spent on counseling by pediatricians to prevent injuries saves $10.
- $1 spent on poison-control center services saves $7 in medical expenses.
- A CDC-funded evaluation study of a regional trauma care system in Portland, Oregon, found a 35% de-

crease in the risk of dying for the severely injured who were treated in the system.

- A smoke detector distribution program in Oklahoma reduced burn-related injuries by 83%.

Because of the variability among the host, agent, and environment at any given time, health care providers cannot always predict or prevent every individual injury. However, health care providers can identify high-risk populations, high-risk products, and high-risk environments. Prevention efforts centered on high-risk groups or settings influence as wide a range of society as possible. Health care providers can pursue prevention in multiple ways. Some strategies have proven successful across the United States and around the world. However, other strategies work in one region but not in another. Before implementing an injury prevention strategy, efforts must center on determining if it will work. Although it is not necessary to "reinvent the wheel," health care providers may need to modify a prevention strategy to improve its chances of success. Methods for doing this are examined in the following section.

Concepts of Injury Prevention

Goal

The goal of injury prevention programs is to bring about a change in knowledge, attitude, and behavior on the part of a preidentified segment of society. Simply providing information to potential victims is not enough to prevent injury. A program must be implemented in a manner that will influence society's attitude and most importantly change behavior. Any change in behavior will hopefully be long term. This task is monumental but not insurmountable.

Opportunities

Prevention strategies can be arranged according to their effect on the injury event. They coincide with the temporal phases of the Haddon Matrix. Preevent interventions, known as primary interventions, strive to prevent the injury from occurring. Actions intended to keep intoxicated drivers off the road, lower speed limits, and install traffic lights are designed to prevent crashes from occurring. Event phase interventions are intended to reduce injury severity by softening the blow of injuries that occur. Wearing safety belts, installing cushioned dashboards in vehicles, and enforcing child safety seat laws are means to reduce the severity of crashes. Postevent interventions provide a means

to improve the likelihood of survival for those who are injured. Encouraging physical fitness, designing fuel systems for vehicles that do not explode on impact, and implementing high-quality EMS systems are intended to reduce the recovery time for persons who are injured.

Prehospital systems have traditionally limited their involvement to the postevent phase. Countless lives have been saved as a result. However, because of the limitations inherent in waiting until injury has occurred, the best results have not been achieved. EMS systems must look at entering the injury cycle earlier. Using the Haddon Matrix, EMS systems can identify opportunities to collaborate with other public health and public safety organizations to prevent injuries from occurring or to soften their blow.

Potential Strategies

No single strategy provides the best approach to injury prevention. The most effective option or options depends on the type of injury being studied. However, Haddon developed a list of 10 generic strategies designed to break the chain of injury-producing events at numerous points (Figure 1-6). These strategies represent ways that release of uncontrolled energy can be prevented or at least reduced to amounts the body can better tolerate. Figure 1-6 presents countermeasures that can be enacted in the preevent, event, and postevent phases and are directed towards the host, agent, or environment. This list should not be considered complete but it may serve as a starting point to help figure out the most effective options for the particular problem under study.

Most injury prevention strategies are either "active" or "passive." Passive strategies require little or no action on the part of the individual. Sprinkler systems and vehicle air bags are examples. Active strategies require the cooperation of the person being protected in order to work. Examples include manual seatbelts and choosing to wear a motorcycle helmet. Passive measures are generally more effective because people do not have to consciously do anything to take advantage of the protection. Nonetheless, they are usually harder to implement because they can be expensive or require legislative or regulatory action. Sometimes a combination of active and passive strategies is the best option.

Strategy Implementation

Three common approaches to implementing an injury prevention strategy have become known as the Three Es of Injury Prevention—Education, Enforcement, and Engineering.

STRATEGY	POSSIBLE COUNTERMEASURES
Prevent the initial creation of the hazard	• Do not produce firecrackers, three-wheeled all-terrain vehicles, or various poisons • Eliminate spearing in high school football
Reduce the amount of energy contained in the hazard	• Limit the horsepower of motor vehicle engines • Package toxic drugs in smaller, safer amounts • Reduce speed limits • Mandate public transportation to reduce the number of vehicles on the road • Limit the temperature of tap water in homes through regulators at the water heater • Limit the muzzle velocity of guns • Limit the amount of gunpowder in firecrackers
Prevent the release of a hazard that already exists	• Store firearms in locked containers • Close pools and beaches when no lifeguard is on duty • Make bathtubs less slippery • Childproof containers for all hazardous household drugs and chemicals • Limit cell phone use in vehicles to hands-free models • Require safety shields on rotating farm machinery • Improve vehicle handling
Modify the rate or spatial distribution of the hazard	• Use seatbelts • Provide antilock brakes • Use short cleats on football shoes so feet rotate rather than transmit sudden force to the knees • Require vehicle air bags • Provide hydraulic bumpers on vehicles • Provide safety nets to protect workers from falls • Wear flame-retardant pajamas
Separate in time or space the hazard from that which is to be protected	• Provide pedestrian overpasses at high-volume traffic crossings • Keep roadsides clear of poles and trees • Do not have play areas near unguarded bodies of water • Install bike paths • Spray pesticides at a time when people are not around • Install sidewalks • Route trucks carrying hazardous materials along low-density roads
Separate the hazard from that which is to be protected by a material barrier	• Install fencing around all sides of swimming pools • Provide protective eyewear for racquet sports • Build highway medians • Build protective shields around hazardous machinery • Install guard rails between sidewalks and roads • Install reinforced panels in vehicle doors • Require EMS personnel to place used needles directly into a sharps box
Modify the basic nature of the hazard	• Provide air bags in motor vehicles • Provide collapsible steering columns • Provide breakaway poles • Make crib slats too narrow to strangle a baby • Adopt breakaway baseball bases • Install nonslip surfaces in bathtubs • Round the corners of cabinetry in the patient compartment of ambulances
Make what is to be protected more resistant to the hazard	• Encourage calcium intake to reduce osteoporosis • Encourage musculoskeletal conditioning in athletes • Prohibit alcohol sales and consumption near recreational water areas • Treat medical conditions, such as epilepsy, to prevent episodes that can result in burns, drownings, and falls • Earthquake-resistant building codes in susceptible areas
Begin to counter the damage already done by the hazard	• Provide emergency medical care • Employ system to route injured persons to appropriately trained prehospital care providers • Develop school protocols for responding to injury emergencies • Provide first-aid training to residents • Automatic sprinkler systems
Stabilize, repair, and rehabilitate the object of the damage	• Develop rehabilitation plans at an early stage of injury treatment • Make use of occupational rehabilitation for paraplegics

Figure 1-6   Basic strategies for injury countermeasures. (The examples listed above are for illustrative purposes only and are not necessarily the official recommendations of PHTLS, the National Association of EMTs, and the American College of Surgeons.)

EDUCATION

Educational strategies are meant to impart information. To be effective, the target audience must embrace its newfound knowledge with enough enthusiasm to alter behavior in the manner prescribed by the program. Because the audience is required to do something, education is an active countermeasure. The target audience may be individuals who engage in high-risk activities, policymakers who have the authority to then enact further prevention legislation or regulation, or prehospital care providers learning to become active participants in injury prevention. The NAS/NRC white paper is an example of an education initiative.

Education once was the primary means of implementing prevention programs because society felt that most injuries were simply the result of human error. While this is true to a certain extent, they failed to recognize the role that energy and the environment play in causing injury. Nonetheless, education is still commonly used and is probably the easiest of the three strategies to implement.

Education strategies have not met with overwhelming success for several reasons. The target audience may never hear the message. If the message is heard, some may reject it outright or not embrace it enough to alter behavior. Those who embrace it may do so sporadically or with declining enthusiasm over time. However, education still can be particularly useful in reducing injury in four areas:

1. *Teaching young children basic safety behaviors and skills that stay with them later in life.* Examples might include what to do when a smoke detector sounds an alarm, calling 9-1-1 for help in an emergency, or fastening seat belts.
2. *Teaching about certain types and causes of injury and for certain age groups.* Education may be the only strategy available for these groups.
3. *Altering the public's perception of risk and acceptable risk to change social norms and attitudes.* This was used regarding drinking and driving and occurs now regarding wearing a helmet when riding a bicycle, scooter, skateboard, or rollerblades.
4. *Promoting policy change and educating consumers to demand safer products.*

As a singular approach to injury prevention, educational programs have had disappointing results. However, when coupled with other forms of implementation strategies, education can be a valuable tool. Education often serves as a starting point to pave the way for enforcement and engineering strategies.

ENFORCEMENT

Enforcement seeks to tap the persuasive power of law to compel adherence to simple but effective prevention strategies. Certain government entities have the power to enact statutes, regulations, and laws in an effort to promote public health, safety, and general welfare even when such actions restrict individual autonomy to a limited degree. Generally, courts tend to uphold injury prevention laws that pose a minimal burden on individuals if they are fairly enforced and the public health benefit is substantial.

Statutory commands can either require or prohibit and they can be directed at individual behavior (people), products (things), or environmental conditions (places):

- Legal requirements that apply to people are mandatory seat belt, child restraint, and helmet use laws.
- Prohibitions that apply to people are drunk driving laws, speed limits, and making assaultive behavior a crime.
- Legal requirements that apply to things include design and performance standards, such as the federal Motor Vehicle Safety Standards.
- Prohibitions that apply to things include restrictions on dangerous animals and flammable fabrics.
- Legal requirements that apply to places include the installation of breakaway signposts along highways and fencing around swimming pools.
- Prohibitions that apply to places include the outlawing of rigid structures along highways and firearms in airport terminals.

Enforcement is also an active countermeasure because people must obey the law to benefit from it. Enforcement typically has wide application because laws apply to all members of society within a given jurisdiction. The effectiveness of enforcement initiatives depends on the willingness of society to obey and the feasibility and visibility of its enforcement. The target audience may be less likely to comply if they feel that the directive infringes on personal freedom, they have little chance of getting caught, or they will not face consequences of violating the law. Because society as a whole tends to obey laws or at least stay within narrow limits around them, enforcement is often more effective than education. Enforcement in tandem with education appears to produce better results than either initiative alone.

ENGINEERING

Often the most effective means of injury prevention are those in which destructive energy release is permanently separated from the host. Passive countermeasures accomplish this goal with little or no effort on the part of the individual. Engineering strategies strive to build injury prevention into products or environments so that the host does not have to act differently to be protected. Engineering strategies help the people who actually need them, and they do so every time. Measures such as automatic sprinkler systems in buildings, flotation hulls in boats, and EMS systems have all been proven to save lives with little or no effort on the part of the host.

Engineering seems to be the perfect answer to injury prevention. It is passive, effective, and usually the least disruptive of the Three Es. Unfortunately, it is often the most expensive to implement. Designing safety into a product usually makes it more expensive and may require legislative or regulatory initiation. The price may be more than the manufacturer is willing to absorb or the customer is willing to pay. Society dictates how much safety it wants built into a product and how much it is willing to pay. Enforcement and engineering strategies should be preceded with education initiatives. The most effective countermeasures may be those that incorporate all three implementation strategies.

Public Health Approach

Much has been learned about injury and injury prevention. Unfortunately, a wide discrepancy exists between what is known about injury and what is being done about it. EMS systems must help close that gap. Injury is a complex problem in all societies of the world. A single person or single agency cannot prevent it. A public health approach has demonstrated success in dealing with other diseases and is making progress with injury prevention as well.

A public health approach creates a community-based coalition to combat a community-based disease through a four-step process:

1. Surveillance
2. Risk factor identification
3. Intervention evaluation
4. Implementation

The coalition is composed of experts from such diverse fields as epidemiology, the medical community, schools of public health, public health agencies, community advocacy programs, economics, sociology, and criminal justice. EMS systems have an important place in a public health approach to injury prevention. Being part of a coalition to improve playground safety may not have

the immediate effect of providing care at the scene of a horrific vehicle crash, but the results will be much more widespread.

SURVEILLANCE

Surveillance is the process of collecting data. Collection of population-based data on the community in question aids in discovery of an injury's true magnitude and effect on the community. A community can be a neighborhood, city, county, state, or even the entire nation. Because injury patterns may differ from country to country and even region to region, successful intervention strategies from one community may not produce similar results in another. Support for the program, proper allocation of resources, and even knowing who to include on the interdisciplinary team depends on understanding the scope of the problem.

The following are several sources of information available to a community:

- Mortality data
- Hospital admission and discharge statistics
- Medical records
- Trauma registries
- Police reports
- EMS run sheets
- Insurance reports

However, these data may contain only segments of the entire injury event, making accurate determinations sometimes difficult. The health care provider may need to establish a unique surveillance system to capture the most useful information.

RISK FACTOR IDENTIFICATION

After a problem is identified and researched, it is necessary to know who is at risk to direct a prevention strategy at the correct population. Shotgun approaches to injury prevention are less successful than targeted ones. Identification of causes and risk factors determines who is injured; what kinds of injuries are sustained; and where, when, and why those injuries occur. To ensure that a risk factor is a determinant in the cause of the injury, it may be necessary to compare a group with the risk factor with a group without the risk factor. Sometimes a risk factor is an obvious cause, such as the presence of alcohol in fatal vehicles crashes. At other times, research is required to discover the true risk factors involved in injury events. EMS systems can serve as the eyes and ears of public health at the scene of injuries to identify actual risk factors that no one else may be able to uncover. Risk factors can be charted on a Haddon Matrix as they are properly identified.

INTERVENTION EVALUATION

As risk factors become clear, intervention strategies begin to emerge. Haddon's list of 10 injury prevention strategies serves as a starting point (see Figure 1-6). When considering possible interventions, a health care provider must give attention to the values of the community (sociocultural environment), the target population (host), and the cost of implementation. Even though communities have different characteristics, with modification an injury prevention initiative from one community may work in another. Once a potential intervention has been selected, a pilot program using one or more of the Three Es may give indications of the success of full-scale implementation.

IMPLEMENTATION

The final step in the public health approach is implementation and evaluation of the intervention. Detailed implementation procedures are prepared so others interested in implementation of similar programs will have a guide to follow. Collection of evaluation data measures the effectiveness of a program. Three questions may help determine the success of a program:

1. Have attitudes, skills, or judgment changed?
2. Has behavior changed?
3. Does behavioral change lead to a favorable outcome?

The public health approach provides a proven means to combat a disease process. Through a multidisciplinary, community-based effort, it is possible to identify the who, what, where, when, and why of an injury problem and develop a plan of action. EMS systems need to play a much more substantial role to help close the gap between what is known about injury and what is being done about it.

Evolving Role of EMS

Traditionally, the prehospital care provider's role in health care focuses almost exclusively on postevent, one-on-one treatment of the individual. Little emphasis is placed on understanding the causes of the injuries or what a prehospital care provider could do to prevent them. As a result, patients may return to the same environment only to be injured again. In addition, information that could aid in the development of a community-wide prevention program to keep others from being injured in the first place may not be documented and therefore may remain unavailable to other sectors of public health.

Public health approaches health care from a different direction. It is proactive, working to determine how to alter the host, agent, and environment to prevent injuries. Through coalitions that conduct surveillance and implement interventions, public health works to develop community-wide prevention programs. The *EMS Agenda for the Future* envisions closer ties between EMS systems and public health that would make both sectors of health care more effective.

Prehospital care providers can take a more active role in development of community-wide injury prevention programs. EMS systems enjoy a unique position in the community. With over 600,000 providers in the United States alone, basic and advanced prehospital care providers are widely distributed at the community level. Prehospital care providers enjoy a credible reputation in the community, making them high-profile role models. In addition, they are readily welcomed into homes and businesses. All phases of the public health approach to injury prevention will benefit from an EMS presence.

One-on-One Interventions

EMS systems do not have to give up their one-on-one approach to patient care to conduct valuable injury prevention interventions. The one-on-one approach makes EMS systems uniquely able to conduct injury prevention initiatives. Prehospital care providers can bring injury prevention messages directly to high-risk individuals. One indicator of a successful educational program is that the information is received with enough enthusiasm to change behavior. Prehospital care providers can use their role model status to deliver important prevention messages. Implicitly, people look up to role models, listen to what they have to say, and emulate what they do.

On-scene prevention counseling takes advantage of a "teachable moment." A teachable moment is one in which the patient who does not require critical medical interventions or family members may be in a state that makes them more susceptible to what a role model says. The prehospital care provider may think of the on-scene time as wasted when it becomes apparent that little or no medical interventions are necessary. However, this may be the best time to deliver primary prevention.

Not every call allows for injury prevention counseling. Serious and life-threatening calls require concentration on acute care. However, as many as 95% of ambulance calls are non–life threatening. A significant proportion require minor, if any, treatment. One-on-one prevention counseling may be appropriate during these noncritical calls.

Patient interactions are typically short encounters, especially ones that require little or no treatment. However, they provide enough time to discuss and/or demonstrate to patients and family members practices that may prevent an injury in the future. A role model that discusses the importance of replacing a burned-out light bulb and removing a slippery throw rug in a dimly lit hallway may prevent a fall by an elderly resident. Prehospital care providers have an attentive audience during the ride to a hospital. Prevention is a more valuable topic to discuss than the weather or the local sports team. Teachable moments take 1 to 2 minutes to complete and do not interfere with treatment or transport.

Educational programs have been developed to train prehospital care providers to administer injury prevention counseling on-scene. These types of programs must be further developed and evaluated to discover which are the most valuable and therefore worthy of inclusion in the primary education of a prehospital care provider.

Community-Wide Interventions

The public health approach to injury prevention is community based and involves a multidisciplinary team. The EMS system has the expertise to be a valuable member of that team. Community-wide prevention strategies depend on data to properly address the who, what, when, where, and why of an injury problem. Multiple sources of information as described previously provide the needed data. Prehospital care providers, perhaps more than any other team member, have the opportunity to see a patient interact with his or her environment. This may allow identification of a high-risk individual, high-risk attitude, or high-risk behavior that is not present by the time the patient arrives at the emergency department.

The prehospital care provider can use documentation acquired en route to a medical facility in two ways:

1. It can be used immediately by emergency personnel who receive the patient. Emergency room physicians and nurses are also being called upon to improve and increase their role in injury prevention. Their "teachable moment" can reinforce and supplement the prehospital care provider's on-scene counseling if they know what has already been discussed or demonstrated.
2. Others in public health can use injury data provided by prehospital care providers retrospectively to help develop a comprehensive, community-wide injury prevention program.

Prehospital care providers do not commonly practice documentation to help build a community-wide prevention program. Knowing what to acquire and when to document information beneficial to the development of community-wide prevention programs requires opening a dialogue with other members of the public health team. Leaders in the EMS system need to build a coalition with public health to develop policies that promote complete documentation of injuries.

Injury Prevention for EMS Providers

In a prehospital service, employees are not only the most valuable asset but the most expensive. The service, community, and most importantly, the employee benefit when the employee remains uninjured. An in-house effort may be an excellent choice to conduct an injury prevention program through a public health approach. The community (e.g., the ambulance service) is small, there is 100% access to it, and surveillance is easier because the ambulance service has access to many of the data sources it may need. Identification of risk factors is simplified because the target audience consists of fellow employees. Gaining evaluation information should be almost immediate, which allows for midcourse correction. Outcome data collection should be readily available as well.

Kinnane and colleagues mention in-house prevention programs that utilize education, enforcement, and engineering implementation strategies. The wide variability of the programs demonstrates the dangers involved in EMS systems and the need for prevention initiatives. It also demonstrates the variability among EMS communities. Even though all EMS services are similar, individual services (communities) have different risk factors and different prevention priorities.

Education programs as described previously enhance wellness, prevent back injury, and increase awareness of the potential for violent patients. Enforcement programs introduced mandatory fitness programs and establishment of protocols to deal with violent patients. Engineering initiatives dealt with increasing seat belt use in the back of the ambulance by evaluating the position of equipment and location of the seat and reducing back injury through pre-employment screening and physical strengthening.

A small scale, in-house injury prevention program may reap rewards beyond the obvious and most important outcome of improved employee health. Small successes lay the groundwork for participation in larger, more complicated endeavors. They provide a valuable on-the-job learning tool about injury prevention for all employees. In addition, in-house prevention programs provide an introduction of the EMS service to other public health agencies in the community that assist in in-house program implementation and evaluation.

Summary

Trauma is the most neglected current epidemic. Although EMS systems have progressed dramatically in the management of injuries since the 1966 publication of the NAS/NRC "white paper," the health care industry has failed to measurably decrease the incidence of injuries. Over 146,000 people die as a result of injuries each year in the United States alone despite the development of highly evolved EMS systems. EMS providers are in a unique position to influence injury morbidity and mortality rates through prevention. This position has been recognized, and the role of EMS personnel in illness and injury prevention is evolving.

EMS personnel must integrate knowledge, skills, and tools used in public health into the practice of the EMS profession. This is an opportunity for EMS systems to significantly affect the health of all individuals. The advancement of EMS systems in injury prevention depends on the adoption of this new role by each individual prehospital care provider. Prehospital care providers must have knowledge and skills in injury prevention, believe in its importance, commit to the effort, and serve as an advocate to their peers.

Scenario Solution

Six months earlier:

Mark and Pam have been frustrated at the incidence of intentional and unintentional injuries in their district. They have noticed that since the implementation of community policing in their district, the number of crime-related injuries has been reduced. After a discussion of their observation, Mark and Pam write a proposal to the director of their EMS system for a community-based EMS program in their district. Mark and Pam become highly visible in the community and establish rapport with the residents, taking every opportunity to discuss injury prevention. Although they enjoy working this way, Mark and Pam feel that they need to address some specific, wide-spread problems and develop the following program.

With permission from their director, Mark and Pam arrange to work with police and fire units in the area to reduce injuries to bicycle riders. Bicycle officers from the police department will give bicycle safety courses along with local EMS providers. Fire stations in the area start a program for neighborhood children to bring their bicycles to the station for inspection, repair, and maintenance. Mark and Pam write a grant proposal and receive $1500 from a local charitable organization to purchase bicycle helmets for area children. Mark and Pam realize that although knowledge and equipment are important factors in injury prevention, they do not guarantee compliance. They solicit the involvement of a local chain of convenience stores to provide coloring books on safety for local EMS, police, and fire personnel to distribute to children to reinforce bicycle safety and promote other safe behaviors. Most importantly, children seen wearing their helmets and riding safely are always praised.

An analysis of data 6 months later reveals a 45% reduction in bicycle-related injuries in the community.

Review Questions

Answers are provided on p. 414.

1. Which of the following is a common element in all injuries?
   a. Energy transfer
   b. Lack of engineering controls
   c. An uneducated victim
   d. High-risk behavior

2. A driver who falls asleep behind the wheel represents which part of the disease triangle?
   a. Environment
   b. Agent
   c. Host
   d. Mechanism

3. Which of the following is a useful instrument for identifying factors responsible for injuries?
   a. Fick Principle
   b. Cushing's Triad
   c. Revised Trauma Score
   d. Haddon Matrix

4. A supplemental restraint system (air bag) in a vehicle is an example of intervention in which phase of an injury?
   a. Event phase
   b. Preevent phase
   c. Collateral event phase
   d. Postevent phase

5. Which of the following is NOT one of the common approaches to implementing an injury prevention strategy?
   a. Education
   b. Enforcement
   c. Engineering
   d. Economics

6. In which activity/activities of the public health approach to injury prevention is the involvement of EMS appropriate?
   a. Risk factor identification
   b. Surveillance
   c. Implementation
   d. All of the above

REFERENCES

Christoffel T, Gallagher SS: *Injury prevention and public health: practical knowledge, skills, and strategies*, Gaithersburg, Md, 1999, Aspen.

Kellerman AL, Hutson HR: Injury control. In Schwartz GR: *Principles and practice of emergency medicine*, Philadelphia, 1992, Lea & Febiger.

Kellerman AL, Todd KH: Injury control. In Tintinelli JE, Kelen GD, Stapczynski JS, editors: *Emergency medicine: a comprehensive study guide*, New York, 1999, McGraw-Hill.

Kinnane JM, Garrison HG, Coben JH, Alonzo-Serra HM: Injury prevention: is there a role for out-of-hospital emergency medical services? *Acad Emerg Med* 4:306, 1997.

Martinez R: Injury control: a primer for physicians, *Annals of Emerg Med* 19:1, 1990.

National Academy of Sciences/National Research Council: *Accidental death and disability: the neglected disease of modern society*. Washington, DC, 1966, NAS/NRC.

National Center for Health Statistics: *Health, United States, 1996-1997 and injury chartbook*, Hyattsville, Md, 1997, NCHS.

National Center for Health Statistics: *Health, United States, 2000 with adolescent health chartbook*, Hyattsville, Md, 2000, NCHS.

National Center for Injury Prevention and Control: *Fact book for the year 2000: working to prevent and control injury in the United States*, 2000. Available at www.cdc.gov/ncipc/pub-res/FactBook/default.htm (accessed 05/01).

National Committee for Injury Prevention and Control: *Injury prevention: meeting the challenge*, New York, 1989, Oxford University Press (Published as a supplement to the *Am J Prev Med* 5:4, 1989).

National Highway Traffic Safety Administration, US Department of Health and Human Services, Health Resources and Services Administration, Maternal and Child Health Bureau: *Emergency medical services agenda for the future*, Washington, DC, 1999, The Administration.

Todd KH: *Accident's aren't: proposal for evaluation of an injury prevention curriculum for EMS providers: a grant proposal to the National Association of State EMS Directors*, Atlanta, 1998, Department of Emergency Medicine, Emory University School of Medicine.

Waller JA: *Injury control: a guide to the causes and prevention of trauma*, Lexington, Mass, 1985, Lexington Books.

World Health Organization: *Injury: a leading cause of the global burden of disease*, Geneva: 2001, WHO. Available at www.who.int/violence_injury_prevention/injury/burden.htm (accessed 05/01).

Chapter 2

Kinematics of Trauma

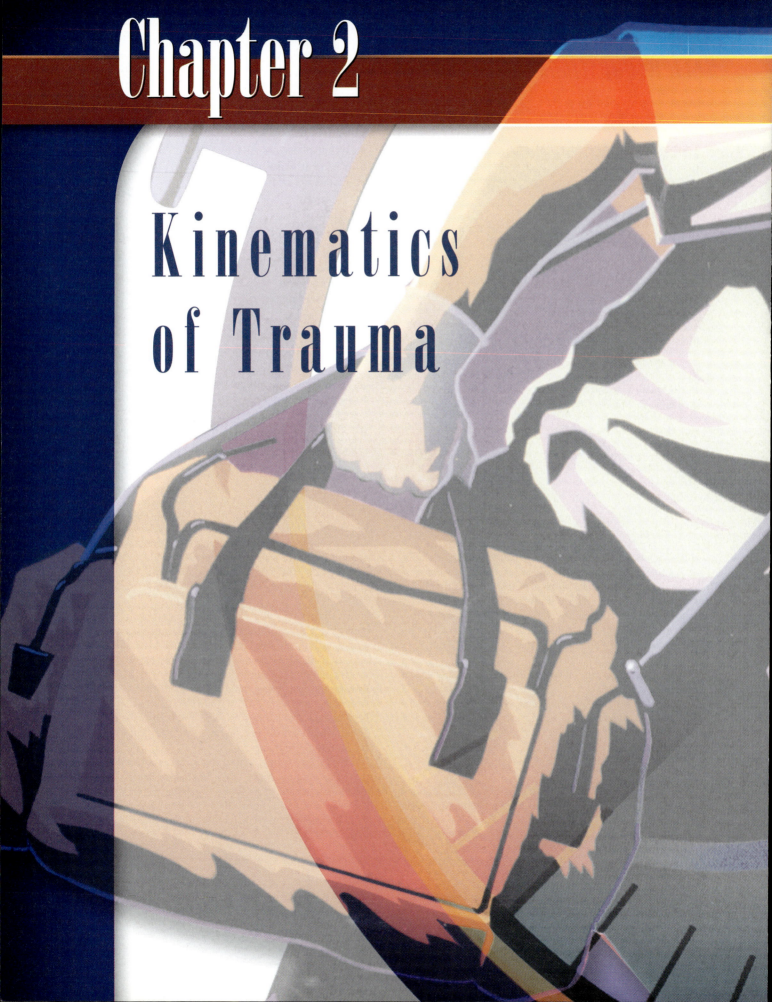

Chapter Objectives

At the completion of this chapter, the reader should be able to do the following:

- Define energy and force as they relate to trauma.
- Relate the laws of motion energy to the kinematics of trauma.
- Relate the exponential change in kinetic energy as a result of increased speed to the potential for injury.
- Given the description of a motor vehicle crash, use kinematics to predict the likely injury pattern for an unrestrained occupant.
- Associate the principles of energy exchange involved in a given situation to the pathophysiology of the head, spine, thorax, and abdomen resulting from that exchange.
- Anticipate specific injuries and their causes as related to interior and exterior vehicle damage.
- Describe the function of vehicle occupant restraint systems.
- Describe the physics of penetrating injuries.
- Relate the laws of motion and energy to mechanisms other than motor vehicle crashes (e.g., blasts, falls).
- Integrate principles of the kinematics of trauma into patient assessment.

Scenario

It is about 5:00 PM on Sunday evening and Matt is driving home from college looking forward to a spring break full of surfing and sun. As he approaches the intersection of a relatively busy highway he is thinking about all the fun he will have over the next week. Suddenly he hears the screech of brakes and realizes that he has passed through a red light. There is a loud crash and he feels terrible pain in his left side.

Paramedics are dispatched to the scene. Upon arrival at the scene of a two-vehicle crash, the paramedics find one vehicle with moderate front-end damage and another one, Matt's vehicle, with severe driver's side damage and about 2 feet of passenger compartment intrusion. Although the driver of the vehicle with front-end damage is ambulatory at the scene, Matt is lying on his right side across the front seat.

Based on this information, can you predict the potential injuries to Matt's head, neck, chest, abdomen, spine, pelvis, and extremities?

Unexpected traumatic injuries are responsible for more than 146,000 deaths in the United States each year. Vehicle collisions accounted for 41,000 deaths and over 3 million injured persons in 1999. Outside the United States, other countries have an equal or even greater problem. Successful management of trauma patients depends on identification of injuries or potential injuries and good assessment skills. However, even with good assessment skills, a prehospital care provider may miss many injuries if he or she does not suspect them. A prehospital care provider may overlook an injury simply because of not knowing where to look. Even if obvious injuries are treated, injuries that are not obvious can be fatal because they are not managed at the scene. Knowing where to look and how to assess for injuries is as important as knowing what to do after finding injuries. A complete, accurate history of a traumatic incident and proper interpretation of this information can allow the prehospital care provider to predict most of a patient's injuries before examining the patient.

Based on the principles of injury prevention, the medical care of a trauma patient can be divided into three phases—precrash, crash, and postcrash. The term *crash* does not necessarily mean a vehicular crash. The crash of a vehicle into a pedestrian, a missile (bullet) into the abdomen, or a construction worker into the asphalt after a fall are all crashes. In each case, energy is exchanged between a moving object and the tissue of the trauma victim or between the moving trauma victim and a stationary object.

- The *precrash phase* includes all of the events that precede the incident, such as the ingestion of alcohol or drugs. Conditions that predate the incident are also part of the precrash phase, such as a patient's acute or preexisting medical conditions (and medications to treat those conditions) or a patient's state of mind. Typically, young trauma patients do not have chronic illnesses. However, with older patients, medical conditions that are present before the trauma occurs can cause serious complications in the prehospital management of the patient and can significantly influence the outcome. For example, the elderly driver of a vehicle that has struck a utility pole may have chest pain indicative of a myocardial infarction (heart attack). Did the driver hit the utility pole and have a heart attack, or did he have a heart attack and then strike the utility pole?

- The *crash phase* begins at the time of impact between one moving object and a second object. The second object can be moving or stationary and can be either an object or a human being. Three impacts occur in most traumas: (1) the impact of the two objects, (2) the impact of the occupants, and (3) the impact of the vital organs inside the occupants. For example, when a vehicle strikes a tree, the first impact is the collision of the vehicle into the tree. The second impact is the occupant of the vehicle striking the steering wheel or windshield. If the patient is restrained, an impact occurs between the occupant and the seatbelt. The third impact is between the patient's internal organs and his or her chest wall or abdominal wall. The directions in which the energy exchange occurs, the amount of energy that is exchanged, and the effect that these forces have on the patient are all important considerations for a prehospital provider.

- During the *postcrash phase*, the prehospital care provider uses the information gathered during the crash and precrash phases to manage a patient. This phase begins as soon as the energy from the crash is absorbed and the patient is traumatized. The onset of the complications of life-threatening trauma can be slow or fast (or these complications can be prevented or significantly reduced) depending in part on the action taken by the prehospital care provider. In the postcrash phase the prehospital care provider's understanding of the kinematics of trauma, the index of suspicion regarding injuries, and strong assessment skills all become crucial to the outcome of the patient.

To understand the effects of the forces that produce bodily injury, the prehospital care provider must understand two components—energy and anatomy.

Energy

The first step in obtaining a history is to evaluate the events that occurred at the crash scene (Figure 2-1). For example, in a motor vehicle crash (MVC), what does the scene look like? Who hit what and at what speed? How long was the stopping time? Were the victims restrained by seat belts? Did the air bag deploy? Were the children restrained properly in seats, or were they unrestrained and thrown about the vehicle? Were occupants thrown from the vehicle? Did they strike objects? If so, how many objects? These and many other questions must be answered if the prehospital care provider is to understand the exchange of forces that took place and translate this information into a prediction of injuries and appropriate patient care.

The process of surveying the scene to determine what injuries might have resulted from the forces and motion involved is called *kinematics*. Because kinematics is based on fundamental principles of physics, an understanding of the pertinent laws of physics is necessary.

Laws of Energy and Motion

Newton's first law of motion states that a body at rest will remain at rest and a body in motion will remain in mo-

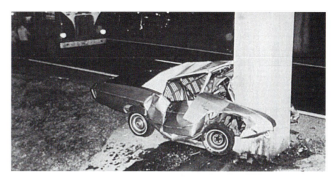

Figure 2-1   Evaluating the scene of an incident is critical. Such information as direction of impact, passenger compartment intrusion, and amount of energy exchange provides insight into the possible injuries of the occupants. This photograph was in the first edition of this text and, although an older model vehicle, continues to show the concept of mechanism of injury.

tion unless acted upon by an outside force. The motorcycle in Figure 2-2 was stationary until the energy from the engine moved it along the dirt track. Once in motion, although it leaves the ground, it remains in motion until it hits something or returns to the ground and the brakes are applied. The same is true of the person sitting in the front seat of a vehicle. Even if the vehicle hits a tree and stops, the unrestrained person continues in motion until he or she hits the steering column, dashboard, and/or windshield. The impact with these objects stops the forward motion of the torso or head. The internal organs of the person remain in motion until they hit the chest wall or abdominal wall, halting the forward motion.

Why does the sudden starting or stopping of motion result in trauma and injury to an individual? The *law of conservation of energy* states that energy cannot be created or destroyed but can be changed in form. The motion of the vehicle is a form of energy. When the motion starts or stops, the energy changes to another form. It may take on the form of mechanical, thermal, electrical, or chemical energy.

An example of energy changing form when motion is stopped is when a driver brakes and the vehicle decelerates. The energy of motion is converted into the heat of friction (thermal energy) by the brake pads on the brake drums and by the tires on the roadway. Similarly, the mechanical energy of a vehicle crashing into a wall is dissipated by the bending of the frame or other parts of the vehicle. The energy remaining is transferred to the occupants and their internal organs.

Kinetic energy is a function of an object's weight and speed. A victim's weight and mass are the same thing.

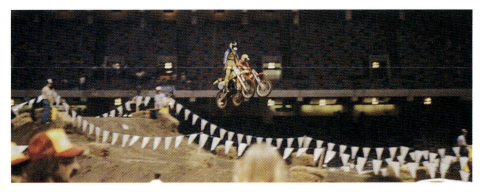

Figure 2-2 A motorcycle going over a jump does not suddenly stop when it loses contact with the ground. The momentum of the motorcycle and the previously existing energy carry the motorcycle and rider forward unless something obstructs the motion.

Likewise, speed and velocity are the same. The relationship between weight and speed as it affects kinetic energy is as follows:

Kinetic energy = ½ of the mass times the velocity squared, or

$$KE = \tfrac{1}{2}mv^2$$

Thus the kinetic energy involved when a 150 lb (68 kg) person travels at 30 mph (48 km/hr) is calculated as follows:

$$KE = \frac{150}{2} \times 30^2$$
$$KE = 67{,}500 \text{ units}$$

For the purpose of this discussion, no specific physical unit of measure (such as foot-pounds or joules) is given. The formula is used merely to illustrate the change in energy. As just shown, a 150 lb (68 kg) person traveling at 30 mph (48 km/hr) would have 67,500 units of energy converted to another form when he or she stops. This change takes the form of damage to the vehicle and injury to the person in it, unless the energy dissipation can take some less harmful form, such as on a seat belt or into an air bag.

Which factor, however, has the greatest effect on the amount of kinetic energy produced: mass or velocity? Consider a 160 lb (72 kg) person traveling at 30 mph (48 km/hr):

$$KE = \frac{160}{2} \times 30^2$$
$$KE = 72{,}000 \text{ units}$$

Returning to the previous example of a 150 lb (68 kg) person and increasing the speed by 10 mph (16 km/hr), the kinetic energy is as follows:

$$KE = \frac{150}{2} \times 40^2$$
$$KE = 120{,}000 \text{ units}$$

These calculations show how increasing the velocity (speed) increases the rate of production of kinetic energy much more than increasing the mass. Much greater damage will occur in a high-speed crash than in a crash at a slower speed. Differences in mass (weight) among occupants of the same vehicle have relatively little effect on their vulnerability to injury. For example, a small child and a 200 lb (90 kg) adult differ greatly in size and weight. If they are both in a vehicle traveling at 55 mph (88 km/hr), the most significant determinant of the amount of force applied to them is their common speed—not their weight difference.

Another example is that the impact of the steering column against the chest of the driver in a 35 mph (56 km/hr) collision would be equivalent to a standing person having a telephone pole driven into his or her chest at the same speed.

Another important factor in a crash is the stopping distance. Before a crash, the driver is moving at the same speed as the vehicle. At the split second of the crash, the vehicle and driver both decelerate to a speed of zero. This deceleration force is transmitted to the driver's body. If the stopping distance is increased, the force of deceleration is decreased and the resulting damage is proportionately decreased.

This inverse relationship between stopping distance and injury also applies to falls. A person has a better

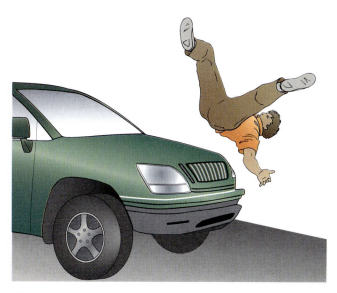

Figure 2-3   The energy exchange from a moving vehicle to a pedestrian crushes tissue and imparts speed and energy to the pedestrian to knock the victim away from the point of impact. Injury to the patient can occur at the point of impact as the pedestrian is hit by the vehicle and as the pedestrian is thrown to the ground or into another vehicle.

chance of surviving a fall if he or she lands on a compressible surface, such as deep powder snow. The same fall terminating on a hard surface, such as concrete, can produce more severe injuries. The compressible material (i.e., the snow) increases the stopping distance and absorbs at least some of the energy rather than allowing all of the energy to be absorbed by the body. The result is decreased injury and damage to the body. This principle also applies to other kinds of crashes. For example, a vehicle that hits an unyielding bridge abutment will be more seriously damaged than a vehicle that hits another vehicle from behind. In the latter example, both vehicles absorb a significant amount of the energy, thus reducing the amount of energy that must be absorbed by the occupants. In addition, an unrestrained driver will be more severely injured than a restrained driver. The restraint system, rather than the body, will absorb a significant portion of the damage energy.

Therefore once an object is in motion and has a specific energy of motion, to come to a complete rest the object must lose all of its energy by converting the energy to another form or transferring it to another object. For example, if a vehicle strikes a pedestrian, the pedestrian is knocked away from it (Figure 2-3). The vehicle is slowed by the impact, but this reduced velocity is transferred to the pedestrian, resulting in injury. Loss of motion of a moving object translates into tissue damage to the victim.

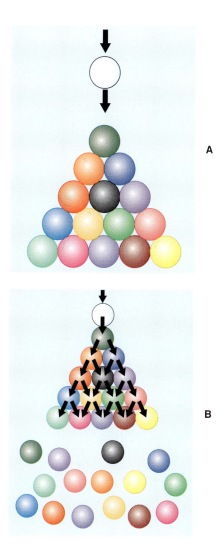

Figure 2-4   **A,** The energy of a cue ball is transferred to each of the other balls. **B,** The energy exchange pushes the balls apart, or creates a cavity.

Cavitation

The basic mechanics of energy exchange are relatively simple. Driving a cue ball down the length of a pool table into the racked balls at the other end transfers the energy of the cue ball to each of the racked balls (Figure 2-4). The cue ball gives up its energy and slows or even stops. The other balls take on this energy as motion and move away from the impact point. The same kind of energy exchange occurs when a bowling ball rolls down the alley, hitting the set of pins at the other end. The pool balls and bowling pins are knocked out of their positions. The same thing happens when a moving object strikes the human body or when the human body is in motion and strikes a stationary object. The tissue of the human body is

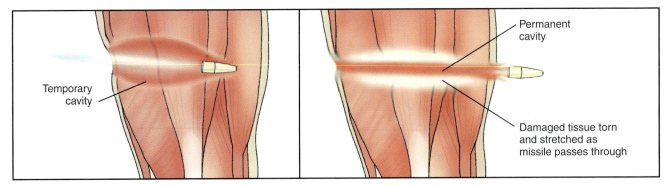

Figure 2-5 Damage to tissue is greater than the permanent cavity that remains from a missile injury. The faster or heavier the missile, the larger the temporary cavity and the greater the zone of tissue damage.

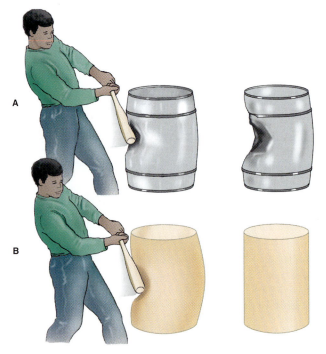

Figure 2-6 A, Swinging a baseball bat into a steel drum leaves a dent, or cavity, in its side. B, Swinging a baseball bat into a piece of foam leaves no visible cavity.

knocked out of its normal position, creating a hole. This process is called *cavitation*.

Two types of cavities are created. A temporary cavity forms at the time of impact, but depending on the elasticity of the tissue, it can return to its previous position. This cavity may not be visible when the prehospital or hospital provider examines the patient later. A temporary cavity is caused by stretch. A permanent cavity also forms at the time of impact and is caused by compression or tearing of tissue. It is also caused partly by stretch, but because it does not rebound to its original shape, it can be seen later (Figure 2-5).

The size difference between the two cavities is related to the elasticity of the tissue involved. For example, forcefully swinging a baseball bat into a steel drum leaves a dent, or cavity, in its side. Swinging the same baseball bat with the same force into a similarly sized and shaped mass of foam rubber will leave no dent once the bat is removed (Figure 2-6). The difference is elasticity—the foam rubber is more elastic than the steel drum. The human body is more like the foam rubber than the steel drum. If a person punches a fist into another person's abdomen, he or she would feel it go in. However, when the person pulls the fist away, a dent is not left. Similarly, a baseball bat swung into the chest will leave no obvious cavity in the thoracic wall, but it would cause damage. A complete history of the incident will allow the prehospital care provider to determine the approximate size of the cavity at the time of impact to accurately predict injuries.

Energy Exchange

As the body collides with an object, the number of tissue particles affected by the impact determines the amount of energy exchange and therefore the resulting amount of damage. The number of tissue particles affected is determined by the density of the tissue and by the surface area of the impact.

DENSITY

The more dense a tissue (measured in particles per volume), the greater the number of particles that will be hit by a moving object. Driving a fist into a feather pillow and driving a fist at the same speed into a brick wall will produce different effects on the hand. The fist absorbs more energy colliding with the dense brick wall than with the less dense feather pillow.

Simplistically, the body has three different types of tissue densities—air (lung and intestine), water (muscle and most solid organs such as liver and spleen), and bone. Therefore injury will depend on which type of organ is impacted.

FRONTAL SURFACE AREA

Wind exerts pressure on a hand when it is extended out of the window of a moving vehicle. When the palm of the hand is horizontal and parallel to the direction of the flow through the wind, some backward pressure is exerted on the front of the hand (fingers) as the particles of air strike the hand. Rotating the hand 90 degrees to a vertical position places a larger surface area into the wind; thus more air particles make contact with the hand, increasing the amount of force on it. The surface area can be modified by the size of the object, its motion within the body, and fragmentation.

Blunt and Penetrating Trauma

Trauma is generally classified as either blunt or penetrating. However, the energy exchange and the injury produced are similar in both types of trauma. The only real difference is penetration of the skin. If an object's entire energy is concentrated on one small area of skin, the skin likely will tear and the object will enter the body and create a more concentrated energy exchange. This can result in greater destructive power to one area. A larger object whose energy is dispersed over a much larger area of skin may not penetrate the skin. The damage will be distributed over a larger area of the body, and the injury pattern will be less localized.

Energy exchange is directly related to the density and size of the frontal area at the point of contact between the object and the victim's body. In blunt trauma, injuries are produced as the tissues are compressed, decelerated, or accelerated. In penetrating trauma, injuries are produced as the tissues are crushed and separated along the path of the penetrating object. Both types create a cavity, forcing the tissues out of their normal position.

Blunt trauma creates both shear tears and cavitation. The cavitation is frequently only a temporary cavity and is directed away from the point of impact. Penetrating trauma creates both a permanent and a temporary cavity. The energy of a rapidly moving object with a small frontal surface area will be concentrated in one area and may exceed the tensile strength of the tissue and penetrate it. The temporary cavity that is created will spread away from the pathway of this missile in both frontal and lateral directions.

Blunt Trauma

In blunt trauma, two forces are involved in the impact—shear and compression. Shear is the result of one organ or structure (or part of an organ or structure) changing speed faster than another organ or structure (or part of an organ or structure). Compression is the result of an organ or structure (or part of an organ or structure) being directly squeezed between other organs or structures. Injury can result from any type of impact, such as MVCs (vehicle or motorcycle), pedestrian collisions with vehicles, falls, sports injuries, or blast injuries. All of these mechanisms are discussed separately, followed by the results of this energy exchange on the specific anatomy in each of the body regions.

MOTOR VEHICLE CRASHES

Many kinds of blunt trauma occur, but MVCs—including motorcycle crashes—are the most common. In 1999, 86% of fatalities were vehicle occupants. The remaining 14% were pedestrians, cyclists, and other nonoccupants (National Highway Traffic Safety Administration [NHTSA], 1999). MVCs can be divided into five types:

1. Frontal impact
2. Rear impact
3. Lateral impact
4. Rotational impact
5. Rollover

Although each pattern has variations, accurate identification of the five patterns will provide insight into other similar types of crashes.

In MVCs and other rapid-deceleration mechanisms, such as snowmobile, motorcycle, and boating crashes and falls from heights, three collisions occur: (1) the vehicle collides with an object or with another vehicle, (2) the unrestrained occupant collides with the inside of the vehicle, and (3) the occupant's internal organs collide with one another or with the wall of the cavity that contains them.

An example is a vehicle hitting a tree. The first collision occurs when the vehicle strikes the tree. Although the vehicle stops, the unrestrained driver keeps moving forward (consistent with Newton's first law of motion). The second collision occurs when the driver hits the steering wheel and windshield. Although the driver stops moving forward, many internal organs keep moving (Newton's first law again) until they strike another organ or cavity wall or are suddenly stopped by a ligament, fascia, vessel, or muscle. This is the third collision.

Each of these collisions causes a different kind of damage, and each must be considered separately in analyzing the incident. One easy way to estimate the injury pattern to the occupant is to look at the vehicle and determine which of the five types of collisions occurred.

The occupant receives the same kind and amount of force as the vehicle. The energy exchange will be similar and will take place in a similar direction.

Frontal Impact. In a frontal impact (or "head-on" collision) involving a motor vehicle, such as a vehicle hitting a brick wall, the first collision occurs when the vehicle hits the wall, resulting in damage to the front of the vehicle. The amount of damage to the vehicle indicates the approximate speed of the vehicle at the time of impact. For example, a severely damaged vehicle was probably moving at a high speed and will probably contain severely injured victims.

Although the vehicle suddenly ceases to move forward in a frontal impact, the occupant, if unrestrained and therefore not slowed with the vehicle, continues to move and will follow one of two possible paths—either up-and-over or down-and-under.

Up-and-Over Path. In this sequence, the body's forward motion carries it up and over the steering wheel (Figure 2-7). The head is usually the lead body portion striking the windshield or windshield frame. The chest or abdomen collides with the steering wheel. If the chest strikes the steering wheel, serious injury to the thoracic cage, soft tissues, or organs can occur. If the abdomen strikes it, compression injuries can occur, most often to the solid abdominal organs (kidneys, liver, pancreas, and spleen). Hollow organs are also susceptible to injury.

The kidneys, spleen, and liver are also subject to shear injury as the abdomen strikes the steering wheel

and abruptly stops. An organ may be torn from its normal anatomic restraints and supporting tissues. For example, the continued forward motion of the kidneys after the vertebral column has stopped moving may cause tears in the renal vessels near the points at which they join the inferior vena cava and the descending aorta. These great vessels adhere so tightly to the posterior abdominal wall and vertebral column that the continued forward motion of the kidneys can stretch the renal vessels to the point of rupture.

As the body continues to rotate forward and upward, the chest strikes the steering wheel or dashboard. The victim will have compression injuries to the anterior chest, which may include broken ribs, flail chest, pulmonary contusion, myocardial contusion, or damage to the great vessels. If the impact is low on the chest wall, rupture of the higher solid abdominal organs (liver and spleen) can occur.

The head is also a point of impact. When the forward motion of the head stops, the momentum of the still-moving torso following it must be absorbed. One of the most easily bent or fractured parts of the body lies between the head and the torso—the cervical spine.

Down-and-Under Path. In a down-and-under path, the occupant continues to move downward into the seat and forward into the dashboard or steering column (Figure 2-8). The importance of understanding kinematics is illustrated by what happens to the knee in this pathway. The foot, if planted on the floor panel or on the brake pedal with a straight knee, can twist as the continued

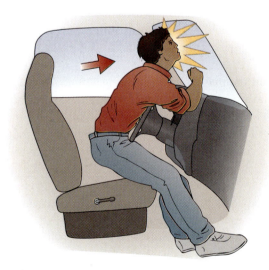

Figure 2-7 The configuration of the seat and the position of the occupant can direct the initial force on the upper torso with the head as the lead point.

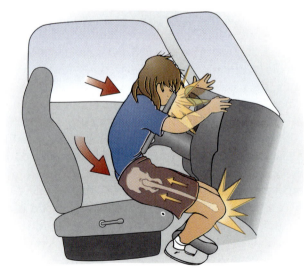

Figure 2-8 The occupant and the vehicle travel forward together. The vehicle stops, and the unrestrained occupant continues forward until something stops that motion.

torso motion angulates and fractures the ankle joint. In most cases the knees bend and strike the dashboard.

The knee has two possible impact points against the dashboard—the tibia and the femur (Figure 2-9). If the tibia hits the dashboard and stops first, the femur remains in motion and overrides it. A dislocated knee, with torn ligaments, tendons, and other supporting structures, can result. Because the popliteal artery lies in close proximity to the knee joint, dislocation of the joint is frequently associated with injury to the vessel. The popliteal artery may be completely disrupted, or more commonly, the lining of the artery (intima) may be damaged (Figure 2-10). In either case, a blood clot may form in the injured vessel, resulting in significantly decreased blood flow to the leg tissues below the knee.

Early recognition of a popliteal artery injury and prompt surgical repair restores blood flow to the calf and foot and significantly decreases the subsequent need for an amputation. If a delay in either identifying the injury or performing corrective surgery occurs, the lack of perfusion results in severely ischemic tissue. If perfusion to this tissue is not reestablished within about 6 hours, amputation is often necessary. Such delays could occur because the prehospital care provider fails to consider the kinematics of the injury or because he or she overlooks important clues during his or her assessment of the patient.

Although most of these patients have evidence of injury to the knee, an imprint on the dashboard where the knee impacted is a key indicator that significant energy was focused on this joint and adjacent structures (Figure 2-11). Unless a prehospital care provider observes the dents in the dashboard and recognizes their significance, he or she may not suspect this injury and thus not report it to the physicians at the receiving facility.

When the femur is the point of impact, the energy is absorbed on the bone shaft, which can then break (Figure 2-12). The continued forward motion of the pelvis onto the femur that remains intact can override the femur's head, resulting in a posterior dislocation of the acetabular joint (Figure 2-13).

After the knees impact, the upper body may rotate forward into the steering column or dashboard. The victim may then sustain many of the same injuries described previously for the up-and-over pathway.

Rear Impact.   Rear impact collisions occur when a slower moving or stationary object is struck from behind by a vehicle moving at a faster rate of speed. In these collisions, the energy of the impact is converted to acceleration. The greater the difference in the speed of the two

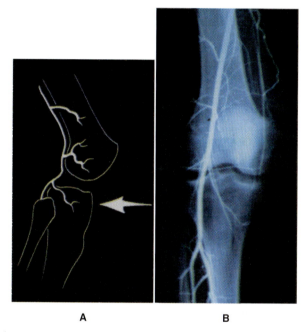

A   B

Figure 2-10   The popliteal artery lies in close proximity to the joint, tightly tied to the femur above and tibia below. Separation of these two bones stretches, kinks, and/or tears the artery.

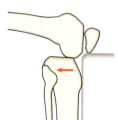

Figure 2-9   The knee has two possible impact points in a motor vehicle crash—the femur and the tibia.

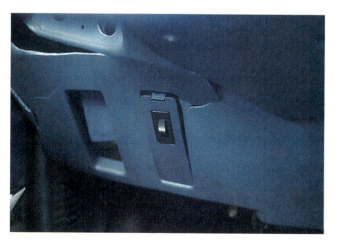

Figure 2-11   The impact point of the knee on the dashboard indicates both a down-and-under pathway and a significant absorption of energy along the lower extremity.

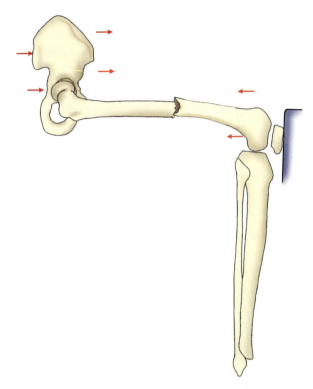

Figure 2-12   When the femur is the point of impact, the energy is absorbed on the bone shaft, which can then break.

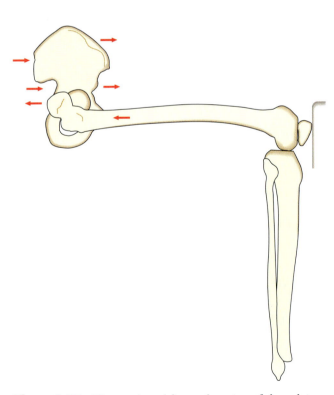

Figure 2-13   The continued forward motion of the pelvis onto the femur can override the femur's head, resulting in a posterior dislocation of the acetabular joint.

vehicles, the greater the force of the initial impact and the more energy available to create damage.

Upon impact, the vehicle in front is accelerated forward, like a bullet discharged from a gun. Everything that is attached to the frame will also move forward, as does everything in contact with the vehicle. If the headrest is not positioned to move the head with the torso, then the body in contact with the vehicle is accelerated out from underneath the head. This results in hyperextension of the neck over the top of the headrest. Tearing of the neck's ligaments and supporting anterior structures can result (Figure 2-14).

If the headrest is up, the head moves with the seat (Figure 2-15). If the vehicle is allowed to move forward

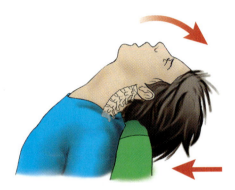

Figure 2-14   A rear impact collision forces the torso forward. If the headrest is improperly positioned, the head is hyperextended over the top of the headrest.

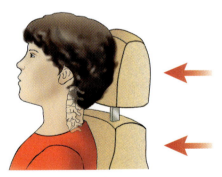

Figure 2-15   If the headrest is up, the head moves with the torso and neck injury is prevented.

If it can be proved that the victim's headrest was not properly positioned when the neck injury occurred, some courts consider reducing the liability of the party at fault in the crash on the grounds that the victim's negligence contributed to the injuries (contributory negligence). Similar measures have been considered in cases of failure to use occupant restraints.

without interference until it slows to a stop, the occupant will probably not be injured. However, if the vehicle strikes another vehicle or object or if the driver slams on the brakes and stops suddenly, the occupants will continue forward, following the characteristic pattern of a frontal impact collision. The collision then involves two impacts—rear and frontal. The double impact increases the likelihood of injury. When dealing with this kind of MVC, the prehospital care provider should look for two sets of injuries: (1) those caused by the rear impact and (2) those caused by the secondary, frontal impact.

Lateral Impact.   Lateral impact collisions occur when a vehicle is struck from the side. The vehicle that is hit is propelled away from the impact in the direction of the impact. The side of the vehicle or the door is thrust against the side of the occupant. The occupant may then be injured in three ways: (1) by impact with the vehicle (Figure 2-16), (2) by impact with other unrestrained passengers, and (3) by the door's projection into the passenger compartment as it is bent inward (Figure 2-17). Injury caused by the vehicle's movement is less severe if the occupant is restrained and moves with the vehicle.

Four body regions can sustain injury in a lateral impact:

1. *Neck.* The torso can move out from under the head. Lateral flexion and rotation can fracture or dislocate the cervical vertebrae (Figure 2-18).
2. *Head.* The head can impact the frame of the door.
3. *Chest.* Compression of the thoracic wall can result in fractured ribs on the side of the impact (Figure 2-19), pulmonary contusion, shear injuries to the aorta

(25% of aortic shear injuries occur in lateral impact collisions), or injury to other solid organs. The clavicle can be compressed and fractured (Figure 2-20).
4. *Abdomen/Pelvis.* The intrusion compresses and fractures the pelvis and pushes the head of the femur through the acetabulum (Figure 2-21). Occupants on the driver's side are vulnerable to splenic injuries because the spleen is on the left side of the body, whereas those on the passenger side are more likely to receive an injury to the liver.

When the vehicle is moved by the force of the impact, it reacts as if the vehicle is suddenly moved out from under its occupants. In this case, the use of seat belts will reduce the severity of injury. Because of the lap belt, the occupant begins lateral motion with the vehicle and is "pulled" away from the impact point. The head is supported by the spine but in an off-center position. The center of gravity is forward and superior to the point of support. As the trunk is pushed laterally by the side impact, the tendency of the head to remain in its original position until pulled by the neck (according to Newton's first law of motion) will produce both lateral flexion and rotation of the cervical spine (see Figure 2-18).

During a lateral impact crash, the occupants are also subject to injury from a secondary collision with other passengers, such as when the head of one occupant strikes the head or shoulder of another occupant. The presence of an injury on the side of the patient opposite the side hit by the other vehicle should alert the prehospital provider to check the adjacent occupant for injuries resulting from the collision of the two persons. Another form of secondary collision can occur when the occupants of the vehicle are projected and strike the opposite

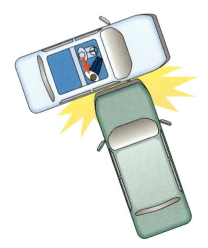

Figure 2-16   Lateral impact of the vehicle pushes the entire vehicle into the unrestrained passenger. A restrained passenger moves laterally with the vehicle.

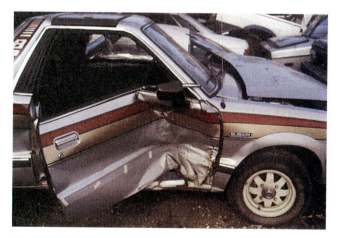

Figure 2-17   Intrusion of the side panels into the passenger compartment provides another source of injury.

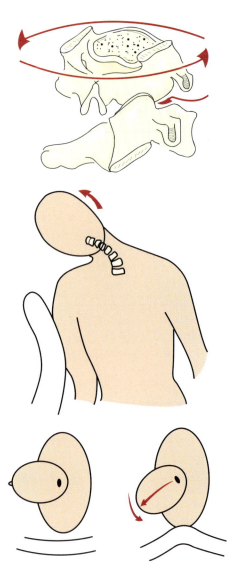

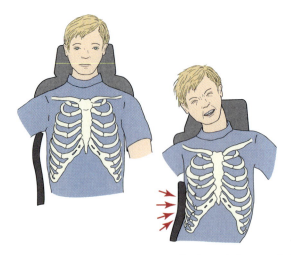

Figure 2-19   Compression against the lateral chest and abdominal wall can fracture ribs and injure the underlying spleen, liver, and kidney.

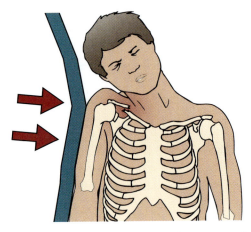

Figure 2-18   The center of gravity of the skull is anterior and superior to its pivot point between the skull and cervical spine. During a lateral impact, when the torso is rapidly accelerated out from under the head, the head turns toward the point of impact, both in the lateral and anterior-posterior angles. Such motion separates the vertebral bodies from the side of opposite impact and rotates them apart. Jumped facets, ligaments, tears, and lateral compression fractures result.

side of the vehicle from the initial collision point. Near side impacts produce more injuries than far side impacts.

Rotational Impact.   Rotational impact collisions occur when one corner of a vehicle strikes an immovable object, the corner of another vehicle, or a vehicle moving slower or in the opposite direction of the first vehicle. Following Newton's first law of motion, this corner of the vehicle will stop while the rest of the vehicle continues its forward motion until all of its energy is completely transformed.

Figure 2-20   Compression of the shoulder against the clavicle produces midshaft fractures of this bone.

Rotational impact collisions result in injuries that are a combination of those seen in frontal and lateral impact collisions—the victim continues to move forward and then is hit by the side of the vehicle (as in a lateral collision) as the vehicle rotates around the point of impact. *More severe injuries are seen in the victim closest to the point of impact.*

Rollover.   During a rollover, a vehicle may undergo several impacts at many different angles, as may the occupant's body and internal organs (Figure 2-22). Injury and damage can occur with each of these impacts. The prehospital care provider can almost never predict the injuries that these victims receive. In rollover collisions a

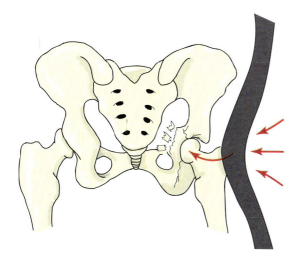

Figure 2-21   Lateral impact on the femur pushes the head through the acetabulum or fractures the pelvis.

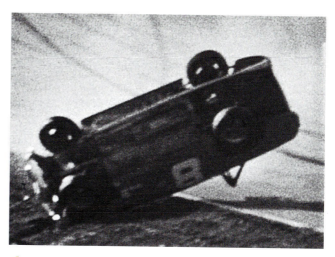

Figure 2-22   During a rollover, the unrestrained occupant can be wholly or partially ejected out of the vehicle or can bounce around inside the vehicle. This action produces multiple and somewhat unpredictable injuries that are usually severe.

restrained patient often sustains shearing-type injuries because of the significant forces created by a rolling vehicle. The forces are similar to the forces of a spinning carnival ride. Although the occupants are held secure by restraints, the internal organs still move and can tear at the connecting tissue areas. More serious injuries occur as a result of being unrestrained. In most cases the occupants are ejected from the vehicle as it rolls and either are crushed as the vehicle rolls over them or sustain injuries from the impact with the ground. If the occupants are ejected onto the roadway, they can be struck by oncoming traffic.

Restraints.   In the injury patterns described previously, the victims were assumed to be unrestrained, as are most vehicle occupants in the United States (67% in a 1999 NHTSA report). Ejection from vehicles accounted for approximately 25% of the 41,000 vehicular deaths in 1999. About 75% of passenger vehicle occupants who were totally ejected were killed. One out of thirteen ejection victims sustains a spine fracture. After ejection from a vehicle, the body is subjected to a second impact as the body strikes the ground (or another object) outside the vehicle. This second impact can result in injuries that are even more severe than the initial impact. The risk of death for ejected victims is six times greater than for those who are not ejected. Clearly, seat belts (restraints) save lives.

The NHTSA reports that 49 states and the District of Columbia have safety belt legislation. In 1999, over 11,000 lives were saved by the use of these restraining devices. Over 123,000 lives have been saved since 1975. If all occupants wore restraints, the total lives saved for 1999 would have been over 20,000.

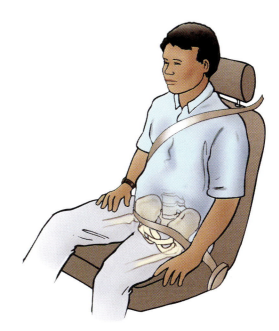

Figure 2-23   A properly positioned seat belt is located below the anterior superior iliac spine on each side, above the femur, and is tight enough to remain in this position. The bowl-shaped pelvis protects the soft intraabdominal organs.

What occurs when the victims are restrained? If a seat belt is positioned properly, the pressure of the impact is absorbed by the pelvis and the chest, resulting in few, if any, serious injuries (Figure 2-23). The proper use of restraints transfers the force of the impact from the patient's body to the restraint belts and restraint system. With restraints, injuries are not life threatening, or at least the chance of receiving life-threatening injuries is greatly reduced.

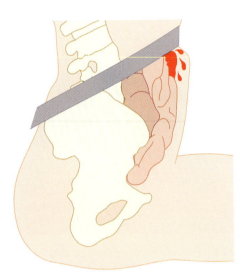

Figure 2-24   A seat belt that is incorrectly positioned above the brim of the pelvis allows the abdominal organs to be trapped between the moving posterior wall and the belt. Injuries to the pancreas and other retroperitoneal organs as well as blowout ruptures of the small intestine and colon result.

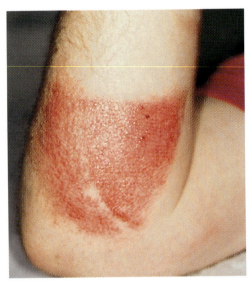

Figure 2-25   Abrasions of the forearm are secondary to rapid expansion of the air bag when the hands are tight against the steering wheel. (*From McSwain NE Jr, Paturas JL: The basic EMT: comprehensive prehospital patient care, ed 2, St Louis, 2001, Mosby.*)

Restraints must be worn properly to be effective. An improperly worn restraint may not protect against injury in the event of a crash, and it may even cause injury. When lap belts are worn loosely or are strapped above the anterior iliac crests, compression injuries of the soft abdominal organs can occur. Compression injuries of the soft intraabdominal organs (spleen, liver, and pancreas) result from compression between the seat belt and the posterior abdominal wall (Figure 2-24). Increased intraabdominal pressure can cause diaphragmatic rupture and herniation of abdominal organs. Anterior compression fractures of the lumbar spine can also occur as the upper and lower parts of the torso pivot over the restrained T12, L1, and L2 vertebrae. Lap belts should also not be worn alone. Many occupants of vehicles still place the diagonal strap under the arm and not over the shoulder.

As mandatory seat belt usage laws are passed, injuries caused by improperly worn restraints have become more frequent, and the prehospital care provider must evaluate for these injuries. However, because a seat belt is being used, even if improperly, the overall severity of the injuries will be lessened, and the number of fatal crashes will be significantly reduced.

Air Bags.   Air bags should always be used in combination with seat belts for maximum protection. Originally, front-seat driver and passenger air bag systems were designed to cushion the forward motion of only the front-seat occupant. They absorbed energy slowly by increasing the body's stopping distance. They are extremely effective in the first collision of frontal and near-frontal impacts (the 65% to 70% of crashes that occur within 30 degrees of the headlights). Because many air bags deflate immediately after the impact, they are not effective in multiple impact collisions or rear impact collisions. An air bag deploys and deflates within 0.5 seconds. If a vehicle veers into the path of an oncoming vehicle or off the road into a tree, no air bag protection is left. Because front air bags are of little or no use in lateral and rollover collisions, several manufacturers have now developed side-impact air bags. Although these seem to be effective in crash tests at the time of publication of this text, a significant reduction in injuries has not yet been documented.

When air bags deploy, they can produce minor but noticeable injuries that the prehospital care provider must manage. These include abrasions of the arms, chest, and face (Figure 2-25); foreign bodies to the face and eyes; and injuries caused by the occupant's eyeglasses (Figure 2-26). Air bags that do not deploy can still be dangerous to both the patient and the prehospital care provider. Air bags should be deactivated by an extrication specialist trained to do so properly and safely.

MOTORCYCLE CRASHES

Motorcycle crashes account for a significant number of the motor vehicle deaths each year. The laws of physics are the same, but the mechanism of injury varies slightly from automobile and truck crashes. This variance occurs in each of the following types of impacts—head-on, angular, or ejection.

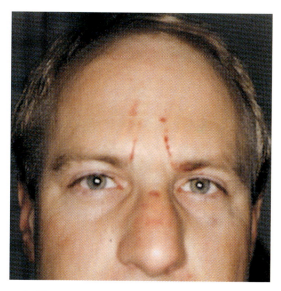

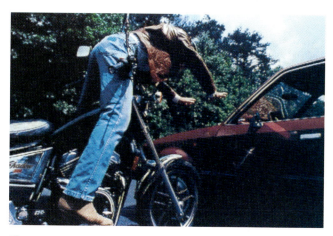

Figure 2-27   The position of a motorcycle driver is above the pivot point of the front wheel as the motorcycle impacts an object head on.

Figure 2-26   Expansion of the air bag into eyeglasses produces abrasions. (*From McSwain NE Jr, Paturas JL: The basic EMT: comprehensive prehospital patient care, ed 2, St Louis, 2001, Mosby.*)

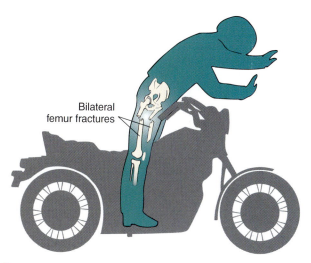

Bilateral femur fractures

Figure 2-28   The body travels forward and over the motorcycle, impacting the thighs and the femurs into the handlebars. The driver can also be ejected.

Front-seat passenger air bags have been shown to be dangerous to children and small adults, especially when children are placed in incorrect positions in the front seat or with incorrectly installed child car seats. As of October 1999, the NHTSA reported 146 air-bag–related deaths. In nearly every incident, the proximity to the air bag was the issue. Children 12 years of age and younger should always be in the proper restraint device for their size and should be in the back seat. The impact of a deploying air bag striking a rear facing child seat could result in injury or death to the child.

Drivers should always be at least 10 inches (25 cm) from the air bag cover, and front seat passengers should be at least 18 inches (45 cm) away. In most cases, when the proper seating arrangements and distances are used, air bag injuries are limited to simple abrasions.

Head-On Impact.   A head-on collision into a solid object stops the forward motion of a motorcycle (Figure 2-27) because the motorcycle's center of gravity is above and behind the front axle, which is the pivot point in such a collision. The motorcycle will tip forward, and the rider will crash into the handlebars. The rider may receive injuries to the head, chest, abdomen, or pelvis depending on which part of the anatomy strikes the handlebars. If the rider's feet remain on the pegs of the motorcycle and the thighs hit the handlebars, the forward motion will be absorbed by the midshaft femur, commonly resulting in bilateral femur fractures (Figure 2-28).

Angular Impact.   In an angular impact collision, the motorcycle hits an object at an angle. The motorcycle will then collapse on the rider or cause the rider to be crushed between the motorcycle and the object struck. Injuries to the upper or lower extremities can occur, resulting in fractures and/or extensive soft tissue injury (Figure 2-29). Injuries can also occur to organs of the abdominal cavity as a result of energy exchange.

Ejection Impact.   In an ejection impact collision, the rider is thrown from the motorcycle like a missile. The rider will continue in flight through the air until his or her head, arms, chest, abdomen, or legs strike another object, such as a motor vehicle, a telephone pole, or the road. Injury will occur at the point of impact and will

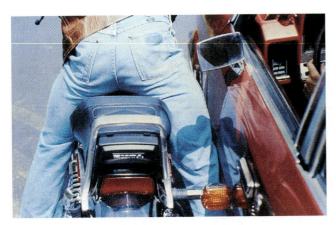

Figure 2-29   If the motorcycle does not hit an object head on, it collapses like a pair of scissors, trapping the rider's lower extremity between the object impacted and the motorcycle.

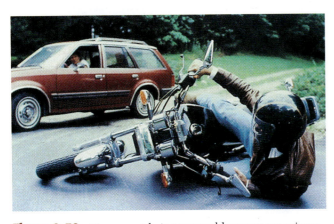

Figure 2-30   To prevent being trapped between two pieces of steel (motorcycle and vehicle), the rider "lays the bike down" to dissipate the injury. This often causes abrasions (road rash) as the rider's speed is slowed on the asphalt.

radiate to the rest of the body as the energy is absorbed. As with the occupant ejected from a motor vehicle, the potential for serious injury is high for this essentially unprotected rider.

Injury Prevention.   "Laying the bike down" is a protective maneuver used by professional racers and some street bikers to separate themselves from the motorcycle in an impending crash (Figure 2-30). The rider turns the motorcycle sideways and drags his or her inside leg on the ground. This action slows the rider more than the motorcycle so that the motorcycle will move out from under the rider. The rider will then slide along on the pavement but will not be trapped between the motorcycle and the object it hits. These riders usually get abrasions (road rash) and minor

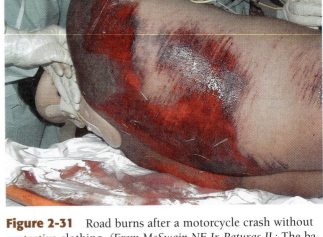

Figure 2-31   Road burns after a motorcycle crash without protective clothing. *(From McSwain NE Jr, Paturas JL: The basic EMT: comprehensive prehospital patient care, ed 2, St Louis, 2001, Mosby.)*

fractures but avoid the severe injuries associated with the other kinds of impacts (Figure 2-31).

Protection for motorcyclists includes boots, leather clothing, and helmets. Of the three, the helmet affords the best protection. It is built like the skull—strong and supportive externally and energy-absorbent internally. The helmet's skull-like structure absorbs much of the impact, thereby decreasing injury to the face, skull, and brain. The helmet provides only minimal protection for the neck but does not cause neck injuries. Failure to use helmets has been shown to increase head injuries by more than 300%. Most states that have passed mandatory helmet legislation have found an associated reduction in motorcycle incidents. For example, Louisiana had a 60% reduction in head injuries in the first 6 years after passing a helmet law.

PEDESTRIAN INJURY

Two patterns commonly seen in pedestrian versus motor vehicle crashes demonstrate different injury patterns. The difference is associated with the age group of the victim—adult or child. When adults see that they are about to be struck by an oncoming vehicle, they try to protect themselves by turning away. Therefore the injuries are frequently lateral or even posterior. Children often face the oncoming vehicle, often resulting in anterior injuries. Because of the variance in heights between a child and an adult relative to the bumper and hood of a vehicle, the striking patterns are also different.

Pedestrian versus motor vehicle crashes have three separate phases, each with its own injury pattern:

1. The initial impact is to the legs and sometimes the hips (Figure 2-32, *A*).

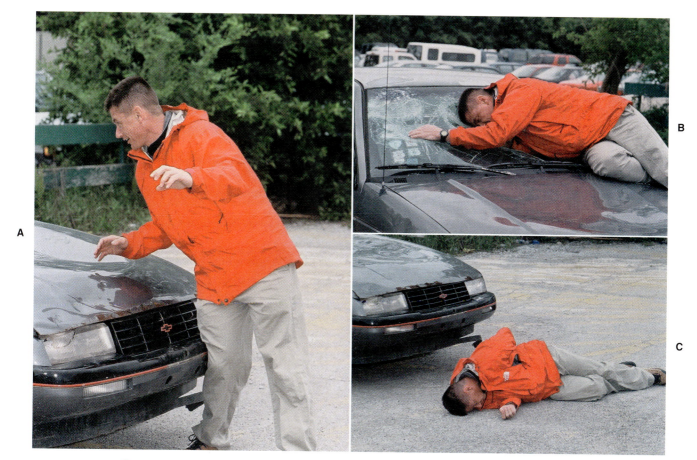

Figure 2-32   A, *Phase 1*. When a pedestrian is struck by a vehicle, the initial impact is to the legs and sometimes to the hips. B, *Phase 2*. The torso of the pedestrian rolls onto the hood of the vehicle. C, *Phase 3*. The pedestrian falls off the vehicle and hits the ground.

2. The torso rolls onto the hood of the vehicle (Figure 2-32, *B*).
3. The victim falls off the vehicle and onto the ground, usually head first, with possible cervical spine trauma (Figure 2-32, *C*).

Adults are usually struck first by the vehicle's bumper in the lower legs, fracturing the tibia and fibula and driving the legs out from under the pelvis and torso. As the victim folds forward, the pelvis and upper femur are struck by the front of the vehicle's hood. As the abdomen and thorax fall forward, they strike the top of the hood. This substantial second strike can result in fractures of the upper femur, pelvis, ribs, and spine and produce serious intraabdominal or intrathoracic damage. Injury to the head and face at this point depends on the victim's ability to protect them with his or her arms. If the victim's head strikes the hood or if the victim continues to move up the hood so that his or her head strikes the windshield, injury to the face, head, and spine can occur.

The third impact occurs as the victim falls off the vehicle and strikes the pavement. The victim can receive a significant blow on one side of the body to the hip, shoulder, and head. Head injury commonly occurs when the victim strikes either the vehicle or the pavement and must always be considered. Similarly, because all three impacts produce sudden, violent movement of the torso, neck, and head, the prehospital care provider must always assume an unstable spine to be present. An evaluation of the mechanism of injury should also include a determination if the victim, after hitting the roadway, was struck again by a second vehicle traveling next to or behind the first.

Children, because they are shorter, are initially struck higher on the body than adults (Figure 2-33, *A*). The first impact generally occurs when the bumper strikes the child's legs (above the knees) or pelvis, damaging the femur or pelvic girdle. The second impact occurs almost instantly afterward when the front of the vehicle's hood continues forward and strikes the child's thorax. The head and face strike the front or top

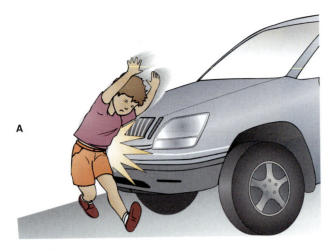

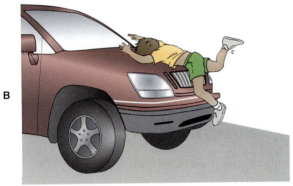

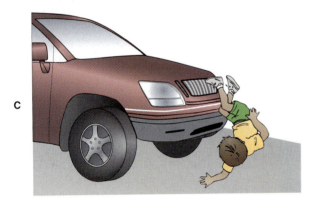

Figure 2-33 **A,** The initial impact on a child occurs when the vehicle strikes the child's upper leg or pelvis. **B,** The second impact occurs when the child's head and face strike the front or top of the vehicle's hood. **C,** A child may not be thrown clear of a vehicle but may be trapped and dragged by the vehicle.

of the vehicle's hood (Figure 2-33, *B*). Because of the child's smaller size and weight, the child may not be thrown clear of the vehicle, as usually happens with an adult. Instead, the child can be dragged by the vehicle while partially under the vehicle's front end (Figure 2-33, *C*). If the child falls to the side, the lower limbs may also be run over by a front wheel. If the child falls backward, ending up completely under the vehi-

cle, almost any injury can occur (e.g., being dragged, struck by projections, or run over by a wheel).

As with an adult, any child struck by a vehicle usually receives some type of head injury. Because of the sudden, violent forces acting on the head, neck, and torso, the prehospital care provider must assume that the child has an unstable spine. Additionally, the force of the impact, which is usually midthoracic, should raise suspicion of significant intrathoracic injury even with children who initially appear asymptomatic. The prehospital care provider should assume that any child who is struck by a vehicle has sustained multisystem trauma, requiring rapid transport to the closest appropriate facility.

Knowing the specific sequence of multiple impacts in pedestrian versus motor vehicle crashes and understanding the multiple underlying injuries that they can produce are key to making an initial assessment and determining the appropriate management of a patient.

FALLS

Victims of falls can also sustain injury from multiple impacts. To properly assess a fall victim, the prehospital care provider should estimate the height of the fall, evaluate the surface on which the victim landed, and determine which part of the body struck first. Victims who fall from greater heights have a higher incidence of injury because their velocity increases as they fall. In general, falls from greater than three times the height of the victim are severe. The kind of surface on which the victim lands, and particularly its degree of compressibility (ability to be deformed by the transfer of energy), also has an effect on stopping distance.

Determining which part of the body hit first is important because it helps the prehospital care provider predict the injury pattern. When victims fall or jump from a height and land on their feet, the pattern that occurs is often called *Don Juan syndrome.* Only in the movies can the character Don Juan jump from a balcony, land on his feet, and walk painlessly away. In real life, bilateral calcaneus (heel bone) fractures, fractures of the ankles, or distal tibia or fibula fractures are often associated with this syndrome. After the feet land and stop moving, the legs are the next body part to absorb energy. Knee fractures, long bone fractures, and hip fractures can result. The body is forced into flexion by the weight of the head and torso, which are still moving, and can cause compression fractures of the spinal column in the thoracic and lumbar areas. Hyperflexion occurs at each concave bend of the S-shaped spine, producing flexion injuries. This victim is often described as breaking his or her "S" (Figure 2-34).

If a victim falls forward onto his or her out-stretched hands, the result can be bilateral Colles' fractures of the wrists. If the victim did not land on his or her feet, the prehospital care provider should assess the part of the body that struck first, evaluate the pathway of energy displacement, and determine the injury pattern.

If the falling victim lands on his or her head with the body almost in line, such as commonly occurs in shallow-water diving injuries, the entire weight and force of the moving torso, pelvis, and legs compress the head and cervical spine. A fracture of the cervical spine can result, just as with the up-and-over pathway of the frontal impact collision.

SPORTS INJURIES

Severe injury can occur during many sports or recreational activities, such as skiing, diving, baseball, and football. These injuries can be caused by sudden deceleration forces or by excessive compression, twisting, hyperextension, or hyperflexion. In recent years, various sports activities have become available to a wide spectrum of occasional, recreational participants who often lack the necessary training and conditioning or the proper protective equipment. Recreational sports and activities include participants of all ages. Sports such as downhill skiing, waterskiing, bicycling, and skateboarding are potentially high-velocity activities. Others sports such as trail biking, all-terrain vehicle (ATV) riding, and snowmobiling can produce velocity deceleration, collisions, and impacts similar to motorcycle crashes or MVCs.

The potential injuries of a victim who is in a high-speed collision and is then ejected from a skateboard, snowmobile, or bicycle are similar to those sustained when a person is ejected from a vehicle at the same speed because the amount of energy is the same. The specific mechanisms of MVCs and motorcycle crashes are described previously in this chapter.

The potential mechanisms commonly associated with each sport are too numerous to list in detail. However, the general principles are the same as for MVCs. While assessing the mechanism of injury, the prehospital care provider should consider the following:

- What forces acted on the victim and how?
- What are the apparent injuries?
- To what object or part of the body was the energy transmitted?
- What other injuries are likely to have been produced by this energy transfer?
- Was protective gear being worn?

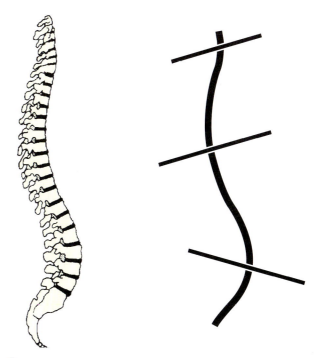

Figure 2-34   As the lower part of the spine stops its forward motion, the continued motion of the upper torso and head compress the spine. This motion tends to produce compression injuries on the side of the concavity and extraction injuries on the side of the convexity.

- Was there sudden compression, deceleration, or acceleration?
- What injury-producing movements occurred (such as hyperflexion, hyperextension, compression, or excessive lateral bending)?

When the mechanism of injury involves a high-speed collision between two participants, such as in a crash between two skiers, reconstruction of the exact sequence of events from eyewitness accounts is often difficult. In such crashes, the injuries sustained by one skier are often guidelines for examination of the other. In general, the prehospital care provider needs to know which part struck what, and what injury resulted from the energy transfer. For example, if one victim sustains an impact fracture of the hip, a part of the other skier's body must have struck with substantial force and therefore must have sustained a similar high-impact injury. If the second skier's head struck the first skier's hip, the prehospital care provider should suspect potentially serious head injury and an unstable spine for the second skier.

Broken or damaged equipment is also an important indicator of injury and must be included in the evaluation of the mechanism of injury. A broken sports helmet is evidence of the force with which it struck. Because skis are made of highly durable material, a broken ski indicates that extreme localized force came to bear even when the mechanism of injury may appear unimpressive. A snowmobile with a severely dented front can indicate the force with which it struck a tree. The presence of a broken stick after an ice hockey skirmish raises the question of whose body broke it, how, and specifically what part of the victim's body was struck by it or fell on it.

The prehospital care provider must take injuries caused by these forces seriously and evaluate the victim thoroughly before moving him or her from the scene. The prehospital care provider should do the following:

- Evaluate the patient for life-threatening injury.
- Evaluate the patient for mechanism of injury. (What happened and exactly how?)
- Determine how the forces that produced injury in one victim may have affected any other person.
- Determine whether protective gear was worn (it may have already been removed).
- Assess damage to equipment. (What are the implications of this damage relative to the patient's body?)
- Assess patient for possible associated injuries.

High-speed falls, collisions, and falls from heights without serious injury are common in many contact sports. The ability of athletes to experience incredible collisions and falls while sustaining only minor injury—which is due largely to impact-absorbing equipment—may cloud a prehospital care provider's assessment. The potential for injury in sports injury victims may be overlooked. By applying the principles of kinematics and carefully considering the exact sequence and mechanism of injury, the prehospital care provider can better recognize those sports collisions in which greater forces than usual came to bear. Kinematics is an essential tool in identifying possible underlying injuries and determining which patients require further evaluation and treatment at a medical facility.

BLAST INJURIES

The incidence of blast injuries increases during warfare, but these injuries are also becoming more common in the civilian world as terrorist activities and hazardous material incidents increase. Blasts may injure 70% of the people in the vicinity, whereas an automatic weapon used against the same size group may injure only 30%. Mines, shipyards, chemical plants, refineries, fireworks firms, factories, and grain elevators are some areas in which explosions are a particular hazard. However, because many volatile materials are transported by truck or rail, and domestic and bottled gas are common household items, an explosion can occur almost anywhere. An explosion can be divided into three phases—primary, secondary, and tertiary (Figure 2-35). Different types of injuries occur during these three phases.

1. *Primary injuries* are caused by the pressure wave of the blast. They usually occur in the gas-containing organs, such as the lungs and the gastrointestinal tract. Primary injuries include pulmonary bleeding, pneumothorax, air emboli, or perforation of the gastrointestinal organs. Pressure waves rupture and tear the small vessels and membranes of the gas-containing organs (cavitation) and may also injure

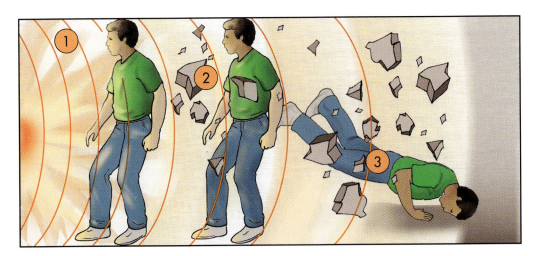

Figure 2-35   Three phases of injury occur during a blast. In the first phase, the pressure wave first reaches the victim. This is followed by the second phase, in which flying debris can become missiles that produce injury. The third phase is when the victim becomes a missile and can be thrown into other objects or the ground.

the central nervous system. These waves may cause severe damage or death without external signs of injury. Burns from the heat wave are also a common primary injury. Burns occur on unprotected body areas that are facing the source of the explosion.

2. *Secondary injuries* occur when the victim is struck by flying glass, falling mortar, or other debris from the blast. Secondary injuries include lacerations, fractures, and burns.

3. *Tertiary injuries* occur when the victim becomes a missile and is thrown against an object. Injury will occur at the point of impact, and the force of the blast will be transferred to other organs of the body as the energy from the impact is absorbed. Tertiary injuries are usually apparent, but the prehospital care provider must look for associated injuries according to the type of impact that occurred. The injuries that occur in the tertiary phase are similar to those sustained in ejections from vehicles and falls from significant heights.

Secondary and tertiary injuries are the most obvious and are usually the most aggressively treated. Primary injuries may be the most severe, but they are often overlooked and sometimes never suspected. Adequate assessment of the various kinds of injuries is vital if the prehospital care provider is to manage the patient properly. Blast injuries often cause severe complications that may result in death if they are overlooked or ignored.

Regional Effects of Blunt Trauma

The prehospital care provider must consider several components in each body region: 1) the external part of the body, usually composed of skin, bone, soft tissue, vessels, and nerves; 2) the internal part of the body, usually vital internal organs; and 3) the injuries produced as a result of shear and compression forces.

HEAD

The only indication that compression and shear injuries have occurred to the patient's head may be a soft tissue injury to the scalp, a contusion of the scalp, or a bull's-eye fracture of the windshield (Figure 2-36).

Compression.   When the body is traveling forward with the head leading the way, as in a frontal vehicular crash or a head-first fall, the head is first to receive the impact and the energy exchange. The continued momentum of the torso then compresses the head. The initial energy exchange occurs on the scalp and the skull. The skull can be compressed and fractured, pushing the broken bony segments of the skull into the brain (Figure 2-37).

Shear.   After the skull stops its forward motion, the brain continues to move forward, becoming compressed against the intact or fractured skull with resultant concussion, contusions, or lacerations. The brain is soft and compressible; therefore its length is shortened. The posterior part of the brain can continue forward, pulling away from the skull which has already stopped moving. Therefore the brain separates from the skull, stretching or breaking (shearing) any vessels in the area (Figure 2-38). Hemorrhage into the epidural, subdural, or subarachnoid space can then result. If the brain separates from the spinal cord, it will most likely occur at the brain stem.

NECK

Compression.   The dome of the skull is fairly strong and can absorb the impact of a collision; however, the cervical spine is much more flexible. The continued pressure from the momentum of the torso toward the stationary skull (Figure 2-39) produces angulation or compression. Hyperextension or hyperflexion of the

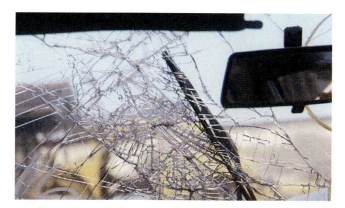

Figure 2-36   A bull's-eye fracture of the windshield is a major indication of skull impact and energy exchange to both the skull and the cervical spine.

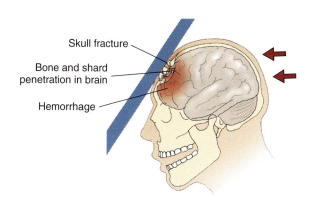

Figure 2-37   As the skull impacts a movable object, pieces of bone are fractured and are pushed into the brain substance.

neck often results in fracture or dislocation of the vertebrae and injury to the spinal cord (Figure 2-40). Direct inline compression crushes the bony vertebral bodies. Both angulation and inline compression can result in an unstable spine.

Shear.   The skull's center of gravity is anterior and cephalad to the point at which the skull attaches to the bony spine. Therefore a lateral impact on the torso when the neck is unrestrained will produce lateral flexion and rotation of the neck (see Figure 2-18). Extreme flexion or hyperextension may also cause stretching injuries to the soft tissues of the neck.

THORAX

Compression.   If the impact of a collision is centered on the anterior part of the chest, the sternum will receive the initial energy exchange. When the sternum stops moving, the posterior thoracic wall (muscles and thoracic spine) and the organs in the thoracic cavity continue to move forward until they hit the sternum.

The continued forward motion of the posterior thorax bends the ribs until their tensile strength is exceeded, and fractured ribs and/or a flail chest can develop (Figure 2-41). This is similar to what happens when a vehicle stops suddenly against a dirt embankment. The frame

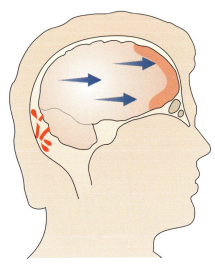

Figure 2-38   As the skull stops its forward motion, the brain continues to move forward. The part of the brain nearest the impact is compressed, bruised, and perhaps even lacerated, while the portion furthest away from the impact is separated from the skull with tearing and lacerations of the vessels involved.

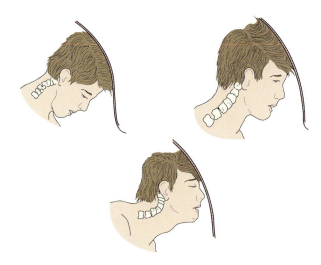

Figure 2-40   The spine can be compressed directly along its own axis or angled either into hyperextension or hyperflexion.

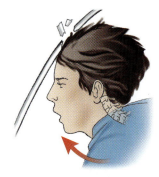

Figure 2-39   The skull frequently stops its forward motion, but the torso does not. Just as the brain compresses within the skull, the torso continues its forward motion until its energy is absorbed. The weakest point of this forward motion is the cervical spine.

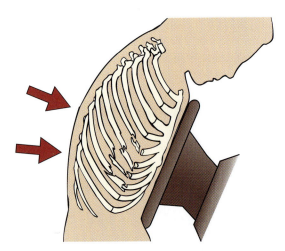

Figure 2-41   Ribs forced into the thoracic cavity by external compression usually fracture in multiple places, producing the clinical condition known as flail chest.

of the vehicle bends, which absorbs some of the energy. The rear of the vehicle continues to move forward until the bending of the frame absorbs all of the energy. In the same way, the posterior thoracic wall continues to move until the ribs absorb all of the energy.

Compression of the chest wall is common with frontal and lateral impacts and produces an interesting phenomenon called the *paper bag effect*, which may result in a pneumothorax. A victim instinctively takes a deep breath and holds it just before impact. This closes the glottis, effectively sealing off the lungs. With a significant energy exchange on impact, the lungs may then burst like a paper bag full of air that is popped (Figure 2-42). The lungs can also become compressed and contused, compromising ventilation.

Compression injuries to the internal structures of the thorax may also include a cardiac contusion, which occurs as the heart is compressed between the sternum and the spine and can result in significant dysrhythmias.

Shear.   The heart, ascending aorta, and aortic arch are relatively unrestrained within the thorax. The descending aorta tightly adheres to the posterior thoracic wall and the vertebral column. The resultant motion is analogous to holding the flexible tubes of a stethoscope just below where the rigid tubes from the earpiece end and swinging the acoustic head of the stethoscope from side to side. As the skeletal frame stops abruptly in a collision, the heart and the initial segment of the aorta continue their forward motion. The shear forces produced

can tear off the aorta at the junction of the portion of free motion and the tightly bound portion (Figure 2-43).

An aortic tear may result in an immediate, complete transection of the aorta. More commonly, aortic tears are only partial, and one or more layers of tissue remain intact. However, the remaining layers are under great pressure, and a traumatic aneurysm often develops, much like the bubble that can form on a weak part of a tire. The aneurysm can eventually rupture within minutes,

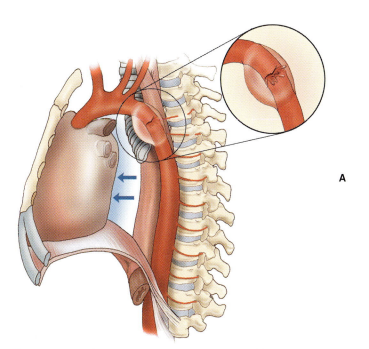

A

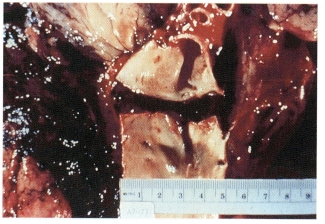

B

Figure 2-42 Compression of the lung against a closed glottis, by impact either on the anterior or lateral chest wall, produces an effect like that of compressing a paper bag when the opening is closed tightly by the hands. The paper bag ruptures, as does the lung.

Figure 2-43 **A,** The descending aorta is a fixed structure that moves with the thoracic spine. The arch, aorta, and heart are freely movable. Acceleration of the torso in a lateral impact collision or rapid deceleration of the torso in a frontal impact collision produces a different rate of motion between the arch-heart complex and the descending aorta. (**A** *from McSwain NE Jr, Paturas JL:* The basic EMT: comprehensive prehospital patient care, *ed 2, St Louis, 2001, Mosby.*) **B,** Tears at the junction of the arch and descending aorta.

hours, or days after the original injury. Approximately 80% of these patients die on the scene at the time of the initial impact. Of the remaining 20%, one third will die within 6 hours, one third will die within 24 hours, and one third will live 3 days or longer. The prehospital care provider must recognize the potential for such injuries and relay this information to the hospital personnel.

ABDOMEN

Compression.   Internal organs pressed by the vertebral column into the steering wheel or dashboard during a frontal impact collision may rupture. The effect of this pressure is similar to the effect of placing the internal organ on an anvil and striking it with a hammer. Solid organs frequently injured in this manner include the pancreas, spleen, liver, and kidneys.

Injury may also result from a buildup of pressure in the abdomen. The diaphragm is a ¼-inch (5 mm) muscle located across the top of the abdomen separating the abdominal cavity from the thoracic cavity. Its contraction causes the pleural cavity to expand for ventilation. The anterior abdominal wall comprises two layers of fascia and one very strong muscle. Three lateral muscle layers have associated fascia, and the lumbar spine and its associated muscles provide strength to the posterior abdominal wall. The multilayered perineum lies inferior to the diaphragm. The diaphragm is the weakest of all of

the walls and structures surrounding the abdominal cavity. It may be torn or ruptured as the intraabdominal pressure increases (Figure 2-44). This injury has four common consequences:

1. The "bellows" effect normally created by the diaphragm as an integral part of breathing is lost.
2. The abdominal organs can enter the thoracic cavity and reduce the space available for lung expansion.
3. The displaced organs can become ischemic from compression of their blood supply.
4. If intraabdominal hemorrhage is present, the blood can also cause a hemothorax.

The diaphragm can be compressed from any direction, but compression most commonly occurs from the direction of the anterior abdominal wall.

Another injury caused by increased abdominal pressure is a rupture of the aortic valve as a result of retrograde blood flow (Figure 2-45). Although this injury is rare, the prehospital care provider should be aware of the possibility. It occurs when a collision with the steering wheel or involvement in another type of incident (e.g., ditch or tunnel cave-in) has produced a rapid increase in intraabdominal pressure. This rapid pressure increase results in a sudden increase of aortic blood pressure. Blood is pushed back (retrograde) against the

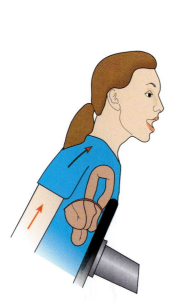

Figure 2-44   With increased pressure inside the abdomen, the diaphragm can rupture.

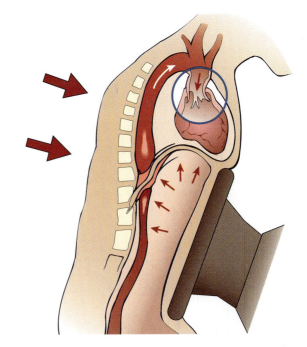

Figure 2-45   Increased intraabdominal pressure can force blood in a retrograde fashion up the aorta and against the aortic valve. The aortic valve may then tear.

aortic valve with enough pressure to cause rupture of the valve cusps.

Shear.   Injury to the abdominal organs occurs at their points of attachment to the mesentery. During a collision, the forward motion of the body stops, but the organs continue to move forward, causing tears at the points of attachment of organs to the abdominal wall. If the organ is attached by a pedicle (a stalk of tissue), the tear can occur where the pedicle attaches to the organ, where it attaches to the abdominal wall, or anywhere along the length of the pedicle (Figure 2-46). Organs that can shear this way are the kidneys, small intestine, large intestine, and spleen.

Another kind of injury that often occurs during deceleration is laceration of the liver caused by its impact with the ligamentum teres. The liver is suspended from the diaphragm but is only minimally attached to the posterior abdomen near the lumbar vertebrae. The ligamentum teres attaches to the anterior abdominal wall at the umbilicus and to the left lobe of the liver in the midline of the body. (The liver is not a midline structure. It lies more on the right than on the left.) A down-and-under pathway in a frontal impact collision or a feet-first fall causes the liver to bring the diaphragm with it as it descends into the ligamentum teres (Figure 2-47). The ligamentum teres will fracture or bisect the liver like a cheese slicer slices cheese.

Pelvic fractures are the result of damage to the external abdomen and may cause injury to the bladder or lacerations of the blood vessels in the pelvic cavity. Approximately 10% of patients with pelvic fractures also have a genitourinary injury.

Penetrating Trauma

PHYSICS OF PENETRATING TRAUMA

The principles of physics discussed at the beginning of this chapter are equally important when dealing with penetrating injuries. As discussed previously, the kinetic energy that a striking object transfers to body tissue is represented by the following formula:

$$KE = \tfrac{1}{2}mv^2$$

Energy cannot be created or destroyed, but it can be changed in form. This principle is important in understanding penetrating trauma. For example, although a lead bullet is in the brass cartridge casing that is filled with explosive powder, the bullet has no force. However, when the primer explodes, the powder burns, producing rapidly expanding gases that are transformed into force. The bullet then moves out of the gun and toward its target.

According to Newton's first law of motion, after this force has acted upon the missile, the bullet will remain at that speed and force until it is acted upon by an outside force. When the bullet hits something, such as a human body, it strikes the individual tissue cells. The energy (speed and mass) of the bullet's motion is exchanged for the energy that crushes these cells and moves them away (cavitation) from the path of the bullet.

Factors that Affect the Size of the Frontal Area.   The larger the frontal area of the moving missile, the greater the number of particles that will be hit; there-

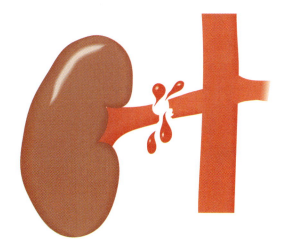

Figure 2-46   Other organs can also tear away from their point of attachment to the abdominal wall. The spleen, kidney, and small intestine are particularly susceptible to these types of shear forces.

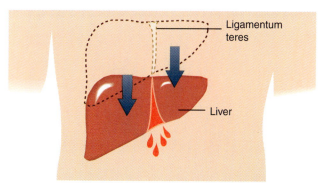

Figure 2-47   The liver is not supported by any fixed structure. Its major support is by the diaphragm, which is freely movable. As the body travels in the down-and-under pathway, so does the liver. When the torso stops but the liver does not, the liver continues downward onto the ligamentum teres, tearing the liver. This is much like pushing a cheese-cutting wire into a block of cheese.

fore the greater the energy exchange that occurs and the larger the cavity that is created. The size of the frontal surface area of a projectile is influenced by three factors—profile, tumble, and fragmentation. Energy exchange or potential energy exchange can be analyzed based on these factors.

Profile.   *Profile* describes an object's initial size and whether that size changes at the time of impact. The profile, or frontal area, of an ice pick is much smaller than that of a baseball bat, which in turn is much smaller than that of a truck. A hollow-pointed missile, if crushed and

> ### Expanding Bullets
>
> A munitions factory in Dum Dum, India manufactured a bullet that expanded when it hit the skin. Ballistic experts recognized this design as one that would cause more damage than is necessary in war; therefore these bullets were prohibited in military conflicts. The Geneva Convention (1880) and the Petersburg Treaty (1899) both affirmed this principle, denouncing these "dum-dum" projectiles and other expanding missiles, such as silver tips, hollow-points, scored-lead cartridges or jackets, and partially jacketed bullets.

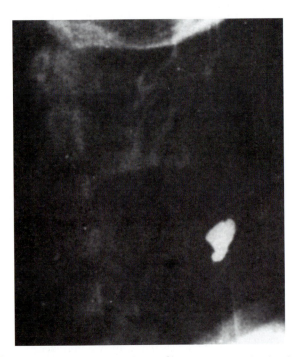

Figure 2-48   Changes in the profile or trauma projection increase the particles hit and therefore the amount of energy dispersal. (*From McSwain NE Jr: Pulmonary chest trauma. In Moylan JA, editor:* Principles of trauma, *New York, 1992, Gower.*)

deformed as a result of striking a body, will have a much larger frontal area than before its shape was changed. A hollow-point bullet flattens and spreads on impact. This change enlarges the frontal area so that it hits more tissue particles and produces greater energy exchange. A larger cavity forms, and more injury results (Figure 2-48).

In general, as a bullet travels through the air after being discharged from a weapon, it will strike fewer air particles and maintain most of its speed if its frontal area is kept small and streamlined by its conical shape. If that missile strikes the skin and becomes deformed, covering a larger area, a much greater energy exchange will occur than if its frontal surface area does not expand.

Tumble.   *Tumble* describes whether the object tumbles and assumes a different angle inside the body than the angle assumed as it entered the body. A wedge-shaped bullet's center of gravity is located nearer to the base than to the nose of the bullet. When the nose of the bullet strikes something, it slows rapidly. Momentum continues to carry the base of the bullet forward, with the center of gravity seeking to become the leading point of the bullet. This movement causes an end-over-end motion, or tumble. As the bullet tumbles, the normally horizontal sides of the bullet become its leading edges, thus striking far more particles than when the nose was the leading edge (Figure 2-49). More energy exchange is produced, and therefore greater tissue damage occurs.

Fragmentation.   *Fragmentation* describes whether the object breaks up after it enters the body. Bullets such as those with soft noses, vertical cuts in the nose, and safety slugs that contain many small fragments increase body damage by breaking apart on impact. The mass of fragments produced comprises a larger frontal area than

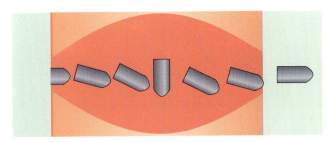

Figure 2-49   The tumble motion of a missile maximizes its damage at 90 degrees.

a single solid bullet, and energy is dispersed rapidly into the tissue. If the missile shatters, it will spread out over a wider area, with two results: 1) more tissue particles will be struck by the larger frontal projection, and 2) the injuries will be distributed over a larger portion of the body because more organs will be struck (Figures 2-50). The multiple pieces of shot from a shotgun blast produce similar results. Shotgun wounds are an excellent example of the fragmentation injury pattern (Figure 2-51).

DAMAGE AND ENERGY LEVELS

The prehospital care provider can estimate damage caused in a penetrating injury by classifying penetrating objects into three categories according to their energy capacity—low-, medium-, and high-energy weapons. Although penetrating trauma is usually confined to gunshot and knife wounds, the prehospital care provider should be prepared to deal with penetrating trauma from impaled objects such as fence posts and street signs in vehicle crashes.

Low-Energy Weapons.   Low-energy weapons include hand-driven weapons such as a knife or ice pick. These missiles produce damage only with their sharp points or cutting edges. Because these are low-velocity injuries, they are usually associated with less secondary trauma (i.e., less cavitation will occur). Injury in these victims can be predicted by tracing the path of the weapon into the body. If the weapon has been removed, the prehospital care provider should identify the type of weapon used and the gender of the attacker whenever possible. Men tend to stab with the blade on the thumb side of the hand and with an upward thrust, whereas women tend to stab downward and hold the blade on the little finger side.

When evaluating a patient with a stab wound, it is important to look for more than one wound. Multiple stab wounds are possible and should not be ruled out until the patient is completely exposed and closely ex-

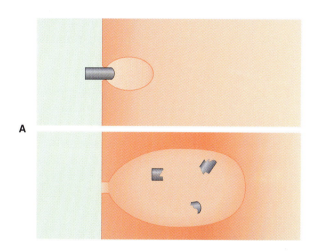

A

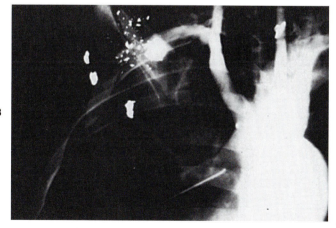

B

Figure 2-50   **A,** A missile that is made of soft lead or another component that breaks up will cause damage over a wider area and create maximum absorption of the energy as many more tissue particles are impacted. **B,** When the missile breaks up into smaller particles, this fragmentation increases its frontal area and increases the energy distribution. (**B** *from McSwain NE Jr: Pulmonary chest trauma. In Moylan JA, editor: Principles of trauma, New York, 1992, Gower.*)

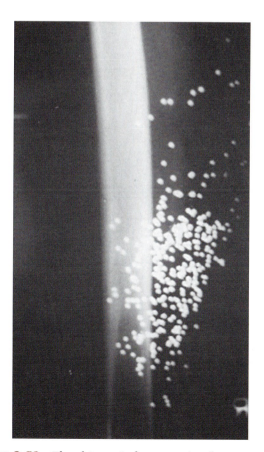

Figure 2-51   The ultimate in fragmentation damage is caused by a shotgun.

amined. This close inspection may take place at the scene, en route to the medical facility, or at the medical facility, depending on the circumstances surrounding the incident and the condition of the patient.

An attacker may stab a victim and then move the knife around inside the body. A simple entrance wound may therefore give the prehospital care provider a false sense of security. The entrance wound may be small, but the damage inside may be extensive. The prehospital care provider cannot determine internal injuries in the field, but he or she must always suspect the possibility, even with seemingly minor injuries. The potential scope of the movement of the inserted blade is an area of possible damage (Figure 2-52).

Evaluation of the patient for associated injury is important. For example, the diaphragm can reach as high as the nipple line on deep expiration. A stab wound to the lower chest can injure intrathoracic as well as intra-abdominal structures.

Medium- and High-Energy Weapons.

Firearms fall into two groups—medium energy and high energy. Medium-energy weapons include handguns and some rifles. As the amount of gunpowder in the cartridge increases, the speed of the bullet and therefore its kinetic energy increases (Figure 2-53).

Medium- and high-energy weapons, in general, damage not only the tissue directly in the path of the missile but also the tissue on each side of the missile's path. The variables of profile, tumble, and fragmentation influence the extent and direction of the injury. The pressure on tissue particles, which are moved out of the direct path of the missile, compress and stretch the surrounding tissue. A temporary cavity is always associated with weapons in the medium-energy classification. This cav-

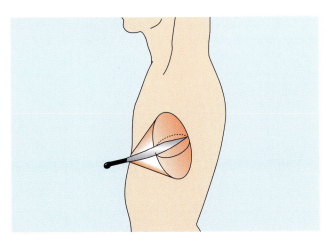

Figure 2-52 The damage produced by a knife depends on the movement of the blade inside the victim.

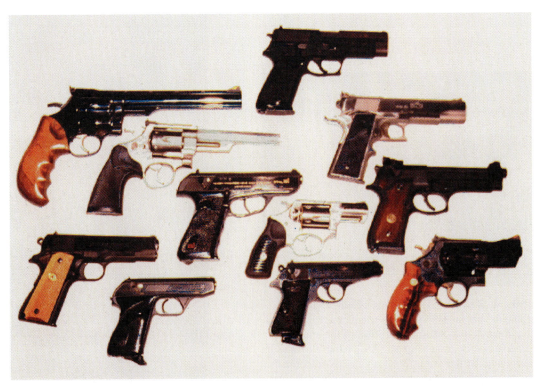

Figure 2-53 Medium-energy weapons are usually guns that have short barrels and contain cartridges with less power. (*From McSwain NE Jr, Paturas JL: The basic EMT: comprehensive prehospital patient care, ed 2, St Louis, 2001, Mosby.*)

ity is usually three to six times the size of the missile's frontal surface area (Figure 2-54).

High-energy weapons include assault weapons, hunting rifles, and other weapons that discharge high-velocity missiles (Figure 2-55). These missiles not only create a permanent track but produce a much larger temporary cavity than lower-velocity missiles. This temporary cavity expands well beyond the limits of the actual bullet track and damages and injures a wider area than is apparent during the initial assessment. Tissue damage is far more extensive with a high-energy penetrating object than with one of medium energy. The vacuum created by this cavity pulls clothing, bacteria, and other debris from the surrounding area into the wound.

A consideration in predicting the damage from a gunshot wound is the range or distance from which the gun (either medium or high energy) is fired. Air resistance slows the bullet; therefore increasing the distance will decrease the velocity at the time of impact and will result in less injury. Most shootings are carried out at close range with handguns, so the probability of serious injury is high.

ENTRANCE AND EXIT WOUNDS

When evaluating the victim of a penetrating trauma, a prehospital care provider should evaluate entrance and exit wounds. Tissue damage will occur at the site of entry into the body, in the path of the weapon's entrance, and upon exit from the body. Knowledge of the victim's position, the attacker's position, and the weapon used is essential in determining the path of injury.

Evaluating wound sites provides valuable information to direct the management of the patient and to relay to the receiving facility. Do two holes in the victim's abdomen indicate that a single missile entered and exited or that two missiles are both still inside the patient? Did the missile cross the midline (usually causing more severe injury) or remain on the same side? In what direction did the missile travel? What internal organs are likely to have been in its path?

Entrance and exit wounds usually produce identifiable injury patterns to soft tissue. An entrance wound from a gunshot lies against the underlying tissue, but an exit wound has no support. The former is a round or oval wound depending on the entry path, and the latter

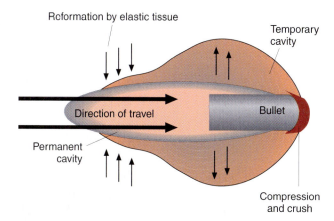

Figure 2-54   A bullet crushes tissues directly in its path. A cavity is created in the wake of the bullet. The crushed part is permanent. The temporary expansion can also produce injury.

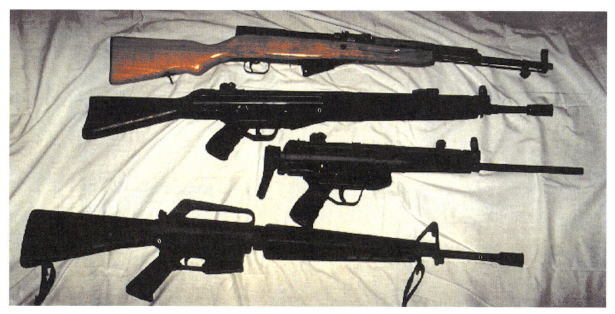

Figure 2-55   High-energy weapons. (*From McSwain NE Jr, Paturas JL:* The basic EMT: comprehensive prehospital patient care, *ed 2, St Louis, 2001, Mosby.*)

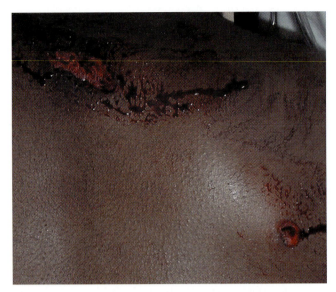

Figure 2-56   The entrance wound is round or oval in shape, and the exit wound is stellate or linear. (*From Mc-Swain NE Jr, Paturas JL: The basic EMT: comprehensive pre-hospital patient care, ed 2, St Louis, 2001, Mosby.*)

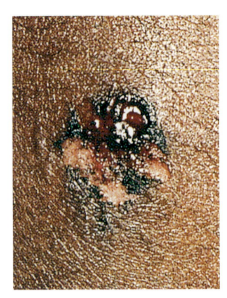

Figure 2-58   Hot gases coming from the end of a muzzle held in close proximity to the skin produce partial- and full-thickness burns on the skin.

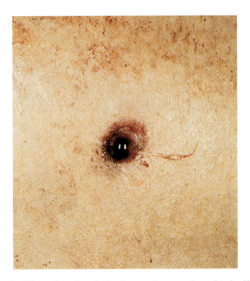

Figure 2-57   The abraded edge indicates that the bullet traveled from top right to bottom left.

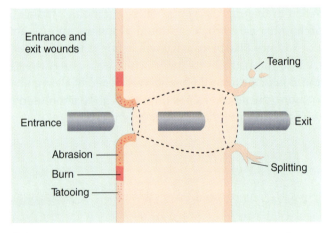

Figure 2-59   Spin and compression on entrance produce round or oval holes. On exit the wound is pressed open.

is a stellate (starburst) wound (Figure 2-56). Because the missile is spinning as it enters the skin, it leaves a small area of abrasion (1 to 2 mm in size) that is black or pink (Figure 2-57). Abrasion is not present on the exit side. If the muzzle was placed directly against the skin at the time of discharge, the expanding gases will enter the tissue and produce crepitus on examination (Figure 2-58). Within 5 to 7 cm the burning gases will burn the skin, at 5 to 15 cm the smoke will adhere to the skin, and inside 25 cm the burning cordite particles will

tattoo the skin with small (1 to 2 mm) burned areas (Figure 2-59).

Regional Effects of Penetrating Trauma

In this section, the injuries sustained by various parts of the body during penetrating trauma are discussed.

HEAD

After a missile penetrates the skull, its energy is distributed within a closed space. Particles accelerating away from the

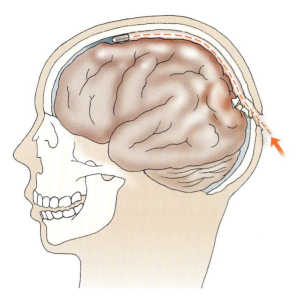

Figure 2-60 The bullet may follow the curvature of the skull. (*From McSwain NE Jr, Paturas JL: The basic EMT: comprehensive prehospital patient care, ed 2, St Louis, 2001, Mosby.*)

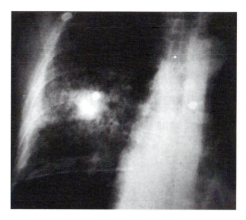

Figure 2-61 Lung damage produced by the cavity at a distance from the point of impact.

missile are forced against the unyielding skull, which cannot expand as skin can. Thus the brain tissue is compressed against the inside of the skull, producing more injury than if it could expand freely. If the forces are strong enough, the skull may explode from the inside out.

A bullet may follow the curvature of the interior of the skull if it enters at an angle and has insufficient force to exit the skull. This path can produce significant damage (Figure 2-60). Because of this characteristic, medium-velocity weapons, such as the 0.22 caliber or 0.25 caliber pistol, have been called the "assassin's weapon."

THORAX

The prehospital care provider must consider three major groups of structures inside the thoracic cavity in evaluating a penetrating injury to the chest—the pulmonary system, vascular system, and gastrointestinal tract.

Pulmonary System. Lung tissue is less dense than blood, solid organs, or bone; therefore a penetrating object does less damage to lung tissue than to other thoracic tissues. Much of the area traversed by the missile is air, fewer particles are hit, and less energy is transferred, so less damage is produced. However, damage to the lungs can be clinically significant (Figure 2-61).

Vascular System. Smaller vessels that are not attached to the chest wall may be pushed aside without significant damage. However, if larger vessels, such as the aorta and

vena cava, are hit, they cannot move aside easily and are more susceptible to damage.

The myocardium stretches as the bullet passes through and then contracts, leaving a smaller defect. The thickness of the muscle may control a low-energy penetration such as a knife or 0.22 caliber bullet, preventing immediate exsanguination and allowing time to get the victim to an appropriate facility.

Gastrointestinal Tract. The esophagus, the part of the gastrointestinal tract that traverses the thoracic cavity, can be penetrated and can leak its contents into the thoracic cavity. The signs and symptoms of such an injury may be delayed for several hours or several days.

ABDOMEN

The abdomen contains structures of three types—air-filled, solid, and bony. Penetration by a low-energy missile may not cause significant damage; only 30% of knife wounds penetrating the abdominal cavity require surgical exploration to repair damage. A medium-energy injury (handgun wound) is more damaging—85% to 95% require surgical repair. However, even with injuries caused by medium-energy missiles, the damage to solid and vascular structures may not produce immediate exsanguination. Often prehospital care providers can temporarily control the hemorrhage and resuscitate the patient by using a pneumatic antishock garment (PASG) and intravenous fluids. This enables them to transport the patient to an appropriate facility in time for effective surgical intervention.

EXTREMITIES

Penetrating injuries to the extremities can include damage to bones, muscles, or vessels. When bones are hit,

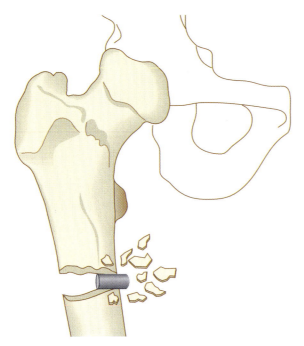

Figure 2-62   Bone fragments become secondary missiles themselves, producing damage by the same mechanism as the original penetrating object.

bony fragments become secondary missiles, lacerating surrounding tissue (Figure 2-62). Muscles often expand away from the path of the missile causing hemorrhage. Blood vessels can be penetrated by the missile, or a near-miss can damage the lining of a blood vessel, causing clotting and obstruction of the vessel within minutes or hours.

Using Kinematics in Assessment

The assessment of a trauma patient must involve knowledge of kinematics. For example, a driver who hits the steering wheel (blunt trauma) will have a large cavity in his or her anterior chest at the time of impact; however, the chest rapidly returns to, or near to, its original shape as he or she rebounds from the steering wheel. If two prehospital care providers examine the patient separately—one who understands kinematics and another who does not—the one without knowledge of kinematics will be concerned only with the bruise visible on the patient's chest. The prehospital care provider who understands kinematics will recognize that a large cavity was present at the time of impact; that the ribs had to bend in for the cavity to form; and that the heart, lungs, and great vessels were compressed by the formation of the cavity. Therefore the knowledgeable provider will suspect injuries to the heart, lungs, great vessels, and chest wall. The other prehospital care provider will not even be aware of these possibilities.

The knowledgeable prehospital care provider will assess the injuries, manage the patient, and initiate transport more aggressively, suspecting serious intrathoracic injuries, rather than reacting to what otherwise appears to be only a minor closed, soft tissue injury. Early identification, adequate understanding, and appropriate treatment of underlying injury will significantly influence whether a patient lives or dies.

Summary

Integrating the principles of the kinematics of trauma into assessment of the trauma patient is the key to discovering otherwise unnoticed and unsuspected injuries. Left unsuspected, undetected, and therefore untreated, these injuries contribute significantly to morbidity and mortality resulting from trauma. A thorough comprehension of the kinematics of trauma is also significant in the prehospital care provider's emerging role in injury prevention. To apply the kinematics of trauma, one must consider both the physics of energy and the effect of the energy of motion on the structures of the body.

Energy cannot be created or destroyed, only changed in form. The kinetic energy of an object, expressed as a function of velocity (speed) and mass (weight), is trans-

ferred to another object on contact. Damage to the object or body tissue impacted is not only a function of the amount of kinetic energy applied to it, but also a function of its ability to tolerate the forces applied to it. The prehospital care provider's knowledge of body structure, combined with clues about the types of forces and amount of energy involved, have a significant predictive value for injuries sustained. The prehospital care provider is in a unique position to observe clues that are not available to hospital personnel.

In applying a critical thinking process to relate kinetic energy to the potential for injury, the prehospital care provider can ask the following questions to interpret and guide the search for clues:

What mechanism of trauma is involved? Is it an impact, blast, fall, or penetrating trauma?

The prehospital care provider can ask the following questions for mechanisms that involve impact, including MVCs, sports injuries, and assaults:

- What type of impact occurred—frontal, lateral, rear, rotational, rollover, or angular?
- Was the victim ejected?
- How many impacts occurred? For example, was an ejected victim then struck by another vehicle? Was the victim of an assault struck multiple times?
- What speeds were involved?
- What was the stopping distance (or time)?
- Was the victim using appropriate protective devices and using them correctly (e.g., seat belts, air bags, helmets, body armor)?
- In field triage, which victims are most likely to have been more severely injured?
- What part or parts of the body impacted another object? For example, was there an up-and-over path that caused the head or chest to impact the vehicle interior? Was the victim of an assault struck with a club, pipe, fists, or other weapon?
- Is the victim an adult or child? How will the pattern of injury vary?

The prehospital care provider can ask the following questions for mechanisms involving falls:

- How far did the victim fall? How does that distance relate to the patient's height?

- On what type of surface did the victim land?
- Did the victim sustain multiple impacts caused by objects in the path of the fall?
- Which part of the victim's body made the initial impact on landing?

The prehospital care provider can ask the following questions for mechanisms involving blasts:

- How close was the victim to the explosion?
- What primary, secondary, and tertiary phase injuries should be suspected?

The prehospital care provider can ask the following questions for penetrating trauma:

- What was the size and gender of the assailant?
- What type of weapon was used?
- What was the angle of injury?
- If a gun was used, is there an indication of the velocity and type of projectile?
- What was the range?

Upon compiling this information, the prehospital care provider must determine the pattern of injury that is likely to have occurred.

Through the use of this knowledge, a prehospital care provider can impact the incidence, morbidity, and mortality rates caused by injuries.

Scenario Solution

When the paramedics reach Matt, he is moaning and has a decreased level of consciousness. He is breathing about 10 times a minute. Based on the mechanism of injury and the findings of their primary survey (initial assessment), the paramedics call a trauma alert, requesting a helicopter for transport, and decide to perform a rapid extrication. The paramedics administer oxygen to Matt at 15 L/min via a nonrebreathing mask and secure him to a longboard with a cervical collar and head blocks in place. As the helicopter approaches, the paramedics start two large bore IVs of normal saline. The flight crew's assessment reveals that Matt has a blood pressure of 80 mm Hg by palpation and a heart rate of 126 beats/min. His ventilatory rate is still 10 breaths/min. The flight crew makes the decision to intubate Matt on the scene. On arrival at the trauma center, the flight crew transfers Matt's care to the trauma team, which begins its assessment and treatment. A bedside ultrasound reveals the presence of blood in the abdominal cavity, and Matt is taken directly to surgery. During the surgery it is discovered that Matt has severely damaged his spleen and left kidney. After 4 hours of surgery Matt is delivered to the intensive care unit. Matt spends 3 days in intensive care and is released from the hospital 6 days after his accident. Matt is seen once a week in the trauma clinic over the next month and experiences an uneventful recovery.

Review Questions

Answers are provided on p. 414.

1. Which of the following events is explained by Newton's first law of motion?
   a. When the tires of a vehicle lock up on braking, the kinetic energy is converted to thermal energy
   b. A projectile entering the body creates both a temporary and a permanent cavity
   c. When a vehicle in a frontal collision comes to a sudden stop, an unrestrained occupant continues moving forward until he or she strikes the vehicle's interior
   d. Penetrating trauma occurs when force is applied to the body in a concentrated area

2. While looking for clues to the kinematics involved at the scene of a frontal vehicle collision, you note that the driver's side of the windshield is "starred." The unrestrained driver was the sole occupant of the vehicle. In addition to a head injury, which of the following injury patterns is most likely to have occurred?
   a. Cervical spine, chest, and abdominal injuries
   b. Chest, abdominal, pelvic, and knee injuries
   c. Thoracic spine, knee, and ankle injuries
   d. Shoulder, cervical spine, and pelvic injuries

3. Which of the following patterns of injury is most likely to occur in the primary phase of an explosion?
   a. Burns, lacerations
   b. Ruptured small bowel, tension pneumothorax
   c. Extremity fractures, cervical spine trauma
   d. Contusions, liver injury

4. The role of air bags is to:
   a. Protect the occupant from ejection
   b. Slow the occupant's rate of deceleration
   c. Accelerate the occupant away from the point of impact
   d. Obstruct the occupant's view of the impact

5. A large sedan traveling at 70 mph (112 km/hr) on the interstate strikes a compact car disabled in the breakdown lane. Which of the following factors is most significant in the severity of injury to the driver of the sedan?
   a. Size of the sedan
   b. Size of the compact car
   c. Speed of the compact car
   d. Speed of the sedan

6. Which of the following factors is LEAST important in determining the path of injury caused by a gunshot?
   a. Shooter's gender
   b. Range from which the bullet was fired
   c. Velocity of the projectile
   d. Fragmentation of the projectile

7. The injury pattern of diaphragmatic rupture; injuries to the spleen, liver, and pancreas; and lumbar spine fracture is best accounted for by the improper placement of which of the following devices in relation to the occupant?
   a. Air bag
   b. Diagonal shoulder strap
   c. Lap belt
   d. Child restraint harness

8. The phenomenon of temporary cavitation can best be described by comparing it to which of the following?
   a. Punching a foam pillow
   b. A cue ball striking the racked balls at the other end of the pool table
   c. Breaking a window with a baseball
   d. Hitting the hood of a vehicle with a large rock

9. Which of the following is NOT true concerning abdominal injuries?
   a. Laceration of the liver may be caused by blunt trauma
   b. Perforation of the intestines may occur with either blunt or penetrating trauma
   c. Abdominal organ injury may occur without penetrating injury or direct impact to the abdomen
   d. Abdominal organ injury only occurs with penetrating trauma and direct impact to the abdomen

10. Upon inspecting a vehicle involved in a frontal collision, the prehospital care provider notes that the dashboard on the driver's side is broken. The prehospital care provider should be suspicious that the victim has sustained which of the following injuries?
   a. Posterior hip dislocation
   b. Knee dislocation
   c. Popliteal artery injury
   d. All of the above

REFERENCES

Alderman B, Anderson A: Possible effect of airbag inflation on a standing child. Proceedings of 18th American Association of Automotive Medicine, September 1974, pp. 15-29.

American College of Surgeons Committee on Trauma: *Advanced Trauma Life Support course*, Chicago, 2002, American College of Surgeons.

Anderson PA, Henley MB, Rivara P, Maier RV: Flexion distraction and chance injuries to the thoracolumbar spine, *J Orthop Trauma* 5(2):153, 1991.

Anderson PA, Rivara FP, Maier RV, Drake C: The epidemiology of seatbelt-associated injuries, *J Trauma* 31(1):60, 1991.

Fackler ML, Surinchak JS, Malinowski JA, Bowen RE: Bullet fragmentation: a major cause of tissue disruption, *J Trauma* 24:35, 1984.

Fackler ML, Surinchak JS, Malinowski JA, Bowen RE: Wounding potential of the Russian AK-47 assault rifle, *J Trauma* 24:263, 1984.

Garrett JW, Braunstein PW: The seat belt syndrome, *J Trauma* 2:220, 1962.

Huelke DF, Mackay GM, Morris A: Vertebral column injuries and lab-shoulder belts, *J Trauma* 38:547, 1995.

Huelke DF, Moore JL, Ostrom M: Air bag injuries and occupant protection, *J Trauma* 33(6):894, 1992.

McSwain NE Jr: Kinematics. In Mattox KL, Feliciano DV, Moore EE, editors: *Trauma*, ed 4, New York, 1999, McGraw Hill.

McSwain NE Jr, Brent CR: Trauma rounds: lipstick sign, *Emerg Med* 21:46, 1989.

National Safety Council: *Accident facts 1994*, Chicago, 1994, NSC.

Oreskovich MR, Howard JD, Compass MK et al: Geriatric trauma: injury patterns and outcome, *J Trauma* 24:565, 1984.

Rutledge R, Thomason M, Oller D et al: The spectrum of abdominal injuries associated with the use of seat belts, *J Trauma* 31(6):820, 1991.

States JD, Annechiarico RP, Good RG et al: A time comparison study of the New York State Safety Belt Use Law utilizing hospital admission and police accident report information, *Accid Anal Prev* 22(6):509, 1990.

Swierzewski MJ, Feliciano DV, Lillis RP et al: Deaths from motor vehicle crashes: patterns of injury in restrained and unrestrained victims, *J Trauma* 37(3):404, 1994.

Sykes LN, Champion HR, Fouty WJ: Dum dums, hollowpoints, and devastators: techniques designed to increase wounding potential of bullets, *J Trauma* 28:618, 1988.

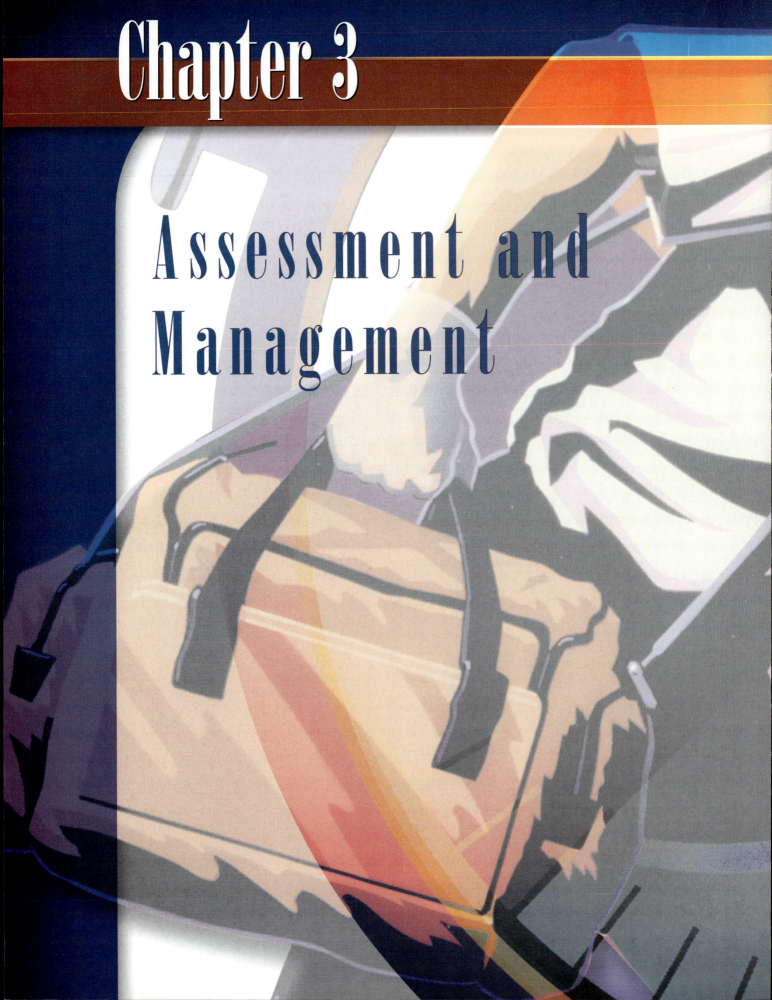

Chapter 3

Assessment and Management

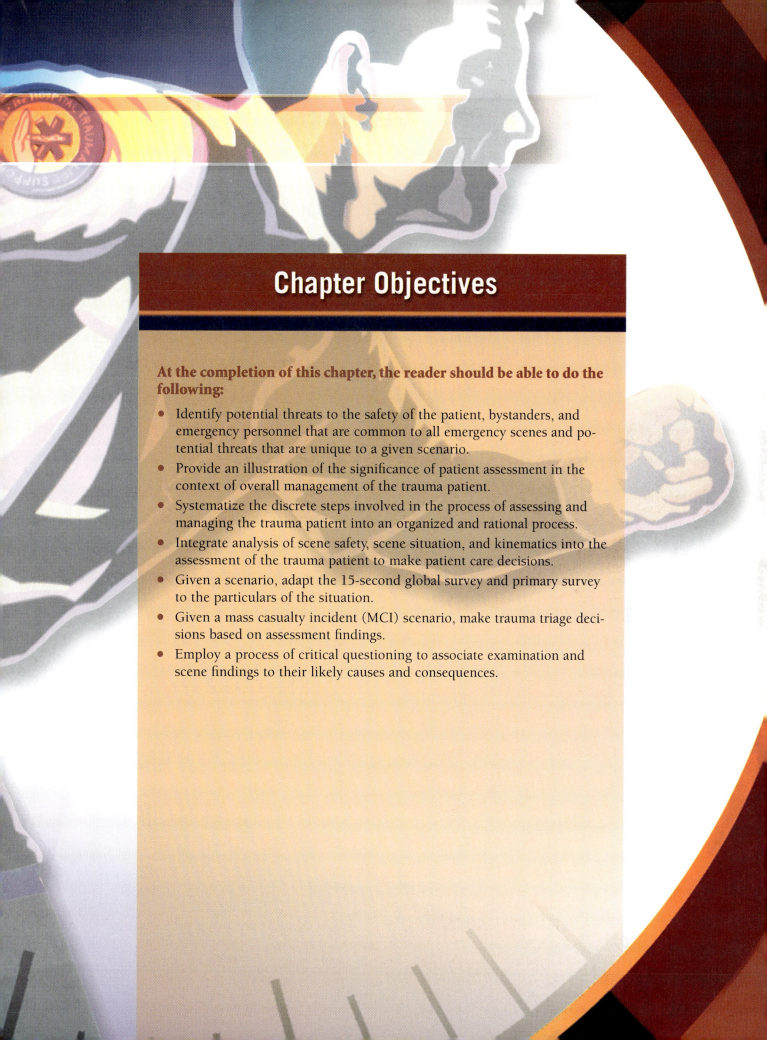

Chapter Objectives

At the completion of this chapter, the reader should be able to do the following:

- Identify potential threats to the safety of the patient, bystanders, and emergency personnel that are common to all emergency scenes and potential threats that are unique to a given scenario.
- Provide an illustration of the significance of patient assessment in the context of overall management of the trauma patient.
- Systematize the discrete steps involved in the process of assessing and managing the trauma patient into an organized and rational process.
- Integrate analysis of scene safety, scene situation, and kinematics into the assessment of the trauma patient to make patient care decisions.
- Given a scenario, adapt the 15-second global survey and primary survey to the particulars of the situation.
- Given a mass casualty incident (MCI) scenario, make trauma triage decisions based on assessment findings.
- Employ a process of critical questioning to associate examination and scene findings to their likely causes and consequences.

Scenario

You are awakened at 4:00 AM on a Saturday to respond to the scene of a person struck by a vehicle. As you get into the ambulance, you notice that it is raining. The temperature is 50° F (10° C). Additional information from dispatch tells you that after hitting the pedestrian, the vehicle crashed into a utility pole. Fluid from the vehicle is leaking onto the street, leaving a sheet on the rain water. Dispatch provides you with the additional information that bystanders report that the patient lost consciousness. On arrival, you detect no additional threats to safety in your scene assessment. Bystanders confirm that they witnessed the patient's loss of consciousness for a period of "several minutes." Approaching the patient, a young adult female, you kneel at her head, observing that she is conscious and her clothes are wet, and you position your hands to provide cervical spine stabilization. In response to your questioning, you discover that the patient's chief complaint is leg pain. Your questioning serves the dual purposes of obtaining the patient's complaint and assessing her ventilatory effort by noting that speech is difficult only because of her chattering teeth. Detecting no shortness of breath, you proceed with further questioning as your partner obtains the patient's vital signs. The patient answers your questions appropriately to establish that she is oriented to person, place, and event.

What have you determined from the patient and scene? Based on kinematics as they relate to pedestrian versus motor vehicle injuries, what are the problems for which you should maintain a high index of suspicion in your assessment? What are your next priorities? How will you proceed with this patient?

Assessment is the cornerstone of excellent patient care. For the trauma patient, as for other critically ill patients, assessment is the foundation upon which all management and transportation decisions are based. The first goal in assessment is to determine a patient's current condition. In doing so, the prehospital care provider can develop an overall impression of a patient's condition and establish baseline values for the status of the patient's respiratory, circulatory, and neurologic systems. The prehospital care provider then rapidly assesses life-threatening conditions and initiates urgent intervention and resuscitation. The prehospital care provider identifies and addresses any conditions that require attention before a patient is moved. If time allows, the prehospital care provider conducts a secondary survey of non–life-or-limb-threatening injuries. Often this occurs during transportation of the patient.

The prehospital care provider performs all of these steps quickly and efficiently, with a goal of minimizing time spent on the scene. Critical patients cannot remain in the field for care other than that needed to stabilize them for transport, unless they are trapped or other complications exist that prevent early transportation. By applying the principles learned in this course, a prehospital care provider can minimize on-scene delay and rapidly move patients to an appropriate medical facility. Successful assessment and intervention require a strong knowledge base of trauma physiology and a well-thought-out plan of management that is carried out quickly and effectively.

The trauma management literature frequently mentions the need to get the trauma patient to definitive surgical care within an absolute minimum amount of time after the onset of the injury. This is because a critical trauma patient who does not respond to initial therapy is most likely bleeding internally. This blood loss will continue until the hemorrhage can be controlled. Except in the instance of the most basic external bleeding, this hemorrhage control can only be accomplished in the operating room (OR).

The following are the primary concerns for assessment and management of the trauma patient in order of importance: (1) airway, (2) ventilation, (3) oxygenation, (4) hemorrhage control, and (5) perfusion. This sequence protects the ability of the body to oxygenate and the ability of the red blood cells (RBCs) to deliver oxygen to the tissues. Hemorrhage control, which is only temporary in the field but permanent in the OR, depends on rapid transportation by the prehospital care providers and the presence of a trauma team that is immediately available upon arrival at the medical facility.

R Adams Cowley, M.D., developed the concept of the "Golden Hour" of trauma. He believed that the time between injury occurrence and definitive care was critical. During this period, when bleeding is uncontrolled and inadequate tissue oxygenation is occurring because of decreased perfusion, damage occurs throughout the body. If bleeding is not controlled and tissue oxygenation is not restored within 1 hour of the injury, the patient's chances of survival plummet.

The Golden Hour is now referred to as the "Golden Period" because some patients have less than an hour to receive care whereas others have more time. A prehospital care provider is responsible for transporting a patient as quickly as possible to a facility where definitive care can be accomplished. To get the trauma patient to definitive care, the prehospital care provider must quickly identify the seriousness of the patient's life-threatening injuries; provide only essential, lifesaving care at the scene; and provide for rapid transportation to an appropriate medical facility. In many urban prehospital systems, the average time between injury and arrival on the scene is 8 to 9 minutes. The prehospital care providers spend another 8 to 9 minutes transporting the patient. If the prehospital care providers spend only 10 minutes on the scene, 30 minutes of the Golden Period will have passed by the time a patient arrives at the receiving facility. Every additional minute spent on the scene is additional time that the patient is bleeding, and valuable time is taken away from the Golden Period. To address this critical trauma management issue, quick, efficient evaluation and management of the patient is the ultimate objective. Scene time should not exceed 10 minutes; the shorter the scene time the better. The longer the patient is kept on scene, the greater the potential for blood loss and death. These time parameters change as delayed extrication, delayed transportation, and other unexpected circumstances arise.

This chapter covers the essentials of patient assessment and initial management in the field. The principles described are identical to those learned in initial basic or advanced provider training programs, although different terminology may occasionally be used. For example, the phrase "primary survey" is used in the Advanced Trauma Life Support (ATLS) and PHTLS programs to describe the patient assessment activity known as "initial assessment" in a U.S. Department of Transportation (DOT) EMT course. What the PHTLS course refers to as the "secondary survey" is essentially the same activity that the basic provider learns as the "focused history and physical examination" of the trauma patient. For the most part, the activities performed in each phase are ex-

Table 3-1 Assessment Terminology	
PHTLS	**EMT national standard curricula**
Scene assessment	Scene size-up
Primary survey	Initial assessment
Secondary survey	Focused history and physical examination
Monitoring and reassessment	Ongoing assessment

actly the same; the various courses simply use different terminology. See Table 3-1 for a comparison of the assessment terminology used in the PHTLS program and the U.S. DOT EMT national standard curricula.

Establishing Priorities

The prehospital care provider has three priorities upon arrival to a scene:

1. Although the prehospital care providers must reach the patients quickly, the first priority for everyone involved at a trauma incident is assessment of the scene. *Scene assessment* involves establishing that the scene is safe and carefully considering the exact nature of the situation. The prehospital care provider may assess the scene safety and situation as he or she approaches the patient; however, the issues identified in this evaluation must be addressed before beginning assessment of individual patients. Although scene assessment is discussed only briefly in this chapter, this should not lead the prehospital care provider to underestimate the importance of this essential aspect of prehospital trauma care.

2. Once the prehospital care providers have performed a brief scene assessment, they should turn their attention to evaluating individual patients. They should begin assessment and management of the patient or patients who have been identified as most critical, as resources allow. Emphasis should be placed on the following in this order: (a) conditions that may result in the loss of life, (b) conditions that may result in the loss of limb, and (c) all other conditions that do not threaten life or limb. Depending on the severity of the injury, the number of injured patients, and the proximity to the receiving facility, the prehospital

care provider may never address the conditions that do not threaten life or limb. Most of this chapter focuses on the *critical thinking* skills required for prehospital care providers to learn to conduct a proper assessment, interpret the findings, and set priorities for proper patient care.

3. The prehospital care provider must recognize the existence of multiple patient incidents and mass casualty incidents (MCIs). In an MCI, the priority shifts from focusing all resources on the most injured patient to saving the maximum number of patients (providing the greatest good to the greatest number). The final part of this chapter addresses these situations and reviews principles of triage.

Scene Assessment (Scene Size-Up)

As all prehospital personnel learn in their initial training courses, patient assessment starts long before arriving at the patient's side. Dispatch begins the process by providing the prehospital care provider with initial information about the incident and the patient, based on bystander reports or information provided by other units first on the scene. Immediately upon arrival a prehospital care provider begins the on-scene information-gathering process by evaluating the scene, observing family members and bystanders, and obtaining a general impression of the scene, all before making contact with the patient.

The scene's appearance creates an impression that influences a prehospital care provider's entire assessment. Correct evaluation of the scene is crucial. The prehospital care provider gathers a wealth of information by simply watching, listening, and cataloging as much information as possible from the environment. The scene often provides information about mechanisms of injury, the preevent situation, and the overall degree of safety.

Scene assessment includes two components:

1. *Safety.* The primary consideration when approaching any scene is the safety of the rescuers. A prehospital care provider should not attempt a rescue unless he or she is trained to do so. A prehospital care provider should not become a victim because he or she will no longer be able to assist other injured people; therefore he or she simply adds to the number of patients and decreases the number of care providers. If the scene is unsafe, the prehospital care provider should stand clear until appropriate personnel have secured the scene.

Scene safety is not just about rescuer safety; patient safety is also of fundamental importance. The prehospital care provider must move any patient in a hazardous situation to a safe area before assessment and treatment can begin. The prehospital care provider evaluates the scene for all possible dangers to ensure that none still exist for either the rescuers or the patient. Threats to patient or rescuer safety may include fire; downed electrical lines; explosives; hazardous materials, including blood or body fluid; traffic; floodwater; weapons (e.g., guns, knives, etc.); or environmental conditions. The prehospital care provider must determine whether family members or other bystanders who are present at the scene may have been the assailant who injured the victim and remain a potential risk to the patient or rescuer.

2. *Situation.* The prehospital care provider should consider several questions to aid in the assessment of the scene situation. What really happened here? Why was help summoned? What was the mechanism of injury (kinematics), and what forces and energies led to the victims' injuries? (See Chapter 2 for a detailed description of kinematics.) How many people are involved, and what are their ages? Are additional EMS units needed for treatment or transport? Is mutual aid needed? Are any other personnel or resources needed, such as from law enforcement, the fire department, or the power company? Is special extrication or rescue equipment needed? Is helicopter transport necessary? Is a physician needed to assist with triage? Could a medical problem be the instigating factor that led to the trauma (e.g., a vehicle crash that resulted from the driver's heart attack)?

Standard Precautions

Another issue within the realm of safety is protection of the prehospital care provider from communicable disease. If a prehospital care provider contracts a disease or condition from a patient, it may prevent him or her from caring for other patients. All health care personnel, including prehospital care providers, are expected to follow standard precautions when interacting with patients. Standard precautions were developed to prevent health care providers from direct contact with patient body substances (e.g., blood, saliva, vomit). The Occupational Safety and Health Administration (OSHA) has developed regulations that mandate employers and their employees to follow standard precautions in the workplace. Items that are included in standard precautions are gloves, gowns, masks, and goggles or clear glasses (for eye protection). Because trauma patients often have external hemorrhage and because blood is an extremely high-risk body fluid, prehospital care providers should wear protective devices as deemed appropriate (as determined by the risk) while tending to patients. Prehospital care providers should follow local regulations or specific employer protocols.

In addition to standard precautions, prehospital care providers should be extremely careful when handling sharp devices (e.g., needles, scalpels, etc.) that are contaminated with a patient's blood or body fluid. Whenever possible, prehospital care providers should have access to devices with built-in protective features.

Primary Survey (Initial Assessment)

In the critical multisystem trauma patient, the priority for the prehospital care provider is the rapid identification and management of life-threatening conditions. More than 90% of trauma patients have simple injuries that involve only one system (e.g., an isolated limb fracture). For these patients, the prehospital care provider has time to be thorough in both the primary and secondary surveys. For the critically injured patient, the prehospital care provider may never conduct more than a primary survey. The emphasis is on rapid evaluation, initiation of resuscitation, and transportation to an appropriate medical facility. This does not eliminate the need for prehospital management; it means that the prehospital care provider must *do it faster, do it more efficiently, and do it en route to the receiving facility.*

Quick establishment of priorities and the initial evaluation of life-threatening injuries must be routine. Therefore the prehospital care provider must memorize the components of the primary and secondary surveys by understanding the logical progression of priority-based assessment and treatment. A prehospital care provider must think about the pathophysiology of a patient's injuries and conditions—he or she cannot waste time trying to remember which priorities are the most important.

The most common basis of life-threatening injuries is lack of adequate tissue oxygenation, which leads to anaerobic (without oxygen) metabolism (energy production). Decreased energy production that occurs with anaerobic metabolism is termed *shock.* Three components are necessary for normal metabolism: (1) oxygenation of the red blood cells (RBCs) in the lung; (2) delivery of RBCs to the cells throughout the body; and (3) off-loading of oxygen to these cells. The activities involved in the primary survey are aimed at identifying and correcting problems with the first two components.

General Impression

The primary survey begins with a simultaneous, or global, overview of the status of a patient's respiratory, circulatory, and neurologic systems to identify obvious significant external problems with oxygenation, circulation, hemorrhage, or gross deformities. When approaching a patient, the prehospital care provider observes whether the patient appears to be moving air effectively, is awake or unresponsive, is holding himself or herself up, and is moving spontaneously. Once at the patient's side, a quick check of the radial pulse allows the prehospital care provider to evaluate the presence, quality, and rate (very fast, very slow, or generally normal) of circulatory activity. The prehospital care provider can simultaneously feel the temperature and moistness of the skin and ask the patient "what happened." The patient's verbal response indicates the overall status of the airway, whether ventilation is normal or labored, and approximately how much air is being moved with each breath. The prehospital care provider can determine the patient's level of consciousness (LOC) and mentation (if the patient responds verbally), the urgency of the situation, and perhaps how many people were involved in the incident. "Where do you hurt?" is a follow-up question that the prehospital care provider can ask while checking the patient's skin color and capillary refilling time. The answer will indicate whether the patient can localize the pain and may help identify the most likely points of injury. The prehospital care provider then scans the patient from head to foot, looking for signs of hemorrhage while gathering all the preliminary data for the primary survey. During this time, the prehospital care provider has taken a quick overall look at the patient, making the first few seconds with the patient a global survey of overall condition and an evaluation of life-threatening possibilities. The prehospital care provider can classify the information according to priorities, categorize the severity of the patient's injuries and condition, and identify which injury or condition needs to be managed first. Within 15 to 30 seconds, the prehospital care provider has gained a general impression of the patient's overall condition.

The general impression establishes whether the patient is presently or imminently in a critical condition and rapidly evaluates the patient's overall systemic condition. The general impression often provides all the information necessary to determine whether additional resources, such as advanced life support (ALS), are required. If helicopter transportation to a trauma facility is appropriate, this is often when the prehospital care provider decides to request the helicopter. Delay in deciding that additional resources are necessary will only extend on-scene time. Early decision-making will ultimately shorten scene time. Once the prehospital care provider gains a general impression of the patient's condition, he or she can rapidly complete the primary survey unless a complication requires more care or evaluation.

The primary survey must proceed rapidly. The following discussion addresses the specific components of the primary survey and the order of priority for optimal patient management.

The following are the five steps involved in the primary survey in order of priority:

A—Airway management and cervical spine stabilization
B—Breathing (ventilation)
C—Circulation and bleeding
D—Disability
E—Expose/Environment

Step A—Airway Management and Cervical Spine Stabilization

AIRWAY

The prehospital care provider should check the patient's airway quickly to ensure that it is patent (open and clear) and that no danger of obstruction exists. If the airway is compromised, the prehospital care provider will have to open it initially using manual methods (trauma chin lift or trauma jaw thrust) and clear blood and body substances if necessary (Figure 3-1). Eventually, as equipment and time become available, airway management can advance to mechanical means (oral airway, nasal airway, or endotracheal intubation) or to transtracheal methods (percutaneous transtracheal ventilation). (See Chapter 4.)

CERVICAL SPINE STABILIZATION

As a prehospital care provider learns in an initial training program, every trauma patient with a significant mechanism of injury is suspected of spinal injury until spinal injury is conclusively ruled out. (See Chapter 9 for a complete list of indications for spinal immobilization.) Therefore when establishing an open airway, the prehospital care provider must remember that a possibility of a cervical spine injury exists. Excessive movement could either aggravate or produce neurologic

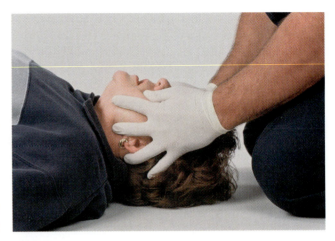

Figure 3-1 If the airway appears compromised, it must be opened while continuing to protect the spine.

damage because bony compression may occur in the presence of a fractured spine. The solution is to ensure that the patient's neck is manually maintained in the neutral position during the opening of the airway and the administration of necessary ventilation. This does not mean that the prehospital care provider cannot or should not apply the necessary airway maintenance procedures just described. Instead, it means that he or she must perform the procedures while protecting the patient's spine from unnecessary movement. When the prehospital care provider has initiated precautions for cervical injury, he or she must immobilize the patient's entire spine. Therefore the patient's entire body must be in line and secured.

Step B—Breathing (Ventilation)

The prehospital care provider must first effectively deliver oxygen to a patient's lungs to initiate the metabolic process. Hypoxia can result from inadequate ventilation of the lungs and lack of oxygenation of the patient's tissues. Once the patient's airway is open, the quality and quantity of the patient's breathing (ventilation) can be evaluated. The prehospital care provider must then do the following:

1. Check to see if the patient is breathing.
2. If the patient is not breathing (apneic), immediately begin assisting ventilations with a bag-valve-mask (BVM) device with supplemental oxygen before continuing the assessment.
3. Ensure that the patient's airway is patent, continue assisted ventilation and prepare to insert an oral or nasal airway, intubate, or provide other means of mechanical airway protection.

Although commonly referred to as the *respiratory rate*, a more correct term is *ventilatory rate*. *Ventilation* refers to the process of inhalation and exhalation, whereas *respiration* best describes the physiologic process of gas exchange between the arteries and the alveoli. This text uses the term *ventilatory rate* rather than *respiratory rate*.

4. If the patient is breathing, estimate the adequacy of the ventilatory rate and depth to determine whether the patient is moving enough air and assess oxygenation. Ensure that the inspired oxygen concentration is 85% or greater.
5. Quickly observe the patient's chest rise, and if the patient is conscious, listen to the patient talk to assess whether he or she can speak a full sentence without difficulty.

Table 3-2   Airway Management Based on Spontaneous Ventilation Rate

Ventilatory rate (breaths/min)	Management
Slow (<12)	Assisted or total ventilation with ≥85% oxygen (FiO_2 ≥0.85)
Normal (12-20)	Observation; consider supplemental oxygen
Too Fast (20-30)	Administration of ≥85% oxygen (FiO_2 ≥0.85)
Abnormally Fast (>30)	Assisted ventilation (FiO_2 ≥0.85)

The ventilatory rate can be divided into five levels:

1. *Apneic.* The patient is not breathing.
2. *Slow.* A very low ventilatory rate may indicate ischemia (decreased supply of oxygen) of the brain. If the ventilatory rate has dropped to 12 breaths/min or less (*bradypnea*), the prehospital care provider must either assist or completely take over the patient's breathing with a BVM device. Assisted or total ventilatory support with the BVM device should include supplemental oxygen that achieves an oxygen concentration of 85% or greater (FiO_2 of 0.85 or greater) (Table 3-2).
3. *Normal.* If the ventilatory rate is between 12 and 20 breaths/min (*eupnea*, a normal rate for an adult), the prehospital care provider should watch the patient closely. Although the patient may appear stable, supplemental oxygen should be considered.
4. *Fast.* If the ventilatory rate is between 20 and 30 breaths/min (*tachypnea*), the prehospital care provider should also watch the patient closely. He or she should determine whether the patient is improving or deteriorating. The drive for increasing the ventilatory rate is increased accumulation of carbon dioxide (CO_2) in the blood or a decreased level of blood oxygen (O_2). When a patient displays an abnormal ventilatory rate, the provider should investigate why. A rapid rate indicates that not enough oxygen is reaching the body tissue. This lack of oxygen initiates anaerobic metabolism (see Chapter 6) and ultimately an increase in CO_2. The body's detection system rec-

ognizes an increased level of CO_2 and tells the ventilatory system to speed up to exhale this excess. Therefore an increased ventilatory rate may indicate that the patient needs better perfusion or oxygenation or both. Administration of supplemental oxygen to achieve an oxygen concentration of 85% or greater (an FiO_2 of 0.85 or greater) is indicated for this patient, at least until the overall status of the patient is determined. The provider should be suspicious of the patient's ability to maintain adequate ventilation and should remain alert for any deterioration in overall condition.
5. *Abnormally fast.* A ventilatory rate above 30 breaths/min (*severe tachypnea*) indicates hypoxia, anaerobic metabolism, or both with a resultant acidosis. The prehospital care provider should immediately begin assisted ventilation with a BVM device with supplemental oxygen that achieves an oxygen concentration of 85% or greater (an FiO_2 of 0.85 or greater). A search for the cause of the rapid ventilatory rate should begin at once. Is this an oxygenation problem or an RBC delivery problem? Once the cause is identified, the prehospital care provider should intervene immediately.

With abnormal ventilation, the prehospital care provider should expose, observe, and palpate the chest rapidly. He or she should auscultate the lungs to identify abnormal, diminished, or absent breath sounds. Injuries that may impede ventilation include tension pneumothorax, spinal cord injuries, or traumatic brain injuries. These injuries should be identified during the primary survey and required ventilatory support initiated at once.

When assessing the trauma patient's ventilatory status, the prehospital care provider must assess the ventilatory depth as well as the rate. A patient can be breathing at a normal ventilatory rate of 16 breaths/min but have a greatly decreased ventilatory depth. Conversely, a patient can have a normal ventilatory depth but an increased or decreased ventilatory rate. The ventilatory depth and rate combine to produce the total minute ventilation of the patient (see Chapter 4).

Step C—Circulation and Bleeding

Assessing for circulatory system compromise or failure is the next step in caring for the trauma patient. Oxygenation of the RBCs without delivery to the tissue cells is of no benefit to the patient. In the primary survey of a trauma patient, the prehospital care provider must identify and control external hemorrhage. The prehospital care provider can then obtain an adequate overall estimate of the cardiac output and perfusion status.

HEMORRHAGE CONTROL

The prehospital care provider must identify and control external hemorrhage in the primary survey. Hemorrhage control is included in circulation because if gross bleeding is not controlled as soon as possible, the potential for the patient's death increases dramatically. The three types of external hemorrhage are as follows:

1. *Capillary bleeding* is caused by abrasions that have scraped open the tiny capillaries just below the skin's surface. Usually capillary bleeding will have slowed or even stopped before the arrival of prehospital care.
2. *Venous bleeding* is from deeper within the tissue and is usually controlled with a small amount of direct pressure. Venous bleeding is usually not life-threatening unless the injury is severe and/or blood loss is not controlled.
3. *Arterial bleeding* is caused by an injury that has lacerated an artery. This is the most important and most difficult type of blood loss to control. It is characterized by spurting blood that is bright red in color. Even a small, deep arterial puncture wound can produce life-threatening arterial blood loss.

The prehospital care provider should control hemorrhage according to the following steps:

1. *Direct pressure.* Direct pressure bleeding control is exactly what the name implies—applying pressure to the site of bleeding. The prehospital care provider

accomplishes this by placing a dressing (such as a 4 × 4 gauze) or abdominal pads directly over the site and applying pressure. Applying direct pressure will require all of one provider's attention, preventing him or her from continuing patient care. However, if bleeding is not controlled, it will not matter how much oxygen or fluid the patient receives. The oxygen and fluid will simply be lost through the wound.
2. *Elevation.* If the prehospital care provider cannot control blood loss with direct pressure, he or she should elevate the extremity. Because of gravity, blood can have a hard time "climbing" up an extremity. Caution must be exercised when elevating an extremity with a suspected fracture or dislocation.
3. *Pressure points.* The prehospital care provider can also control blood loss by applying deep pressure to the artery proximal to the wound. This is an attempt to obstruct blood from flowing to the wound, therefore decreasing the blood lost from the wound, by using manual pressure to occlude the artery. The main pressure points on the body are the brachial artery, which impedes blood flow to the forearm; the axillary artery, for more proximal upper-extremity hemorrhage; the popliteal artery, which impedes blood flow to the leg; and the femoral artery in the groin, for more proximal lower-extremity hemorrhage.
4. *Tourniquets.* The prehospital care provider should only use tourniquets if no other alternative is available and he or she cannot stop the blood loss using other methods. *Use of a tourniquet is a last resort.* Refer to Chapter 16 for combat use of tourniquets.

Hemorrhage control is a priority. Rapid control of blood loss is one of the most important goals in the care of a trauma patient. The primary survey cannot advance unless hemorrhage is controlled.

In cases of external hemorrhage, application of direct pressure will control most major hemorrhage until the prehospital care provider can move the patient to a location where an OR and adequate equipment are available. The prehospital care provider must initiate hemorrhage control and maintain it throughout transport. He or she may require assistance to accomplish both ventilation and bleeding control.

If the prehospital care provider suspects internal hemorrhage, he or she should quickly expose the patient's abdomen to inspect and palpate for signs of injury. The provider should also palpate the pelvis because a pelvic fracture is a major source of intraabdominal bleeding. Pelvic fractures are managed with rapid transport, use of a PASG, and rapid, warm intravenous fluid replacement.

Many causes of hemorrhage are not easy to control outside the hospital. The prehospital treatment is rapid delivery of the patient to a facility equipped and staffed for rapid control of hemorrhage in the OR (e.g., a trauma center, if available).

PERFUSION

The prehospital care provider can obtain the patient's overall circulatory status by checking the pulse; skin color, temperature, and moisture; and capillary refilling time.

Pulse. The prehospital care provider evaluates the pulse for presence, quality, and regularity. The presence of a palpable peripheral pulse also provides a rough estimate of blood pressure. A quick check of the pulse reveals whether the patient has tachycardia, bradycardia, or an irregular rhythm. It can also reveal information about the systolic blood pressure. If a radial pulse is not palpable in an uninjured extremity, the patient has likely entered the decompensated phase of shock, a late sign of the patient's critical condition. In the primary survey, determination of an exact pulse rate is not necessary. Instead, a gross estimate is rapidly obtained and assessment moves on to other gross evaluations. The actual pulse rate is obtained later in the process. If the patient lacks a palpable carotid or femoral pulse, then he or she is in cardiopulmonary arrest (Box 3-1).

Skin
Color. Adequate perfusion produces a pinkish hue to the skin. Skin becomes pale when blood is shunted away from an area. Bluish coloration indicates incomplete oxygenation. Pale coloration is associated with poor perfusion. The bluish color is due to lack of blood or oxygen to that region of the body. Skin pigments can often make this determination difficult. Examination of the color of nail beds and mucous membranes serves to overcome this challenge because these changes in color usually first appear in the lips, gums, or fingertips.

Temperature. As with overall skin evaluation, skin temperature is influenced by environmental conditions. Cool skin indicates decreased perfusion, regardless of the cause. The prehospital care provider usually assesses skin temperature by touching the patient with the back of the hand; therefore an accurate determination can be difficult with gloves donned. Normal skin temperature is warm to touch, neither cool nor extremely hot. Normally the blood vessels are not dilated and do not bring the heat of the body to the surface of the skin.

Moisture. Dry skin indicates good perfusion. Moist skin is associated with shock and decreased perfusion. This decrease in perfusion is due to blood being shunted to the core organs of the body through the vasoconstriction of peripheral vessels.

Capillary Refilling Time. The prehospital care provider checks capillary refilling time by pressing over the nail beds. This removes the blood from the visible capillary bed. The rate of return of blood to the beds (refilling time) is a tool in estimating blood flow through this most distal part of circulation. A capillary refilling time of greater than 2 seconds indicates that the capillary beds are not receiving adequate perfusion. However, capillary refilling time by itself is a poor indicator of shock because it is influenced by so many other factors. For example, peripheral vascular disease (arteriosclerosis), cold temperatures, the use of pharmacologic vasodilators or constrictors, or the presence of neurogenic shock can skew the result. It becomes a less useful check of cardiovascular function in these instances. Capillary refilling time maintains a place in evaluation of circulatory adequacy; however, the prehospital care provider should always use it in conjunction with other physical examination findings (just as one uses other indicators such as blood pressure).

Step D—Disability
Having evaluated and corrected, to the extent possible, the factors involved in delivering oxygen to the lungs and circulating it throughout the body, the next step in the primary survey is assessment of cerebral function, which is an indirect measurement of cerebral oxygenation. The goal is to determine the patient's LOC and ascertain the potential for hypoxia.

The prehospital care provider should consider a belligerent, combative, or uncooperative patient hypoxic until proven otherwise. Most patients want help when their lives are medically threatened. If a patient refuses help, one must question the reason. Why does the patient feel threatened by the presence of a prehospital care provider on the scene? If the patient appears threatened by the situation, the provider should establish rapport and gain the patient's trust. If nothing in the situation seems to be threatening, one must consider that the source is physiological and identify and treat reversible conditions. During the assessment, the

Box 3-1

Traumatic Cardiopulmonary Arrest

Cardiopulmonary arrest resulting from trauma differs from that resulting from medical problems in three significant ways:

1. Most medical cardiac arrests are the result of either a respiratory problem, such as a foreign body airway obstruction, or a cardiac dysrhythmia that EMS personnel may be able to treat fairly easily. Cardiac arrest resulting from injury most often results from exsanguination or, less commonly, a problem incompatible with life, such as a devastating brain or spinal cord injury, and cannot be appropriately resuscitated in the field.

2. Medical arrests are best managed with attempts at stabilization at the scene (e.g., removal of an airway foreign body or defibrillation). In contrast, traumatic cardiopulmonary arrest is best managed with immediate transport to a facility that offers immediate blood and emergent surgery.

3. Because of the differences in etiology and management, patients with traumatic cardiopulmonary arrest in the prehospital setting have an extremely low likelihood of survival. Less than 4% of trauma patients who require cardiopulmonary resuscitation (CPR) in the prehospital setting survive to be discharged from the hospital, with most studies documenting that victims of penetrating trauma have a slightly increased chance of survival over those of blunt trauma. Of the small percentage of patients who are discharged from the hospital alive, many sustain significant neurologic impairment.

In addition to the extremely low survival rate, resuscitation attempts in patients who are extremely unlikely to survive put prehospital care providers at risk from exposure to blood and body fluids and injuries sustained in motor vehicle crashes during transport. Such unsuccessful attempts at resuscitation may divert resources away from patients who are viable and have a greater likelihood of survival. Because of these reasons, the prehospital care provider must exercise judgment regarding the decision to initiate resuscitation attempts for victims of traumatic cardiopulmonary arrest. While specific decisions regarding resuscitation of patients with traumatic cardiopulmonary arrest should be established on a local level, the National Association of EMS Physicians and the American College of Surgeons Committee on Trauma have endorsed the following guidelines:

- For victims of blunt trauma, resuscitation efforts may be withheld if the patient is pulseless and apneic upon arrival of EMS.
- For victims of penetrating trauma, resuscitation efforts may be withheld if there are no signs of life (pupillary reflexes, spontaneous movement, or organized cardiac rhythm on ECG greater than 40 per minute).
- Resuscitation efforts are not indicated when the patient has sustained an obviously fatal injury (such as decapitation) or when evidence exists of dependent lividity, rigor mortis, and decomposition.
- Termination of resuscitation should be considered in trauma patients with an EMS-witnessed cardiopulmonary arrest and 15 minutes of unsuccessful resuscitation and CPR.
- Termination of resuscitation should be considered for patients with traumatic cardiopulmonary arrest that would require transport of greater than 15 minutes to reach an emergency department or trauma center.
- Victims of drowning, lightning strike, or hypothermia, or those in whom the mechanism of injury does not correlate with the clinical situation (suggesting a nontraumatic cause), deserve special consideration before a decision is made to withhold or terminate resuscitation.

---

provider should determine from the history whether the patient lost consciousness at any time since the injury occurred, what toxic substances might be involved, and whether the patient has any preexisting conditions that may produce a decreased LOC or aberrant behavior.

A decreased LOC should alert a prehospital care provider to four possibilities:

1. Decreased cerebral oxygenation (due to hypoxia and/or hypoperfusion)
2. Central nervous system injury
3. Drug or alcohol overdose
4. Metabolic derangement (diabetes, seizure, cardiac arrest)

The Glasgow Coma Scale (GCS) is a tool used for determining LOC. It is a quick, simple method for determining cerebral function and is predictive of patient outcome, especially the best motor response. It also provides a baseline of cerebral function for serial neurologic evaluations. The GCS is divided into three sections: (1) *E*ye opening, (2) best *V*erbal response, and (3) best *M*otor response (EVM). The prehospital care provider assigns the patient a score according to the *best* response to each component of the EVM (Figure 3-2). For example, if a patient's right eye is so severely swollen that the patient cannot open it, but the left eye opens spontaneously, then the patient receives a "4" for the best eye movement. If a patient lacks spontaneous eye opening, the provider should use a verbal command ("Open your eyes!"). If the patient does not respond to a verbal stimulus, a painful stimulus, such as nail bed pressure with a pen or squeezing of the axillary tissue, can be applied.

The prehospital care provider can examine the patient's verbal response using a question such as, "What happened to you?" If the patient is fully oriented, he or she will supply a coherent answer. Otherwise, the patient's verbal response is scored as confused, inappropriate, unintelligible, or absent. If a patient is intubated, the GCS score contains only the eye and motor scales and a "T" is added to note the inability to assess the verbal response, such as "8T".

The third component of the GCS is the motor score. The prehospital care provider should give the patient a simple, unambiguous command, such as "Hold up two fingers!" or "Show me a hitchhiker's sign!" A patient who squeezes or grasps the finger of a provider may simply be demonstrating a grasping reflex and not purposefully following a command. If the patient fails to follow a command, a painful stimulus, as noted previously, should be used and the patient's *best* motor response should be scored. A patient who attempts to push away a painful stimulus is considered to be localizing. Other possible responses to pain include withdrawal from the stimulus, abnormal flexion (decorticate posturing) or extension (decerebrate posturing) of the upper extremities, or absence of motor function.

The maximum GCS score is 15, indicating a patient with no disability, whereas the lowest score of 3 is generally an ominous sign. A score of less than 8 indicates a major injury, 9 to 12 a moderate injury, and 13 to 15 a minor injury. A GCS score of ≤ 8 is an indication for intubating a patient. The prehospital care provider can easily calculate the score and should include it in the verbal report to the receiving facility as well as the patient care record.

If a patient is not awake, oriented, and able to follow commands, the prehospital care provider should assess the pupils quickly. Are the pupils equal and round, reactive to light (PEARRL)? Are the pupils equal to each other? Is each pupil round and of normal appearance, and does it appropriately react to light by constricting, or is it unresponsive and dilated? A GCS score of less than

Eye Opening	Points
Spontaneous eye opening	4
Eye opening on command	3
Eye opening to painful stimulus	2
No eye opening	1
Best Verbal Response	
Answers appropriately (oriented)	5
Gives confused answers	4
Inappropriate response	3
Makes unintelligible noises	2
Makes no verbal response	1
Best Motor Response	
Follows command	6
Localizes painful stimuli	5
Withdrawal to pain	4
Responds with abnormal flexion to painful stimuli (decorticate)	3
Responds with abnormal extension to pain (decerebrate)	2
Gives no motor response	1
Total	

Figure 3-2   Glasgow Coma Scale (GCS).

14 in combination with an abnormal pupil examination can indicate the presence of a life-threatening traumatic brain injury (see Chapter 8).

The prehospital care provider can also describe the patient's LOC using the acronym AVPU, which stands for the following:

A—Alert
V—Responds to verbal stimulus
P—Responds to painful stimulus
U—Unresponsive

Although AVPU is quicker to assess than the GCS, it provides less useful information. Because the GCS is a key assessment performed in the emergency department and throughout a patient's hospital stay, the prehospital care provider should use it in the prehospital setting to provide important baseline information. Although the GCS is more complicated to remember than AVPU, repeated practice will make this crucial assessment second nature.

Step E—Expose/Environment

An early step in the assessment process is to remove a patient's clothes because exposure of the trauma patient is critical to finding all injuries (Figure 3-3). The saying that "the one part of the body that is not exposed

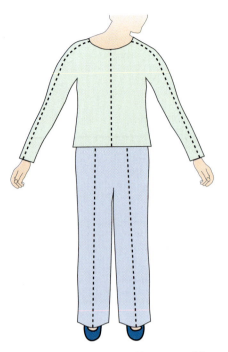

Figure 3-3   Clothing can be quickly removed by cutting as indicated by the dotted lines.

will be the most severely injured part" may not always be true, but it is true often enough to warrant a total body examination. Also, blood can collect in and be absorbed by clothing and thereby go unnoticed. When the prehospital care provider has seen the patient's entire body, he or she should recover the patient to conserve body heat. Although it is important to expose a trauma patient's body to complete an effective assessment, hypothermia is a serious problem in the management of a trauma patient. Only what is necessary should be exposed to the outside environment. Once inside the warm EMS unit, the provider can complete the examination and then recover the patient as quickly as possible.

The amount of the patient's clothing that should be removed during an assessment varies depending on the conditions or injuries found. A general rule is to remove as much clothing as necessary to determine the presence or absence of a condition or injury. The prehospital care provider should not be afraid to remove clothing if it is the only way to properly complete assessment and treatment. On occasion, patients can sustain multiple mechanisms of injury, such as experiencing a motor vehicle crash after having been shot. Potential life-threatening injuries may be missed if the patient is inadequately examined. Injuries cannot be treated if they are not first identified.

Simultaneous Evaluation

In discussing the process of patient assessment, management, and decision-making, the information must be presented in a linear format (i.e., step A followed by step B followed by step C, etc.). Although presentation of information in this manner makes explanation easier and perhaps makes the concepts easier for a student to understand, that is not how the real world functions. The prehospital care provider's brain is like a computer that can receive input from several sources at once (cerebral multitasking). The brain can assess data received simultaneously. The brain is also capable of prioritizing the information from all input sources, sorting them in such a way that orderly decision-making follows.

The brain can gather most data in about 15 seconds. Simultaneous processing of this data and appropriate prioritization of the information by the prehospital care provider identifies the component that he or she must manage first. Although the ABCDE approach described in this chapter may not necessarily be the order in which the prehospital care provider collects or receives the information, it does serve to establish priorities for management.

The primary survey addresses life-threatening conditions. The secondary survey of the patient identifies possible limb-threatening injuries as well as other less significant problems.

Resuscitation

Resuscitation describes treatment steps taken to correct life-threatening problems as identified in the primary survey. PHTLS assessment is based on a "treat as you go" philosophy, wherein treatment is initiated as each threat to life is identified, or at the earliest possible moment.

Limited Scene Intervention

The prehospital care provider manages airway problems as the top priority. If the airway is open but the patient is not breathing, the prehospital care provider initiates ventilatory support. Ventilatory support should include administration of high concentrations of oxygen (oxygen concentration of 85% [an FiO_2 of 0.85] or greater) as early as possible. If the patient is exhibiting signs of ventilatory distress and lowered levels of air exchange, ventilatory assistance is needed by way of a BVM. The provider identifies cardiac arrest during the assessment of circulation and initiates chest

Box 3-2

Critical Trauma Patient

Limit scene time to 10 minutes or less when any of the following life-threatening conditions are present:

- Inadequate or threatened airway
- Impaired ventilation as demonstrated by the following:
  —Abnormally fast or slow ventilatory rate
  —Hypoxia (Spo$_2$ <95 even with supplemental oxygen)
  —Dyspnea
  —Open pneumothorax or flail chest
  —Suspected pneumothorax
- Significant external hemorrhage or suspected internal hemorrhage
- Abnormal neurologic status
  —GCS score ≤13
  —Seizure activity
  —Sensory or motor deficit
- Penetrating trauma to the head, neck, or torso, or proximal to elbow and knee in the extremities
- Amputation or near amputation proximal to the fingers or toes
- Any trauma in the presence of the following:
  —History of serious medical conditions (e.g., coronary artery disease, chronic obstructive pulmonary disease, bleeding disorder)
  —Age >55 years
  —Hypothermia
  —Burns
  —Pregnancy

The prehospital care provider should consider the use of a PASG for the patient with circulatory insufficiency caused by trauma because it is an effective device for restoring the perfusion of the heart, brain, and lungs when a low circular blood volume exists. Some research suggests that a PASG may be particularly useful when the patient's systolic blood pressure is below 60 mm Hg. In addition, application of a PASG may control suspected intraperitoneal, retroperitoneal, or pelvic hemorrhage.

compressions, if appropriate. The provider also controls exsanguinating hemorrhage. In a patient with adequate airway and breathing, the provider should rapidly correct hypoxia and shock (anaerobic metabolism), if present.

Transport

If life-threatening conditions are identified during the primary survey, the patient should be rapidly packaged after initiating limited field intervention. Transport of critically injury trauma patients to the closest appropriate facility should be initiated as soon as possible (Box 3-2). Unless extenuating circumstances exist, the provider should limit the scene time to 10 minutes or less for these patients. The provider must realize that limiting

scene time and initiation of rapid transport to the closest appropriate facility, preferably a trauma center, are fundamental aspects of prehospital trauma resuscitation.

Fluid Therapy

Another important step in resuscitation is the restoration of the cardiovascular system to an adequate perfusing volume as quickly as possible. Because blood is usually not available in the prehospital setting, lactated Ringer's is the preferred solution for trauma resuscitation. In addition to sodium and chloride, lactated Ringer's solution contains small amounts of potassium, calcium, and lactate and is an effective volume expander. Crystalloid solutions, such as lactated Ringer's, do not replace the oxygen-carrying capacity of the lost RBCs or the lost platelets that are necessary for clotting and bleeding control. Therefore rapid transportation of a severely injured patient to an appropriate facility is an absolute necessity.

En route to the receiving facility, the prehospital care provider should place two large-bore (14 or 16 gauge) intravenous catheters in the forearm or antecubital veins, if possible. In general, central intravenous lines (subclavian, internal jugular, or femoral) are not appropriate for the field management of trauma patients. If time and other factors permit, the prehospital care provider should administer 1 to 2 L of warm (if possible) lactated Ringer's solution during transport.

Starting an intravenous line at the scene only prolongs on-scene time and delays transport. As addressed previously in this chapter, the definitive treatment for the trauma patient can only be accomplished in the hospital. For example, a patient with an injury to the spleen who is losing 50 mL of blood per minute will continue to bleed at that rate for each additional minute that delays arrival in the OR. Initiating IVs on the scene in lieu of early transportation will not only increase blood loss, but it may also decrease the patient's chance of survival.

Exceptions exist, such as entrapment, when a patient simply cannot be moved immediately. Also, aggressive and continual volume replacement is not a substitute for manual hemorrhage control.

Basic Provider Level

At the basic provider level, the key steps in resuscitating a critically injured trauma patient include immediate control of major external hemorrhage; rapid packaging of the patient for transportation; and quickly initiated, rapid but safe transport of the patient to the closest appropriate facility. If transportation time is prolonged, it may be appropriate to call for aid from a nearby ALS service that can intercept the basic unit en route. Helicopter evacuation to a trauma center is another option. Both the ALS service and the flight service will allow advanced airway management, ventilatory management, and earlier fluid replacement.

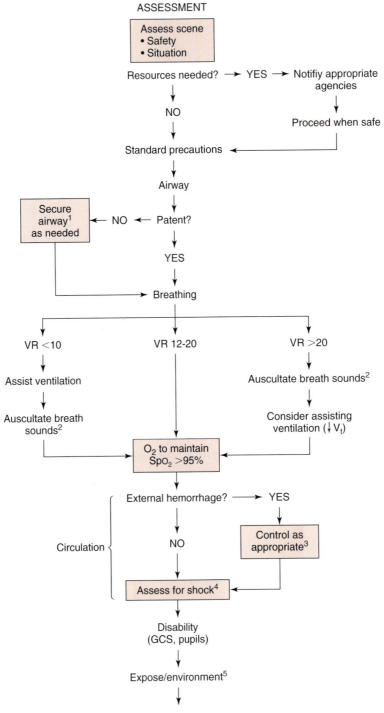

Continued

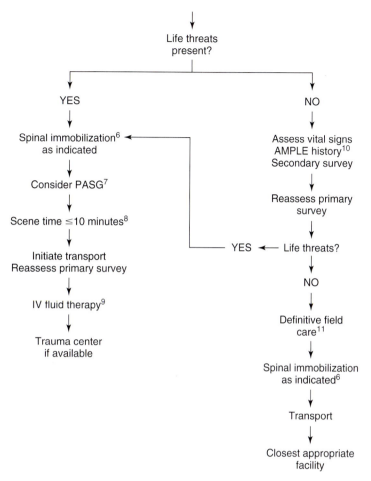

Notes for Assessment Algorithm

[1]Follow Airway Management algorithm.

[2]Consider pleural decompression only if ALL are present:
- Diminished or absent breath sounds
- Increased work of breathing or difficulty ventilating with bag-valve-mask
- Decompensated shock/hypotension (SBP <90 mm Hg)
**Consider bilateral pleural decompression only if patient is intubated.

[3]External hemorrhage control:
- Direct pressure/pressure dressing
- Elevation, unless contraindicated
- Pressure points
- Tourniquet

[4]Shock: tachycardia; cool, diaphoretic, pallorous skin; anxiety; absence of peripheral pulses.

[5]Quick check for other life-threatening conditions; cover patient to preserve body heat.

[6]See Indications for Spinal Immobilization algorithm.

[7]PASG should be considered for: SBP <60 mm Hg; suspected pelvic fracture; suspected intraperitoneal hemorrhage; suspected retroperitoneal hemorrhage with decompensated shock (SBP <90 mm Hg).

[8]Scene time should be limited to 10 minutes or less for patients with life-threatening injuries unless extenuating circumstances exist.

[9]Initiate two large-bore IV lines; administer 1- to 2-liter bolus of LR or NS if shock is present.

[10]AMPLE: allergies, medications, past medical/surgical history, last meal, events leading up to injury.

[11]Splint fractures and dress wounds as needed.

Secondary Survey (Focused History and Physical Examination)

The secondary survey is a head-to-toe evaluation of a patient. The prehospital care provider must complete the primary survey, identify and treat all life-threatening injuries, and initiate resuscitation before beginning the secondary survey. The objective of the secondary survey is to identify injuries or problems that were not identified during the primary survey. Because a well-performed primary survey will identify all life-threatening conditions, the secondary survey, by definition, deals with less serious problems. Therefore the prehospital care provider should transport a critical trauma patient as soon as possible after conclusion of the primary survey and should not hold the patient in the field for either IV initiation or a secondary survey.

The secondary survey uses a "look, listen, and feel" approach to evaluate the skin and everything it contains. Rather than looking at the entire body at one time, returning to listen to all areas, and finally returning to palpate all areas, the prehospital care provider "searches" the body. The prehospital care provider identifies injuries and correlates physical findings region-by-region, beginning at the head and proceeding through the neck, chest, and abdomen to the extremities, concluding with a detailed neurologic examination. The following phrases capture the essence of the entire assessment process:

See, don't just look
Hear, don't just listen
Feel, don't just touch

The definition of the word *see* is "to perceive with the eye" or "to discover," whereas *look* is defined as "to exercise the power of vision." *Listen* is defined as "to monitor without participation," and *hear* is defined as "to listen with attention." While examining the patient, the prehospital care provider should use all information available to formulate a patient care plan. The prehospital care provider should do more than just provide the patient with transport; he or she should do everything possible to ensure survival of the patient.

See

- Examine all the skin of each region.
- Be attentive for external hemorrhage or signs of internal hemorrhage, such as marked tenseness of an extremity or an expanding hematoma.

- Make note of soft tissue injuries, including abrasions, burns, contusions, hematomas, lacerations, and puncture wounds.
- Make note of any masses or swelling or deformation of bones that should not be present.
- Make note of abnormal indentations on the skin and the skin's color.
- Make note of anything that does not "look right."

Hear

- Make note of any unusual sounds when the patient inhales or exhales.
- Make note of any abnormal sounds when auscultating the chest.
- Verify whether the breath sounds are equal in both lung fields.
- Auscultate over the carotid arteries and other vessels.
- Make note of any unusual sounds (bruits) over the vessels that would indicate vascular damage.

Feel

- Carefully move each bone in the region. Note whether this produces crepitus, pain, or unusual movement.
- Firmly palpate all parts of the region. Note whether anything moves that should not, whether anything feels "squishy," where pulses are felt, whether pulsations are felt that should not be present, and whether all pulses are present.

Vital Signs

The prehospital care provider must continually reevaluate the quality of the pulse and ventilatory rates and the rest of the components of the primary survey because significant changes can occur rapidly. The provider should measure quantitative vital signs and evaluate motor and sensory statuses in all four extremities as soon as possible, although this is normally not accomplished until the conclusion of the primary survey. Depending on the situation, a second provider may obtain vital signs while the first provider completes the primary survey to avoid further delay. However, exact "numbers" for pulse rate, ventilatory rate, and blood pressure are not critical in the initial management of the patient with severe multisystem trauma. Therefore the measurement of the exact numbers can be delayed until completion of the essential steps of resuscitation and stabilization.

A set of complete vital signs includes blood pressure, pulse rate and quality, ventilatory rate including breath sounds, and skin color and temperature. The prehospital care provider should evaluate and record a complete set of vital signs every 3 to 5 minutes, as often as possible, or at the time of any change in condition or a medical problem.

AMPLE History

The prehospital care provider should perform a quick history on the patient. This information should be documented on the patient care report and passed on to the medical personnel at the receiving facility. The mnemonic AMPLE serves as a reminder for the key components:

- *Allergies.* Primarily to medications
- *Medications.* Prescription and nonprescription drugs that the patient takes regularly
- *Past medical and surgical history.* Significant medical problems for which the patient receives ongoing medical care; also includes prior surgeries
- *Last meal.* Many trauma patients will require surgery, and recent food intake increases the risk of aspiration during induction of anesthesia
- *Events.* Events leading up to the injury

Head

Visual examination of the head and face will reveal contusions, abrasions, lacerations, bone asymmetry, hemorrhage, bony defects of the face and supportive skull, and/or abnormalities of the eye, eyelid, external ear, mouth, and mandible. The prehospital care provider does the following during a head examination:

- Searches thoroughly through the patient's hair for the presence of any soft tissue injuries

- Checks pupil size for reactivity to light, equality, accommodation, roundness, or irregular shape
- Carefully palpates the bones of the face and skull to identify crepitus, deviation, depression, or abnormal mobility (this is extremely important in the nonradiographic evaluation for head injury)

Figure 3-4 reviews the normal anatomic structure of the face and skull.

Neck

Visual examination of the neck for contusions, abrasions, lacerations, and deformities will alert the prehospital care provider to the possibility of underlying injuries. Palpation may reveal subcutaneous emphysema of a laryngeal, tracheal, or pulmonary origin. Crepitus of the larynx, hoarseness, and subcutaneous emphysema compose a triad classically indicative of laryngeal fracture. Lack of tenderness of the cervical spine may help rule out cervical spine fractures (when combined with strict criteria), whereas tenderness may frequently indicate the presence of a fracture, dislocation, or ligamentous injury. The prehospital care provider should perform such palpation carefully, ensuring that the cervical spine remains in a neutral inline position. Figure 3-5 reviews the normal anatomy of the neck.

Chest

Because the thorax is strong, resilient, and elastic, it can absorb a significant amount of trauma. Close visual examination of the chest for deformities, areas of paradox-

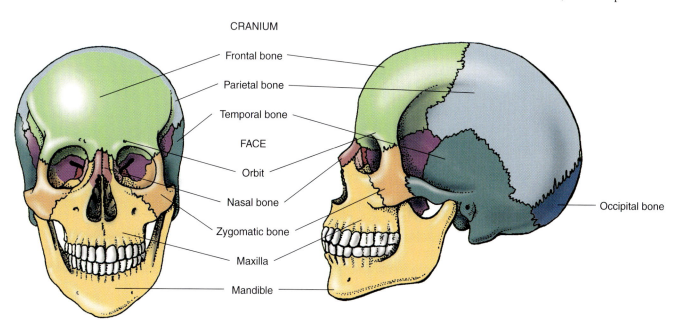

Figure 3-4   Normal anatomic structure of the face and skull.

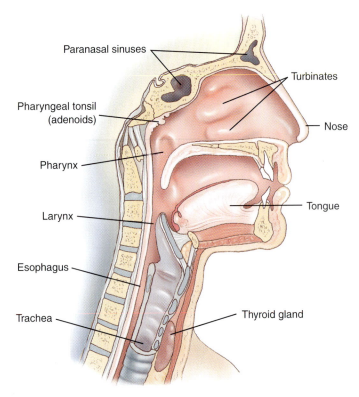

Figure 3-5   Normal anatomy of the neck.

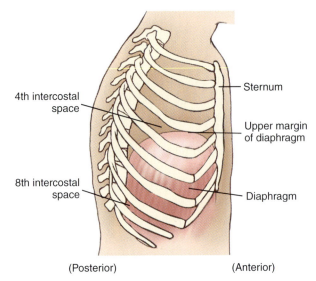

Figure 3-6   Lateral view of diaphragm position at full expiration.

ical movement, contusions, and abrasions is necessary to identify underlying injuries. Other signs for which the prehospital care provider should watch closely include splinting and guarding, unequal bilateral chest excursion, and intercostal, suprasternal, or supraclavicular bulging or retraction.

For example, a contusion over the sternum may be the only indication of a cardiac injury. A stab wound near the sternum may indicate a cardiac tamponade. A line traced from the fourth intercostal space anteriorly to the sixth intercostal space laterally to the eighth intercostal space posteriorly defines the upward excursion of the diaphragm at full expiration (Figure 3-6). A penetrating injury that occurs below this line or whose pathway may have taken it below this line should be considered to have traversed both the thoracic and abdominal cavities.

Except for the eyes and hands, the stethoscope is the most important instrument a prehospital care provider can use for chest examination. A patient will most often be in a supine position so that only the anterior and lateral chest is available for auscultation. A prehospital care provider should learn to recognize normal and decreased breath sounds with a patient in this position. A small area of rib fractures may indicate a severe underlying pulmonary contusion. Any type of compression injury to the chest can result in a pneumothorax (Figure 3-7). Diminished or absent breath sounds indicate a possible pneumothorax, tension pneumothorax, or hemothorax. Crackles heard posteriorly (when the patient is logrolled) or laterally may indicate pulmonary contusion. Cardiac tamponade is characterized by distant heart sounds; however, these may be difficult for the prehospital care provider to ascertain given the commotion at the scene or road noise during transport. The prehospital care provider should also feel the thorax for subcutaneous emphysema.

Abdomen

The prehospital care provider initiates abdominal examination, as with the other parts of the body, by visual evaluation. Abrasions and ecchymosis indicate the possibility of underlying injury. The prehospital care provider should examine the abdomen, near the umbilicus, carefully for a telltale transverse contusion, which suggests that an incorrectly worn seat belt has caused underlying injury. Almost 50% of patients with this sign will have an intestinal injury. Lumbar spine fractures may also be associated with the "seat belt sign."

Examination of the abdomen also includes palpation of each quadrant to evaluate tenderness, abdominal muscle guarding, and masses. When palpating, the prehospital care provider should note whether the abdomen is soft and whether rigidity or guarding are present. There is no need to continue palpating after discovering abdominal tenderness or pain. Additional information will not alter prehospital management, and the only out-

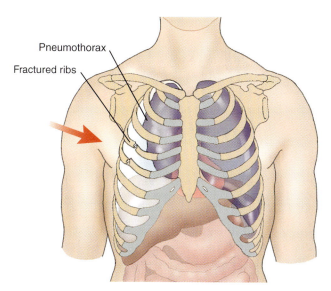

Pneumothorax

Fractured ribs

Figure 3-7   A compression injury to the chest can result in a rib fracture and a subsequent pneumothorax.

comes of a continued abdominal examination are further discomfort to the patient and delay of transportation to the receiving facility. Similarly, auscultation of the abdomen adds virtually nothing to the assessment of a trauma patient.

Pelvis

The prehospital care provider evaluates the pelvis by observation and palpation. The prehospital care provider should visually examine for abrasions, contusions, lacerations, open fractures, and signs of distention. Pelvic fractures can produce massive internal hemorrhage, resulting in rapid deterioration of a patient's condition.

The pelvis is palpated only once for instability as part of the secondary survey. Since palpation can aggravate hemorrhage, the prehospital care provider should not repeat this examination step. Palpation is accomplished by gently applying first anterior to posterior pressure with the heels of the hands on the symphysis pubis and then medial pressure to the iliac crests bilaterally, evaluating for pain and abnormal movement. The provider should suspect hemorrhage with any evidence of instability.

Back

The back of the torso should be examined for evidence of injury. This is best accomplished when logrolling the patient for placement onto the long backboard. Breath sounds can be auscultated over the posterior thorax, and the spine should be palpated for tenderness and deformity.

Extremities

The prehospital care provider should begin examination of the extremities with the clavicle in the upper extremity and the pelvis in the lower extremity and proceed toward the most distal portion of each extremity. Each individual bone and joint should be evaluated by visual examination for deformity, hematoma, or ecchymosis and by palpation to determine the presence of crepitus, pain, tenderness, or unusual movements. Any suspected fracture should be immobilized until radiographic confirmation of its presence or absence is possible. The provider should also check circulation and motor and sensory nerve function at the distal end of each extremity. If an extremity is immobilized, pulses, movement, and sensation should be rechecked after splinting.

Neurologic Examination

As with the other regional examinations described, the prehospital care provider conducts the neurologic examination in the secondary survey in much greater detail than in the primary survey. Calculation of the GCS score, evaluation of motor and sensory function, and observation of pupillary response are all included. When examining a patient's pupils, the prehospital care provider should check for equality of response as much as for equality of size. A significant portion of the population has pupils of differing sizes as a normal condition (anisocoria). However, even in this situation, the pupils should react to light in a similar manner. Pupils that react at differing speeds to the introduction of light are considered to be unequal. Unequal pupils in an unconscious trauma patient may indicate increased intracranial pressure or pressure on the third cranial nerve, caused by either cerebral edema or a rapidly expanding intracranial hematoma (Figure 3-8). Direct eye injury can also cause unequal pupils.

A gross examination of sensory capability and response will determine the presence or absence of weakness or loss of sensation in the extremities and will identify areas that require further examination. The prehospital care provider must immobilize the entire length of the spine and thus the entire patient. Use of a long backboard, cervical collar, head pads, and straps is required. The prehospital care provider must not immobilize the head only. If the body is not immobilized, a shift in the patient's body caused by lifting or ambulance movement will cause the body to move and not the head, potentially causing further injury to the spinal cord. Protection of the entire spinal cord is required at all times.

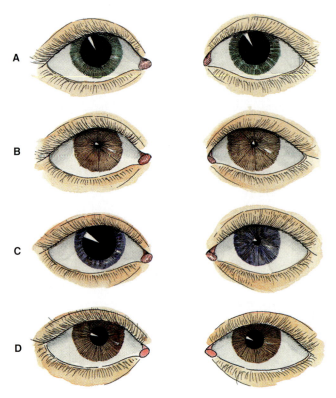

Figure 3-8 **A**, Pupil dilation. **B**, Pupil constriction. **C**, Unequal pupils. **D**, Normal pupils.

Definitive Care in the Field

Included in assessment and management are the skills of packaging, transportation, and communication. Definitive care is the end phase of patient care. The following are examples of definitive care:

- For a patient with cardiac arrest, definitive care is defibrillation with resultant normal rhythm; cardiopulmonary resuscitation (CPR) is just a holding pattern until defibrillation can be accomplished.
- For a patient in a diabetic hypoglycemic coma, definitive care is intravenous glucose and a return to normal blood glucose levels.
- For a patient with an obstructed airway, part of the definitive care is the jaw thrust and assisted ventilation.
- For the patient with severe bleeding, definitive care is hemorrhage control and resuscitation from shock.

In general, definitive care for the trauma patient can only be provided in the OR. Anything that delays the administration of that definitive care will lessen the patient's chance for survival. The care given to the trauma patient in the field is like CPR for the cardiac arrest patient. It keeps the patient alive until something definitive can be done. For the trauma patient, the care given in the field is frequently only temporizing—buying additional minutes to reach the OR.

Packaging

As discussed previously, the prehospital care provider should suspect spinal injury in all trauma patients. Therefore when indicated, stabilization of the spine should be an integral component of packaging the trauma patient. If time is available, the prehospital care provider should do the following:

- Carefully stabilize extremity fractures using specific splints.
- If the patient is in critical condition, immobilize all fractures as the patient is stabilized on a long backboard ("trauma" board).
- Bandage wounds as necessary and appropriate.

Transport

Transportation should begin as soon as the patient is loaded and stabilized. As discussed previously in this chapter, delay at the scene to start an IV line or to complete the secondary survey only extends the period of time before the receiving facility can administer blood and control hemorrhage. Continued evaluation and further resuscitation occur en route to the receiving facility. *For some critically injured trauma patients, initiation of transport is the most important aspect of definitive care in the field.*

A patient whose condition is not critical can receive attention for individual injuries before transportation, but even this patient should be transported rapidly before a hidden condition becomes critical.

The Trauma Score (TS), originally developed by surgeon Howard Champion and colleagues, is a good predictor of survival of blunt trauma patients. The Revised Trauma Score (RTS), published in 1989, eliminated two components of the older TS and is equally useful in predicting survival from serious injury. The RTS is composed of scores for the GCS, systolic blood pressure, and ventilatory rate (Figure 3-9). Each of these three components is assigned a value from 4 (best) to 0 (worst). The combined score indicates the patient's condition. The lowest possible combined score, 0, is obviously the most critical; the highest, 12, is the least critical. The com-

		Score	Start of Transport	End of Transport
A. Ventilatory rate	10-29/min	4		
	>29/min	3		
	6-9/min	2		
	1-5/min	1		
	0	0		
B. Systolic blood pressure	>89 mm Hg	4		
	76-89 mm Hg	3		
	50-75 mm Hg	2		
	1-49 mm Hg	1		
	No pulse	0		
C. Glasgow Coma Scale score	13-15 =	4		
	9-12 =	3		
	6-8 =	2		
	4-5 =	1		
	<4 =	0		
Trauma score total = A+ B + C				

Figure 3-9   Revised Trauma Score. A trauma score can be numerically calculated en route to the hospital. Such information is extremely helpful in preparing to manage a patient. (*Adapted from Champion HR, Sacco WJ, Copes WS et al: A revision of the Trauma Score, J Trauma 29(5):624, 1989.*)

bined score is valuable to analyze the care given to a patient, but it is not necessarily a prehospital triage tool. In many prehospital systems, the score is calculated and recorded at the receiving facility based on information provided in the radio report, but prehospital care providers are neither required nor expected to compute it before arrival.

The Triage Decision Scheme published by the American College of Surgeons Committee on Trauma is more useful than the RTS in making prehospital patient triage decisions (Figure 3-10). In some systems the Triage Decision Scheme is used in the process of determining the most appropriate receiving facility for a trauma patient. However, like any schematic tool, it should be used as a guideline and not as a replacement for good judgment. The Triage Decision Scheme divides triage into three prioritized steps that will assist in the decision as to when it is best to transport a patient to a trauma center, if available: (1) physiologic criteria, (2) anatomic criteria, and (3) mechanism of injury (kinematics). Following this scheme results in overtriage (not all patients taken to the trauma center will actually need a trauma center level of care), but this outcome is better than undertriage (patients needing a trauma center level of care and are taken to nontrauma centers). Medical directors or local medical control boards should establish local protocols to familiarize prehospital field personnel with trauma centers.

The prehospital care provider should choose a receiving facility according to the severity of the patient's injury. In simple terms, the patient should be transported to the closest appropriate facility (i.e., the closest facility most capable of managing the patient's problems). If the patient's injuries are severe or indicate the possibility of continuing hemorrhage, the provider should take the patient to a facility that will provide definitive care as quickly as possible (i.e., a trauma center if available).

For example, if an ambulance responds to a call in 8 minutes and the prehospital team spends 6 minutes on the scene to properly package and load the patient into the transporting unit, 14 minutes of the Golden Period have passed. The closest hospital is 5 minutes away, and the trauma center is 14 minutes away. On arrival at the trauma center the surgeon is in the emergency department with the emergency physician and the entire trauma team. The OR is staffed and ready. After 10 minutes in the emergency department for resuscitation and necessary radiographs and blood work, the patient is taken to the OR. The total time since the incident is now 38 minutes. In comparison, the closest hospital has an available emergency physician, but the surgeon and OR team are out of the hospital. The patient's 10 minutes in the emergency department for resuscitation could stretch to 45 minutes by the time the surgeon arrives and examines the patient. Another 30 minutes could elapse

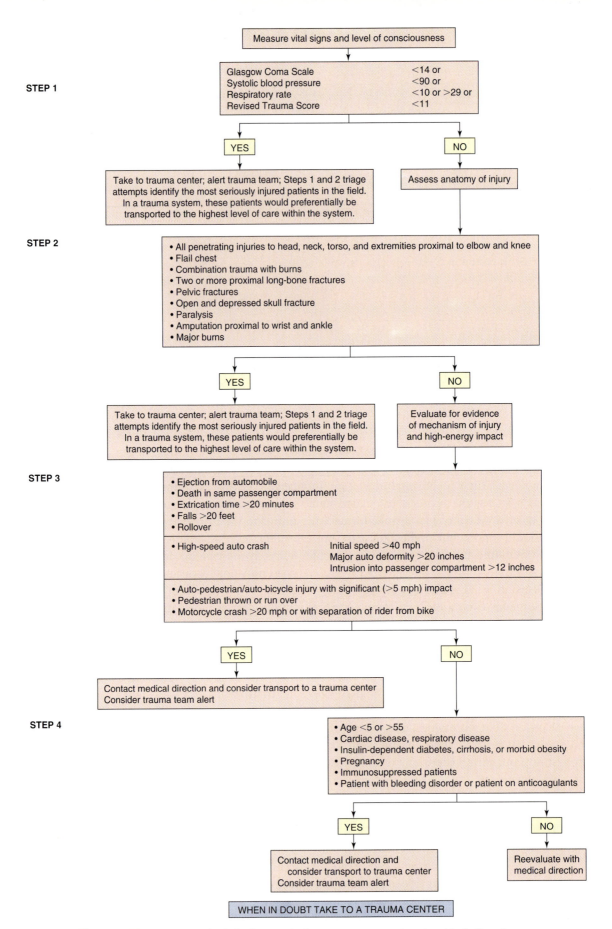

Figure 3-10   Deciding which facility to which to transport a patient is critical. Situations that will most likely require an in-house trauma team are detailed in the Triage Decision Scheme. (*From American College of Surgeons Committee on Trauma:* Resources for optimal care of the injured patient: 1999, *Chicago, 1998, American College of Surgeons.*)

while waiting for the OR team to arrive once the surgeon has examined the patient and decided to operate. The total time is 94 minutes, or 2½ times longer than the first scenario. The 9 minutes saved by the shorter ambulance ride actually cost 57 minutes, during which operative management could have been started and hemorrhage control achieved.

Obviously, in a rural community the transport time to an awaiting trauma team may be 45 to 60 minutes or even longer. In this situation, the closest hospital with an on-call trauma team is the appropriate receiving facility.

Another aspect in the transportation decision is the transportation method. Some systems offer an alternative option of air transportation. Air medical services may offer a higher level of care than ground units. Air transportation may also be quicker and smoother than ground transportation in some circumstances. As mentioned previously in this chapter, if air transportation is available in a community, the prehospital care provider should anticipate its use early in the assessment process to benefit the patient.

Monitoring and Reassessment (Ongoing Assessment)

After the primary survey and initial care are complete, the prehospital care provider should continue to monitor the patient, reassess vital signs, and repeat the primary survey several times while en route to the receiving facility, or at the scene if transport is delayed. Continual reassessment of the points in the primary survey will help ensure that unrecognized compromise of vital functions does not occur. The provider should pay particular attention to any significant change in a patient's condition and reevaluate management if the patient's condition changes. Furthermore, the continued monitoring of a patient helps reveal conditions or problems that may have been overlooked during the primary survey. Often the patient's condition will be obvious, and looking at and listening to the patient provides much information. How the information is gathered is not as important as ensuring that all the information is gathered. Reassessment should be conducted as quickly and thoroughly as possible.

Communication

The prehospital care provider should begin communication with medical direction and the receiving facility as soon as possible. The information transmitted about a patient's condition, management, and the expected time of arrival will give the receiving facility time to prepare. The prehospital team should also transmit information about the mechanism of injury, the characteristics of the scene, the number of patients, and other pertinent facts to allow the receiving facility staff to best coordinate its resources and meet each patient's needs.

Equally important is the written prehospital care report (PCR). A good PCR is valuable for two reasons:

1. It gives the receiving facility staff a thorough understanding of the events that occurred and of the patient's condition should any questions arise after the prehospital care providers have left.
2. It helps ensure quality control throughout the prehospital system by making case review possible.

For these reasons, the prehospital care provider should fill out the PCR accurately and completely and provide it to the receiving facility. The report should stay with the patient; the report is of little use if it does not arrive until hours or days after the patient arrives.

The PCR often becomes a part of the patient's medical record. It is a legal record of what was found and what was done and can be used as part of a legal action. The report is considered to be a complete record of the injuries found and the actions taken. "If it is not on the report, it was not done" is a good adage to remember. The prehospital care provider should record in the report all that he or she knows, has seen, and has done to the patient. Another important reason for providing a copy of the PCR to the receiving facility is that most trauma centers maintain a "trauma registry," a database of all trauma patients admitted to their facility. The prehospital information is an important aspect of this database and may aid in valuable research.

The prehospital care provider must also verbally transfer responsibility for a patient ("sign off," "report off," or "transfer over") to the physician or nurse who takes over the patient's care at the receiving facility. This verbal report is typically more detailed than the radio report and less detailed than the written record, providing an overview of the significant history of the incident, the action taken by the prehospital care providers, and the patient's response to this action. The report must highlight any significant changes in the patient's condition that have taken place since transmitting the radio report. Transfer of important prehospital information further emphasizes the team concept of patient care.

Pain Management

Pain management (analgesia) is often used in the pre-hospital setting for pain caused by angina or myocardial infarction. Traditionally, pain management has had a limited role in the management of trauma patients, primarily because of the concern that side effects (decreased ventilatory drive and vasodilation) of narcotics may aggravate preexisting hypoxia and hypotension. This concern has resulted in some patients with appropriate indications, such as an isolated limb injury or spinal fracture, being denied pain relief. The prehospital care provider should consider pain management in such situations, particularly if prolonged transport occurs, provided that signs of ventilatory impairment or shock are not present.

Chapter 10 devotes a section to pain management as it relates to isolated extremity injuries and fractures. Morphine sulfate is typically the agent of choice and should be titrated intravenously in 1 to 2 mg increments until some degree of pain relief is obtained or a change in the patient's vital signs occurs. The prehospital care provider should monitor pulse oximetry and serial vital signs if any narcotics are administered to a trauma patient. Sedation with an agent such as a benzodiazepine should be reserved for exceptional circumstances, such as a combative intubated patient, because the combination of a narcotic and benzodiazepine may result in respiratory arrest. Prehospital personnel should collaborate with their medical control to develop appropriate protocols.

Abuse

A prehospital care provider is often the first person on the scene, allowing him or her to observe a potentially abusive situation. A prehospital care provider inside a house can relay what is at the scene to the receiving facility, allowing the appropriate services in the area to be alerted. The prehospital care provider is usually the first, and sometimes the only, person to suspect and relay information about this silent danger.

Anyone at any age can be a potential abuser or victim of abuse. A pregnant woman, infant, toddler, child, adolescent, young adult, middle-age adult, and older adult are all at risk for abuse. Several different types of abuse exist, including physical, psychological (emotional), and financial. Abuse may occur by commission, in which a purposeful act results in an injury (physical abuse or sexual abuse), or by omission (e.g., neglectful care of a dependent). This chapter does not discuss all types of abuse; its purpose is to introduce the reader to general

characteristics and to heighten a prehospital care giver's awareness and suspicion of abuse.

General characteristics of a potential abuser include dishonesty, the "story" not correlating with the injuries, a negative attitude, and abrasiveness with prehospital personnel. General characteristics of the abused patient include quietness, not wanting to elaborate on details of the incident, constant eye contact or lack of eye contact with someone at the scene, and minimization of their own injuries. Abuse, abusers, and the abused can take many different forms, and prehospital care providers must keep suspicion high if the scene and the story do not correlate. The prehospital care provider must relay his or her suspicion and any information to the proper authorities.

Triage

Triage is a French word meaning "to sort." In the prehospital environment, triage is used in two different contexts:

1. Sufficient resources are available to manage all patients. In this case, the most severely injured patients are treated and transported first while those with lesser injuries are treated and transported later.
2. Triage is used as a method to deal with MCIs in which the number of patients exceeds the immediate capacity of on-scene resources. The objective in triage is to ensure survival of the largest possible number of injured patients. Patients are sorted into categories for patient care. In an MCI, patient care must be rationed because the number of patients exceeds the available resources. Relatively few prehospital care providers ever experience an MCI with 80 to 120 simultaneously injured persons, but many will be involved in MCIs with 10 to 20 patients, and rare is the prehospital veteran who has not managed an incident with 2 to 10 patients.

The purpose of triage is to salvage the greatest possible number of patients given the circumstances and resources available. The prehospital care provider must make decisions about who to manage first. The usual rules about saving lives do not apply in MCIs. In a choice between a patient with a catastrophic injury, such as severe traumatic brain injury, and a patient with an acute intraabdominal hemorrhage, the proper course of action in an MCI is to manage first the salvageable patient—the one with the abdominal hemorrhage. Treating the severe head trauma patient first will probably result in the loss of both patients—the head trauma patient because he or she may not be salvageable and the abdominal hemorrhage patient because time, equipment, and personnel spent managing the unsalvageable patient keep the salvageable patient from getting the simple care needed to survive until definitive surgical care is available.

In a triage MCI situation, the catastrophically injured may need to be considered second priority with treatment delayed until more help and equipment become available. These are difficult circumstances, but a prehospital care provider must respond quickly and properly. A medical care team should not make efforts to resuscitate a traumatic cardiac arrest patient with little or no chance of survival while three other patients die because of airway compromise or external hemorrhage. The "sorting scheme" most often used divides patients into five categories based on need of care and chance of survival:

1. *Immediate.* Patients whose injuries are critical but who will require only minimal time or equipment to manage and who have a good prognosis for survival. An example is a patient with a compromised airway or massive external hemorrhage.

2. *Delayed.* Patients whose injuries are debilitating but who do not require immediate management to salvage life or limb. An example is a patient with a long bone fracture.

3. *Expectant.* Patients whose injuries are so severe that they have only a minimal chance of survival. An example is a patient with a 90% full-thickness burn and thermal pulmonary injury.

4. *Minimal.* Patients, often called the "walking wounded," who have minor injuries that can wait for treatment or who may even assist in the interim by comforting other patients or helping out as litter bearers.

5. *Dead.* Patients who are unresponsive, pulseless, and breathless. In a disaster, resources rarely allow for attempted resuscitation of arrested patients.

Summary

In the care of the trauma patient, a missed problem is a missed opportunity to potentially aid in an individual's survival. A patient's chance for survival of traumatic injuries depends on the immediate identification and mitigation of conditions that interfere with tissue perfusion. The identification of these conditions requires a systematic, prioritized, logical process of collecting information and acting on it. This process is referred to as patient assessment. Patient assessment begins with scene assessment and includes the formation of a general impression of the patient; a primary survey; and when the patient's condition and availability of additional EMS personnel permit, a secondary survey. The prehospital care provider analyzes the information obtained through this process and uses it as the basis for patient care and transport decisions.

Life depends on adequate perfusion—the circulation of oxygenated blood to the tissues of the body and the release of oxygen to the cells of the tissues. Impairment of perfusion must occur during the patient's Golden Period, the length of which depends on the degree of impairment. After the simultaneous determination of scene safety and a general impression of the situation, the prehospital care provider directs priorities of patient assessment at the patency of the patient's airway, the ventilatory status, and the circulatory status. Once the prehospital care provider has responded to these immediate threats to the patient's life, further assessment is necessary to identify the patient's neurologic status and the presence of other injuries. This primary survey follows the ABCDE format for evaluation of the patient's airway, breathing, circulation, disability (initial neurologic examination), and exposure (removing the patient's clothing to discover additional significant injuries).

Although the sequential nature of language limits the ability to describe the simultaneity of these actions, the prehospital care provider must understand the primary survey of the patient as a process of actions that occur at the same time. For a patient with any impairment or potential for impairment of perfusion, the prehospital care provider will quickly intervene in a "find and fix" fashion for immediate threats to the patient's life. Once the prehospital care provider manages the patient's airway and breathing and controls exsanguinating hemorrhage, he or she packages the patient and begins transportation without additional treatment at the scene. The prehospital care provider must understand the limitations of the field management of trauma and make his or her goal the safe, expedient delivery of the patient to definitive care.

Scenario Solution

You have been on the scene for 1 minute, yet you have obtained a great deal of important information to guide the further assessment and treatment of the patient. In the first 15 seconds of patient contact, you have developed a general impression of the patient, determining that resuscitation is not necessary. With a few simple actions you have evaluated the A, B, C, and D of the initial assessment. The patient spoke to you without difficulty, indicating that her airway is open and she is breathing with no signs of distress. At the same time, with an awareness of the mechanism of injury, you have stabilized the cervical spine. You have noted no obvious bleeding, your partner has assessed the radial pulse, and you have observed the patient's skin color, temperature, and moisture. These findings indicate no immediate threats to the patient's circulatory status. Additionally, you have simultaneously found no initial evidence of disability because the patient is awake, is alert, and answers questions appropriately. This information, along with information about the speed of the vehicle at the time of impact and the damage to the vehicle at the point of impact, will help you determine the need for additional resources, the type of transportation indicated, and to what type of facility you should deliver the patient.

Now that you have completed these steps and no immediate life-saving intervention is necessary, you will proceed with step E of the primary survey early in the evaluation process and then obtain vital signs. You will expose the patient to look for additional injuries and bleeding that may have been concealed by clothing, then cover the patient to protect her from the environment. During this process, you will perform a more detailed examination, noting less serious injuries. The next steps you will take are packaging the patient, including splinting extremity injuries and bandaging wounds if time allows; initiating transportation; and communicating with medical direction and/or the receiving facility. During the trip to the hospital, you will continue to reevaluate and monitor the patient. Your knowledge of kinematics and the patient's witnessed loss of consciousness will generate a high index of suspicion for traumatic brain injury, lower-extremity injuries, and injuries to the chest and abdomen. In an ALS system, IV access will be established en route to the receiving facility.

Review Questions

Answers are provided on p. 414.

1. You are called to the scene of a "man down on the sidewalk, unknown reason" at the intersection of two busy streets. As you approach the scene, you note that the patient has received some type of trauma and is bleeding from the head and is not moving as you approach. What will be your first action as you arrive on the scene?
   a. Determine whether the patient can speak
   b. Control the bleeding from the patient's head
   c. Ensure scene safety
   d. Protect the patient from the environment

2. Asking the patient questions will help the prehospital care provider assess which of the following?
   a. Airway
   b. Mechanism of injury

   c. Disability
   d. All of the above

3. Stabilization of the cervical spine should occur simultaneously with which of the following steps in assessment of the trauma patient?
   a. Determination of GCS
   b. Neurologic examination
   c. Secondary survey examination
   d. Airway assessment

4. When caring for a trauma patient with an immediate threat to life, which of the following is the most appropriate time to obtain a complete set of vital signs?
   a. En route or after the primary survey if time and number of personnel permit
   b. During the primary survey, to assess circulatory status

c. Before packaging the patient
d. Before the primary survey, to determine the need for resuscitation

5. Which of the following patients should be transported to a trauma center?
   a. An adult who has fallen from a 7-foot ladder
   b. A 15 year old with burns to both hands
   c. A 40 year old who was ejected from a vehicle on impact
   d. A 73 year old with emphysema who has a deformity of the left forearm

6. Upon the primary survey of a 29-year-old male involved in a motorcycle crash, you find that his ventilatory rate is abnormally rapid and each ventilation is very shallow. You have simultaneously noted cyanosis of the patient's lips. Which of the following should be your next step?
   a. Assess the patient's circulatory status
   b. Control exsanguinating hemorrhage
   c. Insert an airway adjunct
   d. Auscultate the lungs

7. The purpose of assessing the conscious trauma patient's radial pulse in the primary survey is to do which of the following?
   a. Estimate the rate and quality of the pulse
   b. Determine the need for a PASG
   c. Determine the exact pulse rate
   d. Distract the patient while you count his ventilations

8. Your patient is a 16-year-old female who has been found lying in an alley in a high-crime area of the city. She appears to have been beaten with a piece of pipe found lying nearby. The patient responds to painful stimuli, has a patent airway, and is breathing with adequate depth at a rate of approximately 30 breaths/min. You can find no source of significant external bleeding. A quick check of her radial pulse reveals a very rapid heart rate with a weak and thready quality. Which of the following actions should you perform next?
   a. Start an IV of lactated Ringer's solution
   b. Apply a PASG
   c. Expose the patient for a secondary survey
   d. Check for evidence of abdominal injury

9. You are on the scene of a chartered bus that exited onto a tightly curved interstate ramp too quickly and rolled several times down an embankment. A quick scene assessment indicates at least 40 injured people. At least 12 of these people appear to be critically injured. You expect only four ambulances to respond within the next 45 minutes. The only helicopter service with less than an hour response time is out of service for maintenance. You are at the side of a 69-year-old male who was ejected and is trapped under the bus from the chest down. He is unresponsive with agonal ventilations and a weak, slow carotid pulse. Based on the available information, you would triage this patient into which of the following categories?
   a. Expectant
   b. Immediate
   c. Delayed
   d. Minimal

REFERENCES

Anonymous: Initial assessment and management. In Committee on Trauma, American College of Surgeons: *Advanced Trauma Life Support course for physicians*, Chicago, 2002, American College of Surgeons.

Champion HR, Sacco WJ, Copes WS et al: A revision of the Trauma Score, *J Trauma* 29:623, 1989.

Committee on Trauma, American College of Surgeons: *Resources for optimal care of the injured patient: 1999*, Chicago, 1998, American College of Surgeons.

Gardner JS, Hospital Infection Control Practices Advisory Committee, Centers for Disease Control and Prevention: *Guidelines for isolation precautions in hospitals*, 1996. Available at wonder.cdc.gov/wonder/prevguid/p0000419/p0000419.asp.

McSwain NE Jr, Paturas JL: *The basic EMT: comprehensive prehospital patient care*, ed 2, St Louis, 2001, Mosby.

National Association of EMS Physicians: Air medical dispatch: guidelines for scene response, *Prehosp Disaster Med* 7(1):75, 1992.

National Association of EMS Physicians, American College of Surgeons Committee on Trauma: *Termination of resuscitation in prehospital traumatic cardiopulmonary arrest* (in press).

Sanders MJ: *Mosby's paramedic textbook*, ed 2, St Louis, 2000, Mosby.

Teasdale G, Jennett B: Assessment of coma and impaired consciousness: a practical scale, *Lancet* 2:81, 1974.

Wong DL et al: *Whaley and Wong's nursing care of infants and children*, ed 4, St Louis, 1991, Mosby.

SUGGESTED READING

Rinnert KJ: A review of infection control practices, risk reduction, and legislative regulations for blood-borne disease: applications for emergency medical services, *Prehosp Emerg Care* 2(1):70, 1998.

Rinnert KJ, O'Connor RE, Delbridge T: Risk reduction for exposure to blood-borne pathogens in EMS: National Association of EMS Physicians, *Prehosp Emerg Care* 2(1):62, 1998.

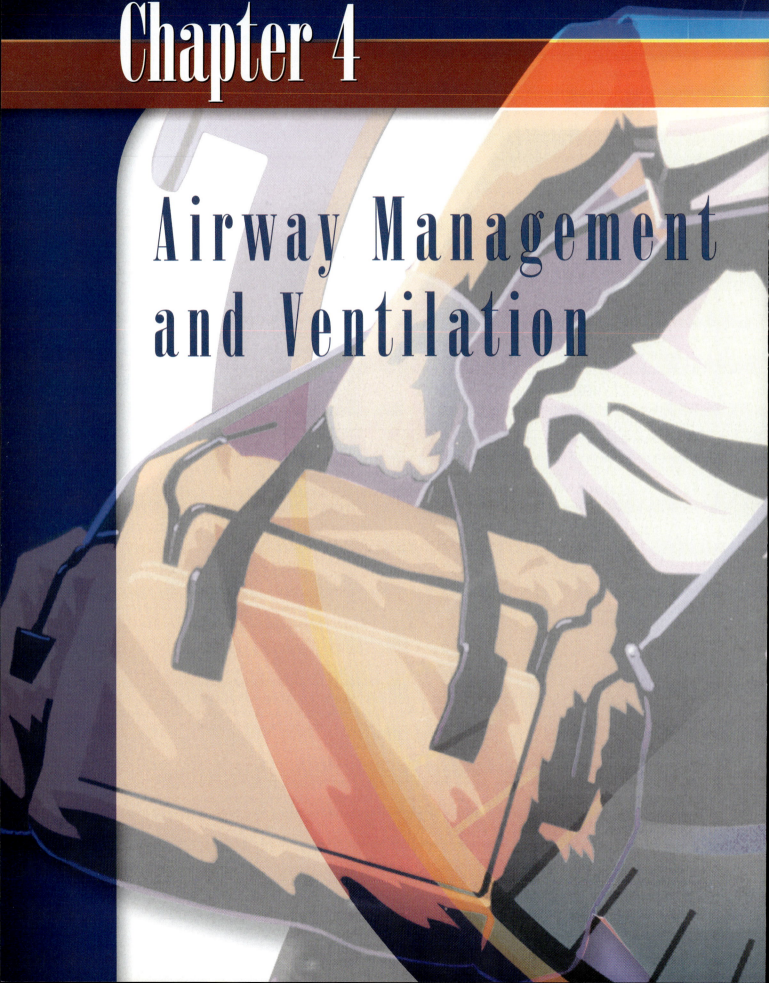

Chapter 4

Airway Management and Ventilation

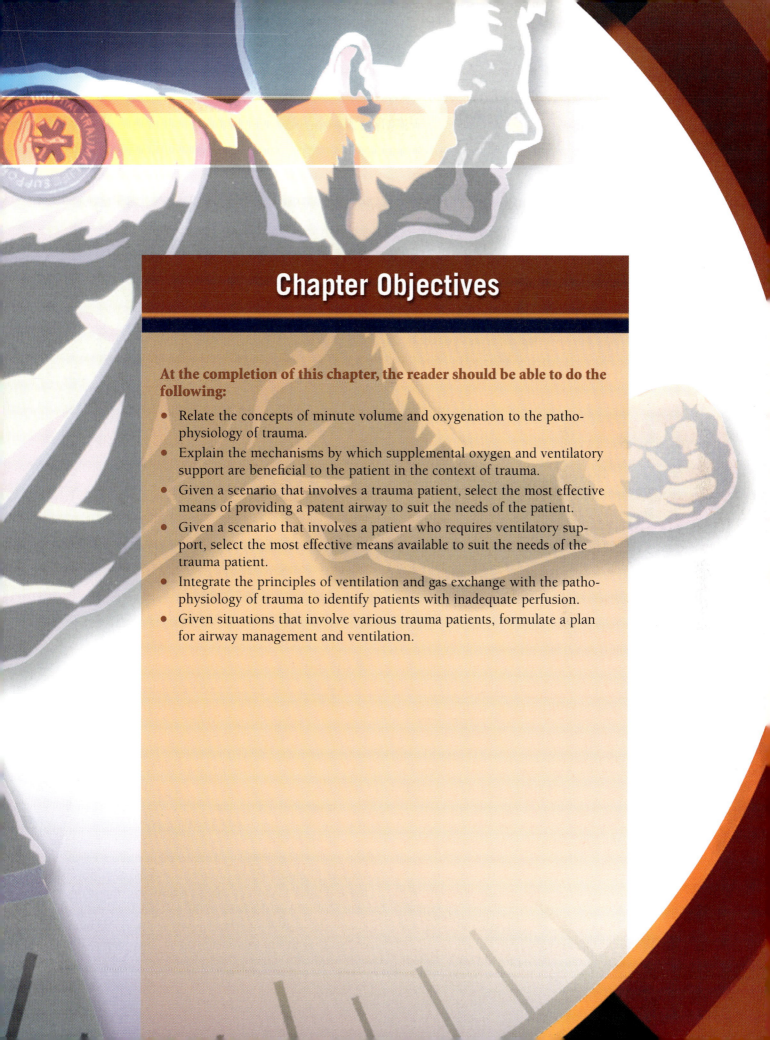

Chapter Objectives

At the completion of this chapter, the reader should be able to do the following:

- Relate the concepts of minute volume and oxygenation to the pathophysiology of trauma.
- Explain the mechanisms by which supplemental oxygen and ventilatory support are beneficial to the patient in the context of trauma.
- Given a scenario that involves a trauma patient, select the most effective means of providing a patent airway to suit the needs of the patient.
- Given a scenario that involves a patient who requires ventilatory support, select the most effective means available to suit the needs of the trauma patient.
- Integrate the principles of ventilation and gas exchange with the pathophysiology of trauma to identify patients with inadequate perfusion.
- Given situations that involve various trauma patients, formulate a plan for airway management and ventilation.

Scenario

You are dispatched to a motor vehicle crash. On arrival, you observe that an SUV has struck a tree with the driver's side of the vehicle. The entire driver's side of the vehicle has sustained substantial damage. The driver of the SUV, a 30-year-old male, is lying in the grass approximately 30 feet (9 meters) from the incident site. Fire department first responders have logrolled the patient onto a long backboard and applied a cervical collar. They report that the patient has been unresponsive since their arrival. Periorbital ecchymosis (raccoon eyes) is already present. You observe bleeding from both nares and the right ear. Frequent suctioning is required to maintain a patent airway. Ventilations are irregular and snoring sounds are audible. The patient's skin is pale, and cyanosis is present around the lips.

What indicators of airway compromise are evident in this patient? What other information, if any, would you seek from witnesses or the first responders? Describe the sequence of actions you would take to manage this patient before and during transport.

Airway management plays a prominent role in the management of trauma patients. Its importance is recognized even more now than in years past. Studies carried out during the Championship Auto Racing Team (CART) auto racing circuit have demonstrated that patients with head injuries may undergo a period of apnea within the first 5 minutes after impact. Although this apnea lasts only a short time and spontaneous ventilation usually resumes quickly, the apnea has a major influence on patient outcome. In one 3-year period after the CART introduced an emergency response team, no major complications from head injuries occurred because the patient was ventilated during this period of apnea. The theoretical benefit is decreasing the brain edema that is a result of the anoxic events (see Chapters 6 and 8).

Cerebral oxygenation and oxygen delivery to other parts of the body provided by adequate airway management and ventilation remain the most important components of prehospital patient care. Because techniques and adjunct devices are changing and will continue to change, the well-informed prehospital provider must continually keep abreast of these changes.

The respiratory system serves three primary functions:

1. The system provides oxygen to the red blood cells, which carry the oxygen to all the cells in the body.
2. In aerobic metabolism, the cells use this oxygen as fuel to produce energy.
3. The system removes carbon dioxide from the body.

Inability of the respiratory system to provide oxygen to the cells or of the cells to use the oxygen supplied can quickly lead to death. Failure to eliminate carbon dioxide can lead to coma.

Anatomy

The respiratory system is composed of the upper airway and the lower airway, including the lungs (Figure 4-1). Each part of the system plays an important role in ensuring gas exchange—the process by which oxygen enters the bloodstream and carbon dioxide is removed.

Upper Airway

The airway system is an open path that leads atmospheric air through the nose, mouth, pharynx, trachea, and bronchi to the alveoli. With each breath, the average adult takes in approximately 500 mL of air. The airway system holds up to 150 mL of air that never actually reaches the alveoli to participate in the critical gas exchange process. The space in which this air is held is known as *dead space*. The air inside the space is not available to the body to be used for oxygenation.

The upper airway consists of the nasal cavity and the oral cavity (Figure 4-2). Air entering the nasal cavity is warmed, humidified, and filtered to remove impurities. Beyond these cavities is the area known as the *pharynx*, which runs from the back of the soft palate to the upper end of the esophagus. The pharynx is composed of muscle lined with mucous membranes. The pharynx is divided into three discrete sections—the *nasopharynx* (the

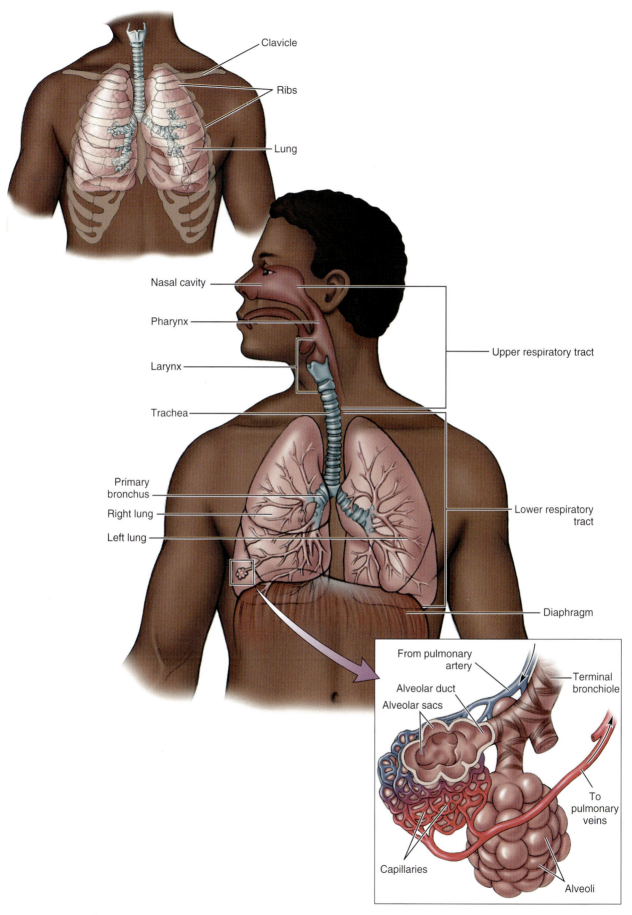

Figure 4-1 Organs of the respiratory system: upper respiratory tract and lower respiratory tract. (*From Herlihy B, Maebius WK: The human body in health and disease, Philadelphia, 2000, WB Saunders.*)

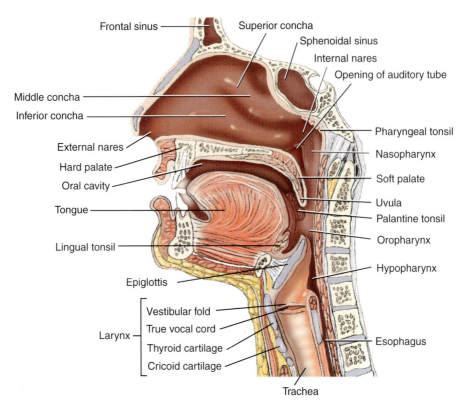

Frontal sinus
Superior concha
Sphenoidal sinus
Internal nares
Opening of auditory tube
Middle concha
Inferior concha
External nares
Hard palate
Oral cavity
Tongue
Lingual tonsil
Epiglottis
Pharyngeal tonsil
Nasopharynx
Soft palate
Uvula
Palantine tonsil
Oropharynx
Hypopharynx
Larynx
Vestibular fold
True vocal cord
Thyroid cartilage
Cricoid cartilage
Esophagus
Trachea

Figure 4-2   Sagittal section through the nasal cavity and pharynx viewed from the medial side.

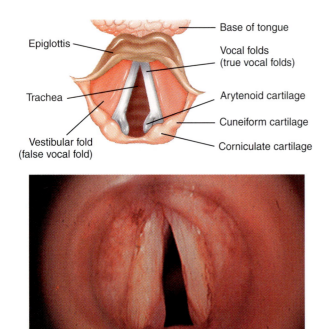

Epiglottis
Trachea
Vestibular fold (false vocal fold)
Base of tongue
Vocal folds (true vocal folds)
Arytenoid cartilage
Cuneiform cartilage
Corniculate cartilage

Figure 4-3   The vocal cords viewed from above, showing their relationship to the paired cartilages of the larynx and the epiglottis. (Bottom, *Custom Medical Stock photo, from Thibodeau GA: Structure and function, ed 9, St Louis, 1992, Mosby.*)

upper portion), the *oropharynx* (the middle portion), and the *hypopharynx* (the distal end of the pharynx).

Below the pharynx are the esophagus, which leads to the stomach, and the trachea, at which point the lower airway begins. Above the trachea is the larynx (Figure 4-3), which contains the vocal cords, and the muscles that make them work, housed in a strong cartilaginous box. The vocal cords are folds of tissue that meet in the midline. The false cords, or vestibule fold, block the free passage of air and force the airflow through the vocal cords. Supporting the cords posteriorly is the arytenoid cartilage. Directly above the larynx is a leaf-shaped structure called the *epiglottis*. Acting like a gate, the epiglottis directs air into the trachea and solids and liquids into the esophagus.

Lower Airway

The lower airway consists of the trachea, its branches, and the lungs. On inspiration, air travels through the upper airway and into the lower airway before reaching the lungs, where the actual gas exchange occurs (Figure 4-4). The trachea divides into the right and left mainstem bronchi. Each of the mainstem bronchi subdivides into several primary bronchi and then into bronchioles. Bronchioles (very small bronchial tubes) terminate at the alve-

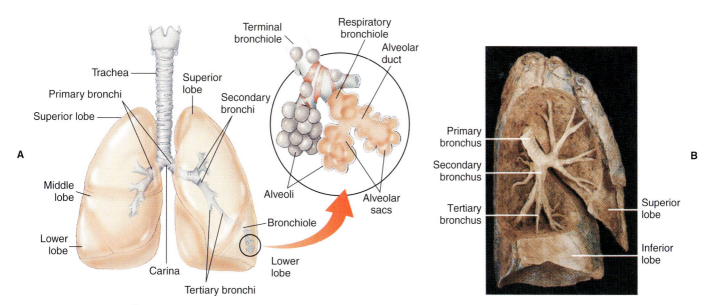

Figure 4-4   **A**, Drawing of the trachea and lungs. Inset shows enlargement of a terminal bronchiole and its associated alveoli. **B**, Branching of the bronchi in the left lung.

oli, which are tiny air sacs surrounded by capillaries. The alveoli are the site of gas exchange where the respiratory and circulatory systems meet.

Physiology

With each breath, air is drawn into the lungs. When atmospheric air reaches the alveoli, oxygen moves from the alveoli, across the alveolar-capillary membrane, and into the red blood cells (RBCs). The circulatory system then delivers the oxygen-carrying RBCs to the body tissues, where oxygen is used as fuel for metabolism.

As oxygen is transferred from inside the alveoli to the RBCs, carbon dioxide is exchanged in the opposite direction, from the plasma to the alveoli. Carbon dioxide, which is carried in the plasma, not in the RBCs, moves from the bloodstream, across the alveolar-capillary membrane, and into the alveoli, where it is eliminated during exhalation (Figure 4-5). Upon completion of this exchange, the oxygenated RBCs and plasma with a low carbon dioxide level return to the left side of the heart to be pumped to all the cells in the body.

Once at the cell, the oxygenated RBCs deliver their oxygen, which the cells then use as fuel for aerobic metabolism. Carbon dioxide, a byproduct of aerobic metabolism, is released into the blood plasma. Deoxygenated blood returns to the right side of the heart. The blood is pumped to the lungs, where it is again supplied with oxygen and the carbon dioxide is eliminated by diffusion.

The alveoli must be constantly replenished with a fresh supply of air that contains an adequate amount of oxygen. This replenishment of air, known as *ventilation*, is essential for the elimination of carbon dioxide. Ventilation is measurable. The size of each breath, called the *tidal volume*, multiplied by the ventilatory rate for 1 minute equals the minute volume:

Minute volume =
Tidal volume × Ventilatory rate per minute

During normal resting ventilation, about 500 mL of air is taken into the lungs. As mentioned previously, part of this volume, 150 mL, remains in the airway system as dead space and does not participate in gas exchange. If the tidal volume is 500 mL and the ventilatory rate is 14 breaths/min, then the minute volume can be calculated as follows:

Minute volume = 500 mL × 14 breaths/min
Minute volume = 7000 mL/min, or 7 L/min

Therefore, at rest, about 7 liters of air must move in and out of the lungs each minute to maintain adequate carbon dioxide elimination and oxygenation. If the minute volume falls below normal, the patient has inadequate ventilation, a condition called *hypoventilation*. Hypoventilation leads to a buildup of carbon dioxide in the body. Hypoventilation is common when head or chest trauma causes an altered breathing pattern or an inability to move the chest wall adequately. For example, a patient with rib fractures who is breathing quickly and shallowly because of the pain of the injury may

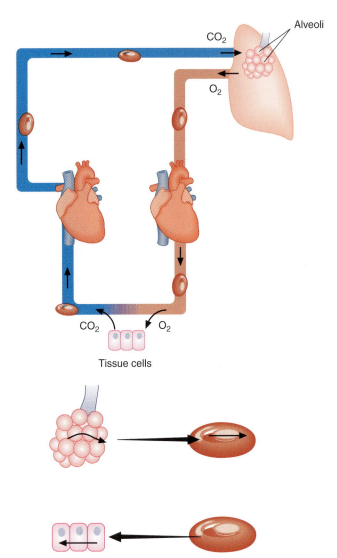

Figure 4-5 Oxygen moves into the red blood cells from the alveoli. The oxygen is transferred to the tissue cell on the hemoglobin molecule. After leaving the hemoglobin molecule, the oxygen travels into the tissue cell. Carbon dioxide travels in the reverse direction but not on the hemoglobin molecule. It travels in the plasma as carbon dioxide.

have a tidal volume of 100 mL and a ventilatory rate of 40 breaths/min. This patient's minute volume can be calculated as follows:

Minute volume = 100 mL × 40 breaths/min
Minute volume = 4000 mL/min, or 4 L/min

If 7 L/min is necessary for adequate gas exchange in a nontraumatized person at rest, then 4 L/min is far below what the body requires to effectively eliminate carbon dioxide, indicating hypoventilation. Further-

more, 150 mL of air is necessary to overcome dead space. If tidal volume is 100 mL, oxygenated air will never reach the alveoli. If left untreated, this hypoventilation will quickly lead to severe distress and ultimately death.

In the previous example the patient is hypoventilating even though the ventilatory rate is 40 breaths/min. The prehospital care provider must consider both ventilatory rate and depth when evaluating a patient's ability to exchange air. A common mistake is assuming that any patient with a fast ventilatory rate is hyperventilating. A much better judge of ventilatory status is the amount of carbon dioxide elimination. The effect of carbon dioxide elimination on metabolism is discussed with the Fick principle and aerobic and anaerobic metabolism in Chapter 6.

Prehospital assessment of ventilatory function must include an evaluation of how well a patient is taking in, diffusing, and delivering oxygen. Without proper intake and processing of oxygen, anaerobic metabolism will begin. In addition, effective ventilation must also be accomplished. A patient may accomplish ventilation completely, partially, or not at all. Prehospital care providers must act aggressively to assess and manage inadequacies in both oxygenation and ventilation.

Oxygenation and Ventilation of the Trauma Patient

The oxygenation process within the human body involves three phases:

1. *External respiration* is the transfer of oxygen molecules from the atmosphere to the blood. All alveolar oxygen exists as free gas; therefore each oxygen molecule exerts pressure. Increasing the percentage of oxygen in the inspired atmosphere will increase alveolar oxygen tension.
2. *Oxygen delivery* is the result of an oxygen transfer from the atmosphere to the RBC during ventilation and the transportation of these RBCs to the tissues via the cardiovascular system. This process primarily involves cardiac output, hemoglobin concentration, and oxyhemoglobin saturation. The volume of oxygen consumed by the body in 1 minute is known as *oxygen consumption*. In a sense, one could describe the RBCs as the body's "oxygen tankers." These tankers move along the vascular system "highways" to "off-load" their supply of oxygen at the body's distribution points, the capillary beds.

3. *Internal respiration* is the movement, or diffusion, of oxygen between the RBCs into the tissue cells. Metabolism normally occurs via glycolysis and the Kreb's cycle to produce energy and remove the byproducts of carbon dioxide and water. Because the actual exchange of oxygen between the RBCs and the tissues occurs in the thin-walled capillaries, oxygen available for consumption will be decreased if FiO$_2$ (fraction of inspired oxygen) is low (interruption in supply) or if circulation to the capillary beds is compromised (road blocked). The tissues cannot consume adequate amounts of oxygen if adequate amounts of oxygen are not available.

Adequate oxygenation depends on all three of these phases. Although the ability to assess tissue oxygenation in prehospital situations is improving rapidly, all trauma patients must receive appropriate ventilatory support with supplemental oxygen to ensure that hypoxia is corrected or averted entirely.

Pathophysiology

Trauma can affect the respiratory system's ability to adequately provide oxygen and eliminate carbon dioxide in the following ways:

1. Hypoventilation can result from loss of ventilatory drive, usually because of decreased neurologic function.
2. Hypoventilation can result from obstruction of airflow through the upper and lower airways.
3. Hypoventilation can be caused by decreased expansion of the lungs.
4. Hypoxia can result from decreased diffusion of oxygen across the alveolar-capillary membrane.
5. Hypoxia can be caused by decreased blood flow to the alveoli.
6. Hypoxia can result from the inability of the air to reach the capillaries, usually because the alveoli are filled with fluid or debris.
7. Hypoxia can be caused at the cellular level by decreased blood flow to the tissue cells.

The first three ways involve hypoventilation as a result of the reduction of minute volume. If left untreated, hypoventilation results in carbon dioxide buildup, acidosis, and eventually death. Management involves improving the patient's ventilatory rate and depth by correcting existing airway problems and assisting ventilation.

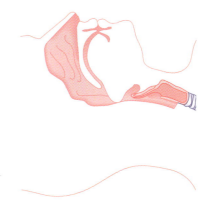

Figure 4-6   In an unconscious patient the tongue has lost its muscle tone and falls back into the hypopharynx, occluding the airway and preventing passage of oxygen into the trachea and lungs.

The following sections discuss the first two causes of inadequate ventilation—decreased neurologic function and mechanical obstruction. The third cause, a reduction in minute volume as a result of decreased pulmonary expansion, is discussed in more detail in Chapter 5. The last three causes are discussed in Chapter 6.

Decreased Neurologic Function

Decreased minute volume can be caused by two clinical conditions related to decreased neurologic function—flaccidity of the tongue and a decreased level of consciousness (LOC).

Flaccidity of the tongue associated with a reduced LOC allows the tongue to fall into a dependent position (toward the lowest area of the body). If a patient is supine, the base of the tongue will fall backward and occlude the hypopharynx (Figure 4-6). To prevent the tongue from occluding the hypopharynx, the prehospital care provider should manage the airway of any supine patient with a diminished LOC, regardless of whether signs of ventilatory compromise exist. Such patients may also require periodic suctioning. A decreased LOC will also affect ventilatory drive and may reduce the rate of ventilation, the volume of ventilation, or both. This reduction in minute volume may be temporary or permanent.

While covering auto racing events, the CART medical staff identified one crucial aspect of neurologically based temporary loss of ventilatory drive as a prehospital care concern. Ventilatory drive temporarily ceases within the first 4 to 5 minutes after a brain injury occurs. The resulting hypoxic injury to the brain can, in some cases, lead to permanent brain damage. If treated rapidly and aggressively, permanent brain injury can be avoided.

Recognition and treatment of hypoxia may be the most important factor in the prevention of permanent brain damage.

Mechanical Obstruction

Another cause of decreased minute volume is mechanical airway obstruction. The source of these obstructions may be neurologically influenced or purely mechanical in nature. Neurologic insults that alter the LOC may disrupt the "controls" that normally hold the tongue in an anatomically neutral (nonobstructing) position. If these "controls" are compromised, the tongue falls rearward, occluding the hypopharynx (see Figure 4-6).

Management of purely mechanical airway obstructions can challenge prehospital personnel. Foreign bodies in the oral cavity may become lodged and create occlusions in the hypopharynx or the larynx. Crush injuries to the larynx and edema of the vocal cords must be considered. Foreign bodies may originate from either the external environment or from within the patient's body. Patients with facial injuries present with two of the most common foreign bodies obstructions, blood and vomit. The prehospital care provider must clear these body fluids from the airway immediately.

Foreign bodies in the airway can be objects that were in the patient's mouth at the time of the injury, such as false teeth, chewing gum, tobacco, real teeth, and bone. Outside materials, such as glass from a broken windshield or any object that is near the patient's mouth at the time of injury, can also potentially threaten airway patency. Upper and lower airway obstructions can also be caused by bone or cartilage collapse as a result of a fractured larynx or trachea, by a mucous membrane avulsed from the hypopharynx or tongue, or by facial damage in which blood and fragments of bone and tissue create an obstruction.

Management

Airway Control

Ensuring a patent airway is the first priority of trauma management and resuscitation, and nothing is more crucial in prehospital airway management than appropriate assessment of the airway. Regardless of the manner in which the airway is managed, the prehospital care provider must keep the possibility of a cervical spine injury in mind. The use of any of these methods of airway control requires simultaneous stabilization of the cervical spine in a neutral position until the patient has been completely immobilized. Refer to Chapter 9 for more information about spinal immobilization.

ESSENTIAL SKILLS

Every prehospital care provider must have excellent command of a set of fundamental airway management skills. For prehospital care providers with limited training, these techniques may represent the full extent of their ability to manage an airway. However, if carefully applied, these skills will serve to maintain an airway and greatly decrease the risk of a patient dying from asphyxia. Even prehospital care providers who have been trained in more advanced airway techniques must maintain their ability to perform these essential skills as they provide an acceptable alternative when more advanced techniques fail.

Manual Clearing of the Airway.   The first step in airway management should be a quick visual inspection of the oropharyngeal cavity. Foreign material, such as pieces of food, or broken teeth and blood may be found in the mouth of a trauma patient. The prehospital care provider should use gloved fingers to sweep this material out of the mouth.

Manual Maneuvers.   In unresponsive patients, the tongue becomes flaccid, falling back and blocking the hypopharynx (see Figure 4-6). The tongue is the most common cause of airway obstruction. The prehospital care provider can easily use manual methods to clear this type of obstruction because the tongue is attached to the mandible (jaw) and moves forward with it. Any maneuver that moves the mandible forward will pull the tongue out of the hypopharynx:

- *Trauma jaw thrust.* In cases of suspected head, neck, or facial trauma, the prehospital care provider should maintain the cervical spine in a neutral inline position. The trauma jaw thrust maneuver allows the prehospital care provider to open the airway with little or no movement of the head and cervical spine (Figure 4-7). The mandible is thrust forward by placing the thumbs on each zygoma (cheekbone), placing the index and long fingers on the mandible, and at the same angle, pushing the mandible forward.

- *Trauma chin lift.* The trauma chin lift maneuver is ideally used to relieve a variety of anatomic airway obstructions in patients who are breathing spontaneously (Figure 4-8). The chin and lower incisors are grasped and then lifted to pull the mandible forward. The prehospital care provider must wear gloves to avoid body fluid contamination.

AIRWAY MANAGEMENT

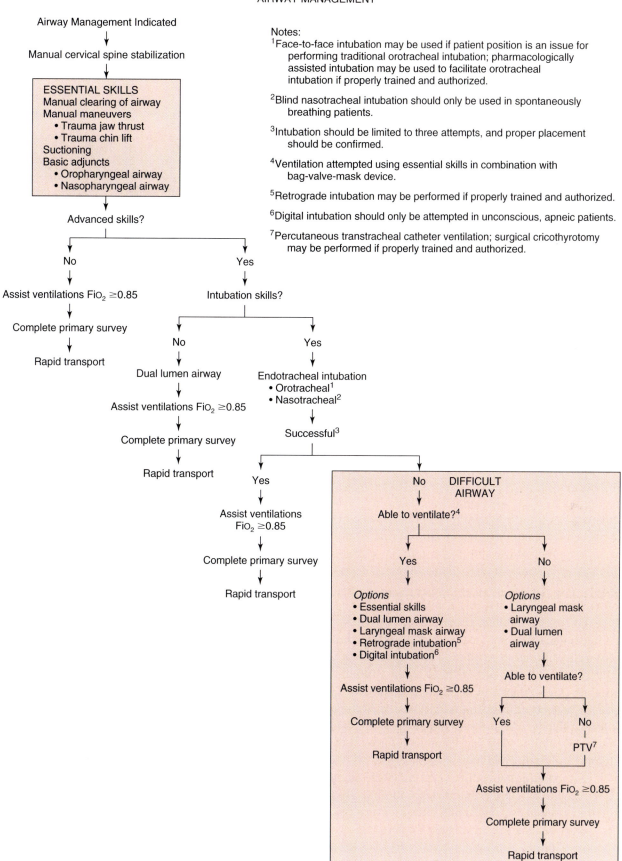

Notes:
[1]Face-to-face intubation may be used if patient position is an issue for performing traditional orotracheal intubation; pharmacologically assisted intubation may be used to facilitate orotracheal intubation if properly trained and authorized.

[2]Blind nasotracheal intubation should only be used in spontaneously breathing patients.

[3]Intubation should be limited to three attempts, and proper placement should be confirmed.

[4]Ventilation attempted using essential skills in combination with bag-valve-mask device.

[5]Retrograde intubation may be performed if properly trained and authorized.

[6]Digital intubation should only be attempted in unconscious, apneic patients.

[7]Percutaneous transtracheal catheter ventilation; surgical cricothyrotomy may be performed if properly trained and authorized.

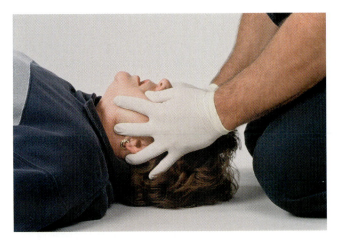

Figure 4-7   Trauma jaw thrust. The thumb is placed on each zygoma with the index and long fingers at the angle of the mandible. The mandible is lifted superiorly.

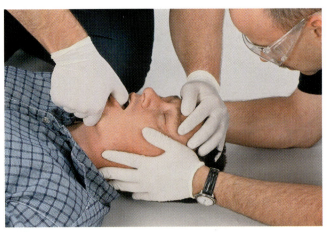

Figure 4-8   Trauma chin lift. The chin lift performs a function similar to that of the trauma jaw thrust. It moves the mandible forward by moving the tongue.

Both of these techniques result in movement of the lower mandible anteriorly (upward) and slightly caudal (toward the feet), pulling the tongue forward, away from the posterior airway, and opening the mouth. The trauma jaw thrust pushes the mandible forward, whereas the trauma chin lift pulls the mandible. The trauma jaw thrust and the trauma chin lift are modifications of the conventional jaw thrust and chin lift. The modifications allow the prehospital care provider to protect the patient's cervical spine while opening the airway by displacing the tongue from the posterior pharynx.

Suctioning.   A trauma patient may not be capable of effectively clearing the buildup of secretions, vomitus, blood, or foreign objects from the trachea. Providing suction is an important part of maintaining a patent airway.

The most significant complication of suctioning is that suctioning for prolonged periods of time will produce hypoxemia that may manifest as a cardiac abnormality, such as initial tachycardia. Preoxygenation of the trauma patient will help prevent hypoxemia. In addition, during an extended period of suctioning, cardiac dysrhythmias may occur from arterial hypoxemia, leading to myocardial hypoxemia and vagal stimulation secondary to tracheal irritation. True vagal stimulation may lead to profound bradycardia and hypotension.

When suctioning an endotracheal tube, the suction catheter should be made of soft material to limit trauma to the tracheal mucosa and to minimize frictional resistance. It must be long enough to pass the tip of the artificial airway (20 to 22 inches [50 to 55 cm]) and should have smooth ends to prevent mucosal trauma. The soft

catheter will probably not be effective in suctioning copious amounts of foreign material or fluid from the pharynx of a trauma patient, in which case the device of choice will be one with a tonsil-tip design.

While suctioning a patient who is intubated, aseptic procedures are vital, and the prehospital care provider should implement the following basic technique:

1. Preoxygenate the trauma patient with 100% oxygen (FiO_2 of 1.0).
2. Insert the catheter without suction. Suctioning is continued for up to 15 to 30 seconds.
3. Reoxygenate the patient and ventilate for at least 5 assisted ventilations.

The trauma patient who has yet to be intubated may require aggressive suctioning of the upper airway. Far larger amounts of blood and vomit can be in the airway upon EMS arrival than a suction unit can quickly clear. If this is the case, cervical spine stabilization should be undertaken and the patient rolled onto his or her side; gravity will then assist in clearing the airway. A rigid suction device should be used to clear the oropharynx.

Basic Adjuncts.   When manual airway maneuvers are unsuccessful at correcting an anatomic airway obstruction, the use of an artificial airway is the next step.

Oropharyngeal Airway.   The most commonly used artificial airway is the oropharyngeal airway (OPA) (Figure 4-9). The OPA is inserted in either a direct or inverted fashion.

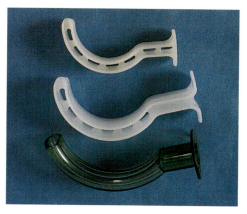

Figure 4-9   Oropharyngeal airways. (*From McSwain NE Jr, Paturas JL:* The basic EMT: comprehensive prehospital patient care, *ed 2, St Louis, 2001, Mosby.*)

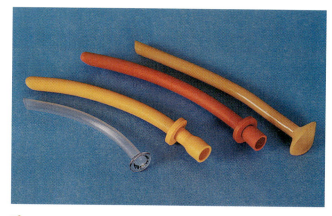

Figure 4-10   Nasopharyngeal airways. (*From McSwain NE Jr, Paturas JL:* The basic EMT: comprehensive prehospital patient care, *ed 2, St Louis, 2001, Mosby.*)

Indications
- Patient who is unable to maintain his or her airway
- To prevent an intubated patient from biting an endotracheal tube

Contraindications
- Patient who is conscious or semiconscious

Complications
- Because it stimilates the gag reflex, use of the OPA may lead to gagging, vomiting, and laryngospasm in patients who are conscious.

Nasopharyngeal Airway.   The nasopharyngeal airway (NPA) is a soft, rubberlike (latex) device that is inserted through one of the nares and then along the curvature of the posterior wall of the nasopharynx and oropharynx (Figure 4-10).

Indications
- Patient who is unable to maintain his or her airway

Contraindications
- No need for an airway adjunct

Complications
- Bleeding caused by insertion may be a complication

Dual Lumen Airways.   Dual lumen airways offer prehospital care providers a functional alternative airway. Many jurisdictions allow the use of these devices because minimal training is required to achieve competency. Prehospital care providers with advanced airway skills should consider these devices to be a useful back-up airway in instances where endotracheal intubation attempts are unsuccessful, even when rapid sequence intubation has been attempted. The greatest single advantage of these airways is that they may be inserted independent of the patient's position, which may be especially important in trauma patients with a high suspicion of cervical injury. The use of these airways is typically limited to patients 16 years of age or older who are at least 5 feet tall.

Indications
- *Basic providers.* If the provider is trained and authorized, the primary airway device for an unconscious trauma patient who lacks a gag reflex and is apneic or ventilating at a rate of less than 10 breaths/min
- *Advanced providers.* Alternative airway device when the provider is unable to perform endotracheal intubation and cannot easily ventilate the patient with a bag-valve-mask (BVM) device and an OPA or NPA

Contraindications
- Intact gag reflex
- Known esophageal disease
- Recent ingestions of caustic substances

Complications
- Gagging and vomiting, if gag reflex is intact
- Damage to the esophagus
- Hypoxia if ventilated using the wrong lumen

ENDOTRACHEAL INTUBATION

Of all of the emergency and trauma care intervention skills performed by prehospital care providers, endotracheal intubation is one of the most important and can

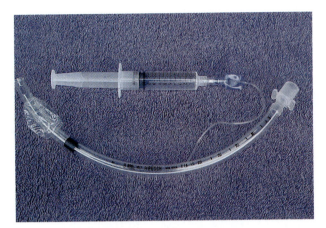

Figure 4-11 Endotracheal tube.

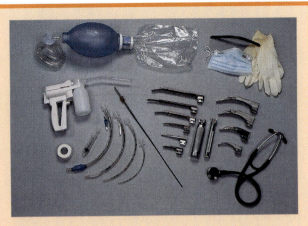

Figure 4-12 Equipment for endotracheal intubation. (*From McSwain NE Jr, Paturas JL:* The basic EMT: comprehensive prehospital patient care, *ed 2, St Louis, 2001, Mosby.*)

have a dramatic effect on a trauma patient's outcome. Endotracheal intubation is the most desirable method for achieving maximum control of the airway in trauma patients who are either apneic or require assisted ventilation (Figure 4-11). Endotracheal intubation is the prefered method of airway control because it does the following:

- Isolates the airway
- Allows for ventilation with 100% oxygen (FiO_2 of 1.0)
- Eliminates the need to maintain an adequate mask-to-face seal
- Significantly decreases the risk of aspiration (vomitus, foreign material, or blood)
- Facilitates deep tracheal suctioning
- Prevents gastric insufflation
- Provides an additional route for medication administration

Indications
- Patient who is unable to protect his or her airway
- Patient with significant oxygenation problem, requiring administration of high concentrations of oxygen
- Patient with significant ventilatory impairment, requiring assisted ventilations

Contraindications
- Lack of training in technique
- Lack of proper indications
- Close proximity to receiving facility (relative contraindication)

Complications
- Hypoxemia from prolonged intubation attempts
- Trauma to the airway with resultant hemorrhage
- Right mainstem bronchus intubation
- Esophageal intubation

As with any advanced life support skill, prehospital care providers must have the proper equipment. The standard components of an intubation kit should include the following {Figure 4-12}:
- Laryngoscope with adult- and pediatric-sized straight and curved blades
- Extra batteries and spare light bulbs
- Suction machine
- Adult- and pediatric-sized endotracheal tubes
- Stylet
- 10 mL syringe
- Water-soluble lubricant
- Magill forceps
- End-tidal detection device (ETDD) for end-tidal carbon dioxide detection
- Tube-securing device

- Vomiting leading to aspiration
- Loose or broken teeth
- Injury to the vocal cords
- Conversion of a cervical spine injury without neurologic deficit to one with neurologic deficit

Alternative Methods. The prehospital care provider may select from several alternative methods for performing endotracheal intubation. The method of choice depends on such factors as the patient's needs, the level of urgency (i.e., orotracheal vs. nasotracheal), patient positioning (face-to-face), or training and scope of practice (pharmacologically assisted intubation). Regardless of the method selected, the patient's head and neck should be stabilized in a neutral position during the procedure and until spinal immobilization is completed. In general, the provider should not attempt to place an endotracheal tube more than three times. At that point a back-up technique should be considered.

Orotracheal Intubation.   Orotracheal intubation involves placing an endotracheal tube into the trachea through the mouth. The nontrauma patient is often placed in a "sniffing" position to facilitate intubation. Because this position hyperextends the cervical spine at C1-C2 (the second most common site for cervical spine fractures in the trauma patient) and hyperflexes it at C5-C6 (the most common site for cervical spine fractures in the trauma patient), it should not be used for trauma patients (Figure 4-13).

Nasotracheal Intubation.   In conscious trauma patients or in those with an intact gag reflex, the prehospital care provider may have difficulty accomplishing endotracheal intubation. If spontaneous ventilations are present, the provider may attempt blind nasotracheal intubation (BNTI) only if the benefit outweighs the risk. When performing BNTI the patient *should* be breathing for the provider to ensure that the tube is more easily passed through the vocal cords. Extreme caution should be exercised when attempting nasotracheal intubation in the presence of midface trauma or fractures. Advancing the tube in a superior direction, rather than directly posterior, and using significant force when resistance is encountered may lead to passage of the tube into the cranial vault with damage to the brain. This is an extremely rare event that can be prevented by use of proper technique. Apnea is a relative contraindication specific to BNTI. In general, no stylet is used when BNTI is performed.

Face-to-Face Intubation.   Face-to-face intubations are indicated when standard trauma intubation techniques cannot be used because of the inability of the rescuer to assume the standard position at the head of the trauma patient. These situations may include but are not limited to the following:

- Vehicle entrapment
- Pinning of the patient in rubble

Pharmacologically Assisted Intubation.   Intubation using pharmacologic agents may occasionally be required to facilitate endotracheal tube placement in injured patients. In skilled hands, this technique can facilitate effective airway control when other methods fail

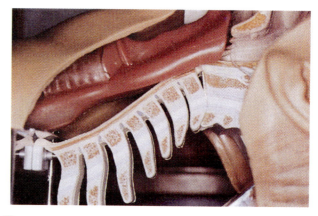

Figure 4-13   Placing the patient's head in the sniffing position provides ideal visualization of the larynx through the mouth. However, such positioning hyperextends the patient's neck at C1 and C2 and hyperflexes it at C5 and C6. These are the two most common points of fracture of the cervical spine.

or are otherwise not acceptable. To maximize the effectiveness of this procedure and ensure patient safety, personnel using drugs to assist with intubation must be familiar with applicable local protocols, medications, and indications for use of the technique. The use of drugs to assist with intubation, particularly rapid sequence intubation (RSI), is not without risk. Pharmacologically assisted intubation is a procedure of necessity, not convenience. Pharmacologically assisted intubation falls into two categories:

1. *Intubation using sedatives or narcotics.* Medications such as diazepam, midazolam, fentanyl, or morphine are used alone or in combination, with the goal being to relax the patient enough to permit intubation but not to abolish protective reflexes or breathing.
2. *Rapid sequence intubation (RSI) using paralytic agents.* The patient is chemically paralyzed after first being sedated. This provides complete muscle paralysis but removes all protective reflexes and causes apnea. Studies of this method of airway management have generally been positive with intubation success rates reported in the mid-90% range and with relatively few complications.

However, pharmacologically assisted intubation of any type requires time to accomplish. In every trauma patient for whom the prehospital care provider considers pharmacologically assisted intubation, he or she must carefully weigh the benefits of securing an airway against the additional time spent on the scene to perform the procedure.

Indications
- Any patient who requires a secure airway and is difficult to intubate because of uncooperative behavior (as induced by hypoxia, traumatic brain injury, hypotension, or intoxication) is a candidate for this procedure.

Relative Contraindications
- Availability of an alternative airway (e.g., dual lumen)
- Severe facial trauma that would impair or preclude successful intubation
- Neck deformity or swelling that complicates or precludes placement of a surgical airway
- Known allergies to indicated medications
- Medical problems that would preclude use of indicated medications
- Inability to intubate

Complications
- Inability to insert the endotracheal tube in a sedated or paralyzed patient no longer able to protect his or her airway or breathe spontaneously; patients who are medicated and then cannot be intubated require prolonged BVM ventilation until the medication wears off
- Development of hypoxia or hypercarbia during prolonged intubation attempts
- Aspiration
- Hypotension; virtually all of the drugs have a side effect of decreasing blood pressure. Patients who are

Table 4-1   Common Drugs Used for Pharmacologically Assisted Intubation

Drug	Dose (adult)	Dose (pediatric)	Indication	Complications/Side effects
PRETREATMENT				
Oxygen	High flow Assist ventilation as needed to achieve oxygen saturation of 100% if possible	High flow Assist ventilation as needed to achieve oxygen saturation of 100% if possible	All patients undergoing pharmacologic assisted intubation	
Lidocaine	1.5 mg/kg	1.5 mg/kg IV	Brain injury	Seizure
Atropine		0.01-0.02 mg/kg IV	Pediatric intubation, prevention of bradycardia and excess secretions	Tachycardia
INDUCTION OF SEDATION				
Midazolam (Versed)	0.1-0.15 mg/kg up to 0.3 mg/kg IV	0.1-0.15 mg/kg up to 0.3 mg/kg IV	Sedation	Respiratory depression/apnea, hypotension
Fentanyl (Sublimaze)	2-3 μg/kg IV	1-3 μg/kg IV	Sedation	Respiratory depression/apnea, hypotension, bradycardia
Etomidate	0.2-0.3 mg/kg IV	Not approved for patients <10 years of age	Sedation, induced anesthesia	Apnea, hypotension, vomiting
CHEMICAL PARALYSIS				
Succinylcholine	1-2 mg/kg	1-2 mg/kg	Muscle relaxation and paralysis (short duration)	Hyperkalemia, muscle fasciculations
Vecuronium	0.1 mg/kg	0.1 mg/kg	Muscle relaxation and paralysis (intermediate duration)	Hypotension
Pancuronium (Pavulon)	0.04-0.1 mg/kg	0.04-0.1 mg/kg	Muscle relaxation and paralysis (long duration)	Tachycardia, hypertension, salivation

mildly or moderately hypovolemic but compensating may have a profound drop in their blood pressure associated with the intravenous administration of these drugs. Caution must always be exercised whenever the use of medications for intubation is considered (Table 4-1).

Verification of Endotracheal Tube Placement. Once intubation has been performed, specific efforts must be taken to ensure that the tube has been properly placed in the trachea. An improperly positioned endotracheal tube, if unrecognized for only a brief period, may result in profound hypoxia with resultant brain injury (hypoxic encephalopathy) and even death. Therefore the prehospital care provider must make reasonable efforts to ensure proper placement. Techniques to verify intubation include the use of both clinical assessments and adjunctive devices. Clinical assessments include the following:

- Direct visualization of the tube passing through the vocal cords
- Presence of bilateral breath sounds (auscultate laterally below the axilla) *and* absence of air sounds over the epigastrium
- Visualization of the chest rising and falling during ventilation
- Fogging (water vapor condensation) in the endotracheal tube on expiration

---

Sample Protocol for RSI

1. Ensure availability of required equipment.
   a. Oxygen supply
   b. Bag-valve-mask of appropriate size and type
   c. Nonrebreather mask
   d. Laryngoscope with blades
   e. Endotracheal tubes
   f. Surgical and alternative airway equipment
   g. RSI medications
   h. Materials or devices to secure the endotracheal tube after placement
   i. Suction equipment
2. Ensure that a minimum of one, but preferably two, patent IV lines is present.
3. Preoxygenate the patient using a nonrebreathing mask or bag-valve-mask with 100% oxygen. Preoxygenation for 3 to 4 minutes is preferred.
4. Apply cardiac and pulse oximetry monitors.
5. If the patient is conscious, strongly consider the use of sedative agents.
6. Consider the administration of sedative agents and lidocaine in the presence of potential or confirmed traumatic brain injury (TBI).
7. After administration of paralytic agents, use the Sellick (cricoid pressure) maneuver to decrease the potential for aspiration.
8. Confirm tube placement immediately after intubation. Continuous electrocardiogram (ECG) and pulse oximeter monitoring is required during and after RSI. Reconfirm tube placement periodically throughout transport and each time the patient is moved.
9. Use repeat doses of paralytic agents as needed to maintain paralysis.

PROCEDURE

1. Assemble the required equipment.
2. Ensure the patency of the IV lines.
3. Preoxygenate the patient with 100% oxygen for approximately 3 to 4 minutes if possible.
4. Place the patient on ECG and pulse oximeter monitors.
5. Administer a sedative, such as midazolam, if appropriate.
6. In the presence of confirmed or potential TBI, administer lidocaine, 1.5 mg/kg, 2 to 3 minutes before administration of a paralytic agent.
7. Give pediatric patients atropine, 0.01-0.02 mg/kg, 1 to 3 minutes before paralytic administration to minimize the vagal response to intubation.
8. Administer a short-acting paralytic agent, such as succinylcholine IV. Paralysis and relaxation should occur within 30 seconds.
   a. Adult: 1 to 2 mg/kg
   b. Pediatric: 1 to 2 mg/kg
9. Insert an endotracheal tube. If initial attempts are unsuccessful, precede repeat attempts with preoxygenation.
10. Confirm the endotracheal tube placement.
11. If repetitive attempts to achieve endotracheal intubation fail, consider placement of an alternative or surgical airway.
12. Use doses of a long-acting paralytic agent, such as vecuronium, to continue paralysis.
    a. Initial dose: 0.1 mg/kg IV push
    b. Subsequent doses: 0.01 mg/kg every 30-45 min (Requirements vary with individual patients.)

Unfortunately, none of these techniques is 100% reliable *by itself* for verifying proper tube placement. Therefore prudent practice involves assessing and documenting *all* of these clinical signs, if possible. On rare occasions, because of difficult anatomy, visualization of the tube passing through the vocal cords may not possible. In a moving vehicle (ground or aeromedical), engine noise may make auscultation of breath sounds nearly impossible. Obesity and chronic obstructive pulmonary disease (COPD) may interfere with the ability to see chest movement during ventilation.

Adjunctive devices include the following:

- Esophageal detector device
- Carbon dioxide monitoring
- Colorimetric carbon dioxide detector
- End-tidal carbon dioxide monitoring (capnography)
- Pulse oximetry

As with the clinical assessments, none of these adjuncts is 100% accurate in all patients. In a patient with a perfusing rhythm, end-tidal carbon dioxide monitoring (capnography) serves as the "gold standard" for determining endotracheal placement of an airway in the operating room. This technique should be used in the prehospital setting if it is available. Patients in cardiopulmonary arrest do not generate carbon dioxide, and therefore neither colorimetric detectors nor capnography may be useful in patients who lack a perfusing cardiac rhythm.

Because none of these techniques is universally reliable, all of the clinical assessments noted previously should be performed, unless impractical, followed by use of at least one of the adjunctive devices. Because of the cost of performing capnography, most EMS systems require a combination of clinical assessments and a colorimetric carbon dioxide detector or esophageal detector device. In any instance, if any of the techniques used to verify proper placement suggest that the tube may not be properly positioned, the tube should be immediately removed and reinserted, with placement reverified. All of the techniques used to verify tube placement should be noted on the patient care report.

Securing the Endotracheal Tube. Once endotracheal intubation has been performed and proper placement verified, the depth of tube insertion at the central incisors (front teeth) should be noted. Next, the endotracheal tube must be secured in place. The most common method used is to tape the tube to the patient's face. Unfortunately, blood and secretions often prevent the tape from adhering satisfactorily, allowing movement and potential dislodging of the endotracheal tube. Several commercially available products exist that may serve to adequately secure the airway. Ideally, if sufficient personnel are present, someone should be assigned the task of manually holding the tube in proper position to ensure that it does not move.

Continuous pulse oximetry should be considered *necessary* for all patients who require endotracheal intubation. Any decline in the pulse oximetry reading (SpO_2), or development of cyanosis, should prompt the prehospital care provider to reverify that the tube remains in the trachea. Additionally, an endotracheal tube may also become dislodged during any movement of the patient. Tube placement should be reverified *after every move of a patient,* such as logrolling to a long backboard or carrying the patient down a staircase.

BACK-UP TECHNIQUES

If the advanced prehospital care provider has not succeeded in properly placing an endotracheal tube in three attempts, he or she should reassess the ability to manage the airway using the essential skills described previously and ventilating with a BVM device. *If the receiving facility is reasonably close, these techniques may be the most prudent option for airway management when faced with a brief transport time.* If the closest appropriate facility is more distant, then one of the following back-up techniques may be considered.

Retrograde Intubation. In the prehospital setting, retrograde tracheal intubation (RI) is potentially useful because the presence of blood or secretions does not hinder insertion as it may in more traditional intubation methods. RI, although comparatively time-consuming, is a less invasive (and less risky) procedure than surgical cricothyrotomy when the cervical spine is properly stabilized and when orotracheal or nasotracheal intubation attempts have failed.

RI is a fairly straightforward procedure. The prehospital care provider inserts a needle (large enough to accommodate the guide wire) into the caudal aspect of the cricothyroid membrane. A guide wire is advanced through the needle into the oropharynx. An endotracheal tube is then advanced over the guide wire and into the oropharynx. When resistance at attempts to further advance the tube is encountered, the guide wire is then pulled completely out of the neck and the endotracheal tube is advanced as the guide wire exits the neck. Because these procedures are often difficult to perform expediently, RI is generally not recommended for use in apneic patients.

Indications

- Patients in whom endotracheal intubation failed but for whom ventilations can be assisted with a BVM device

Relative Contraindications

- Apneic patient
- Close proximity to receiving facility
- Insufficient training

Complications

- Damage to the vocal cords and larynx
- Bleeding at the puncture site
- Esophageal intubation
- Hypoxia or hypercarbia during the procedure

Digital Intubation. Digital, or tactile, intubation was a precursor to the current use of laryngoscopes for endotracheal intubation. Essentially, the intubator's fingers act in a fashion similar to a laryngoscope blade by manipulating the epiglottis and acting as a guide for placement of the endotracheal tube.

Indications

- Patients in whom endotracheal intubation failed but for whom ventilations can be assisted with a BVM device
- When intubation equipment is in short supply or fails
- When the airway is obscured or blocked because of large volumes of blood or vomitus
- Entrapment with inability to perform face-to-face intubation

Contraindications

- Any patient who is not comatose and may bite the intubator's fingers (a dental clamp or bite stick may be used to hold the patient's mouth open)

Complications

- Esophageal intubation
- Lacerations or crush injuries to the prehospital care provider's fingers
- Hypoxia or hypercarbia during the procedure
- Damage to the vocal cords

Laryngeal Mask Airway. The laryngeal mask airway (LMA) is another alternative for unconscious or seriously obtunded adult and pediatric patients. The device consists of an inflatable silicone ring attached diagonally to a silicone tube (Figure 4-14). When in-

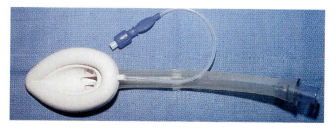

Figure 4-14 Laryngeal mask airway.

serted, the ring creates a low pressure seal between the LMA and the glottic opening without direct insertion of the device into the larynx.

Advantages of the LMA include the following:

- The device is designed for blind insertion. Direct visualization of the trachea and vocal cords is unnecessary.
- With proper cleaning and storage, the LMA can be reused multiple times.
- Disposable LMAs are now available.
- The LMA is available in a range of sizes to accommodate both pediatric and adult patient groups.

One limitation of the LMA is the high initial acquisition cost. Prehospital use of the LMA has thus far been more prevalent in Europe than in North America. A recent development is the introduction of an "intubating LMA." This device inserts like the original LMA, but a flexible endotracheal tube is then passed though the LMA, intubating the trachea. This secures the airway without the need to visualize the vocal cords.

Indications

- Device for use when unable to perform endotracheal intubation and the patient cannot be ventilated using a BVM device

Contraindications

- When endotracheal intubation can be performed
- Insufficient training

Complications

- Aspiration because it does not completely prevent regurgitation and protect the trachea
- Laryngospasm

Percutaneous Transtracheal Ventilation. In rare instances, a trauma patient's airway obstruction cannot be relieved by the methods previously discussed. In these situations, a needle tracheostomy may be performed using a percutaneously placed catheter.

Advantages of percutaneous transtracheal ventilation (PTV) include the following:

- Ease of access (landmarks usually easily recognized)
- Ease of insertion
- Minimal equipment required
- No incision necessary
- Minimal education required

Indications
- When all other alternative methods of airway management fail or are impractical and the patient cannot be ventilated with a BVM device

Contraindications
- Insufficient training
- Lack of proper equipment
- Ability to secure airway by another technique described previously or ability to ventilate with a BVM device

Complications
- Hypercarbia from prolonged use (carbon dioxide elimination not as effective as with other methods of ventilation)
- Damage to surrounding structures, including the larynx, thyroid gland, carotid arteries, jugular veins, and esophagus

Surgical Cricothyrotomy. Surgical cricothyrotomy involves the creation of a surgical opening in the cricothyroid membrane, which lies between the larynx and the cricoid cartilage. In most patients, the skin is very thin in this location, making it amenable to immediate access to the airway. This should be considered a technique of "last resort" in prehospital airway management.

The use of this surgical airway in the prehospital arena is controversial. Proficient endotracheal intubation skills should minimize the need to even consider its use. *Surgical cricothyrotomy should never be the initial airway control method.* Insufficient data exist at this time to support a recommendation that surgical cricothyrotomy be established as a national standard for routine use for prehospital airway management. Local protocols should govern the implementation of surgical cricothyrotomy.

Indications
- Massive midface trauma precluding the use of a BVM device

- Inability to control the airway using less invasive maneuvers
- Ongoing tracheobronchial hemorrhage

Contraindications
- Any patient who can be safely intubated, either orally or nasally
- Patients with laryngotracheal injuries
- Children under 10 years of age
- Patients with acute laryngeal disease of traumatic or infectious origin
- Insufficient training

Complications
- Prolonged procedure time
- Hemorrhage
- Aspiration
- Misplacement or false passage of the endotracheal tube
- Injury to neck structures or vessels
- Perforation of the esophagus

CONTINUOUS QUALITY IMPROVEMENT

The service medical director or his or her designate should individually review all out-of-hospital uses of medications for intubation or invasive airway techniques. Specific points should include the following:

- Adherence to protocol and procedures
- Proper indications for the use of medications
- Proper documentation of drug dosage routes and monitoring of the patient during and after intubation
- Confirmation of tube placement procedures
- Outcome and complications

Ventilatory Devices

All trauma patients must receive appropriate ventilatory support with supplemental oxygen to ensure that hypoxia is corrected or averted entirely. In deciding which method or equipment to use, prehospital care providers should consider the following devices and their respective oxygen concentrations (Table 4-2).

MASKS

Regardless of which mask the prehospital care provider chooses to support ventilation of the trauma patient, he or she must consider several issues. The ideal mask has a good fit; is equipped with a one-way valve; is made of a transparent material; has an oxygen insufflation port (15 to 22 mm); and is available in infant, pediatric, and adult sizes. Mouth-to-mask ventilation satisfactorily delivers adequate tidal volumes by ensuring a tight face seal even when performed by those who do not use the skill often.

BAG-VALVE-MASK

The BVM consists of a self-inflating bag and a nonrebreathing device; it can be used with basic or advanced artificial airways. Most of the BVM devices currently on the market have a volume of 1600 mL and can deliver an oxygen concentration of 90% to 100%. Some models have a built-in colorimetric carbon dioxide detector. However, a *single* provider attempting to ventilate with a BVM may create poor tidal volumes because it is difficult to create a tight face seal and squeeze the bag adequately. A prehospital care provider must continually practice this skill to ensure that his or her technique is effective so that the trauma patient receives adequate ventilatory support.

MANUALLY TRIGGERED (OXYGEN-POWERED) DEVICES

Manually triggered devices can deliver oxygen concentrations of 100%. Because the prehospital care provider cannot feel compliance of the chest during the ventilation process, he or she must take care not to overinflate the lung. Maintaining a tight face seal with this device is easy because the trigger mechanism requires only one hand to operate. Complications may include gastric distention, lack of tactile feel for inflation, overinflation of the lung, barotrauma, and lung rupture. These devices should not be used in the field except in unusual circumstances.

Evaluation

PULSE OXIMETRY

Over the past few years, usage of pulse oximetry has increased in the prehospital environment. Appropriate use of pulse oximetry devices allows prehospital care providers to detect early pulmonary compromise or cardiovascular deterioration before physical signs are evident. Pulse oximeters are particularly useful in prehospital applications because of their high reliability, portability, ease of application, and applicability across all age ranges and races (Figure 4-15).

Pulse oximeters provide measurements of arterial oxyhemoglobin saturation (SpO_2) and pulse rate. SpO_2 is determined by measuring the absorption ratio of red and infrared light passed through tissue. A small microprocessor correlates changes in light absorption caused by the pulsation of blood through vascular beds to determine arterial saturation and pulse rate. Normal SpO_2 is between 93% and 95%. When SpO_2 falls below 90%, severe compromise of oxygen delivery to the tissues is most likely present.

To ensure accurate pulse oximetry readings, the prehospital care provider should follow these general guidelines:

- Use the appropriate size and type of sensor.
- Ensure proper alignment of sensor light.
- Ensure that sources and photo detectors are clean, dry, and in good repair.
- Avoid sensor placement on grossly edematous sites.

Table 4-2	Ventilatory Devices and Oxygen Concentration	
Device procedure	**Liter flow (LPM)**	**Oxygen concentration***
WITHOUT SUPPLEMENTAL OXYGEN		
Mouth-to-mouth	N/A	16%
Mouth-to-mask	N/A	16%
Bag-valve-mask (BVM)	N/A	21%
WITH SUPPLEMENTAL OXYGEN		
Nasal cannula	1-6	24%-45%
Mouth-to-mask	10	50%
Simple face mask	8-10	40%-60%
BVM without reservoir	8-10	40%-60%
Partial rebreather mask	6	60%
Simple mask with reservoir	6	60%
BVM with reservoir	10-15	90%-100%
Nonrebreather mask with reservoir	10-15	90%-100%
Demand valve	Source	90%-100%

*Percentages indicated are approximate.

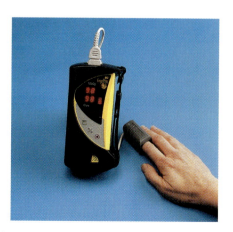

Figure 4-15   Pulse oximeter. (*From Sanders MJ: Mosby's paramedic textbook, ed 2, St Louis, 2000, Mosby.*)

Common problems that can produce inaccurate SpO_2 measurement include the following:

- Excessive motion
- Moisture in SpO_2 sensors
- Improper sensor application and placement
- Poor patient perfusion or vasoconstriction from hypothermia
- Anemia

In a critical trauma patient, pulse oximetry may be less than accurate because of poor capillary perfusion status. Therefore pulse oximetry is only a valuable addition to the prehospital care provider's "tool box" when combined with a thorough knowledge of trauma pathophysiology and strong assessment and intervention skills.

CAPNOGRAPHY

Capnography, or end-tidal carbon dioxide ($ETCO_2$) monitoring, has been used in critical care units for years. Recent advances in technology have allowed smaller more durable units to be produced for prehospital use (Figure 4-16). Capnography measures the partial pressure of carbon dioxide ($ETCO_2$) in a sample of gas. If this sample is taken at the end of exhalation, it correlates closely to arterial $PaCO_2$.

Most critical care units within the hospital setting use the mainstream technique. This technique places a sensor directly into the "main stream" of the exhaled gas. In the patient being ventilated with a BVM, the sensor is placed between the BVM and the endotracheal tube. In the critical patient, the $PaCO_2$ is generally 2 to 5 mm Hg higher than the $ETCO_2$. (A normal $ETCO_2$ reading in a critical trauma patient is between 30 and 40 mm Hg). Although these readings may not be totally reflective of the

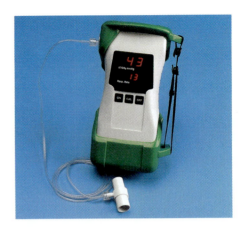

Figure 4-16 Handheld end-tidal carbon dioxide detector. (*From Sanders MJ: Mosby's paramedic textbook, ed 2, St Louis, 2000, Mosby.*)

patients $PaCO_2$, maintaining readings between normal levels will, in most cases, be beneficial to the patient.

Although capnography correlates closely to $PaCO_2$, certain conditions will cause variations in accuracy. These conditions are commonly seen in the prehospital environment and include severe hypotension, high intrathoracic pressure, and any increase in dead space ventilation, such as with a pulmonary embolism.

Continuous capnography provides another tool in the prehospital management of a trauma patient, but the prehospital care provider should look at all information about a patient. Capnography should be used as a tool to monitor endotracheal tube placement and to continuously monitor patient status during transport. The prehospital care provider should base initial transport decisions on physical and environmental conditions. He or she should not take time to place the patient on monitors if the patient is losing blood.

Summary

The trauma patient is susceptible to various mechanisms by which ventilation and gas exchange may be impaired. Injuries of the chest, airway obstruction, central nervous system injury, and hemorrhage can all result in inadequate tissue perfusion. A prehospital care provider must understand the pathophysiology of inadequate tissue perfusion and the mechanisms by which it occurs to recognize the patient in need of airway management and ventilatory support.

The quality and timeliness with which the prehospital care provider delivers airway care in the field directly affects a patient's long-term outcome and length of hospital stay. Therefore the first action in caring for any patient, once the scene assessment is complete, is to assess the status of airway and breathing. Aggressive airway management is the highest priority of care of the trauma patient. To achieve this, the prehospital care provider must continually practice airway management skills and stay abreast of new information, techniques, and technology related to airway management.

Scenario Solution

Physical evidence at the scene suggests that the driver has likely been subjected to kinetic forces capable of creating life-threatening injuries. The position of the patient suggests that multiple impacts have occurred.

The driver exhibits several signs of airway compromise and ventilatory insufficiency. His ventilations are sonorous and irregular, he has an altered level of consciousness, and he requires frequent suctioning. Bleeding from the nares and ears and the early presence of "raccoon eyes" strongly suggest the presence of a basilar skull fracture. The primary survey indicates a rapidly deteriorating patient who requires aggressive airway care and rapid transport.

First responder personnel should already be administering oxygen with ventilatory assistance via a BVM. If this has not been done, you should begin oxygen therapy immediately. You should continue ventilatory support and cervical spine stabilization while preparing for endotracheal intubation. You must be careful to ensure that the airway remains clear and that manual ventilations are effective.

You should orally intubate the patient with an appropriately sized endotracheal tube. Cervical spine stabilization must continue before, during, and after the intubation attempt. Once you place the endotracheal tube, you must ensure proper positioning of the endotracheal tube via auscultation of breath sounds, the use of an esophageal intubation detector, end-tidal capnometry (if available), or another adjunctive device. You should thoroughly suction the patient before transport and as often as needed thereafter.

After you completely immobilize the patient and secure the endotracheal tube, initiate transport without delay. You may establish intravenous access while the patient is en route to a trauma receiving facility. Take care to maintain the effectiveness of immobilization efforts, and frequently reassess the patient's condition. To ensure proper activation of the receiving facility's trauma response, early notification from the scene or during transport is necessary. Upon arrival at the trauma center, concisely convey all pertinent information regarding the incident, the patient, and your medical interventions to the receiving physician or other appropriate trauma team member.

Review Questions

Answers are provided on p. 414.

1. Adequacy of ventilation is expressed as which of the following?
   a. Tidal volume
   b. Ventilatory rate
   c. Minute volume
   d. Alveolar volume

2. Which of the following may result in hypoventilation?
   a. Decreased blood flow to the alveoli
   b. Decreased diffusion of gases across the alveolar-capillary membrane
   c. Decreased blood flow to the tissues
   d. Decreased expansion of the lungs

3. Which of the following devices, when properly inserted, prevents aspiration of gastric contents?
   a. Endotracheal tube
   b. Laryngeal mask airway
   c. Both of the above
   d. None of the above

4. Which of the following is NOT an advantage of retrograde intubation?
   a. Can be performed quickly in the apneic patient
   b. Is less invasive than surgical cricothyroidotomy
   c. Can be performed in the presence of blood or secretions in the upper airway
   d. Does not require direct laryngoscopy

5. Complications of manually triggered oxygen-powered devices include all of the following EXCEPT:
   a. Gastric distention
   b. Limited ventilatory volume
   c. Barotrauma of the lung

   d. Inability to assess lung compliance

6. Which of the following is the primary disadvantage of bag-valve-mask (BVM) ventilation?
   a. Difficulty achieving adequate tidal volume
   b. Difficulty achieving adequate ventilatory rate
   c. Difficulty achieving high oxygen concentration

   d. Difficulty assessing lung compliance

7. How does ET_{CO_2} correlate with Pa_{CO_2}?
   a. 5 mm higher
   b. 5 mm lower
   c. 20 mm higher
   d. 20 mm lower

REFERENCES

Advanced Trauma Life Support, Committee on Trauma, American College of Surgeons: *Airway and ventilatory management*, Chicago, 2002, Author.

Falcone RE, Herron H, Dean B, Werman H: Emergency scene endotracheal intubation before and after the introduction of a rapid sequence induction protocol, *Air Med J* 15:163, 1996.

Frame SB, Simon JM, Kerstein MD, McSwain NE Jr: Percutaneous transtracheal catheter ventilation (PTCV) in complete airway obstruction: a canine model, *J Trauma* 29:774, 1989.

Gerich TG, Schmidt U, Hubrich V et al: Prehospital airway management in the acutely injured patient: role of surgical cricothyrotomy revisited, *J Trauma* 45:312, 1998.

Jacobson LE, Gomez GA, Sobieray RJ et al: Surgical cricothyroidotomy in trauma patients: analysis of its use by paramedics in the field, *J Trauma* 41:15, 1996.

Krisanda TJ, Eitel DR, Hess D et al: An analysis of invasive airway management in a suburban emergency medical services system, *Prehospital Disaster Med* 7:121, 1992.

O'Connor RE, Swor RA: Verification of endotracheal tube placement following intubation, *Prehosp Emerg Care* 3: 248, 1999.

Sloane C, Vilke GM, Chan TC et al: Rapid sequence intubation in the field versus hospital in trauma patients, *J Emerg Med* 19:259, 2000.

Walls RM, Luten RC, Murphy MF, Schneider RE, editors: *Manual of emergency airway management*, Philadelphia, 2000, Lippincott Williams and Wilkins.

SUGGESTED READING

Fortune JB, Judkins DG, Scanzaroli D et al: Efficacy of prehospital surgical cricothyrotomy in trauma patients, *J Trauma* 42:832, 1997.

Hardwick WC, Bluhm D: Digital intubation, *J Emerg Med* 1:317, 1983.

Iserson KV: Blind nasotracheal intubation, *Ann Emerg Med* 10:468, 1981.

McNamara RM: Retrograde intubation of the trachea, *Ann Emerg Med* 16:680, 1987.

O'Connor RE, Megargel RE, Schnyder ME et al: Paramedic success rate for blind nasotracheal intubation is improved with the use of an endotracheal tube with directional tip control, *Ann Emerg Med* 36:328, 2000.

Oswalt JL, Hedges JR, Soifer BE, Lowe DK: Analysis of trauma intubations, *Am J Emerg Med* 10:511, 1992.

Winchell RJ, Hoyt DB: Endotracheal intubation in the field improves survival in patients with severe head injury, *Arch Surg* 132:592, 1997.

Specific Skills

Airway Management and Ventilation Skills

Manual Inline Stabilization

Principle: To maintain the cervical spine in a neutral and inline position until the patient is completely immobilized.

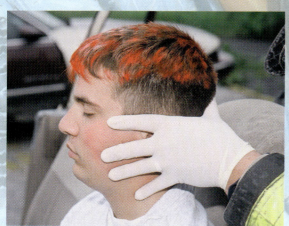

Behind

From behind the patient, the prehospital care provider places his or her hands over the patient's ears without moving the patient's head. The thumbs are placed against the posterior aspect of the patient's skull. The little fingers are placed just under the angle of the mandible. The remaining fingers are spread on the flat lateral planes of the patient's head. Pressure is applied in such a manner as to maintain the head in a stable position. If the head is not in a neutral inline position, the provider slowly moves the head until it is, unless contraindicated (see Chapter 9). The provider brings his or her arms in and rests them against the seat, headrest, or torso for additional support.

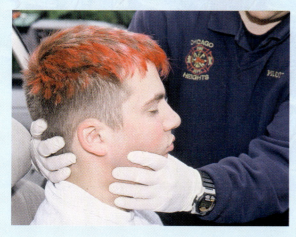

Side

Standing at the side of the patient, the prehospital care provider passes his or her arm over the patient's shoulder closest to the provider and cups the back of the patient's head with his or her hand, being careful not to move the patient's head. The thumb and first finger of one hand are placed on either side of the patient's face. The thumb and finger should rest in the notch formed where the patient's teeth and maxilla join. Enough pressure is supplied to support and stabilize the patient's head. If the patient's head is not in an inline neutral position, the provider slowly moves the head until it is, unless contraindicated (see Chapter 9). The provider braces his or her elbows on the patient's torso for additional support.

Specific Skills

Front

Standing directly in front of the patient, the prehospital care provider places his or her hands on both sides of the patient's head as shown. The little fingers are placed at the posterior aspect of the patient's skull. One thumb is placed in the notch between the patient's upper teeth and the maxilla on each cheek. The remaining fingers are spread on the flat lateral planes of the patient's head. Pressure is applied in such a manner as to maintain the head in a stable position. If the patient's head is not in a neutral inline position, the provider slowly moves the head, unless contraindicated (see Chapter 9). The provider brings his or her arms in and braces the elbows against the patient's torso for additional support.

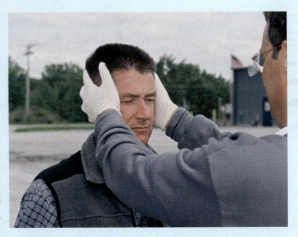

Note: The provider can also use this method when kneeling alongside the thorax of a supine patient and facing toward his or her head.

Supine Patient

The prehospital care provider positions himself or herself above the supine patient's head, either kneeling or lying. The hands are placed on either side of the patient's head, covering the patient's ears with the palms. The fingers are spread in a fashion to stabilize the patient's head with the fingers pointing toward the patient's feet (caudal). The fourth and fifth digits of each hand should wrap around the posterior portion of the patient's skull. The elbows and forearms can be rested on either the ground or the provider's knees for additional support.

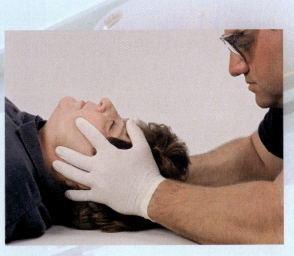

Trauma Jaw Thrust

Principle: To open the airway without moving the cervical spine.

In both the trauma jaw thrust and the trauma chin lift, manual neutral inline stabilization of the head and neck is maintained while the mandible is moved anteriorly (forward). This maneuver moves the tongue forward, away from the hypopharynx, and holds the mouth slightly open.

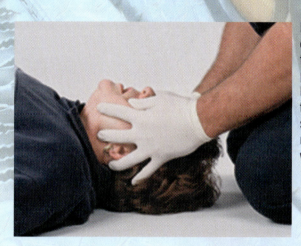

From a position above the patient's head, the prehospital care provider positions his or her hands on either side of the patient's head, fingers pointing caudad (toward the patient's feet). Depending on the size of the provider's hands, the fingers are spread across the face and around the angle of the patient's mandible. Gentle, equal pressure is applied with these digits to move the patient's mandible anteriorly (forward) and slightly downward (toward the patient's feet).

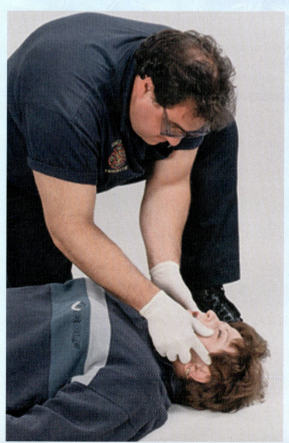

The trauma jaw thrust can also be performed while positioned beside the patient, facing toward the patient's head. The provider's fingers point cephalad (toward the top of the patient's head). Depending on the size of the provider's hands, the fingers are spread across the face and around the angle of the patient's mandible. Gentle, equal pressure is applied with these digits to move the patient's mandible anteriorly (forward) and slightly downward (toward the patient's feet).

Trauma Chin Lift

Principle: To open the airway without moving the cervical spine.

From a position above the patient's head, the patient's head and neck are moved into a neutral inline position and manual stabilization is maintained. A provider positions himself or herself at the patient's side between the patient's shoulders and hips, facing the patient's head. With the hand closest to the patient's feet, the provider grasps the patient's teeth or the lower mandible between his or her thumb and first two fingers beneath the patient's chin. The provider now pulls the patient's chin anteriorly and slightly caudad, elevating the mandible and opening the mouth.

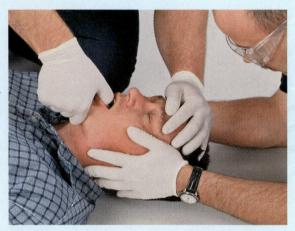

Bag-Valve-Mask Ventilation

Principle: The preferred method of providing assisted ventilation.

Ventilation using a bag-valve-mask (BVM) system has an advantage over other ventilatory support systems because it gives a prehospital care provider feedback by the feel of the bag (compliance). Positive feedback ensures the operator of successful ventilations; changes in the feedback indicate a loss of mask seal, the presence of a pathologic airway, or a thoracic problem interfering with the delivery of successful ventilations. This "feel" and the control it provides also make the BVM suitable for assisting ventilations. The BVM's portability and ability for immediate use make it useful for immediate delivery of ventilations upon identification of the need.

However, without supplemental oxygen, a BVM provides an oxygen concentration of only 21% (Fio_2 of 0.21); as soon as time allows, an oxygen reservoir and high-concentration supplemental oxygen should be connected to the BVM. When oxygen is connected without a reservoir, the Fio_2 will be limited to 0.50 or less; with a reservoir, the Fio_2 is ≥0.85.

If the patient being ventilated is unconscious without a gag reflex, a properly sized OPA should be inserted before attempting to ventilate with the BVM. If the patient has an intact gag reflex, a properly sized NPA should be inserted before attempting to assist ventilations.

Various BVM devices are available, including disposable single-patient-use models that are relatively inexpensive. Different brands have varying bag, valve, and reservoir designs. All of the parts used should be of the same model and brand since these parts are usually not safely interchangeable.

BVM units are available in adult, pediatric, and neonatal sizes. Although an adult bag can be used with the properly sized pediatric mask in an emergency, use of the correct bag size is recommended as a safe practice. Adequate ventilations of an adult patient are achieved when a minimum of 800 mL/breath is delivered (1000 to 1200 mL/breath is preferred).

When ventilating with any positive-pressure device, inflation should stop once the chest has risen maximally. When using the BVM, the chest should be visualized for maximum inflation and the bag felt to recognize any marked increased resistance in the bag when lung expansion is at its maximum. Adequate time for exhalation is needed (1:3 ratio between time for inhalation and time for exhalation). If enough time is not allowed, "stepped breaths" occur, providing a greater volume of inspiration than expiration. Stepped breaths produce poor air exchange and result in hyperinflation, increased pressure, opening of the esophagus, and gastric distention.

Single Provider Method

On many occasions, it is difficult for a single provider to maintain a proper mask seal and provide adequate ventilations when using a BVM device. In ideal situations, at least two prehospital care providers should be used to provide ventilations with a BVM. However, in most prehospital conditions, multiple experienced and trained providers may not be readily available. In these situations a single provider must provide adequate ventilatory support to a patient until additional help arrives or until the patient is delivered to the appropriate facility.

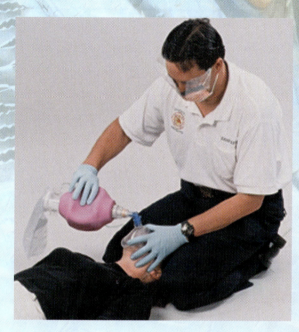

The prehospital care provider kneels above the patient's head providing manual stabilization of the patient's head and neck in a neutral inline position with his or her knees. After insertion of an airway adjunct, the mask is fitted over the patient's nose and mouth and held in place with firm downward pressure while keeping the airway open. This can be accomplished by placing the third, fourth, and fifth fingers around the mandible and applying slight upward pressure, wrapping the thumb and first finger around the mask at the mask and bag attachment point forming a "C." Either adequate hand pressure is used or the bag is pressed against one's own body (e.g., the thigh) to squeeze the air or oxygen from the bag and into the patient's lungs.

Two Provider Method

Two or more prehospital care providers performing ventilations with a BVM device is easier than one. One provider can focus his or her attention on maintaining an adequate mask seal while the other provides good delivery volume by using both hands to squeeze (deflate) the bag.

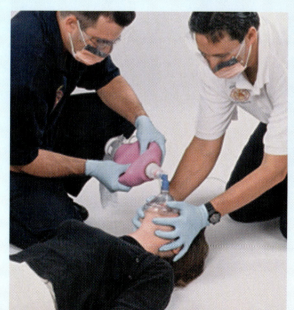

One provider kneels above the patient's head and maintains manual stabilization of the patient's head and neck in a neutral inline position. The facemask is placed over the patient's nose and mouth, and the mask is held in place with the thumbs on the lateral portion of the mask while pulling the mandible up into the mask. The other fingers provide the manual stabilization and maintain a patent airway. A second provider kneels at the side of the patient and squeezes the bag with both hands to inflate the lungs. If an adequate volume (minimum of 800 mL/breath) cannot be provided, the second provider should attempt to deflate the bag against his or her body.

Specific Skills

Oropharyngeal Airway

Principle: An adjunct used to mechanically maintain an open airway in a patient without a gag reflex.

The oropharyngeal airway (OPA) is designed to hold the patient's tongue anteriorly out of the pharynx. The OPA is available in various sizes and must be properly sized to the patient to ensure a patent airway. *Use of an OPA placed in the hypopharynx is contraindicated in patients who have an intact gag reflex.*

Two methods for insertion of the OPA are effective—the tongue jaw lift insertion method and the tongue blade insertion method. Regardless of which method is used, one provider must stabilize the patient's head and neck in a neutral inline position while a second provider measures and inserts the OPA.

Tongue Jaw Lift Insertion Method

One provider brings the patient's head and neck into a neutral inline position and maintains stabilization while opening the patient's airway with a trauma jaw thrust maneuver. A second provider selects and measures for a properly sized OPA. The accompanying illustration shows a workable method for measuring the OPA (the first provider's hands have been removed for clarification). The distance from the corner of the patient's mouth to the ear lobe is a good estimate for proper size.

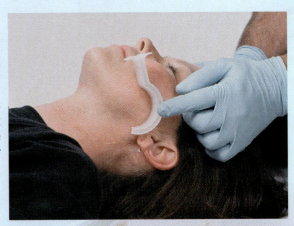

The patient's airway is opened with the chin lift maneuver. The OPA is turned so the distal tip is pointing toward the top of the patient's head (flanged end pointing toward the patient's head) and tilted toward the mouth opening (the first provider's hands have been removed for clarification).

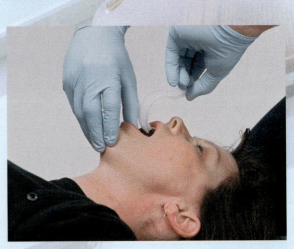

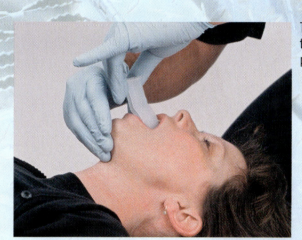

The OPA is inserted into the patient's mouth and rotated to fit the contours of the patient's anatomy (the first provider's hands have been removed for clarification).

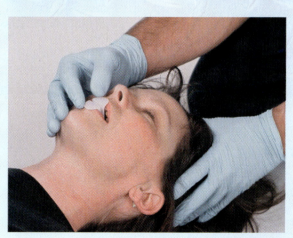

The OPA is rotated until the inside curve of the OPA is resting against the tongue and holding it out of the posterior pharynx. The flanges of the OPA should be resting against the outside surface of the patient's teeth (the first provider's hands have been removed for clarification).

Specific Skills

Tongue Blade Insertion Method

The tongue blade insertion method is probably a safer method because it eliminates the accidental tearing or puncturing of gloves or the skin by sharp, pointed, or broken teeth. This method also eliminates the possibility of being bitten if the patient's level of consciousness (LOC) is not as deep as previously assessed or if any seizure activity occurs.

The first provider brings the patient's head and neck into a neutral inline position and maintains stabilization while opening the patient's airway with the trauma jaw thrust maneuver. A second provider selects and measures for a properly sized OPA. The second provider pulls the patient's mouth open by the chin and places a tongue blade into the patient's mouth to move the tongue forward in place and keep the airway open. With the flanged end pointing toward the patient's head and the distal tip pointing into the patient's mouth, the second provider continues to insert the OPA following the curvature of the airway until the flanged end of the OPA rests against the outside surface of the patient's teeth.

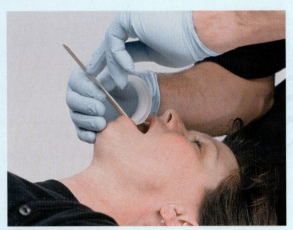

Nasopharyngeal Airway

Principle: An adjunct used to mechanically maintain an open airway in a patient with or without a gag reflex.

The nasopharyngeal airway (NPA) is a simple airway adjunct that provides an effective way to maintain a patent airway in patients who may still have an intact gag reflex. When properly sized, most patients will tolerate the NPA. NPAs are available in a range of diameters (internal diameters of 5 to 9 mm), and the length varies appropriately with the size of the diameter. NPAs are usually made of a flexible rubber-like material. Ridged NPAs are not recommended for field use.

The first provider brings the patient's head and neck into a neutral inline position and maintains stabilization while opening the patient's airway with the trauma jaw thrust maneuver. A second provider examines the patient's nostrils with a light and selects the one that is the largest and least deviated or obstructed (usually the right nostril). The second provider selects the appropriately sized NPA for the patient's nostril, a size slightly smaller in diameter than the size of the nostril opening (frequently the diameter of the patient's little finger). The length of the NPA is also important. The NPA must be long enough to supply an air passage between the patient's tongue and the posterior pharynx. An acceptable method for measuring the NPA for proper length is shown in the accompanying illustration (the first provider's hands have been removed for clarification). The distance from the patient's nose to the ear lobe is a good estimate for proper size.

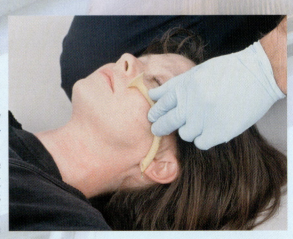

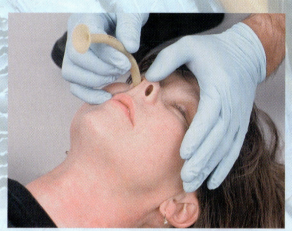

The distal tip (nonflanged end) of the NPA is lubricated liberally with a water-soluble jelly and slowly inserted into the nostril of choice. Insertion should be in an anterior-to-posterior direction along the floor of the nasal cavity, not in a superior-to-inferior direction. If resistance is met at the posterior end of the nostril, a gentle back-and-forth rotation of the NPA between the fingers will usually aid in passing beyond the turbinate bones of the nasal cavity without damage. Should the NPA continue to meet with resistance, the NPA should not be forced past the obstruction but rather should be withdrawn, and the distal tip should be re-lubricated and inserted into the other nostril. (The first provider's hands have been removed for clarification.)

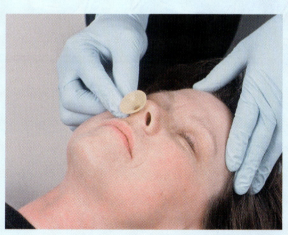

The second provider continues insertion until the flange end of the NPA is next to the anterior nares or until the patient gags. If the patient gags, the NPA is withdrawn slightly. (The first provider's hands have been removed for clarification.)

Specific Skills

Dual Lumen Airway

Principle: A mechanical device used for opening and maintaining an airway when unable to intubate.

The dual lumen airway provides prehospital care providers with a functional alternative airway. These combination airways are an acceptable prehospital field device and typically do not require extensive training to achieve competency. The airway's greatest advantage is that it can be inserted independent of the patient's position ("blindly" inserted), which may be especially important in trauma patients with high suspicion of cervical injury. The indications for placement of a dual lumen airway are the same as for the placement of any airway—the necessity of obtaining a patent airway in a patient. Each manufacturer of the dual lumen airway will identify age and size requirements pertinent to their airway. The provider should always follow the manufacturer's recommendations for size selection, contraindications, and specific insertion procedures.

Like any other invasive airway, the patient is preoxygenated with a high concentration of oxygen using a simple airway adjunct or manual airway procedure before insertion of a dual lumen airway.

As with any other piece of medical equipment, the dual lumen should be inspected and each part tested before insertion. The distal end of the airway should be lubricated with a water-soluble lubricant.

Note: The Combitube is used in the following illustrations for demonstration purposes only. Other brands of dual lumen airways are also effective.

The provider stops ventilations and removes all other airway adjuncts. If the patient is supine, the tongue and lower jaw are lifted upward with one hand (chin lift). The distal end of the tube is inserted (tearing the cuff when inserting the airway past broken teeth or dental appliances should be avoided). The Combitube is inserted until the marker rings line up with the patient's teeth.

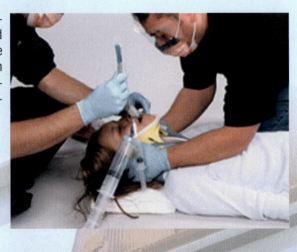

Using the large syringe, the the pharyngeal cuff is inflated with 100 mL of air and the syringe is removed. The device should seat itself in the posterior pharynx just behind the hard palate.

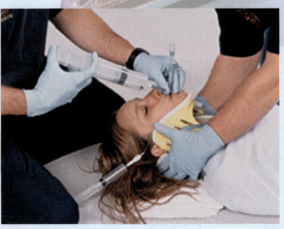

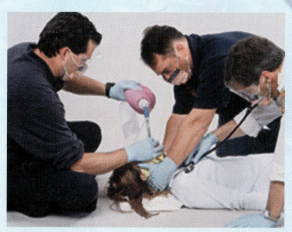

Using the small syringe, the distal cuff is inflated with 15 mL of air and the syringe is removed. Typically the balloon will be placed (inflated) in the patient's esophagus. The provider begins ventilation through the esophageal tube (generally marked with a #1). If auscultation of breath sounds is positive and gastric insufflation is negative, the provider continues ventilation through the esophagus tube.

If auscultation of breath sounds is negative and gastric insufflation is positive, the provider immediately ventilates via the shortened tracheal tube (generally marked with a #2), after which reauscultation of breath sounds and gastric sounds is done to affirm proper tube placement. The provider continues to ventilate the patient and initiate immediate transport to an appropriate facility.

All esophageal airways require the patient to have no gag reflex. If the patient regains consciousness and begins to gag or vomit, the provider must remove these devices immediately. Extubation of esophageal airways nearly always causes vomiting or regurgitation. Consequently, suction equipment must be readily available when the device is removed. Standard precautions must be observed.

Specific Skills

Visualized Orotracheal Intubation of the Trauma Patient

Principle: To secure a definitive airway without manipulating the cervical spine.

Visualized orotracheal intubation of the trauma patient is done with the patient's head and neck stabilized in a neutral inline position. Orotracheal intubation while maintaining manual inline stabilization requires additional training and practice beyond that for intubation of nontrauma patients. Like all skills, training requires observation, critique, and certification intially and at least twice a year by the medical director or designate.

In hypoxic trauma patients who are not in cardiac arrest, intubation should not be the initial airway maneuver. The provider should only perform intubation after he or she has preoxygenated the patient with a high concentration of oxygen using a simple airway adjunct or manual maneuver. Contact with the deep pharynx when intubating a severely hypoxic patient without preoxygenation can easily produce vagal stimulation, resulting in a dangerous bradycardia.

The provider should not interrupt ventilation for more than 20 seconds when intubating the patient. Ventilation should never be interrupted for more than 30 seconds for any reason.

Visualized orotracheal intubation is extremely difficult in conscious patients or patients with an intact gag reflex. The provider should consider use of topical anesthesia or paralytic agents after additional training, protocol development, and approval by the EMS medical director.

For the novice provider, the use of a straight laryngoscope blade tends to produce less rotary force (pulling the patient's head toward a "sniffing" position) than that produced by the use of a curved blade. However, because the success rate of intubation is often related to the provider's comfort with a given design, the style of blade selection for the laryngoscope must remain a matter of individual preference.

Note: The cervical collar will limit forward motion of the mandible and complete opening of the mouth. Therefore after adequate spinal immobilization is ensured, the cervical collar is removed, manual stabilization of the cervical spine is held, and intubation is attempted.

Before attempting intubation, the providers should assemble and test all required equipment and follow standard precautions. The first provider kneels at the patient's head and ventilates the patient with a BVM and high-concentration oxygen. The second provider, kneeling at the patient's side, provides manual stabilization of the patient's head and neck.

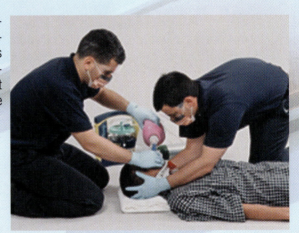

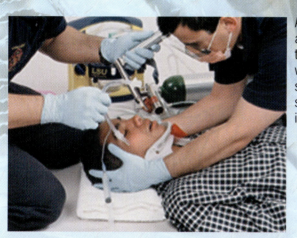

After preoxygenation, the first provider stops ventilations and grasps the laryngoscope in his or her left hand and the endotracheal (ET) tube (with syringe attached to pilot valve) in his or her right hand. If a stylet is used, this should have been inserted when the equipment was inspected and tested. The distal end of the stylet should be inserted just short of the ET tube's distal opening.

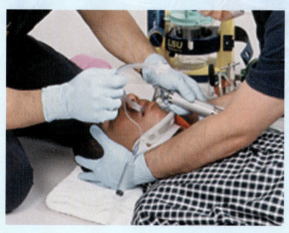

The laryngoscope blade is inserted into the right side of the patient's airway to the correct depth, sweeping toward the center of the airway while observing the desired landmarks.

Specific Skills

4 After identification of desired landmarks, the ET tube is inserted between the patient's vocal cords to the desired depth. The laryngoscope is then removed while holding the ET tube in place; the depth marking on the side of the ET tube is noted. If a malleable stylet has been used, it should be removed at this time.

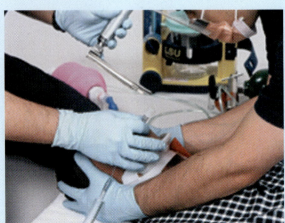

5 The pilot valve is inflated with enough air to complete the seal between the patient's trachea and the cuff of the ET tube (usually 8 to 10 mL of air), and the syringe is removed from the pilot valve. The first provider attaches the bag-valve system with a reservoir attached to the proximal end of the ET tube, and ventilation is resumed while observing the rise of the patient's chest with each delivered breath. Manual stabilization of the patient's head and neck is maintained throughout the process. Bilateral breath sounds and absence of air sounds over the epigastrium and other indications of proper ET tube placement are checked. Once tube placement is confirmed, the ET tube is secured in place. Although the use of tape or other commercially available devices is adequate in controlled situations in which the patient is not moved, the best way to guard against displacement of the ET tube in the prehospital situation is to physically hold onto the tube at all times.

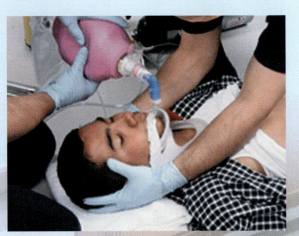

Alternative Methods for Orotracheal Intubation of the Trauma Patient

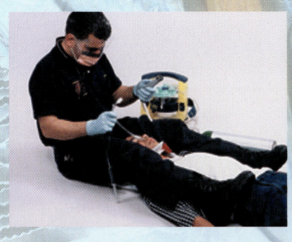

Alternative Positioning

An alternative method to perform orotracheal intubation is for a prehospital care provider to provide stabilization of the patient's head and neck while performing the intubation. the prehospital care provider sits on the ground above the patient's head, places his or her legs over the top of the patient's shoulders, holding the patient's head and neck in a neutral inline position with the inner thighs. While placing the laryngoscope into the patient's airway, the provider leans back, lifts the mandible without lifting the patient's head with the laryngoscope, and observes for desired landmarks. After identification of desired landmarks, the provider introduces the ET tube into the airway and confirms placement.

Another alternative method is for the prehospital care provider to kneel above the patient's head, scooting forward until the patient's head is between his or her knees. Lateral pressure is applied to the patient's head to maintain stabilization of the head and neck in a neutral inline position. The provider leans back after inserting the laryngoscope into the patient's airway to the desired depth, without lifting forward or upward with the laryngoscope, and observes for the desired landmarks.

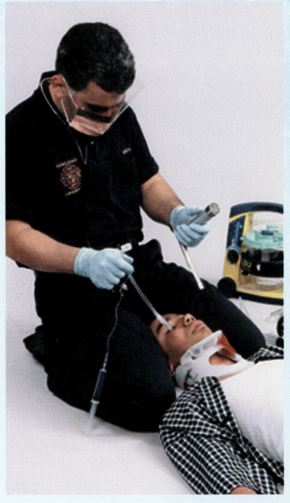

Specific Skills

Face-to-Face Orotracheal Intubation

Principle: An alternative method of securing a definitive airway when patient positioning limits use of traditional methods.

Situations may arise in the prehospital setting in which the provider cannot take a position above the patient's head to initiate endotracheal intubation in a traditional manner. The face-to-face method for intubation is a viable option in these situations. The basic concepts of intubation still apply with face-to-face intubation—preoxygenate the patient with a BVM and high-concentration oxygen before attempting intubation, maintain manual stabilization of the patient's head and neck throughout the intubation, and do not interrupt ventilation for longer then 20 to 30 seconds at a time.

While manual stabilization of the patient's head and neck in a neutral inline position is held, the prehospital care provider positions himself or herself in front of the patient, "face-to-face." The laryngoscope is held in the right hand with the blade on the patient's tongue. The blade moves the tongue down and out rather than up and out. The patient's airway is opened with the left hand, and the laryngoscope is placed into the patient's airway.

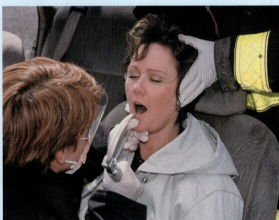

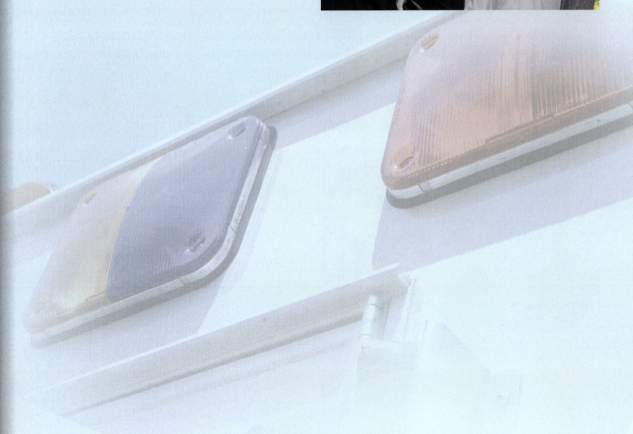

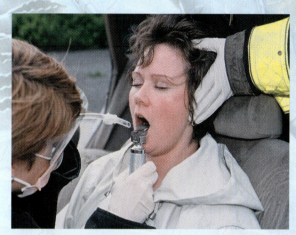

After the laryngoscope blade is placed in the patient's airway, the desired landmarks are found. Looking into the airway from a position above the open airway provides the best view.

Specific Skills

After identification of desired landmarks, the ET tube is passed between the patient's vocal cords to the desired depth with the left hand. The cuff is inflated with air to form the seal, and the syringe is removed. A bag-valve device is attached, and placement of the ET tube is confirmed.

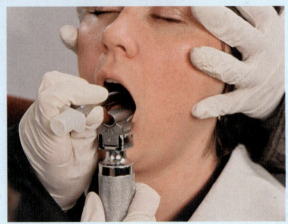

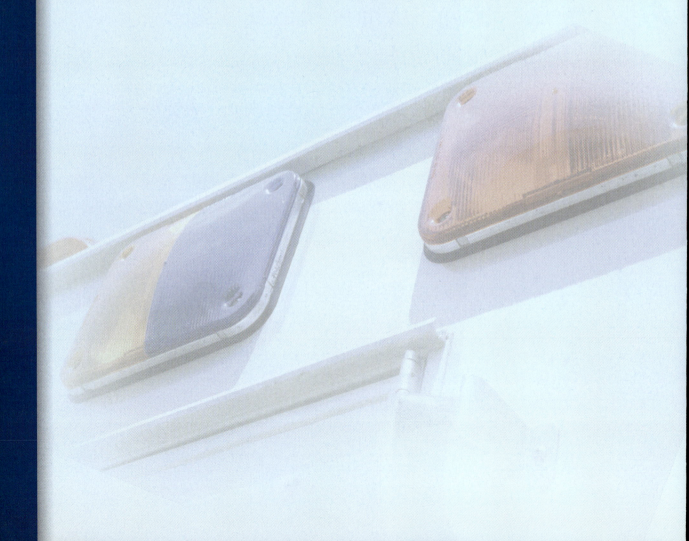

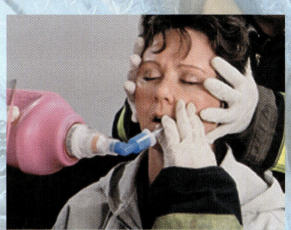

After confirmation of ET tube placement, the patient is ventilated while holding onto the ET tube and maintaining manual stabilization of the patient's head and neck. The ET tube should then be secured into place.

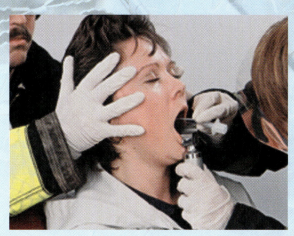

An alternative method for face-to-face intubation is to hold the laryngoscope in the left hand and place the ET tube with the right hand. This method may block the visualization of the lower airway as the ET tube is placed.

Specific Skills

Blind Nasotracheal Intubation

Principle: To secure a definitive airway without manipulating the cervical spine.

This technique depends on the patient's spontaneous ventilation to ensure proper alignment when passing the ET tube between the vocal cords and into the trachea. Therefore blind nasotracheal intubation is limited to use with spontaneously breathing patients and in an environment that allows for the hearing and feeling of air exchange at the external (proximal) end of the ET tube.

This technique should only be attempted by personnel qualified in endotracheal intubation and who, after practice, have demonstrated their ability to their medical director or his or her designate.

Before attempting blind nasotracheal intubation, the prehospital care provider should gather all required equipment and check for proper operating condition. Using a light source, the patient's nostrils are inspected and the largest one with the least deviation or obstructions is selected. The appropriately sized ET tube is one slightly smaller than the diameter of the nostril. The distal end of the ET tube should be lubricated with a generous amount of a water-soluble lubricant before insertion. Use of a stylet during nasotracheal intubation requires more than casual experience.

 Manual stabilization of the patient's head and neck in a neutral inline position is held while a second prehospital care provider is positioned above the patient and preoxygenates the patient with high-concentration oxygen and BVM-assisted ventilation.

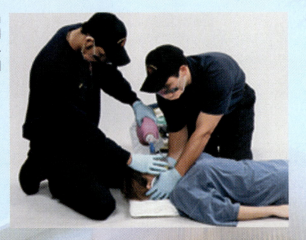

The ET tube is taken in one hand. The other hand applies slight superior traction to the tip of the patient's nose. This traction will help ensure that the tube follows the anatomy of the nasal airway. The tube is placed into the patient's nostril (usually the right one) in an anterior-to-posterior direction (from the nose to the back of the head).

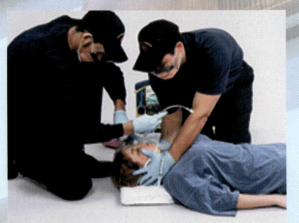

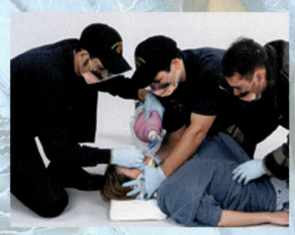

The prehospital care provider should place his or her ear over the proximal (external) opening of the ET tube and listen for breathing sounds. The ET tube is passed down the hypopharynx until the breath sounds are the loudest. At this point, progress is paused until the next inhalation begins. With a quick motion, the tube is passed through the vocal cords. If breath sounds stop, the tube has gone into the esophagus. The tube is then withdrawn until breath sounds are heard loudly again, and another attempt is made.

After passing the ET tube to the desired depth, the cuff is inflated with enough air to create a seal and the syringe is removed. Tube placement is confirmed, the ET tube is secured with tape and manual holding, and ventilation with a BVM and high-concentration oxygen is begun.

Verification of Endotracheal Tube Placement

Once intubation has been performed, specific efforts must be taken to ensure that the tube has been properly placed in the trachea. An improperly positioned endotracheal tube, if unrecognized for only a brief period, may result in profound hypoxia with resultant brain injury (hypoxic encephalopathy) and even death. Therefore the prehospital care provider must make reasonable efforts to ensure proper placement. Techniques to verify intubation include the use of both clinical assessments and adjunctive devices. Clinical assessments include the following:

- Direct visualization of the tube passing through the vocal cords
- Presence of bilateral breath sounds (auscultate laterally below the axilla) *and* absence of air sounds over the epigastrium
- Visualization of the chest rising and falling during ventilation
- Fogging (water vapor condensation) in the endotracheal tube on expiration

Unfortunately, none of these techniques is 100% reliable *by itself* for verifying proper tube placement. Therefore prudent practice involves assessing and documenting *all* of these clinical signs, if possible. On rare occasions, because of difficult anatomy, visualization of the tube passing through the vocal cords may not be possible. In a moving vehicle (ground or aeromedical), engine noise may make auscultation of breath sounds nearly impossible. Obesity and chronic obstructive pulmonary disease (COPD) may interfere with the ability to see chest movement during ventilation.

Adjunctive devices include the following:

- Esophageal detector device
- Carbon dioxide monitoring
- Colorimetric carbon dioxide detector
- End-tidal carbon dioxide monitoring (capnography)
- Pulse oximetry

As with the clinical assessments, none of these adjuncts is 100% accurate in all patients. In a patient with a perfusing rhythm, end-tidal carbon dioxide monitoring (capnography) serves as the "gold standard" for determining endotracheal placement of an airway in the operating room. This technique should be used in the prehospital setting if it is available. Patients in cardiopulmonary arrest do not generate carbon dioxide, and therefore neither colorimetric detectors nor capnography may be useful in patients who lack a perfusing cardiac rhythm.

Because none of these techniques is universally reliable, all of the clinical assessments noted previously should be performed, unless impractical, followed by use of at least one of the adjunctive devices. Because of the cost of performing capnography, most EMS systems require a combination of clinical assessments and a colorimetric carbon dioxide detector or esophageal detector device. In any instance, if any of the techniques used to verify proper placement suggest that the tube may not be properly positioned, the tube should be immediately removed and reinserted, with placement reverified. All of the techniques used to verify tube placement should be noted on the patient care report.

Specific Skills

Percutaneous Transtracheal Ventilation

Principle: A method of providing oxygenation to a patient who cannot be intubated or ventilated with a BVM.

All parts except the needle, tank, and regulator should be modified as needed, preassembled, and packaged for ready availability in the field. This will ensure successful assembly. When this technique is needed, time will be of the essence. The equipment should be ready to use, requiring only connection to the regulator and needle. The prehospital care provider can use a commercially available product that contains all of the necessary equipment. If this is not available, the following equipment is required:

- Syringe: 10 to 30 mL
- To allow for inflation and deflation of the lung while there is constant flow from the oxygen source, some type of bypass is necessary. The following are two examples:
    1. A hole approximately 40% of the circumference of the oxygen delivery tube, cut in the side, that can be occluded by the thumb
    2. A plastic "T" or "Y" connector of a size compatible with the oxygen tubing used and connected to the oxygen source with a length of standard universal oxygen tubing
- A short piece of tubing that will fasten over the lower end of the "T" or "Y" and snugly fit into the hub of the needle (this leaves one opening of the "T" or "Y" connector free with nothing attached to it)
- An oxygen tank with a regulator that has a 50 psi delivery pressure at its supplemental oxygen nipple
- Strips of ½-inch adhesive tape

The patient should be in the supine position while manual inline stabilization is maintained.

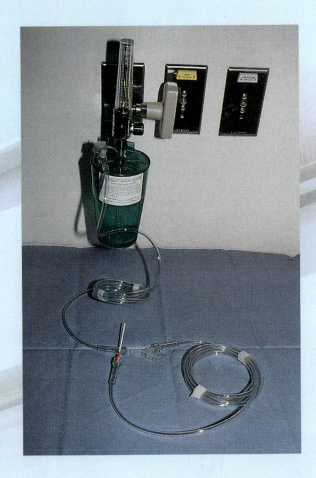

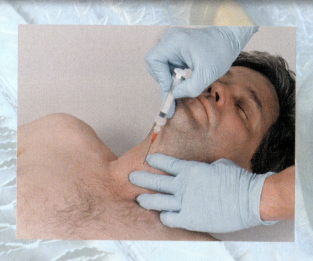

The larynx and trachea are stabilized with the fingers of one hand. The needle, attached to the syringe, is placed midline over the cricothyroid membrane or directly into the trachea at a slightly downward angle. As the needle is inserted into the trachea, the plunger of the syringe is withdrawn to create a negative pressure. Once the needle enters into the trachea, air will be sucked into the syringe, confirming that the tip of the needle is properly located. The needle is advanced an additional centimeter, and then the syringe is removed from the needle. The inner needle is removed, leaving the catheter in place. The provider quickly forms a loop with adhesive tape around the needle or the hub of the catheter and places the ends of tape on the patient's neck to secure the airway. The provider should use caution when securing the catheter to prevent kinking the catheter.

The oxygen delivery tube with a vent is connected to the hub of the needle while the hand that initially stabilized the trachea is moved to hold the needle in place. Ventilation is begun by occluding the opening of the tubing assembly with the thumb for 1 second. The patient's chest may or may not rise to indicate that inhalation is occurring. To stop the flow of oxygen into the lungs, the thumb is removed from the opening.

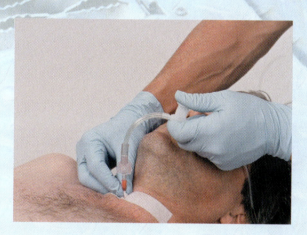

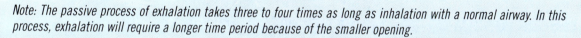

Note: The passive process of exhalation takes three to four times as long as inhalation with a normal airway. In this process, exhalation will require a longer time period because of the smaller opening.

The patient is oxygenated by alternately closing the hole to provide the positive flow of oxygen for inhalation and opening the same hole to stop the oxygen flow and allow deflation. The proper time sequence for these maneuvers is 1 second of occlusion of the opening for inhalation and 4 seconds of leaving the hole open for passive deflation. This process is continued until a more definitive airway is established.

After percutaneous transtracheal ventilation (PTV) of 45 to 60 minutes, this technique can provide a high $Paco_2$ level because of carbon dioxide retention as a result of the restricted expirations. Therefore the patient should have a more definitive airway established as soon as possible.

Warning: Patients being ventilated using PTV may remain hypoxic and unstable. Prehospital care providers should initiate transportation to a suitable facility without delay because the patient is in urgent need of a more definitive surgical transtracheal procedure (cricothyroidotomy) for adequate ventilation and oxygenation.

Chapter 5

Thoracic Trauma

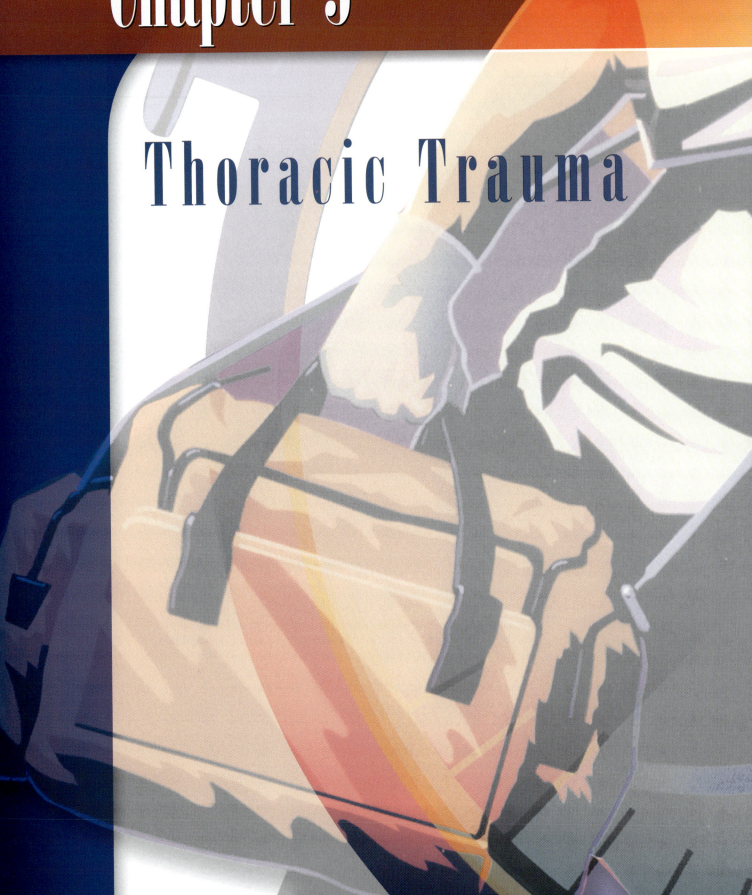

Chapter Objectives

At the completion of this chapter, the reader should be able to do the following:

- Integrate the relationship between thoracic anatomy and the kinematics of trauma with assessment findings to develop an index of suspicion for specific thoracic injuries.
- Explain the physiology of ventilation.
- Describe the pathophysiology, signs and symptoms, and management of the following thoracic injuries:

    Rib fractures

    Flail chest

    Pulmonary contusion

    Pneumothorax (open and closed)

    Tension pneumothorax

    Hemothorax

    Blunt cardiac injury

    Pericardial tamponade

    Tracheal and bronchial rupture

    Aortic rupture

    Traumatic asphyxia

    Diaphragmatic rupture

- Differentiate between patients who require rapid stabilization and transport because of thoracic trauma, and those for whom further on-the-scene assessment and management is appropriate.

Scenario

You are dispatched to the scene of a motor vehicle crash with possible entrapment in a rural location. Your response time will be approximately 20 minutes. En route, first responders from the local volunteer fire service report that they have a 20-year-old male who was the unrestrained driver of a vehicle that has struck a tree head-on. They report that the patient is awake, complaining of chest pain, and trapped in the vehicle. Upon your arrival, fire department personnel have just completed extrication, they are removing the patient from the vehicle on a backboard, and the patient has a cervical collar in place. The scene has been secured before your arrival, and the mechanism of injury is apparent. As you approach the patient, you are able to take a quick look at the interior of the vehicle and find that the windshield is "starred," the steering wheel is bent, and the front seat is collapsed.

Your first priority is to assess the patient. Your general impression of the patient is that he is awake and in respiratory distress. The findings of your simultaneous assessment are that the patient is awake, speaks with difficulty, and has no recollection of the event. He has pale, moist skin; numerous facial lacerations; a rapid ventilatory rate with signs of respiratory distress; and a rapid, bounding radial pulse. As your partner begins the administration of oxygen, further investigation of the patient's ventilatory impairment reveals that the trachea is midline, no jugular venous distention is present, and the patient has diminished breath sounds on the left side with subcutaneous emphysema. The patient has no paradoxical movement of his chest, and his abdomen is soft, nontender, and nondistended.

What is the most likely cause of the patient's respiratory compromise? How do you manage this condition in the field? How does the location of the crash influence your management of the patient? Does the patient have a life-threatening injury? What are your options for transport? Based on the information you have, what other injuries should you suspect?

The reader might appropriately wonder why the thoracic trauma chapter in this text is placed immediately after the airway chapter and before the discussion of shock and fluid replacement. If one recalls the basic approach to the assessment of a trauma patient, the five steps in the primary survey (initial assessment), in order of priority, are airway, breathing, circulation, disability, and expose. Thus the presentation of the information on thoracic trauma after the airway chapter is so the prehospital care provider can learn about and understand the injuries that affect breathing.

Chest injuries are a leading cause of trauma deaths (one out of four) each year, although the vast majority of all thoracic injuries (90% of blunt trauma and 70% to 85% of penetrating trauma) can be managed without surgery. Chest injuries that are missed or go unrecognized because of an incomplete or inaccurate assessment can impair the ventilation or oxygen exchange systems and produce tissue hypoxia (decreased oxygen), hypercarbia (increased CO_2 in the blood), and acidosis (accumulation of acids and decreased pH of the blood). Tissue hypoxia results from inadequate delivery of oxygenated blood to the tissue cells, either from decreased perfusion or decreased oxygenation of the red blood cells (RBCs). Hypercarbia is due to decreased ventilation. Acidosis is usually secondary to anaerobic metabolism by inadequately oxygenated cells.

Various mechanisms, including motor vehicle crashes (MVCs), falls, sports injuries, crush injuries, stab wounds, and gunshot wounds, can cause chest injuries.

Anatomy

The thorax is a hollow cylinder composed of twelve pairs of ribs. Ten pairs articulate posteriorly with the thoracic spine and anteriorly with the sternum via the costal cartilages. The lower two pairs are "floating ribs." A nerve, an artery, and a vein are located along the underside of each rib. Intercostal muscles connect

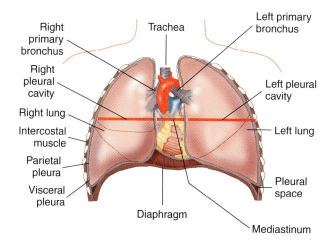

Figure 5-1 The thoracic cavity, including the ribs, intercostal muscles, diaphragm, mediastinum, lungs, heart, great vessels, bronchi, trachea, and esophagus.

each rib to the one above. These muscles, along with the diaphragm, are the primary muscles of ventilation.

The pleurae are thin membranes that consist of two distinct layers. The parietal pleura lines the inner side of the thoracic cavity, and the visceral pleura covers the outer surface of each lung. A small amount of fluid is present between the pleural surfaces of the lung and the inner chest wall. Just as a drop of water between two panes of glass makes it difficult to pull the two panes apart, this pleural fluid creates surface tension between the two pleural membranes and causes them to cling together. In this way, the pleural membranes oppose the natural elasticity and tendency of the lung to collapse. Normally, no space is present between the two pleural membranes; adhesion keeps these layers together. Lack of connection to outside air also keeps them together. If a hole develops in the thoracic wall or the lung, this space fills with air and the lung collapses. This potential space can hold a volume of 3000 mL or more in an adult.

The lungs occupy the right and left halves of the thoracic cavity (Figure 5-1). An area called the *mediastinum* is located in the middle of the thoracic cavity. Within the mediastinum lie all the other organs and structures of the chest cavity—the heart, great vessels, trachea, mainstem bronchi, and esophagus. Any or all of these structures can be injured by thoracic trauma.

Physiology

Mechanics of Ventilation

To fully appreciate the consequences and management of chest injuries, it is important to understand the mechanics

of ventilation. Ventilation is the mechanical process by which air moves from the atmosphere outside the body into the mouth, nose, pharynx, trachea, bronchi, lungs, and alveoli and then out again. Respiration, a cellular process, takes oxygen from the bloodstream and produces energy inside the cells of the body. Respiration includes ventilation. Although the terms *ventilation* and *respiration* are frequently used interchangeably, they represent different levels of function. The patient's ability to get life-sustaining oxygen to the cells of the body depends on both processes—the mechanical one (ventilation) that brings air into the lungs and the biologic one (respiration) that allows the oxygen to reach the cells where it can be used as fuel for the body. This chapter deals primarily with ventilation; Chapter 6, which deals with shock, further discusses the importance of respiration.

During inspiration, the diaphragm and intercostal muscles contract, causing the diaphragm to move downward and the ribs to spread and lift (Figure 5-2, A). This motion increases the volume inside the thoracic cage. Because volume and pressure are inversely proportional in a closed system, the intrathoracic pressure decreases to a level lower than that of the air outside the body, causing air to move into the lungs through the mouth, nose, pharynx, trachea, and bronchi (Figure 5-3).

During expiration (Figure 5-2, B), the diaphragm and intercostal muscles relax, causing the diaphragm to move upward and the ribs to return to their resting position. The intrathoracic volume decreases from that at peak inhalation, while the intrathoracic pressure increases to a level greater than that of the air outside the mouth. The air inside the lungs is forced out of the body through the bronchi, trachea, pharynx, nose, and mouth.

Within the lungs are the alveoli, minute sacs of tissue, each intimately related to a network of capillaries. CO_2 and oxygen diffuse through the walls of the capillaries and alveoli (Figure 5-4).

Neurochemical Control of Respiration

The respiratory center, located in the brain stem, contains chemoreceptor cells that are sensitive to changes in certain chemical levels in the body. These cells in turn stimulate nerve impulses that control inspiration. The chemical to which the respiratory center's chemoreceptor cells normally respond is CO_2.

As a patient's respiratory status deteriorates, anaerobic metabolism occurs and the blood level of carbon dioxide ($PaCO_2$) increases. The chemoreceptors detect the change in the pH of the blood and stimulate the nerve cells to increase the rate and depth of breathing

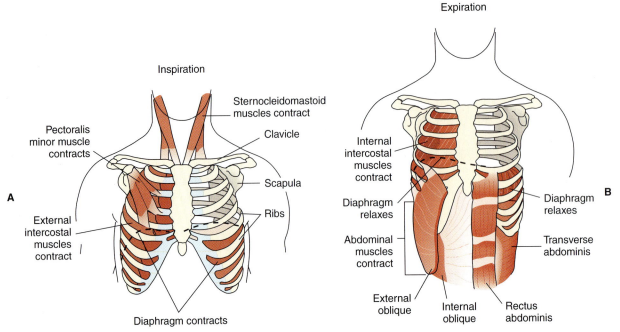

Figure 5-2 **A,** During inspiration, the diaphragm contracts and flattens. Muscles of inspiration, such as the external intercostal, pectoralis minor, and sternocleidomastoid muscles, lift the ribs and sternum, which increases the diameter and volume of the thoracic cavity. **B,** In expiration during quiet breathing, the elasticity of the thoracic cavity causes the diaphragm and ribs to assume their resting positions, which decreases the volume of the thoracic cavity. In expiration during labored breathing, muscles of expiration such as the internal intercostal and abdominal muscles contract, causing the volume of the thoracic cavity to decrease more rapidly.

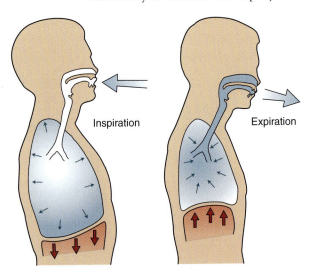

Figure 5-3 When the diaphragm is relaxed and the glottis is open, the pressure inside and outside the lungs is equal. When the chest cavity expands, the intrathoracic pressure decreases and air goes in.

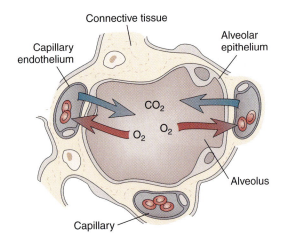

Figure 5-4 The capillaries and alveolus lie in close proximity; therefore oxygen can easily diffuse through the capillary, the alveolar walls, the capillary walls, and the red blood cells. Carbon dioxide can diffuse back in the opposite direction.

to remove the excess CO_2 (Figure 5-5). The CO_2 stimulus can increase ventilation so effectively that the alveoli receive up to 10 times more air than during a normal breath. Some chronic respiratory diseases inhibit the normal elimination of CO_2. The body compensates and becomes accustomed to this increased level of CO_2 in the blood. In this situation, the dominant ventilatory control becomes the level of oxygen in the blood (PaO_2). Located in the aorta and carotid arteries are receptors that react to a PaO_2 below 60 mm Hg

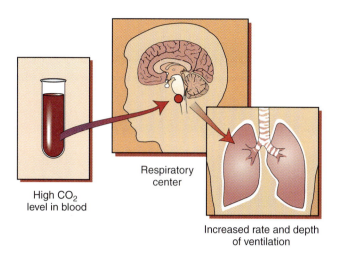

High CO₂ level in blood

Respiratory center

Increased rate and depth of ventilation

Figure 5-5 An increased level of carbon dioxide is detected by nerve cells sensitive to this change, which stimulates the lung to increase both depth and rate of ventilation.

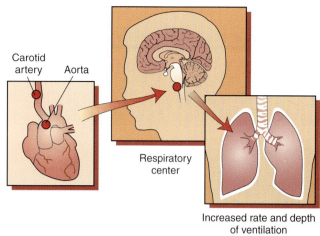

Carotid artery   Aorta

Respiratory center

Increased rate and depth of ventilation

Figure 5-6 Receptors located in the aorta and carotid arteries are sensitive to the oxygen level and will stimulate the lungs to increase air movement into and out of the alveolar sacs.

(Figure 5-6). These receptors alert the brain, causing the ventilatory muscles to increase their activity, producing an increased minute volume (the amount of air exchange that occurs in 1 minute).

During normal nonforced ventilation, about 500 mL of air is exchanged between the lungs and the atmosphere with each breath. This is called the *tidal volume*. After normal inhalation with nonforced inspiratory effort, a total of 3000 mL of air may additionally be inhaled. This is called the *inspiratory reserve volume*. The total volume of air in the lungs after a forced inhalation is called the *total lung capacity*.

Some air always remains trapped in the alveoli and bronchi. This air, approximately 1200 mL, cannot be forcibly exhaled. It is called the *residual volume*. The residual air in the alveoli normally permits the exchange of oxygen and CO_2 in the blood between breathing cycles.

The total ventilation volume expired per minute, termed *minute volume* ($\dot{V}_E$), is equal to the volume of air moved per breath (V_I) multiplied by the breaths/min (f). Under normal resting conditions, the overall ventilation of the lung approximates 6 to 7 L/min. Therefore if the volume of each breath (V_I) equals 500 mL and the rate per minute (f) equals 14, then:

$$\dot{V}_E = V_I \times f$$
$$\dot{V}_E = 500 \text{ mL} \times 14$$
$$\dot{V}_E = 7000 \text{ mL/min, or 7 L/min}$$

Minute volume becomes significant when the patient has an altered breathing pattern. For example, a patient with rib fractures who is breathing fast and shallowly because of the pain and injury may have a V_I of 100 mL at 40 breaths/min, which can soon lead to severe distress:

$$\dot{V}_E = 100 \text{ mL} \times 40$$
$$\dot{V}_E = 4000 \text{ mL/min, or 4 L/min}$$

Thus the patient's ventilation has decreased significantly. This decrease in ventilation may therefore impair respiration and lead to severe distress.

Pathophysiology

Chest injuries can be either penetrating or blunt. Penetrating injuries are caused by forces distributed over a small area that actually penetrate into the chest cavity. Examples are gunshot wounds, stabbings, or falls onto sharp objects. With penetrating trauma, any structure or organ in the chest cavity may be injured. Most often, the organs injured are those that lie along the path of the penetrating object.

In blunt trauma, the forces are distributed over a larger area, and injuries occur from compression and shearing forces. The prehospital care provider should suspect conditions such as pneumothorax, pericardial tamponade, flail chest, pulmonary contusion, and aortic rupture in blunt trauma or when the mechanism of injury involves rapid deceleration. Because of the large number and complexity of these conditions, the pathophysiology, assessment, and management of specific injuries are presented later in this chapter.

Assessment

The signs and symptoms of chest trauma related to the chest wall and lungs are shortness of breath, tachypnea, and chest pain. The pain is usually pleuritic. The pain may occur with motion and may be described as chest tightness or discomfort. Conditions such as pneumothorax, major vascular injuries, or injuries to the esophagus may not produce any symptoms initially. Patients with a hemothorax may show symptoms of blood loss, such as feeling faint or sweaty. The symptoms associated with chest injuries are like symptoms in other injured body areas—when they are present, pathology is indicated. However, a lack of signs or symptoms does not indicate a lack of injury.

Because the organs of ventilation and circulation are located in the chest, major chest injury can produce life-threatening physiologic disturbances. The prehospital care provider should rapidly correlate the presence of shock with the physical examination findings to appropriately intervene and treat that patient. Examination of the chest includes the following:

- *Observation.* A thorough visual examination of the chest can be performed in less than 30 seconds. Observation of the neck and chest may reveal bruises, lacerations, distended neck veins, tracheal deviation, subcutaneous emphysema, open chest wounds, lack of symmetrical chest rise, or paradoxical chest motion. Cyanosis is often a late sign of hypoxia. More importantly, an increasing ventilatory rate could indicate possible hypoxia and respiratory embarrassment.
- *Palpation.* The neck and chest should be palpated for the presence of tenderness, bony crepitus, subcutaneous emphysema, and an unstable chest wall segment. Because of pain, the patient may show "splinting" or try to limit chest motion on inspiration.
- *Auscultation.* The lungs should be auscultated for the presence or absence of breath sounds, the volume inspired, and bilateral symmetry of air movement. Diminished or absent breath sounds on one side of the chest in a trauma patient may indicate air or blood in the pleural space.

Rapid evaluation, initiation of resuscitation, and transport are the keys to the survival of patients with chest injuries.

Management of Specific Injuries

Rib Fractures

Considerable force is required to break ribs. The amount of force needed is indicated by the fact that up to 30% of patients with fractures of the first and second ribs die from associated injuries; as many as 5% of these patients have a ruptured aorta. A single rib fracture occurs when pressure is applied to one specific rib with enough force to exceed the tensile strength of that rib. At the instant of release of the restraining force, the broken end of the rib can travel several centimeters into adjacent structures, such as a lung, causing damage. Although any rib may be fractured, the most common location is the lateral aspect of ribs 3 through 8. These ribs are long, thin, and poorly protected (Figure 5-7). On the other hand, the uppermost ribs, particularly ribs 1 and 2, are short, broad, relatively thick, and well protected by the scapulae, clavicles, and upper chest muscles. This tissue can tear or contuse and result in rupturing of cells, capillaries, and perhaps major vessels. In the case of rib fractures, associated injuries include pulmonary contusion; laceration of the intercostal artery and/or vein with resulting hemothorax, pneumothorax, and hemorrhage; and hematoma formation in the chest wall or in the alveoli and surrounding tissue.

ASSESSMENT

Simple rib fractures alone are rarely life-threatening in adults. The signs and symptoms of fractured ribs include pain with movement, local tenderness, and perhaps bony crepitus. The prehospital care provider can perform gen-

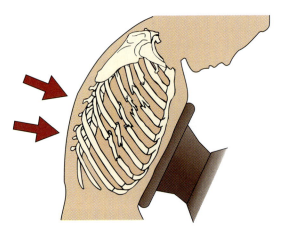

Figure 5-7 Ribs 3 through 8, which are long and thin, are usually fractured by external compression.

tle compression of the chest wall, and often the patient will point to the exact location of the rib fractures as the broken ends of the bone move against each other. Of greater importance is the evaluation and recognition of associated injuries to underlying structures, which may be life-threatening. Fracture of the lower ribs (8 to 12) can be associated with spleen, kidney, or liver injuries.

MANAGEMENT

The initial management of patients with simple rib fractures is pain reduction, most commonly accomplished in the prehospital environment by splinting and minimizing the movement of the fractured ribs. This can be performed by using the patient's arms and a sling and swath. Management should also include patient reassurance and an anticipation of potential complications such as a pneumothorax and hypovolemia. The effectiveness of ventilation and the presence of hypoxemia should also be evaluated. Should ventilation be significantly altered, ventilatory assistance is indicated. Normal ventilations and coughing should be encouraged despite associated pain. This prevents atelectasis (collapse of alveoli or part of the lung), which can lead to pneumonia. Fractured ribs should not be stabilized by taping or using any other firm bandaging or binding that encircles the chest. Such attempts at management can inhibit chest movement, limit ventilation, and lead to atelectasis and pneumonia.

Flail Chest

Flail chest is usually caused by an impact into the sternum or the lateral side of the thoracic wall. In a frontal collision the sternum stops against the steering wheel. The continued forward motion of the posterior thoracic wall bends the ribs until they fracture. In a side impact collision, such as at an intersection, impact will be into the lateral thoracic wall. Flail chest is when two or more adjacent ribs are each fractured in at least two places. The segment of chest wall that is flailed has lost its bony support and attachment to the thoracic cage. This "free" segment will move in the opposite direction from the rest of the chest wall during inspiration and expiration. With inspiration, as the diaphragm moves downward and the ribs elevate and separate, intrathoracic pressure decreases. The combination of the lower pressure in the chest and higher atmospheric pressure outside the chest causes the flail segment to move inward, rather than outward, during inspiration. This motion of the chest is called *paradoxical motion or movement* (Figure 5-8).

During expiration, when the diaphragm moves upward and the ribs come together, intrathoracic pressure increases. The floating segment of the chest wall moves out rather than in. The result of both of these paradoxical movements of the chest wall is decreased ventilation, producing hypoxia and hypercarbia.

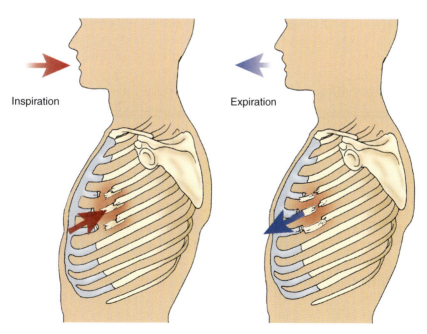

Inspiration   Expiration

Figure 5-8   Paradoxical motion. If stability of the chest wall has been lost by ribs fractured in two or more places, when intrathoracic pressure decreases during inspiration, the external air pressure forces the chest wall in. When intrathoracic pressure increases during expiration, the chest wall is forced out.

Flail chest has four consequences:

1. A decrease in the vital capacity proportional to the size of the flail segment
2. An increase in the labor of breathing
3. Pain produced by the fractured ribs, limiting the amount of thoracic cage expansion
4. Most clinically significant, contusion of the lung beneath the flail segment

The movement of several broken ends of ribs against each other also produces pain. The pain is similar to the pain produced by a single fractured rib, except that it is more severe. Therefore the patient has a greater tendency to splint and does not move air adequately into the lungs.

Compression of the lung can tear tissue, producing hemorrhage into the alveolar walls and the alveolar space and producing a bruise or contusion of the lung. The result is decreased air entry into the lung and decreased transfer of oxygen across the alveolar-capillary membrane and into the red blood cells. This is the most life-threatening consequence of flail chest.

ASSESSMENT

Tenderness and/or bony crepitus elicited by palpation should lead to a closer inspection of that area of the chest wall for paradoxical motion. Paradoxical motion of the chest wall is often extremely difficult to identify. Initially, intercostal muscle spasm may prevent significant paradoxical motion, but as these muscles tire, the flail segment may become more obvious.

Initial and ongoing evaluation of the ventilatory rate should be performed to recognize developing hypoxemia or ventilatory failure. As a patient becomes increasingly hypoxic, the ventilatory rate will gradually increase. Only through careful and repeated determinations of the ventilatory rate will a prehospital care provider identify the subtle changes that indicate that a patient is in trouble. When available, pulse oximetry can be used to help recognize hypoxia; however, it is not a substitute for repeated evaluations of the ventilatory rate.

MANAGEMENT

Several considerations are important in the management of flail chest.

All patients who have an obvious flail segment should be supplied with supplemental oxygen. In some cases, a patient may not respond to supplemental oxygen and will require more aggressive ventilatory support. The key step in the management of a patient with severe respiratory insufficiency secondary to a flail segment is to assist the patient's ventilatory efforts with positive-pressure ventilation by use of a bag-valve-mask (BVM) with supplemental oxygen. Early intubation and positive-pressure ventilation can also be helpful in a significantly compromised patient. Some patients may require intubation in the field, especially if transportation is prolonged.

Assisted ventilation expands the collapsed alveoli in the area of the flail segment and in the area involved when a patient splints. Blood passing through the capillaries that surround the collapsed (nonventilated) alveoli leaves the lung unoxygenated. Providing additional oxygen to the unaffected alveoli, combined with forced expansion of the collapsed alveoli, decreases the amount of oxygen-deprived blood entering the left side of the heart and the aorta. A large percentage of patients with significant flail chest will progress to ventilatory failure and eventually require prolonged ventilatory support.

The use of sand bags to prevent movement in patients with a flail chest decreases aeration of the lungs and promotes alveolar collapse. *This method should no longer be used.*

Pulmonary Contusion

A pulmonary contusion is an area of the lung that has been traumatized to the point where interstitial and alveolar bleeding occur. The amount of interstitial fluid increases in the area between the walls of the capillaries and alveoli, resulting in decreased oxygen transport across the thickened membranes. Hemorrhage into the alveolar sac prevents oxygenation of the affected segment. The mechanism of injury and the presence of associated injuries may be the only indications of a potential pulmonary contusion during the primary survey of a patient.

Pulmonary contusion can be the result of blunt trauma, as in flail chest. It can also result from penetrating trauma. In this scenario, an area of contusion surrounds the pathway that was produced by the cavitation effect of a missile. However, whether the injury was caused by blunt or penetrating trauma, the clinical result is the same—areas of the lung are no longer ventilated. When large areas of the lung are no longer functioning properly, it compounds the significant mechanical problems of a flail chest. A pulmonary contusion produces significant compromise of oxygenation, which is the most serious complication of a flail chest. Even without the associated presence of a flail chest, pulmonary contusion is a common, potentially lethal chest injury. Severe ventilatory failure can develop rapidly in the first 8 to 24 hours.

MANAGEMENT

Patients with contused lungs should be closely monitored with special attention to fluid administration. Any extra fluid will increase the amount of interstitial fluid and further decrease oxygen transport. If the patient is hemodynamically normal, the prehospital care provider should limit intravenous fluid administration to that needed to keep the vein open. Fluids should not be restricted in patients with evidence of compensated or decompensated shock.

As with other traumatic conditions that involve the lungs, appropriate management includes ensuring adequate ventilation and enriched oxygen administration. Pulse oximetry can help guide management if it is available. The prehospital care provider should provide supplemental oxygen to maintain an oxygen saturation above 95%. If the patient cannot maintain adequate ventilation or has preexisting chronic pulmonary disease, an altered level of consciousness, or other major injuries, BVM ventilation should be used and, if required, endotracheal intubation.

Pneumothorax

SIMPLE PNEUMOTHORAX

A simple pneumothorax is caused by the presence of air in the pleural space. This air can come from the outside through an opening in the chest wall, from the inside through a defect in the lung itself, or both. The air separates the two pleural surfaces (the parietal and visceral pleurae), causing the lung on the involved side to collapse as the separation expands (Figure 5-9). As air continues to accumulate and pressure in the pleural space increases, the size of the lung on the affected side continues to decrease. The lung may then either partially or totally collapse.

The large reserve capacity of the ventilatory and circulatory systems usually prevents serious acute consequences from a simple pneumothorax in young and healthy patients. Patients with decreased reserves, such as those with advanced age or cardiopulmonary disease, are more adversely affected.

Assessment.   The signs and symptoms of a pneumothorax can include pleuritic chest pain and difficult and rapid breathing. Decreased or absent breath sounds on the involved side are classic signs. Although percussion for bell tympany is an excellent indicator, it may be

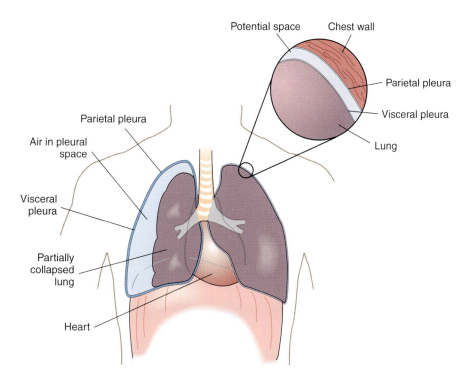

Figure 5-9   Air in the pleural space forces the lung in, decreasing the amount that can be ventilated and therefore decreasing oxygenation of the blood leaving the lung.

difficult to detect in the field. In trauma patients in the prehospital setting, absent or decreased breath sounds with ventilatory distress indicates pneumothorax. When lung collapse is partial, the prehospital care provider may hear reduced or absent breath sounds over the apices and bases of the lung before he or she hears any decrease over the midlung fields. These patients require constant monitoring in anticipation of a developing tension pneumothorax.

Management. High-concentration oxygen (85% or greater, or an FiO_2 of 0.85 or greater) should be administered to patients with a pneumothorax. Assisted ventilation with a BVM may be necessary for patients with a ventilatory rate of either less than 12 or greater than 20 breaths/min or for those who display signs of hypoxia. However, use of positive-pressure ventilation may increase the possibility of a tension pneumothorax. The patient should be transported rapidly and carefully monitored for signs of a tension pneumothorax while en route. Steps should be taken to alleviate any tension pneumothorax that develops. If there is no indication for spinal immobilization and it is required for better patient ventilation, the patient may be transported in a semi-sitting position.

At the basic provider level, rapid transportation must occur as soon as practical in anticipation of a possible tension pneumothorax. If possible, the prehospital care provider should consider interception with an advanced life support (ALS) unit.

OPEN PNEUMOTHORAX

Penetrating wounds to the chest can produce open chest wall injuries (open pneumothorax). These injuries are most often the result of gunshot or knife wounds, but they can also occur from impaled objects, MVCs, and falls. The severity of a chest wall defect is directly proportional to its size. Many small wounds will seal themselves. Some large wounds will be completely open, allowing air to enter and escape the pleural cavity (Figure 5-10). Other wounds function like a ball valve. These wounds allow air to enter when the intrathoracic pressure is negative and block the air's release when the intrathoracic pressure is positive; hence the term "sucking chest wound." These wounds are of particular concern because their management may lead to a tension pneumothorax.

Two sources can leak air into the pleural space—a hole in the chest wall and a hole in the lung or bronchus. Even if an injury to the chest wall is sealed, air leakage from the injury to the lung can contribute to a pneumothorax (Figure 5-11).

Any opening in the chest wall creates a pathway for air to move from the outside environment into the thorax. The negative intrathoracic pressure created during the inspiratory phase of ventilation sucks outside air into the thoracic cavity. This air remains outside the lung on that side of the chest, generally within the pleura. With reduced, if any, air coming through the bronchi to expand the lung and with air accumulating between the pleura outside the lung, the lung is compressed and cannot expand. The oxygen in the air that enters the thorax in this

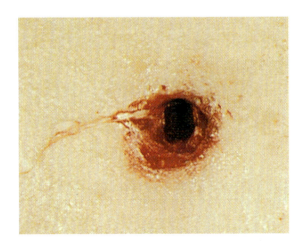

Figure 5-10   A gunshot or stab wound to the chest produces a hole in the chest wall through which air can flow both into and out of the pleural cavity.

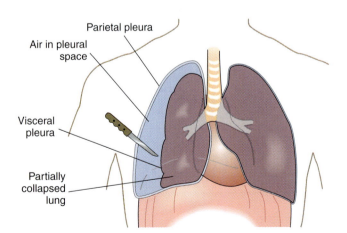

Figure 5-11   Because of the close proximity of the chest wall to the lung, it would be extremely difficult for the chest wall to be injured by penetrating trauma and the lung not to be injured. Stopping the hole in the chest wall does not necessarily decrease air leakage into the pleural space; leakage can come from the lung just as easily.

manner does not enter the lung, cannot become exposed to the alveolar capillaries, and therefore is not diffused into the bloodstream to oxygenate the body cells.

Assessment. Symptoms of an open pneumothorax include pain at the injury site and shortness of breath. The signs may include a moist sucking or bubbling sound as air moves in and out of the pleural space through the chest wall defect.

Management. Management of a patient with an open pneumothorax is first directed at closing the hole in the chest and providing supplemental oxygen. A patient in respiratory distress not responding to this initial management may require positive-pressure ventilation. However, positive-pressure ventilation can rapidly cause a tension pneumothorax when the dressing over an open chest wound is completely sealed. If only three sides of the dressing are taped, an effective vent is created, possibly permitting the spontaneous decompression of a developing tension pneumothorax (Figure 5-12). Closing the wound can be done with Vaseline gauze covered with sterile gauze, or any other type of occlusive dressing secured with tape. Blocking airflow completely with a dressing can produce a tension pneumothorax. Even if a self-venting dressing is applied, the patient with a sealed open chest wound should be carefully monitored for the onset of a tension pneumothorax. If signs of increasing respiratory distress are observed, the patient may be developing a tension pneumothorax, and the dressing should be removed immediately to assist in decompressing the affected side.

TENSION PNEUMOTHORAX

A life-threatening situation arises when a one-way valve is created, allowing air to enter but not leave the pleural space. As the pressure in the pleural space exceeds the outside atmospheric pressure, the physiologic consequences of a simple pneumothorax are magnified. This injury is called a *tension pneumothorax*. Increasing pressure within the pleural space further collapses the lung on the involved side and forces the mediastinum (heart and blood vessels) to the opposite (contralateral) side (Figure 5-13).

Two extremely serious consequences result: (1) ventilation becomes increasingly difficult and (2) the flow of blood into the heart decreases. Ventilation is compromised because not only has the lung collapsed on the injured side, but the lung on the uninjured side is compressed by the shift of mediastinal structures. Normally, the pressure in the great veins leading to the heart is between 5 and 10 mm Hg. As pressure in the pleural space increases, the mediastinum shifts (evidenced by tracheal deviation from the midline), resulting in venous pressures that are higher than normal. This is caused by the increase in intrapleural pressure and kinking of the vena cava, both of which decrease the flow of blood into the heart. This decrease in venous return to the heart results in an overall decrease in cardiac output, and shock ensues.

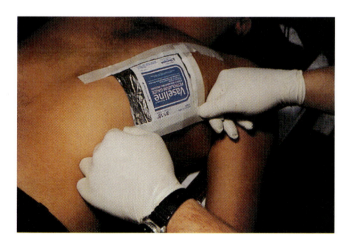

Figure 5-12 Taping a piece of foil or plastic to the chest wall on three sides creates a flutter-valve effect, allowing air to escape from the pleural space but not enter into it.

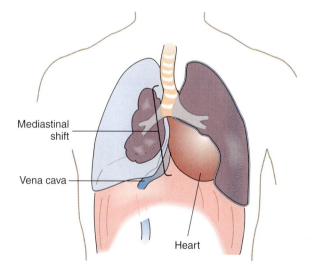

Figure 5-13 Tension pneumothorax. If the amount of air trapped in the pleural space continues to increase, not only is the lung on the affected side collapsed, but the mediastinum is also shifted into the opposite side. The lung on the opposite side then collapses and intrathoracic pressure increases, which decreases capillary blood flow and kinks the vena cava.

Although the following signs are frequently discussed with a tension pneumothorax, many may not be present or are difficult to identify in the field:

- *Tracheal deviation* is usually a late sign. In the neck, the trachea is bound to the cervical spine by fascial and other supporting structures; thus the deviation of the trachea is more of an intrathoracic phenomenon, although it may be felt if it is severe. Tracheal deviation is not often seen in the prehospital environment. Even when it is present, it can be difficult to diagnose by physical examination.
- *Distended neck veins* are described as a classic sign of tension pneumothorax. However, since a patient with a tension pneumothorax may also have lost a considerable amount of blood, distended neck veins may not be prominent. If the patient has a pneumatic antishock garment (PASG) applied, the neck veins may be distended by the device and not by a tension pneumothorax (Figure 5-14).
- *Cyanosis* is difficult to see in the field. Poor lighting, variation in skin color, and dirt and blood associated with trauma often render this sign unreliable.
- *Decreased breath sounds on the injured side.* The most helpful part of the physical examination is checking for decreased breath sounds on the side of the injury. However, to use this sign the prehospital care provider must be able to distinguish between normal and decreased sounds. Such differentiation requires a great deal of practice. Listening to breath sounds during every patient contact will help.
- *Percussion of the chest* is an excellent method for determining the status of the chest cavity in the relative quiet of a hospital. In the noisy prehospital environment this sound is much more difficult to detect. Given the difficulty in obtaining this sign and the time and environment necessary with which to perform it, it is not recommended for field diagnosis of tension pneumothorax.

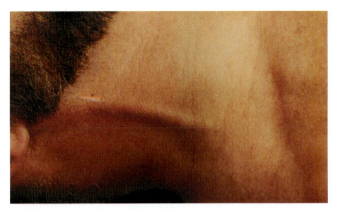

Figure 5-14 Distended neck veins are one indication of an increase in thoracic pressure.

mothorax. The development of a tension pneumothorax is an important concern for any patient who has sustained chest trauma, has been intubated, and requires positive-pressure ventilation. In these cases, a simple pneumothorax can progress to a tension pneumothorax because air is being pushed into the chest with each ventilation. The patient should be monitored constantly for this possibility.

Usual signs and symptoms of a developing tension pneumothorax can be divided into the following stages:

- *Early signs.* Unilateral decreased or absent breath sounds; continued increased dyspnea and tachypnea despite treatment
- *Progressive signs.* Increasing tachypnea and dyspnea, tachycardia and subcutaneous emphysema, increasing difficulty ventilating an intubated patient
- *Late signs.* JVD, tracheal deviation, tympany, signs of acute hypoxia, narrowing pulse pressure, and other signs of increasing decompensated shock

In some cases, the only signs of a developing tension pneumothorax are compromised oxygenation, tachycardia, tachypnea, and unilateral decreased or absent breath sounds.

Management. The management of a patient with a tension pneumothorax involves reducing the pressure in the pleural space.

Penetrating Injury. When a patient has a wound in the chest wall with accompanying signs of a tension pneumothorax, the first step to relieve the increased pressure is to remove the dressing over the wound for a few seconds. If the wound in the chest wall has not

Assessment. The presentation of patients with a tension pneumothorax varies according to how much intrathoracic pressure has developed. Signs and symptoms can be minimal or moderate, whereas in other patients they can be severe. Signs and symptoms of a tension pneumothorax include extreme anxiety, cyanosis, tachypnea, diminished or absent breath sounds on the injured side, bulging of the intercostal muscles, jugular vein distention (JVD), tachycardia, narrow pulse pressure, hypotension, subcutaneous emphysema, and tracheal deviation. Note that in a patient who is hypovolemic from other injuries, JVD may not be present.

Any patient with a simple pneumothorax or hemopneumothorax has a potential to develop a tension pneu-

sealed under the dressing, air will rush out of the wound. Once the pressure has been released, the wound should be resealed with the occlusive dressing. This short release may need to be repeated periodically if pressure again builds up within the chest. If this does not work, needle decompression can be considered. In the rare case that it becomes necessary to keep the defect open to prevent further accumulation of air in the thoracic cavity, assisted ventilation with a BVM and an oxygen concentration of 85% or greater (FiO_2 of 0.85 or greater) is necessary.

Closed Tension Pneumothorax. If the pneumothorax developed without a wound in the chest wall, an advanced prehospital care provider can accomplish decompression of the chest by insertion of a large-bore needle into the pleural space of the affected side. If an advanced provider is not available, the patient should be transported rapidly to an appropriate facility and given a high concentration of oxygen en route. A tension pneumothorax or a potential tension pneumothorax is a life-threatening condition. It requires rapid access to an appropriate facility because needle decompression or dressing removal is only a temporary solution until more definitive care can be provided.

Needle Decompression. Needle decompression carries minimal risk and can greatly benefit the patient by improving oxygenation and circulation. Needle decompression should be performed when the following three criteria are met:

1. Evidence of worsening respiratory distress or difficulty ventilating with a BVM device
2. Decreased or absent breath sounds
3. Decompensated shock (systolic blood pressure <90 mm Hg)

A large-bore (10- to 16-gauge) hollow needle of appropriate length is inserted into the affected pleural space at the second intercostal space in the midclavicular line. The landmark for insertion is the angle of Louis on the sternum, which marks the space between the second and third ribs (Figure 5-15). (See the Thoracic Trauma Skills section at the end of this chapter for the complete needle decompression procedure.)

The midclavicular line is at the midpoint of the clavicle. This area lacks anatomic structures that could be injured during needle decompression. The internal mammary artery is just lateral to the sternal border

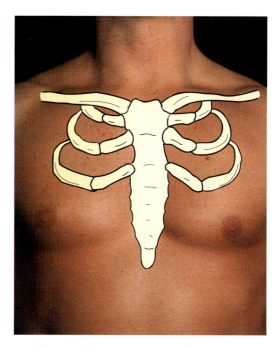

Figure 5-15 Needle decompression of the thoracic cavity is most easily accomplished and produces the least chance for complication if it is done at the midclavicular line through the second intercostal space.

(1 cm), hence the use of the midclavicular line. Since the lung is compressed toward the mediastinum, it will be out of the way if the needle is placed high into the second intercostal space. The nerve, artery, and vein pass just beneath each rib, so the needle should pass just over the top of the third rib. The midclavicular site is preferred over the midaxillary line where chest tubes are inserted. The anterior chest provides better visualization of the needle at the midclavicular line while en route to the hospital and often has less tissue to penetrate with the needle, unlike the midaxillary line where the chest wall can be deep, especially in obese patients. Also, the patient's arm is not strapped down across this area as would be the case if the midaxillary line were chosen. Special situations may require other approaches under the direction of appropriate medical control.

Initially after insertion, air will rush from the needle as the pressure in the chest is relieved. Once the rush of air is noted, the needle should be advanced no further. Needle decompression will convert a life-threatening tension pneumothorax into a non–life-threatening open pneumothorax. The provider should not waste time with a one-way valve. The open pneumothorax created by the needle will not significantly impair a patient's ventilatory effort.

As a general rule, bilateral tension pneumothorax is exceedingly rare in patients who are not intubated and ventilated with positive pressure. The first step in re-assessing the patient is to confirm the location of the en-dotracheal (ET) tube, ensure that it has no kinks or bends causing compression of the tube, and ensure that the tube has not inadvertently moved down into a main-stem bronchus. Extreme caution should be exercised with bilateral needle decompression in patients who are not intubated and ventilated with positive-pressure ventilation.

Hemothorax

Blood in the pleural space constitutes a hemothorax. In adults, the pleural space on each side of the thorax can hold 2500 to 3000 mL of blood. This blood comes from several sources, including torn intercostal vessels, the great vessels, or the lung itself and its vessels. Hypo-volemia (decreased fluid volume) occurs as the blood leaves the cardiovascular space and enters the pleural space. Although a tension hemothorax is an uncommon occurrence, it does happen. A simple hemothorax is much more common, and the clinically critical compo-nent is the associated blood loss (Figure 5-16).

ASSESSMENT

The symptoms of a hemothorax are directly related to blood loss and, to a much lesser extent, the amount of lung collapse and the resulting shortness of breath. De-pending on the magnitude of respiratory and circulatory compromise, as with any hypovolemic condition, a pa-tient may also be confused or anxious. Signs of a hemo-thorax include tachypnea, decreased breath sounds, and clinical signs of shock.

Diminished breath sounds on the same side are found with a hemothorax. Often with penetrating trauma, a pneumothorax is associated with a hemothorax and is called a *hemopneumothorax*.

MANAGEMENT

A patient with a hemothorax is managed by correct-ing the ventilatory and circulatory problems. High-concentration oxygen is administered and ventilations assisted using a BVM (or ET tube as necessary). As with other chest injuries, the patient should be ob-served closely. Hypovolemia and shock are the major physiologic defects and should be treated with intra-venous electrolyte solutions and rapid transport to an appropriate facility where immediate surgical repair can be achieved.

Blunt Cardiac Injury

The heart occupies a large portion of the center of the chest and is situated between the sternum and the tho-racic spine. In severe blunt trauma to the chest, as oc-curs in frontal impact MVCs, the chest first strikes the dashboard or steering wheel and then the heart is crushed between the sternum and spine (Figure 5-17). Several cardiac injuries can result, but the most com-mon injury is myocardial contusion. The cardiac ven-tricles can be forcefully compressed and systolic blood pressure can rise to 800 mm Hg, causing compression of the myocardial wall. This compression can cause cell wall destruction, rupture of the heart wall itself, or damage to the heart valves. The right ventricle is most commonly injured because of its location beneath the sternum.

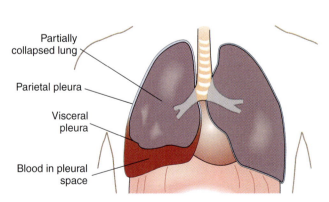

Figure 5-16   Hemothorax. The amount of blood that can accumulate in the thoracic cavity (leading to hypovolemia) is a much more severe condition than the amount of lung com-pressed by this blood loss.

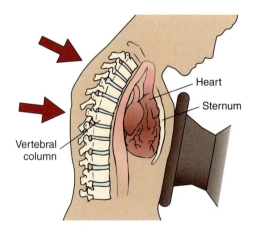

Figure 5-17   The heart can be trapped between the sternum (as the sternum stops against the steering column or dash-board) and the posterior thoracic wall (as the wall continues its forward motion). This can contuse the myocardium.

Three distinct injury patterns can occur with myocardial compressive injury: (1) disturbance in the electrical conducting system of the myocardium caused by a contusion (bruise) to the myocardial wall that can be partial or full thickness, (2) valvular rupture, and (3) rupture of the myocardial wall. The latter condition may lead to rapid exsanguination (massive loss of blood) or pericardial tamponade.

ASSESSMENT

Myocardial contusion is an injury in patients with chest compression. In the field, the prehospital care provider should assume that a patient with significant chest trauma has a bruised myocardium.

Partial- or full-thickness contusions may be indicated by a reduced cardiac output and dysrhythmias; however, signs of these contusions may not be evident at all. When kinematics and other crash and postcrash evaluations indicate this condition but clinical indications are absent, the prehospital care provider should make the receiving facility aware of the possibility. In a frontal impact MVC that includes a bent steering wheel or a collapsed steering column, the prehospital care provider must report these findings.

Patients do not usually exhibit symptoms when they have a myocardial contusion, but a patient may complain of chest discomfort and pain of fractured ribs or bruised muscles. A patient with dysrhythmias may complain of palpitations. Anterior chest tenderness and a bent steering wheel are the most common findings and should be warning signs of possible blunt cardiac injury.

Injuries to the electrical system of the heart may manifest as a variety of dysrhythmias, the most common of which is tachycardia out of proportion to other conditions. Premature ventricular contractions (PVCs) are the second most common, followed by atrial fibrillation. Septal injuries may produce conduction defects in the form of a bundle branch block (BBB), most commonly noted on the right (RBBB). Muscle wall damage is indicated in the field by ST segment elevation or other electrocardiogram (ECG) changes. With valvular rupture, a patient may present with acute signs of heart failure and a loud heart murmur may be noted on auscultation. Myocardial wall rupture produces a pericardial tamponade (discussed later).

MANAGEMENT

Management of patients with blunt cardiac injury includes administration of high-concentration oxygen and monitoring of the patient's pulse. In areas where multiple levels of prehospital response are available and the patient is being treated by basic providers, the providers should consider intersecting with an ALS unit.

If the patient has direct trauma to the chest significant enough to suggest a possible myocardial contusion, the prehospital care provider should place him or her on an ECG monitor, and advanced providers should treat any dysrhythmia pharmacologically. Rapid transportation to an appropriate facility is indicated.

Pericardial Tamponade

The heart is enclosed within a tough, fibrous, flexible, but inelastic membrane called the *pericardium*. A potential space (the pericardial space) exists between the heart and the pericardium. As with the pleural space, a few milliliters of fluid normally occupies and lubricates this space. Blood can enter the pericardial space if myocardial blood vessels are torn by blunt or penetrating trauma or if the myocardium is ruptured or penetrated. This condition, called *hemopericardium*, can lead to pericardial tamponade.

Pericardial tamponade is most frequently associated with stab wounds. Gunshot wounds often create a large enough hole in the pericardium for blood to exit the pericardial space. It can occasionally occur from the rupture of the myocardial chamber. Exsanguination into the chest cavity rather than tamponade is the usual result of gunshot wounds. Exit of blood from the pericardial sac is not possible. The pericardium is an inelastic sac surrounding the heart and, as blood leaks from a wound in the wall of the heart, it fills the sac. As the heart contracts to eject blood during systole, more blood enters the intact pericardial sac. This further compresses the heart and does not allow it to fully expand or refill with blood. This reduces cardiac output and decreases perfusion (Figure 5-18).

ASSESSMENT

A trauma patient with a pericardial tamponade may lack symptoms other than those related to chest injuries and associated shock. In an adult, the pericardial space can hold up to 200 to 300 mL of blood before a cardiac tamponade will occur; however, smaller volumes can still significantly reduce cardiac output.

As the amount of blood in the pericardial sac increases, the heart rate will increase in an attempt to maintain cardiac output. Pulse pressure (the difference between systolic and diastolic pressures) narrows, and a paradoxical pulse may be present. A patient has a paradoxical pulse when the systolic blood pressure drops

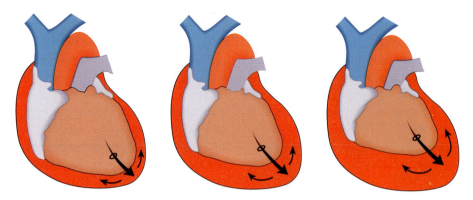

Figure 5-18   Pericardial tamponade. As blood courses from the cardiac lumen into the pericardial space, it limits expansion of the ventricle. Therefore the ventricle cannot fill completely. As more blood accumulates in the pericardial space, less ventricular space is available to accumulate blood and cardiac output is reduced.

more than 10 to 15 mm Hg during each inspiration. The prehospital care provider can clinically determine this blood pressure drop by noting that the radial pulse diminishes or even disappears with inspiration. Because the compressed ventricles have reduced expansion during diastole, only a small amount of blood can enter the heart. Expansion of the pulmonary vascular field during inspiration requires all or almost all of the reduced right heart output. This results in decreased filling of the left heart and reduced left heart output. Back-up of pressure on the right side results in venous pooling and neck vein distention or JVD. Heart sounds may be muffled and distant. Signs of shock appear and progressively worsen. These three findings—elevated venous pressure, shock, and muffled heart sounds—are the classic signs of pericardial tamponade and are known as *Beck's triad.* However, all of these signs are not always present with this condition, especially if the patient is hypovolemic from other injuries.

MANAGEMENT

Patients with pericardial tamponade require rapid, well-monitored transport to an appropriate facility. Delays must not occur in the field. As with any type of shock, intravenous electrolyte infusion may improve cardiac output by increasing venous pressure and should be established during transport.

Management of patients with pericardial tamponade involves removing the pericardial blood and stopping the source of bleeding. Pericardial blood can be removed by use of *needle pericardiocentesis,* a procedure almost exclusively limited to the emergency department. Pericardiocentesis is a temporizing intervention until control of bleeding and surgical repair of the injury can occur in the operating room.

Aortic Rupture

Traumatic aortic rupture usually results from a shear injury. With rapid, high G-force speed change in blunt chest injuries, several events take place. The heart and aortic arch suddenly move either anteriorly or laterally. The heart and aortic arch move away from the descending aorta, which is tightly fixed to the thoracic vertebrae. Severe stress and shear forces occur at the distal portion of the arch where the restrained and unrestrained parts of the aorta meet. If the tensile strength of the aorta is exceeded, these two components can be torn apart (Figure 5-19). The outer layer of tissue surrounding the aorta may remain intact, temporarily preventing immediate exsanguination.

About 80% to 90% of patients with these injuries sustain immediate rupture and complete exsanguination into the left pleural space within the first hour. The remaining patients reach the receiving facility alive. One third of these initial survivors die within 6 hours, another third die in 24 hours, and the other third survive 3 days or longer. Timely surgical repair and hypotension management can prevent most of the deaths of patients who reach the receiving facility alive.

ASSESSMENT

Diagnosis of aortic rupture is extremely difficult. In the hospital, a radiologic study of the aorta (either a computed tomography [CT] scan or an aortogram) is required to make the diagnosis. Although a chest x-ray examination may provide a tool for diagnosis, further diagnostic testing is usually needed.

Information from the scene concerning the magnitude of the trauma can be helpful because up to one third of these patients lack any signs of chest trauma. Patients with unexplained shock and a frontal impact

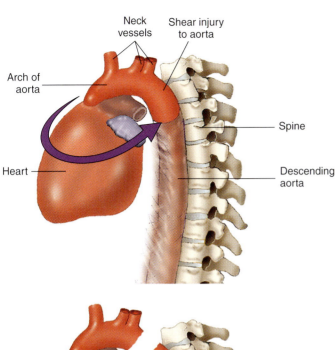

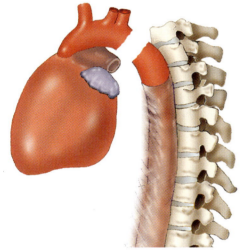

Figure 5-19   The descending aorta is tightly affixed to the thoracic vertebrae. The arch of the aorta and the heart are not attached to the vertebrae. Disruption from shear force usually occurs at the junction of the arch and the descending aorta.

deceleration injury or lateral impact acceleration injury must be suspected of having aortic disruption. In some cases, a difference in pulse quality between the arms and the lower torso or between the left and right arms can be detected. Assessment of both radial and femoral pulses is an important diagnostic step.

MANAGEMENT

Management of patients with aortic rupture involves administration of an oxygen concentration of 85% or greater (FiO₂ of 0.85 or greater) and ventilatory assistance with a BVM when indicated. Immediate transport and communication with the receiving facility are also key factors.

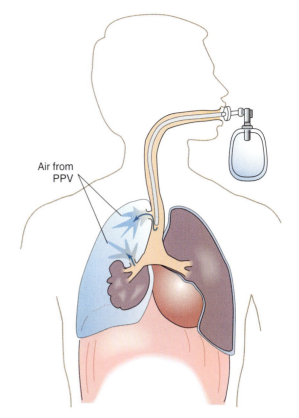

Figure 5-20   Tracheal or bronchial rupture. Positive-pressure ventilation (PPV) can directly force large amounts of air through the trachea or bronchus, rapidly producing a tension pneumothorax.

Tracheal/Bronchial Rupture

Any portion of the tracheal/bronchial tree can be injured by penetrating or blunt trauma. These tears allow rapid movement of air into the pleural space, producing a tension pneumothorax that may be refractive (unresponsive) to decompression (Figure 5-20). Rather than a simple one-time rush of air from needle decompression, air continually flows from the needle. Assisted ventilation frequently worsens the condition of a patient with this type of injury. As air is forced into the lungs, it is forced out of the tear in the bronchus or trachea at the same rate.

ASSESSMENT

Patients with tracheal/bronchial rupture may have severe dyspnea and often cough up bright red blood. Blunt trauma typically ruptures the upper trachea, the larynx, or the major bronchi just beyond the carina. The associated major hemorrhage seen with penetrating trauma is rarely present, but the signs, symptoms, and management are the same as with blunt trauma. With both blunt and penetrating trauma, an associated hemothorax or pneumothorax or an area of subcutaneous emphysema extending supraclavicularly into the neck and face may be present.

MANAGEMENT

Assisted ventilation may be extremely difficult . If assisted ventilation seems to make the patient worse, the prehospital care provider should allow the patient to breathe spontaneously and give supplemental oxygen at a concentration of 85% (an FiO$_2$ of 0.85) or greater. Otherwise, the prehospital care provider should initiate assisted ventilation with a BVM and rapid transportation.

Traumatic Asphyxia

The term *traumatic asphyxia* is a misnomer. Although these patients look like victims of strangulation, the condition has nothing to do with asphyxia. With severe blunt and crushing injuries to the chest and abdomen, a marked increase in intrathoracic pressure occurs. This forces blood backward out of the right side of the heart and into the veins of the upper chest and neck. This pressure is transmitted to capillaries in the brain, head, and neck, producing microrupture.

ASSESSMENT

Patients with traumatic asphyxia present with a bluish discoloration to the face and upper neck. Unless other problems exist, the skin below this area is pink. JVD and swelling or hemorrhage of the conjunctiva may also be present. Most discoloration will resolve within a few days.

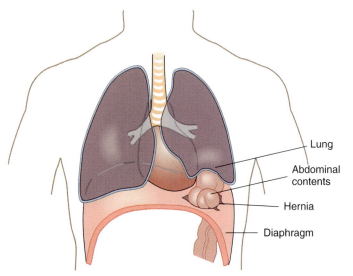

Figure 5-21 Diaphragmatic rupture may cause the bowel or other structures to herniate through the tear, causing partial compression of the lung and respiratory distress.

MANAGEMENT

Because of the forces involved, any of the other injuries mentioned previously may be present. Management of the patient with traumatic asphyxiation includes identifying the condition, providing airway maintenance, and identifying and managing any associated injuries.

Diaphragmatic Rupture

With forceful compression to the abdomen, intra-abdominal pressure may increase enough to tear the diaphragm and allow abdominal contents to enter the thoracic cavity. Penetrating trauma may result in injury to the diaphragm on either side. However, blunt trauma with diaphragmatic rupture on the left side is more commonly recognized. The stomach, spleen, small intestine, and colon can be forced into the thoracic cavity. The space occupied by these organs restricts lung expansion and reduces ventilation. The reduction in ventilation can be severe enough to be life-threatening (Figure 5-21).

Lacerations of the diaphragm can also occur in penetrating trauma because of the change in position of the diaphragm with ventilation. At maximum exhalation, the diaphragm is as high as the fourth intercostal space anteriorly. Therefore any penetrating anterior injury below the nipple line can result in the laceration of the diaphragm.

ASSESSMENT

Diaphragmatic rupture is another extremely difficult condition to diagnose. The patient may have abdominal complaints or may complain of shortness of breath. Upon examination, the prehospital care provider may note decreased breath sounds, particularly over the left chest. In some cases, bowel sounds may be heard in the left chest. If a considerable quantity of abdominal contents is displaced into the chest, the abdomen may have a scaphoid (empty) appearance.

MANAGEMENT

Management of diaphragmatic rupture includes assisted positive-pressure ventilation with a BVM and an oxygen concentration of 85% (an FiO$_2$ of 0.85) or greater. Diaphragmatic rupture can worsen with anything that increases intraabdominal pressure, such as that associated with PASG use. Deterioration of ventilation and oxygenation after inflation of the PASG is an indication that such a condition exists. Diaphragmatic rupture is one of the few situations in which field deflation of the PASG is indicated.

Summary

Chest injuries are particularly significant because of the potential for compromise of respiratory and circulatory function and because chest injuries are frequently associated with multisystem trauma. The prehospital care provider should manage patients with chest injury aggressively and transport them quickly to definitive care. Particular attention should be paid to the administration of oxygen and the need for ventilatory support in any patient suspected of having chest trauma. Signs of tension pneumothorax should be sought because, although quickly lethal if left untreated, a tension pneumothorax can be treated in the field with needle decompression. Because of the high risk of multisystem trauma, especially in blunt chest trauma, the prehospital care provider should consider spinal immobilization and, as with any trauma patient, control hemorrhage. IV access should be obtained en route to the medical facility, and ECG monitoring may give an indication of blunt cardiac injury. Although many chest injuries can be managed nonsurgically, the patient with a chest injury must still be evaluated and managed at an appropriate medical facility.

Scenario Solution

The mechanism of injury, complaint, and physical examination findings are consistent with significant blunt trauma to the thorax. The findings of diminished breath sounds and subcutaneous emphysema of the chest wall indicate a likely pneumothorax, possibly accompanied by a pulmonary contusion. Rapid field identification of the seriousness of these injuries, spinal immobilization, supplemental oxygenation, and expedient transport to a trauma center are the first priorities in this scenario. The patient is at high risk for ventilatory failure, a situation which is compounded by the lengthy transport time. You should consider the appropriateness of air transport. En route to a medical facility, you must monitor the patient's ventilatory status continuously, implement ventilatory assistance if necessary, and institute fluid therapy. In addition to the chest injury, the starred windshield, facial lacerations, and amnesia for the event indicate possible traumatic brain injury and thus cervical spine injury. If the patient's ventilatory status allows and a sufficient number of personnel are available, you should conduct a thorough trauma examination. Although many chest injuries can be treated nonsurgically, the patient still requires assessment and management by a trauma team and therefore should be transported to the closest appropriate facility.

Review Questions

Answers are provided on p. 414.

1. In a patient with a pulmonary contusion, which of following is the primary physiologic mechanism that increases the ventilatory rate?
   a. Increased level of carbon dioxide
   b. Decreased level of carbon dioxide
   c. Increased level of oxygen
   d. Decreased level of oxygen

2. Which of the following is the most likely mechanism of aortic disruption in blunt trauma?
   a. Compression
   b. Penetration
   c. Shearing
   d. Angulation

3. Paradoxical chest wall movement is a sign of which of the following?
   a. Hemothorax
   b. Pericardial tamponade
   c. Bronchial rupture
   d. Flail chest

4. Which of the following is the mechanism by which a tension pneumothorax compromises ventilation and circulation?
   a. Increased intrathoracic pressure
   b. Decreased intrathoracic pressure
   c. Increased intraabdominal pressure
   d. Decreased intraabdominal pressure

5. A fracture of the first or second rib is associated with which of the following?
   a. Application of considerable force
   b. Increased mortality
   c. Aortic rupture
   d. All of the above

6. Which of the following is indicated for the immediate management of an open pneumothorax?
   a. Occlusive dressing
   b. Needle chest decompression
   c. Cricothyroidotomy
   d. Positive-pressure ventilation

7. Your patient is a 45-year-old male who was operating a forklift when it tipped over, trapping him beneath it. The patient was extricated before your arrival. The patient responds to verbal commands with eye opening; has rapid, shallow ventilations; and appears pale with diaphoresis. The patient has no palpable radial pulse but has a weak, rapid carotid pulse. After management is begun, including the use of a PASG, the patient's ventilatory distress becomes markedly worse and he is unresponsive. Which of the following is the most likely cause of the patient's deterioration after the application of the PASG?
   a. Pericardial tamponade
   b. Traumatic asphyxiation
   c. Diaphragmatic rupture
   d. Rupture of the perineum

8. Which of the following is the most common problem associated with hemothorax?
   a. Progression to a tension hemothorax
   b. Bronchial laceration
   c. Hypovolemia
   d. Cardiac dysrhythmia

9. A 16-year-old male has been struck in the anterior neck with a baseball at a high velocity. On your arrival, the patient is responsive only to painful stimulus. He is making inspiratory effort, but ventilation is ineffective. Upon attempting to ventilate the patient via a bag-valve-mask device, you notice the sudden development of subcutaneous air in the neck and realize that it is extremely difficult to ventilate the patient. Even with assisted ventilation, rise and fall of the chest does not occur. What is the next step in the management of this patient?
   a. Assessment of circulatory status
   b. Cricothyroidotomy
   c. Bilateral needle decompression of the chest
   d. Immediate transport without further scene stabilization

10. A 30-year-old female, the unrestrained driver in a significant frontal impact collision, is in severe respiratory distress and is found to have an anterior flail segment. Which of the following is the appropriate way to stabilize the flail segment?
   a. Placing your hand on the flail segment
   b. Placing the patient in a prone position on a backboard
   c. Placing a sand bag on the flail segment
   d. Placing a circumferential bandage around the chest

REFERENCES

American College of Surgeons: Thoracic trauma. In American College of Surgeons Committee on Trauma: *Advanced trauma life support for doctors*, Chicago, 2002, Author.

Barone JE, Pizzi WF, Nealon TF, Richman H: Indications for intubation in blunt chest trauma, *J Trauma* 26:334, 1986.

Eckstein M, Suyehara DL: Needle thoracostomy in the prehospital setting, *Prehosp Emerg Care* 2:132, 1998.

Gervin AS, Fischer RF: The importance of prompt transport in salvage of pateints with penetrating heart wounds, *J Trauma* 22:443, 1982.

Ivatury RR: The injured heart. In Mattox KL, Feliciano DV, Moore EE: *Trauma*, ed 4, New York, 2000, McGraw-Hill, pp 545-558.

Mattox KL, Bickell WH, Pepe PE, et al: Prospective MAST study in 911 patients, *J Trauma* 29:1104, 1989.

Mattox KL, Wall MJ, LeMaire SA: Injury to the thoracic great vessels. In Mattox KL, Feliciano DV, Moore EE: *Trauma*, ed 4, New York, 2000, McGraw-Hill, pp 559-582.

Newman PG, Feliciano DV: Blunt cardiac injury, *New Horizons* 7:26, 1999.

Richardson JD, Spain DA: Injury to the lung and pleura. In Mattox KL, Feliciano DV, Moore EE: *Trauma*, ed 4, New York, 2000, McGraw-Hill, pp 523-524.

SUGGESTED READING:

Barton ED, Epperson M, Hoyt DB et al: Prehospital needle aspiration and tube thoracostomy in trauma victims: a six year experience with aeromedical crews, *J Emerg Med* 13:155, 1995.

Callaham M: Pericardiocentesis in traumatic and nontraumatic cardiac tamponade, *Ann Emerg Med* 13:924, 1984.

Honigman B, Lowenstein SR, Moore EE et al: The role of the pneumatic antishock garment in penetrating cardiac wounds, *JAMA* 266:2398, 1991.

Ivatury RR, Nallathambi MN, Roberge RJ et al: Penetrating thoracic injuries:in-field stabilization vs. prompt transport, *J Trauma* 27:1066, 1987.

Richardson JD, Adams L, Flint LM: Selective management of flail chest and pulmonary contusion, *Ann Surg* 196:481, 1982.

Rozycki GS, Feliciano DV, Oschner MG et al: The role of ultrasound in patients with possible penetrating cardiac wounds: a prospective multicenter study, *J Trauma* 46:542, 1999.

Specific Skills

Thoracic Trauma Skills

Needle Chest Decompression

In patients with increasing intrathoracic pressure from a developing tension pneumothorax, the side of the thoracic cavity that has the increased pressure should be decompressed. If this pressure is not relieved, it will progressively limit the patient's ventilatory capacity and cause inadequate venous return, producing inadequate cardiac output and death.

In cases in which an open pneumothorax has been treated by the use of an occlusive dressing and a tension pneumothorax develops, decompression can usually be achieved through the wound, which provides an existing opening into the thorax. Opening the occlusive dressing over the wound for a few seconds should initiate a rush of air out of the wound as increased pressure in the thorax is relieved.

Once this pressure has been released, the wound is resealed with the occlusive dressing to allow for proper alveolar ventilation and to stop air from "sucking" into the wound. The patient should be monitored carefully and, if any signs of tension reoccur, the dressing should be "burped" again to release the intrathoracic pressure.

Decompression in a closed tension pneumothorax is achieved by providing an opening—a thoracostomy—in the affected side of the chest. Different methods for performing a thoracostomy exist. Because needle thoracostomy is the most rapid method and does not require special equipment, it is the preferred method for use in the field.

Needle decompression carries minimal risk and can greatly benefit the patient by improving oxygenation and circulation. Needle decompression should be performed when the following three criteria are met:
1. Evidence of worsening respiratory distress or difficulty with a BVM device
2. Decreased or absent breath sounds
3. Decompensated shock (systolic blood pressure <90 mm Hg)

Necessary equipment for needle chest compression includes a needle, a syringe, ½-inch adhesive tape, and alcohol swabs. The needles should be large-bore over-the-needle intravenous catheters between 10 gauge and 14 gauge. A 16-gauge catheter can be used if a larger bore is not available.

One prehospital care provider attaches the needle to the syringe while a second provider auscultates the patient's chest to confirm which side has the tension pneumothorax, which is indicated by absent or diminished breath sounds.

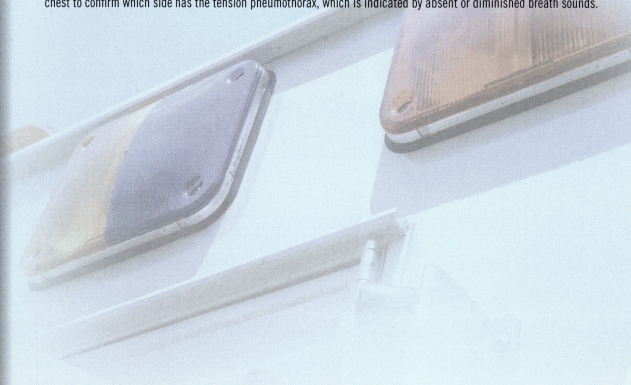

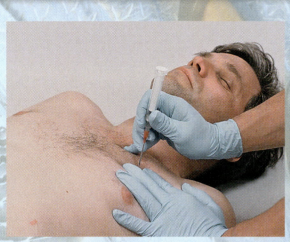

After confirmation of a tension pneumothorax, the anatomic landmarks are located on the affected side (midclavicular line, second or third intercostal space) and the site swabbed with an alcohol wipe. The skin is stretched over the site between the fingers of the nondominate hand. The needle is placed for entrance over the top of the rib. Once the needle enters the thoracic cavity, air will escape. The needle should not be advanced further. The catheter should be left in place, and the needle should be removed, being careful not to kink the catheter. As the needle is removed, a rush of air from the hub of the catheter should be heard. If no air escapes, the catheter should be left in place to indicate that needle decompression of the chest was attempted.

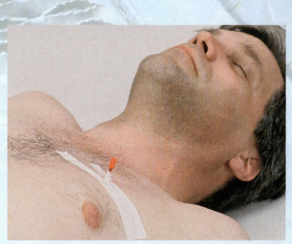

After the needle is removed, the catheter is taped in place with adhesive tape. After securing the catheter, the chest should be auscultated to check for increased breath sounds. The patient should be monitored and transported to an appropriate facility. The provider should not waste time inserting a one-way valve.

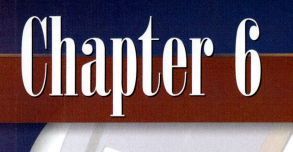

Chapter 6

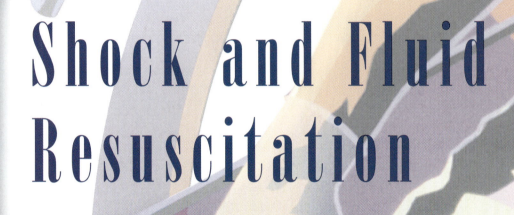

Shock and Fluid Resuscitation

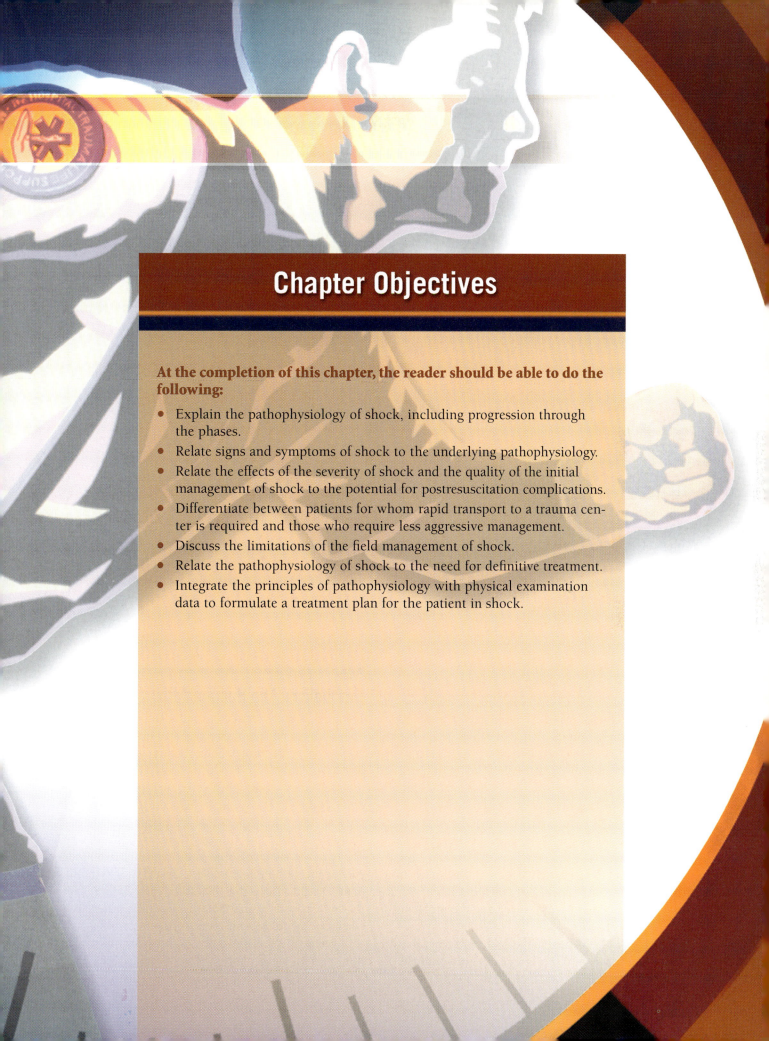

Chapter Objectives

At the completion of this chapter, the reader should be able to do the following:

- Explain the pathophysiology of shock, including progression through the phases.
- Relate signs and symptoms of shock to the underlying pathophysiology.
- Relate the effects of the severity of shock and the quality of the initial management of shock to the potential for postresuscitation complications.
- Differentiate between patients for whom rapid transport to a trauma center is required and those who require less aggressive management.
- Discuss the limitations of the field management of shock.
- Relate the pathophysiology of shock to the need for definitive treatment.
- Integrate the principles of pathophysiology with physical examination data to formulate a treatment plan for the patient in shock.

Scenario

You have arrived on the scene of a late afternoon motor vehicle crash (MVC) at an intersection notorious for serious MVCs. You observe that a compact car has been struck in the driver's side door by a full-sized pickup truck. The pickup has significant front-end damage, and the compact car has about 12 inches (30 cm) of passenger compartment intrusion. All passengers have exited the vehicles on their own before your arrival except the driver of the car.

The driver of the car is a Hispanic woman in her twenties who does not speak English. Unfortunately, neither you nor anyone else on the scene speaks Spanish. You note that the patient is still wearing her seat belt. She is awake, shaky, pale, and diaphoretic. Her ventilatory rate is 24 breaths/min and shallow but nonlabored, and her radial pulse is present but weak, thready, and rapid. The patient's left arm is swollen and deformed, and the upper left quadrant of her abdomen and left flank are tender to palpation. She has a large contusion over her left flank.

Based on the mechanism of injury and physical findings, what injuries might account for the patient's signs and symptoms? What are the steps in field management of this patient? You are 35 minutes away from a trauma center and no air transportation is available. How will this affect the patient's initial resuscitation and eventual outcome?

In 1852, American surgeon Samuel Gross defined *shock* as "a rude unhinging of the machinery of life." Probably no better definition exists to describe the devastating effects of this process on the patient. More recent definitions tend to be concerned with identification of the mechanism of shock and the effects on the patient's homeostasis. They are more specific and perhaps give a better picture of the particular pathophysiology that takes place. A basic tenet of prehospital care is that shock is not defined as low blood pressure, rapid pulse rates, or cool, clammy skin; these are merely systemic manifestations of the entire pathologic process of shock. The correct definition of shock is a widespread lack of tissue perfusion with oxygenated red blood cells (RBCs) that leads to anaerobic metabolism and decreased energy production. The loss of energy production at the cellular level produces the outcome that can lead to the death of the organs involved and subsequently the death of the patient.

For a prehospital care provider to understand this abnormal condition and to prevent and reverse shock, he or she must understand what is happening to the body on a cellular level. A prehospital care provider must understand, recognize, and interpret the normal physiologic responses that the body uses to protect itself from the consequences of shock. Only then can he or she develop a rational approach for managing the problems of the patient in shock.

Shock can kill a patient in the field, emergency department, operating room (OR), or intensive care unit (ICU).

Although health care providers can delay death for several hours to several days or weeks, the most common cause of that death is insufficient early resuscitation. The lack of perfusion of the cells of the body by oxygenated blood produces anaerobic metabolism. Even when some cells are initially spared, death occurs later rather than earlier because the remaining cells are unable to carry out the function of that organ indefinitely. This chapter explains this phenomenon and presents methods to prevent such an outcome.

Anatomy and Physiology

Metabolism: The Human Motor

The human body consists of millions of cells, and each one of these cells requires oxygen to function. The cells take in oxygen and metabolize it through a complicated physiologic process to produce energy. For metabolism to produce energy, cells must have fuel (oxygen and glucose). In the body, oxygen and glucose are mixed to produce energy. The by-products are carbon dioxide (CO_2) and water (H_2O). This process is similar to that of a vehicle engine, in which gasoline and air are mixed to produce energy and carbon monoxide is created as a by-product. *Aerobic metabolism* is the process for energy production in the human body using oxygen. *Anaerobic metabolism* is when energy production occurs without oxygen.

Aerobic metabolism is the body's principal combustion process. It efficiently produces energy using oxygen through a series of chemical reactions known as the *Krebs cycle*. The energy that is produced is stored in a molecule called *adenosine triphosphate* (ATP). ATP is a high-energy molecule that provides energy to the cells.

The body possesses an alternate pathway to produce power—anaerobic metabolism occurs in the absence of oxygen. Anaerobic metabolism is inefficient at producing energy (ATP). Anaerobic metabolism also produces by-products (lactic acid and pyruvic acid), which can cause problems when they accumulate. Anaerobic metabolism is a short-lived, inefficient process (like moving a vehicle with the starter motor and the battery rather than the gasoline engine). If adequate amounts of oxygen do not become quickly available, even this method of energy production fails.

Although a vehicle can be driven when powered only by its battery and electric starting motor if air and gasoline are not available, it would move more slowly and only until the energy in the battery is depleted. The problems with using anaerobic metabolism to power the body are similar to the disadvantages of using a battery to run a vehicle—it can only run for a short time, it does not produce as much energy, it produces by-products that are harmful to the body, and it will eventually lead to irreversible damage to the organ.

If a sufficient number of cells in any one organ die, eventually the entire organ ceases to function. Death does not occur immediately, except in the most extreme cases of lack of oxygen, namely asphyxia. If a large number of cells in an organ die, the organ's function will be significantly reduced and the remaining cells in that organ will have to work even harder than usual to keep the organ functioning. These overworked cells may or may not be able to support the function of the entire organ. Even with some cells remaining, the organ may still die.

An example is a patient who has sustained a heart attack. Blood flow and oxygen are shut off to one portion of the myocardium (heart muscle), and some cells of the heart die. This decreases cardiac output and the oxygen supply to the rest of the heart. In turn, this causes a further reduction in oxygenation of the remaining heart cells. If the remaining cells cannot meet the blood flow needs of the body, heart failure can result. Unless major improvement in cardiac output and oxygenation occur, the patient will not survive. Another example of cell death occurs in the kidneys. When the kidneys are injured or deprived of adequate oxygenated blood, kidney cells begin to die and kidney function decreases. Other cells may be compromised yet continue to function for a while before dying. If enough cells die, the decreased level of function in the kidneys produces an inadequate elimination of

toxic by-products of metabolism, further exacerbating death. As this systemic deterioration continues, more organs die and eventually the organism (the human) dies.

Depending on the organ initially involved, the progression from cell death to organism death can be rapid or delayed. It can take as long as several days to several weeks for trauma-related hypoxia or hypoperfusion to result in a patient's death. The effectiveness of a prehospital care provider's actions to reverse or prevent hypoxia (insufficient oxygen available to meet cell requirements) and hypoperfusion (inadequate blood passing to tissue cells) in the critical prehospital time period may not be immediately apparent. However, these resuscitation measures are unquestionably necessary if the patient is to survive.

The sensitivity of the body's cells to the lack of oxygen varies from organ system to organ system. This sensitivity is called *ischemic* (lack of oxygen) *sensitivity*, and it is greatest in the brain, heart, and lungs. Only 4 to 6 minutes of hypoxia may be necessary before one or more of these vital organs is damaged. Skin and muscle tissues have a significantly longer ischemic sensitivity—as long as 6 to 8 hours. The abdominal organs, namely the kidneys and liver, generally fall between these two groups and are able to survive 45 to 90 minutes of hypoxia (Table 6-1).

Long-term survival of individual organs and the body as a whole requires delivery of important nutrients, such as oxygen and glucose, to the tissue cells. The most important essential substance is oxygen.

Fick Principle

The Fick principle is a description of the components necessary for adequate oxygenation of the body cells (perfusion). The three components are as follows:

1. *On-loading of oxygen to RBCs in the lung.* This requires that the patient's airway be patent; that venti-

Table 6-1   Organ Tolerance to Ischemia

Organ	Warm ischemia time
Heart, brain, lungs	4-6 minutes
Kidneys, liver, gastrointestinal tract	45-90 minutes
Muscle, bone, skin	4-6 hours

lations be of adequate volume, depth, and rate; and that the percentage of oxygen (FiO_2) in the inspired air is adequate. Additionally, adequate diffusion of oxygen across the alveolar membrane in the lung must occur. Processes that may impair this include a pneumothorax, pulmonary contusions, pulmonary edema, aspiration, and airway obstruction.

2. *Delivery of RBCs to tissue cells.* This component requires a sufficient number of RBCs and adequate blood volume. Anything that affects these two factors can severely impair perfusion. A helpful analogy is to think of the RBCs as transport vans, the lungs as oxygen warehouses, the blood vessels as roads and highways, and the body tissue cells as the oxygen's destination. An insufficient number of transport vans, obstructions along the roads and highways, and/or slow transport vans would all contribute to decreased oxygen delivery and the eventual starvation of the tissue cells.

3. *Off-loading of oxygen from RBCs to tissue cells.* The most common problem with off-loading oxygen occurs when edema separates the tissue cells from the capillaries. Another example is carbon monoxide. This poison impairs the ability of the hemoglobin molecule to release oxygen in the body's tissues. Although strictly not a problem of off-loading of oxygen, cyanide toxicity, as occurs from the inhalation of burning plastics, impairs the ability of cells to use oxygen even though adequate amounts may be present.

Prehospital treatment of shock is directed at maintaining the critical components of adequate oxygenation. The goal is to deliver adequate oxygen to produce enough energy to prevent, or reverse, anaerobic metabolism, therefore avoiding cellular death and ultimately patient death. These components should be the major focus of the prehospital care provider and are implemented in the management of the trauma patient by the following actions:

1. Delivering sufficient amounts of oxygen to the alveoli, including airway management, the use of supplemental oxygen, and assisted ventilation
2. Controlling external hemorrhage, recognizing the presence of internal hemorrhage, providing external compression whenever possible, restoring circulating blood volume, and providing rapid transportation to the appropriate medical center for continued care
3. Recognizing the potential for toxic inhalations

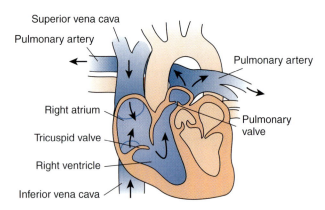

Figure 6-1 With each contraction of the right ventricle, blood is pumped through the lungs. Blood from the lungs enters the left side of the heart, and the left ventricle pumps it into the systemic vascular system.

Cardiovascular System

The cardiovascular system consists of a pump (the heart), the vascular system (a container and complex branching pipeline consisting of arteries, veins, and capillaries through which the blood travels), and circulating fluid (the blood). Malfunctions or deficiencies in any of these three components will result in decreased or absent delivery of oxygen to the cells, even if the oxygenation of RBCs in the lungs is adequate.

HEART

The heart consists of two receiving chambers (atria) and two major pumping chambers (ventricles). The function of the atria is to accumulate and store blood so that the ventricles can fill rapidly, minimizing delay in the pumping cycle. The right atrium receives blood from the veins of the body and pumps it to the right ventricle. With each contraction of the right ventricle, blood is pumped through the lungs for oxygenation (Figure 6-1). The blood from the lungs is returned to the left atrium. From there, blood is pumped into the left ventricle, which then pumps it throughout the arteries of the body (Figure 6-2). Blood is forced through the "container" by the contraction of the left ventricle; a pressure rise occurs in the blood vessels greater than normal resting pressure. This sudden pressure increase in the container produces a pulse wave to push blood through the system. The peak of pressure increase is the systolic blood pressure and represents the force of the blood produced by ventricular contraction (systole). The resting pressure in the vessels between ventricular contractions is the diastolic blood pressure and represents the residual force remaining in the system while the heart is refilling (diastole). This is an indirect estimate of vascular resistance (Figure 6-3). Thus the prehospital

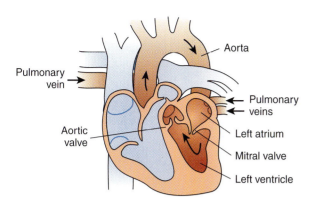

Figure 6-2   Blood returning from the lungs is pumped out of the heart and through the aorta to the rest of the body by left ventricular contraction.

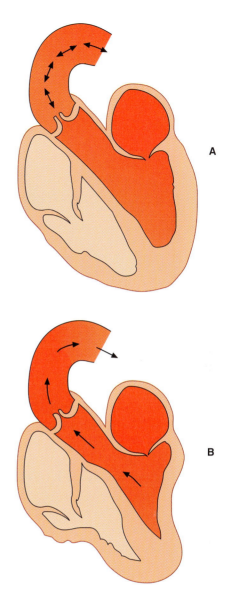

care provider can obtain more information if he or she determines both systolic and diastolic pressures during the secondary survey by auscultating with a stethoscope. However, in some cases the prehospital care provider determines only the systolic pressure using palpation (feeling for a pulse with the fingers). The difference between the systolic and diastolic pressures is called *pulse pressure*.

Another term used in the discussion of shock management but often not emphasized in the prehospital setting is *mean arterial pressure* (MAP). The MAP is the average pressure in the vascular system and is calculated as follows:

MAP = Diastolic pressure + 1/3 Pulse pressure

For example, the MAP of a patient with a blood pressure of 120/80 mm Hg is calculated as follows:

$$\begin{aligned}
\text{MAP} &= 80 + ([120 - 80]/3) \\
&= 80 + (40/3) \\
&= 80 + 13.3 \\
&= 93.3, \text{ rounded to } 93
\end{aligned}$$

Many automatic, noninvasive blood pressure devices report the MAP in addition to the systolic and diastolic pressures.

The amount of fluid pumped into the system with each contraction of the ventricle is called the *stroke volume*, and the amount of blood pumped into the system over 1 minute is called the *cardiac output*. The formula for cardiac output (CO) is as follows:

Cardiac output (CO) =

Heart rate (HR) × Stroke volume (SV)

Figure 6-3   In a relaxed position (diastole), the ventricle fills with blood from the contractions of the atrium. During this time, blood is gradually flowing out of the major vessels as the pressure gradually decreases. During the contraction of the ventricle (systole), a large amount of blood flows into the vascular system, which raises the pressure. Cardiac action and blood flow is demonstrated in **A** and the pulse wave is seen in **B**.

Cardiac output is reported in liters per minute (LPM). Cardiac output is not measured in the prehospital environment. However, understanding cardiac output and its relationship to stroke volume is important in understanding shock management.

For the heart to work effectively, an adequate amount of blood must be present in the vena cava and pulmonary veins to fill the ventricles. Starling's law of the heart is an important concept explaining how this relationship works—the more the ventricles fill, the greater

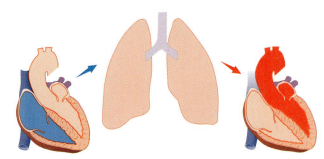

Figure 6-4 Although the heart seems to be one organ, it functions as if it were two. Unoxygenated blood is received into the right heart from the superior and inferior venae cavae and pumped through the pulmonary artery into the lungs. The blood is oxygenated in the lungs, flows back into the heart through the pulmonary vein, and is pumped out of the left ventricle.

the strength of contraction of the heart. This pressure (preload) that fills the heart stretches the myocardial muscle fibers so that ventricular filling is adequate. Significant hemorrhage or relative hypovolemia decreases cardiac preload so that a reduced amount of blood is present and the fibers are not stretched effectively, resulting in a lower stroke volume. If the filling pressure of the heart is too great, the cardiac muscle fibers become overstretched and can fail to deliver a satisfactory stroke volume. This is often the case with congestive heart failure (CHF).

The resistance to blood flow that the left ventricle must overcome to pump blood out into the arterial system is called *afterload*, which can be thought of as a function of the systemic vascular resistance (SVR). As peripheral arterial vasoconstriction increases, the heart has to generate a greater force to pump blood into the arterial system. Conversely, widespread peripheral vasodilation decreases afterload.

The fact that the heart, while being one organ, actually has two subsystems is an important concept in understanding the cardiovascular system. The right atrium, which receives blood from the body, and the right ventricle, which pumps blood to the lungs, are referred to as the *right heart*. The left atrium, which receives blood from the lungs, and the left ventricle, which pumps blood to the body, are referred to as the *left heart*. Preload and afterload of the right heart (pulmonary) and left heart (systemic) pumping systems are important concepts in the discussion and management of shock (Figure 6-4).

The systemic circulation contains more capillaries and a greater length of blood vessels than the pulmonary circulation. Therefore the left heart system works at a higher pressure and bears a greater load than the right

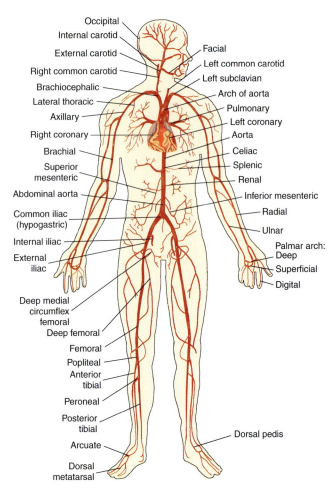

Figure 6-5 Principal arteries of the body.

heart system. Anatomically, the muscle of the left ventricle is thicker and stronger than that of the right ventricle.

Although the two separate systems and two separate pumps exist, they are connected in the body. They share the same electrical system and respond to the same stimuli, from either the internal pacemaker, sympathetic nervous system, hormones, or drug administration. Although they are joined and function as one organ, they are physiologically two separate pumping systems. Separate or together, the actions of one affect the performance of the other and failure of one part frequently results in the failure of the other because they are pumps in series.

BLOOD VESSELS

The blood vessels contain the blood and route it to the various areas and cells of the body. They are the highways of the physiologic process of circulation. The single large exit tube from the heart, the aorta, cannot serve every individual cell in the body and therefore splits into multiple arteries of decreasing size, the smallest of which are the capillaries (Figure 6-5). A capillary may be only one cell wide; therefore oxygen and nutrients carried by RBCs and

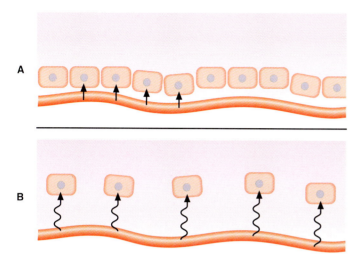

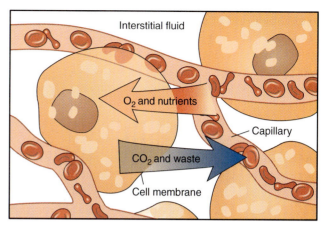

Figure 6-6   **A,** If the tissue cells are close to the capillary, oxygen can easily diffuse into them and carbon dioxide can diffuse out. **B,** If tissue cells are separated from capillary walls by increased edema (interstitial fluid), it is much more difficult for the oxygen and carbon dioxide to diffuse.

Figure 6-7   Oxygen and nutrients diffuse from the red blood cells through the capillary wall, the interstitial fluid, and the cell membrane into the cell. Acid production is a by-product of cellular energy production during the Krebs cycle. By way of the buffer system of the body, this acid is converted into carbon dioxide and travels with the red blood cells and in the plasma to be eliminated from the circulatory system by the lungs.

plasma are able to diffuse easily through the walls of the capillary into the tissue cell (Figure 6-6). Each tissue cell has a membranous envelopment called the *cell membrane.* Interstitial fluid is located between the cell membrane and the capillary wall. The amount of interstitial fluid varies tremendously. If little interstitial fluid is present, the cell membrane and the capillary wall are close together and oxygen can easily diffuse between them (Figure 6-7).

The size of the vascular container is controlled by muscles in the walls of the arteries and arterioles and, to a lesser extent, by muscles in the walls of the venules and veins. These muscles respond to signals from the brain via the sympathetic nervous system, to the circulating hormones epinephrine and norepinephrine, and to other chemicals, such as nitric oxide (NO). These muscle fibers in the walls of the vessels, depending on whether they are being stimulated or allowed to relax, result in either the constriction or dilation of the blood vessels, thus changing the size of the container component of the cardiovascular system.

BLOOD

The fluid component of the circulatory system, the blood, contains not only RBCs but also infection-fighting factors (white blood cells [WBCs] and antibodies), platelets essential for clotting, protein for cellular rebuilding, nutrition in the form of glucose, and other substances necessary for metabolism and survival. The volume of fluid within the vascular system must equal the capacity of the blood vessels if it is to adequately fill the container. Any variance in the size of the vascular system

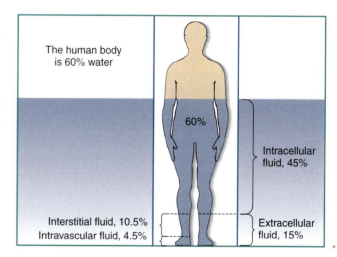

Figure 6-8   Body water represents 60% of body weight. This water is divided into intracellular and extracellular fluid. The extracellular fluid is further divided into interstitial and intravascular fluid.

compared with the amount of blood in the system will affect the flow of blood either positively or negatively.

Human body weight is 60% water, which is the base of all body fluids. A person who weighs 70 kilograms contains approximately 40 liters of water. Body water is present in two components—intracellular and extracellular fluid. Each type of fluid has specific, important properties (Figure 6-8). Intracellular fluid, the fluid within the cells, accounts for approximately 45% of body weight. Extracellular fluid, the fluid outside the cells, can be further classified into two subtypes—interstitial fluid and intravascular fluid. Interstitial fluid, which surrounds the tissue cells and also includes cerebrospinal fluid (found in the brain) and synovial fluid (found in the joints), accounts for approximately 10.5% of body weight. Intravascular fluid, which is found in the vessels and carries the formed components of blood as well as oxygen and other vital nutrients within the blood vessels, accounts for approximately 4.5% of body weight.

A review of some key concepts may be helpful in this discussion of how fluids operate in the body. Cells require a fluid environment, and that fluid must have certain properties and a particular chemical balance to support cellular life. A proper volume of fluid under adequate pressure is essential. Various mechanisms constantly adjust chemical balance, fluid volume, and pressure to achieve homeostasis (a constant, stable, internal environment). Normally, the total volume of water in the body remains constant and the distribution of fluid also remains relatively constant. To maintain these constant conditions, the amount of fluid taken in through the digestive system must equal the amount of fluid lost through the kidneys, lungs, skin, and intestines.

Several mechanisms work to adjust and balance input and output. One way the body maintains this fluid balance is by shifting water from one space to another. When fluid volume drops, the kidneys reduce their output to both reduce water loss and allow the vascular volume to build up again. An individual feels thirsty and is motivated to drink liquids as an additional mechanism to restore fluid volume. In the opposite condition, urine output increases when too much fluid is in the body. A person is normovolemic if fluid balance is normal, hypervolemic if volume is too high, and hypovolemic if volume is too low.

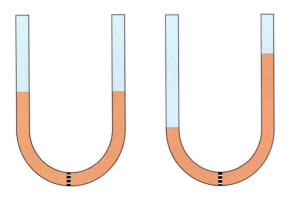

Figure 6-9 A U-tube, in which the two halves are separated by a semipermeable membrane, contains equal amounts of water and solid particles. If a solute that cannot diffuse through the semipermeable membrane is added to one side but not to the other, fluid will flow across to dilute the added particles. The pressure difference of the height of fluid in the U-tube is known as *osmotic pressure*.

The body's systems strive to maintain the life of the cells. When death occurs, it is because the body is no longer able to support cellular life. For cellular life to continue, the fluid environment must be maintained and the cells must be adequately perfused (bathed with oxygenated fluid under appropriate conditions). When oxygen and the other nutrients reach the capillaries, they must be able to move through the capillary membrane into the interstitial fluid that bathes the cells. The oxygen and nutrients must then pass into the cell through the cell membrane. At the same time, the capillaries must be able to transfer CO_2 and other waste products from the tissue cell into the vascular fluid and eventually out of the body. The processes of diffusion and osmosis accomplish this exchange.

Diffusion involves the movement of solutes (substances dissolved in water) across a membrane. Different membranes have different levels of permeability (i.e., different membranes will allow different sizes or types of molecules of the solute to pass through). As noted previously, the body strives to maintain homeostasis, a state of chemical and metabolic balance. Solutes attempt to move from areas in which they are more numerous to areas in which they are less concentrated as part of the homeostatic drive. When a solute encounters a membrane that will not let its molecules pass through, the solute remains on only one side of the membrane. This lack of passage produces a condition in which a greater concentration of that solute is on one side of the membrane (hypertonic state). However, more solute will be on the side of greater pressure, producing a higher pressure (water column) on this side.

On the other hand, water can usually pass through these membranes easily, which will equalize the tonicity on both sides. *Osmosis* is the movement of water across a membrane from an area that is hypotonic (low solute concentration) to an area that is hypertonic (high solute concentration). By diluting the solute concentration on the hypertonic side of the membrane, this movement of water brings both sides to equal solute concentrations. If a membrane will not allow water to pass, the concentration of solutes on the side with the increased number of molecules remains hypertonic, and the concentration on the side with fewer or no molecules is hypotonic.

Pressure is required for the fluid to move not only throughout the circulatory system but also into and out of the cells. Osmotic pressure is produced when differing concentrations of solutes cause fluid to move from the side of lower concentration to the side of higher concentration (Figure 6-9). Osmosis tends to move fluids from the interstitial space, where solute concentrations are lower, to the intravascular space, where concentrations are higher.

Hydrostatic pressure balances osmotic pressure. Hydrostatic pressure can be increased on a body compartment with the use of a constricting band, compression bandage, or tight cast; by increased fluid in a compartment that cannot expand (such as the skull) or in a fascial compartment (such as the lower leg); or by an increase in blood pressure that is maintained by the pumping action of the heart.

Nervous System

The autonomic nervous system directs and controls the involuntary functions of the body, such as respiration, digestion, and cardiovascular function. It is divided into two subsystems, the sympathetic and parasympathetic nervous systems. These systems often work against each other to keep vital body systems in balance.

The sympathetic nervous system produces the fight-or-flight response. This response simultaneously causes the heart to beat faster and stronger, increases the ventilatory rate, and constricts the blood vessels to nonessential organs (skin and gastrointestinal tract), while dilating vessels and improving blood flow to muscles. The goal of this response is to maintain sufficient amounts of oxygenated blood to critical tissues so that an individual can respond to an emergency situation, while shunting blood away from nonessential areas.

However, without some restrictive control, a person's pulse rate and blood pressure could increase too much, overtaxing the heart and killing the individual. The parasympathetic system provides that control. The vagal response of the parasympathetic system slows the heart rate and reduces the force of contractions, maintaining the body in balance.

The medulla is the primary regulatory center of autonomic control of the cardiovascular system. The medulla receives information from specialized areas in the body that "sense" pressure and chemical balance. Chemoreceptors sense changes in chemical balance, and baroreceptors, which sense pressure changes, are located mainly around the carotid artery and aortic arch. When these cells sense an increase in the pressure inside these vessels, a message is sent to the medulla. The cardioinhibitory center of the medulla slows or inhibits cardiac activity by sending impulses through the vagus nerve (cranial nerve X). The parasympathetic stimulation causes a decrease in firing of the sinoatrial (SA) node and slows conduction through the atrioventricular (AV) node. The effect is to slow the heart rate. The combination of decreased heart rate and force of cardiac contraction results in decreased cardiac output and a lowered blood pressure.

The cardioaccelerator center of the medulla increases or accelerates cardiac activity. When the baroreceptors detect a drop in blood pressure or the chemoreceptors detect an increase in acid (hydrogen ion, H^+), this triggers the cardioaccelerator center to activate the sympathetic nervous system. Sympathetic stimulation, through the release of epinephrine (Adrenalin) and norepinephrine, produces many of the classic signs of shock, all as part of a complex compensatory mechanism. The ventilatory rate increases in an effort to overcome hypoxia and hypercarbia. Sympathetic activation causes an increase in the firing of the SA node and increased force of contraction, producing a bounding, rapid heart rate (tachycardia). Peripheral vasoconstriction and sweat production produces the cool, clammy skin, while vasoconstriction of the gastrointestinal tract often leads to nausea and vomiting.

This all occurs in an effort to return blood pressure to normal. As noted in the next section, the body can often compensate for loss of up to 30% of blood volume without becoming hypotensive. Thus *hypotension is a late finding of shock and indicates that the body's compensatory mechanisms have already failed.*

Pathophysiology

Anaerobic Metabolism

As previously stated, when enough oxygen is not present to produce energy by aerobic metabolism, the cells produce only a scant amount of energy via anaerobic metabolism. Anaerobic metabolism is an inefficient process and results in excess production of lactic acid. Shock represents this failure of energy production.

The body attempts to manage the increased production of acid caused by anaerobic metabolism by way of its buffer system. A buffer is a substance that neutralizes or weakens strong acids or bases. In this case, the hydrogen ion (H^+) of the acid joins with sodium bicarbonate (HCO_3^-) to form carbonic acid (H_2CO_3). This in turn breaks down into water (H_2O) and CO_2:

$$H^+ + HCO_3^- \rightarrow H_2CO_3 \rightarrow H_2O + CO_2$$

The brain detects the resulting increase in CO_2, which causes the ventilatory rate to increase. Increasing the ventilatory rate removes more CO_2 from the body. The increased water is removed as the kidneys excrete additional urine in response to the presence of increased acid, a product of anaerobic metabolism, which is always an element of shock. An increased ventilatory rate, along with an increase in the pulse rate and an altered level of consciousness (LOC), is one of the earliest signs of shock (see Chapters 3 and 8).

An increase in the ventilatory rate promotes the increased elimination of CO_2 as just discussed. Increasing the concentration of inspired oxygen (FiO_2) increases the amount of oxygen available to the RBCs to be transported to the tissue cells. These oxygen-depleted tissue cells survive initially by switching to anaerobic metabolism. When more oxygen is available at the cellular level, the cells will revert back to aerobic metabolism.

The effects of a decreased blood supply, decreased oxygenation, and anaerobic metabolism in an organ can be detected by measuring the performance of that particular organ. In trying to resuscitate a patient, each organ should be assessed individually whenever possible to check its level of function. One example is an extremely ischemic heart that develops a slow rate (bradycardia). The heart becomes oxygen depleted and converts to anaerobic metabolism, which depresses automaticity and pumping force. On the other hand, a heart being driven by the brain in response to autonomic stimulation, as in the fight-or-flight response, to increase cardiac output has a rapid rate (tachycardia). The kidneys will either increase or decrease urine output depending on the amount of blood flowing through them. Although urine output is easily measured in the hospital, it is only rarely measured in prehospital situations. Urine output is presented here as another example of what occurs in the body.

The Cardiovascular System in Shock

The container (vascular system) can be artificially divided into three physiologic parts.

1. The blood supply to the heart, brain, and lungs receives the highest priority. The body strives to maintain this part at all costs because its failure would deprive the entire body of circulating oxygenated blood.
2. The blood supply to the liver and kidneys receives the next highest priority.
3. The blood supply to the skin and soft tissues of the extremities and the gastrointestinal tract receives the lowest priority.

When the circulation of oxygenated blood is reduced for any reason, the system of priorities among these three physiologic components of the vascular system takes effect. Blood is shunted away from the lower-priority areas to those areas that are more sensitive to the loss of oxygenated blood and are essential to maintain life. Blood is not shunted away from the heart, brain, or lungs.

When blood pressure drops and circulatory flow decreases, baroreceptors detect the change. Nerves transmit this information to the brain, which in turn sends signals to the sympathetic nervous system to release norepinephrine, causing constriction of the smooth muscles in the peripheral arterioles and venules. This constriction reduces or completely shuts off the flow of blood to the skin and extremities. If this situation continues, blood flow to the abdominal contents will be reduced or shut off. This reduction of blood flow achieved through constriction of the blood vessels results in increased vascular resistance. If the change affects the entire body, it results in increased systemic vascular resistance (SVR). This selective reduction in blood flow has two effects on the body, one helpful and one harmful.

The helpful result is that the vasoconstriction is delayed in the blood vessels that provide circulation to the brain, heart, and lungs. The vasoconstriction and resultant reduced circulation occur in areas of the body that are not immediately essential to preserving life and can tolerate ischemia the longest. Blood is a liquid and follows the laws of physics, flowing along the path of least resistance. The brain, heart, and lungs have less resistance to blood flow compared with other parts of the body where the blood vessels have been constricted. The result is improved circulation to the vital organs and decreased circulation to the rest of the body.

The increased resistance produced by the peripheral vasoconstriction results in an improved blood pressure. The action of cardiotonic substances, such as norepinephrine and epinephrine, increases cardiac output by increasing the volume of fluid and the strength of contractions, adding to the increase in blood pressure. Delivery of oxygen to the tissues by improving RBC oxygenation in the lungs and perfusion of the cells by these RBCs is the goal of shock management. Although blood pressure is one of the most frequently measured functions of the cardiovascular system, it is not the most important factor in the management of shock. In this chapter the discussion is concerned mainly with the perfusion portion of management.

Decreased or absent blood flow will occur on the distal side of the increased vascular resistance. The decreased circulation through the distal capillary beds and decreased blood flow through distal arteries translate into three of the common signs of shock:

1. Loss of normal skin color and temperature
2. Absent or thready distal pulse
3. Delayed capillary refilling time

The decreased blood flow to the skin, abdomen, and extremities also means that these areas receive fewer nutrients and less oxygen than they need. Rather than "starve," these cells convert from aerobic to anaerobic metabolism to survive. The result is a growing state of metabolic acidosis (primarily lactic acid) in the peripheral tissues. This acidosis is entirely related to the tissue cells and has no relationship to the regulation of fluids or electrolytes in the kidney.

If adequate circulation is restored and the peripheral cells receive adequate supplies of nutrients and oxygen, they convert back to aerobic metabolism. At the same time, the toxic by-products of anaerobic metabolism are washed out of the peripheral areas and enter the central systemic circulation, potentially causing systemic metabolic acidosis.

The pathophysiologic process of shock can be theoretically divided into three stages (Figure 6-10):

1. The *ischemic phase* is characterized by reduction of capillary blood flow and conversion to anaerobic metabolism with production of toxic by-products.
2. In the *stagnant phase,* precapillary sphincters open, but postcapillary sphincters remain closed. This results in an increase in hydrostatic pressure within the capillaries. The increased pressure forces fluid out of the capillaries into the interstitial space, contributing to tissue edema (swelling).
3. When the postcapillary sphincters open, the *washout phase* begins. The accumulation of toxic by-products from the first two phases is washed out into the systemic circulation during this third stage. What was once a contained, localized acidosis now becomes a systemic acidosis.

The result of shock is that the heart is forced to function with three handicaps, all of which decrease its efficiency:

1. *Increased afterload.* The increased afterload increases the demand on the heart. An increased myocardial oxygen demand also results because the heart must work harder.

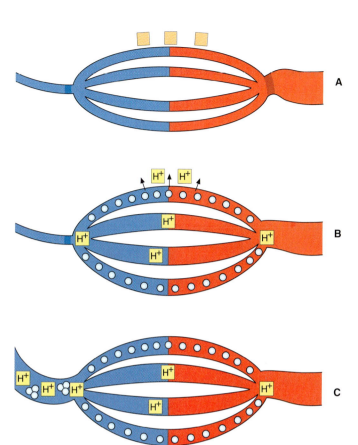

Figure 6-10   The cellular pathophysiologic process of shock is divided into three phases: A, Ischemic. B, Stagnant. C, Washout.

2. *Decreased oxygenation.* The need for oxygen metabolism to produce energy for a harder-working (faster-beating) heart is greater than the amount needed in an easier-working (slower-beating) heart. More work requires more fuel. If the heart must beat faster to overcome the increased afterload, it must have more oxygen. This illustrates the need for adequate oxygenation during any period of cardiac stress to prevent further deterioration into shock.
3. *Lack of available fluid to fill the ventricles during diastole (resting phase).* Ejecting blood from the ventricle when the heart is only half full requires more frequent contractions and produces a lower systolic pressure, and therefore a smaller pulse pressure, than when adequate fluid is available. Cardiac workload increases but produces less output. One sign of worsening shock is a rising diastolic pressure followed by a decline in both systolic and diastolic pressures.

CELLULAR DYSFUNCTION, DEATH, AND EDEMA

The discussion of the pathophysiology of shock up to this point has focused on failure of the cardiovascular system to deliver sufficient quantities of oxygen to the body's tissues and the resultant anaerobic metabolism that produces less energy than that required by the cells. On a cellular level, shock results in many problems that result in abnormal cell function (dysfunction) and, if left uncorrected, cell death. Anaerobic metabolism produces much less energy than aerobic metabolism. Many cellular functions depend on a constant supply of energy. Microscopic pumps and channels in the cell membrane require energy to maintain the internal electrolyte concentrations characteristic of intracellular fluid. When energy is not present, sodium (Na^+), primarily an extracellular ion, enters the cell. Water molecules follow the sodium ions into the cells with resultant cellular swelling. Persistent shock also leads to destruction of the internal cellular structures, including the rupture of lysosomes, structures that contain toxic substances and enzymes. This further interferes with cellular functioning. When damage becomes irreparable, the cells rupture (lyse), releasing potassium, primarily an intracellular ion, into the interstitial fluid.

Trauma that results in severe hypoxia and shock also stimulates the body's inflammatory system, further aggravating the underlying condition. Locally active hormones, called *cytokines*, have many functions that may be both beneficial and detrimental to the recovery of the organism. Some cytokines attract white blood cells (WBCs; leucocytes) to the area of injury. These leucocytes may secrete other substances that cause peripheral vasodilation and cause the capillaries to leak fluid into the interstitial space. This increase in interstitial fluid is edema.

If a large amount of edema is present, the distance between the capillary wall and the cell membrane becomes much greater. Oxygen must diffuse through the capillary wall, then through the interstitial fluid, and finally through the cell membrane. Because of this increased diffusion distance, the ability of oxygen and other nutrients to reach the cells is decreased (see Figure 6-6). More hypoxia results, and the cycle begins all over again, resulting in a downward spiral. Although adequate resuscitation may stop this cycle, sufficient cellular and tissue damage may have occurred to result in dysfunction or failure of vital organs.

If cellular destruction is so widespread that even returning oxygen delivery to normal cannot reverse the process, shock is deemed to be irreversible. Except in the most extreme situations when exsanguination is obvious, irreversible shock cannot be readily identified. Irreversible shock is often only identified when aggressive attempts at managing shock fail and death occurs sometimes days or weeks after the initial insult of hypoxia and decreased energy production.

Causes and Types of Shock

Shock can occur in three ways that are associated with failure of one or more of the components of the cardiovascular system—blood volume (fluid), the vessels (container), or the heart (pump). Hypovolemic shock is due to the loss of blood volume, distributive shock is due to abnormalities of the blood vessels, and cardiogenic shock is due to failure of the heart.

HYPOVOLEMIC SHOCK

When acute blood volume loss occurs through dehydration (loss of plasma) or hemorrhage (loss of plasma and RBCs), the relationship of fluid volume to the size of the container becomes unbalanced. The container retains its normal size, but the fluid volume is decreased. *Hypovolemic shock* is the most common cause of shock encountered in the prehospital environment, and blood loss is by far the most common cause of shock in the management of trauma patients.

When blood is being lost out of circulation, the heart is stimulated to increase cardiac output by increasing the strength and rate of contractions through the release of epinephrine from the adrenal glands. The sympathetic nervous system releases norepinephrine to trigger constriction of the blood vessels to reduce the size of the container and bring it more into proportion with the amount of remaining fluid. Vasoconstriction results in closing of the peripheral capillaries as discussed previously and prompts the switch from aerobic to anaerobic metabolism at the cellular level.

These compensatory defense mechanisms work well up to a point. When defense mechanisms can no longer overcome the volume reduction, a patient's blood pressure drops. A decrease in blood pressure marks the switch from compensated to decompensated shock—a sign of impending death. A patient who has signs of compensation is already in shock, not "going into shock." Unless aggressive resuscitation occurs, the patient who enters decompensated shock has only one more stage of decline left—death.

Hemorrhagic shock (hypovolemic shock resulting from blood loss) can also be categorized into four classes depending on the severity of hemorrhage (Table 6-2):

1. *Class I hemorrhage* represents a loss of up to 15% of blood volume in the adult (up to 750 mL). This

Table 6-2   Classifications of Hemorrhagic Shock

	Class I	Class II	Class III	Class IV
Amount of blood loss (% total blood volume)	<750 mL (<15%)	750-1500 mL (15%-30%)	1500-2000 mL (30%-40%)	>2000 mL (>40%)
Heart rate (beats/min)	Normal or minimally increased	>100	>120	>140
Ventilatory rate (breaths/min)	Normal	20-30	30-40	>35
Systolic blood pressure (mm Hg)	Normal	Normal	Decreased	Markedly decreased
Urine output (mL/hr)	Normal	20-30	5-15	Minimal

Modified with permission from American College of Surgeons: *Committee on Trauma, Advanced Trauma Life Support® for Doctors, Students Course Material,* ed 6, Chicago, 1997, American College of Surgeons, p. 98.

stage has few clinical manifestations. Tachycardia is often minimal, and no measurable changes in blood pressure, pulse pressure, or ventilatory rate occur. Most healthy patients sustaining this amount of hemorrhage do not require fluid resuscitation as long as no further blood loss occurs and the patient is able to drink fluid. The body's compensatory mechanisms restore intravascular fluid.

2. *Class II hemorrhage* represents a loss of 15% to 30% of blood volume (750 to 1500 mL). Most adults are capable of compensating for this amount of blood loss by activation of the sympathetic nervous system. Clinical findings include increased ventilatory rate, tachycardia, and a narrowed pulse pressure. The patient often demonstrates anxiety or fright. Urinary output drops slightly to between 20 and 30 mL/hr in the adult. On occasion, these patients may require blood transfusion; however, most will respond well to crystalloid infusion.

3. *Class III hemorrhage* represents a loss of 30% to 40% of blood volume (1500 to 2000 mL). When blood loss reaches this point, most patients are no longer able to compensate for the volume loss and hypotension occurs. The classic findings of shock are obvious and include tachycardia (heart rate >120 beats/min), tachypnea (ventilatory rate of 30 to 40 breaths/min), and severe anxiety or confusion. Urinary output falls to 5 to 15 mL/hr. Many of these patients will require blood transfusion for adequate resuscitation.

4. *Class IV hemorrhage* represents a loss of over 40% of blood volume (over 2000 mL). This stage of severe shock is characterized by marked tachycardia (heart rate >140 beats/min), tachypnea (ventilatory rate of >35 breaths/min), profound confusion or lethargy,

and a markedly decreased systolic blood pressure, typically in the range of 60 mm Hg. These patients truly have only minutes to live. Survival depends on immediate control of hemorrhage (surgery for internal hemorrhage) and aggressive resuscitation, including blood transfusions.

The definitive management for volume failure is to replace the lost fluid. A dehydrated patient needs fluid replacement with water and salt, whereas a trauma patient who has lost blood needs to have the source of blood loss stopped and the blood replaced. Mild to moderate dehydration can be treated with an electrolyte solution that a conscious patient can drink. An unconscious or severely dehydrated patient should receive the replacement intravenously. Because blood replacement is usually not available in the prehospital environment, trauma patients who have lost blood should undergo measures to control external blood loss and receive an intravenous electrolyte solution and rapid transportation to the hospital where blood and emergent surgery are available.

Shock research has demonstrated that for lost blood, the replacement ratio with electrolyte solution should be 3 liters of replacement for each liter of blood lost. This is because only about one third of the volume of an isotonic crystalloid solution remains in the intravascular space 1 hour after infusing it. For moderate and severe shock, this research has shown that replacement with both a crystalloid solution and blood was better than with blood alone. The use of a limited amount of electrolyte solution before blood replacement is the correct approach. The best crystalloid solution for treating hemorrhagic shock is lactated Ringer's solution. Normal saline (NS) is another isotonic crystalloid solution that can be used for volume replacement, but its use may produce hyperchloremia (marked increase in the blood chloride level).

A pneumatic antishock garment (PASG) may provide short-term assistance with managing severe hemorrhagic shock by increasing vascular resistance, reducing container size, and tamponading abdominal and pelvic hemorrhage. The most important use of the PASG is in intraabdominal and pelvic hemorrhage control in patients with a blood pressure below 60 mm Hg. Use of the PASG is fully explained in the "Management" section of this chapter. However, as the PASG increases the patient's blood pressure, hemorrhage from injury sites outside the confines of the garment may increase.

DISTRIBUTIVE SHOCK

Distributive shock occurs when the vascular container enlarges without a proportional increase in fluid volume. Relatively less fluid will be available for the size of the container. As a result, the amount of fluid available to the heart as preload decreases and cardiac output falls. In most situations, fluid has not been lost from the vascular system. This form of shock is not a case of hypovolemia, where fluid has been lost through hemorrhage, vomiting, or diarrhea; the problem is with the size of the container. For this reason, this condition is sometimes referred to as *relative hypovolemia*. Although some of the presenting signs and symptoms may closely mimic those of hypovolemic shock, the cause of the two conditions is different.

In distributive shock, resistance to flow is decreased because of the relatively larger size of the blood vessels. This reduced resistance decreases the diastolic blood pressure. When this reduced resistance is combined with the reduced preload and therefore a reduced cardiac output, the net result is a decrease in both the systolic and diastolic blood pressures. Although the pressure is decreased, if normal oxygenation has been maintained, the heart rate does not necessarily increase. Tissue oxygenation may remain adequate in some patients.

Distributive shock can result from loss of autonomic nervous system control of the smooth muscles that control the size of the blood vessels or release of chemicals that result in peripheral vasodilation. This loss of control can stem from spinal cord trauma, simple fainting, severe infections, or allergic reactions. Management of distributive shock is directed toward improving oxygenation of the blood and improving or maintaining blood flow to the brain and vital organs.

Neurogenic "Shock". Neurogenic shock occurs when a cervical spine injury damages the spinal cord above

where the nerves of the sympathetic nervous system exit (the thoracolumbar area). Because of the loss of sympathetic control of the vascular system, which controls the smooth muscles in the walls of the blood vessels, the peripheral vessels dilate below the level of injury. The marked decrease in systemic vascular resistance and peripheral vasodilation that occurs as the container for the blood volume increases results in relative hypovolemia. The patient is not hypovolemic, but the normal blood volume insufficiently fills an expanded container. This decrease in blood pressure does not compromise energy production and therefore is *not* shock.

Decompensated hypovolemic shock and neurogenic shock both produce a decreased systolic blood pressure. However, the other vital signs vary significantly, and the treatment for each is also different (Table 6-3). Decreased systolic and diastolic pressures and a narrow pulse pressure characterize hypovolemic shock. Neurogenic shock also displays decreased systolic and diastolic pressures, but the pulse pressure remains normal. Hypovolemia produces cold, clammy, pale, or cyanotic skin and delayed capillary refilling time. In neurogenic shock, the patient has warm, dry skin, especially below the area of injury. The pulse in hypovolemic shock patients is weak, thready, and rapid. Because of unopposed parasympathetic activity on the heart, bradycardia is typically seen rather than tachycardia but the pulse quality may be weak. Hypovolemia produces a decreased LOC, or at least anxiety and often combativeness. In the absence of a traumatic brain injury, the patient with neurogenic shock is alert, oriented, and lucid but has no reflexes.

Neurogenic Shock Versus Spinal Shock

As discussed in this chapter, the term *neurogenic shock* refers to a disruption of the sympathetic nervous system, typically as the result of an injury to the spinal cord, that results in significant dilation of the peripheral arteries. If untreated, this may result in impaired perfusion to the body's tissues. This condition should not be confused with *spinal shock*, a term that refers to an injury to the spinal cord that results in *temporary* loss of sensory and motor function. Thus spinal shock indicates that the spinal cord has been damaged ("shocked") and is not working properly, although one cannot predict when the neurologic deficit will resolve. Strictly speaking, spinal shock does not represent a defect in organ or tissue perfusion. The prehospital care provider should be aware that both neurogenic shock and spinal shock can simultaneously occur in the same patient.

Patients with neurogenic shock may have associated injuries that produce severe hemorrhage. Therefore a patient who has neurogenic shock and signs of hypovolemia, such as tachycardia, should be treated appropriately.

Septic Shock.   Septic shock, seen in patients with life-threatening infections, is another condition that exhibits vascular dilation. Cytokines, which are locally active hormones produced by WBCs responding to the infection, cause damage to the walls of the blood vessels, causing peripheral vasodilation and a leakage of fluid from the capillaries into the interstitial space. Thus septic shock has characteristics of both distributive shock and hypovolemic shock. Preload is diminished because of the vasodilation and loss of fluid, and hypotension occurs when the heart can no longer compensate. Septic shock is virtually never encountered within minutes of an injury; however, the prehospital care provider may be called on to care for a trauma patient in septic shock during an interfacility transfer or if a patient sustains an injury to the gastrointestinal tract and did not promptly seek medical attention.

Psychogenic "Shock".   Psychogenic shock is typically mediated through the parasympathetic nervous system. Stimulation of the tenth cranial nerve (vagus nerve) produces bradycardia. The increased parasympathetic activity may also result in transient peripheral vasodilation and hypotension. If the bradycardia and vasodilation are severe enough, cardiac output falls dramatically, resulting in insufficient blood flow to the brain. Vasovagal syncope (fainting) occurs when the patient loses consciousness. Compared with neurogenic shock, the periods of bradycardia and vasodilation are generally limited to minutes, whereas neurogenic shock may last up to several days. In psychogenic shock patients, normal blood pressure is quickly restored when the patient is placed in a horizontal position. Because it is self-limited, a vasovagal episode is unlikely to result in true "shock" and the body quickly recovers before significant systemic impairment of perfusion occurs.

CARDIOGENIC SHOCK

Cardiogenic shock, or failure of the heart's pumping activity, results from causes that can be categorized as either intrinsic (a result of direct damage to the heart itself) or extrinsic (related to a problem outside the heart).

Intrinsic Causes

- *Heart muscle damage.* Any process that weakens the cardiac muscle will affect its output. The damage may result from an acute interruption of the heart's own blood supply (as in a myocardial infarction from coronary artery disease) or from a direct bruise to the heart muscle (as in a blunt cardiac injury). A recurring cycle will ensue—decreased oxygenation causes decreased contractibility, which results in decreased cardiac output and therefore decreased systemic perfusion. Decreased perfusion results in a continuing decrease in oxygenation and thus a continuation of the cycle. As with any muscle, the cardiac muscle does not work as efficiently when it becomes bruised or damaged.
- *Dysrhythmia.* The development of a cardiac dysrhythmia can affect the efficiency of contractions, resulting in impaired systemic perfusion. Hypoxia may lead to myocardial ischemia and cause dysrhythmias such as premature contractions and tachycardia. Because cardiac output is determined by the stroke volume multiplied by the number of contractions per minute, any dysrhythmia that results in a slow rate of contractions or shortens the left ventricle's fill time (resulting in decreased stroke volume) will impair cardiac output. Blunt cardiac injury may also result in dysrhythmias, the most common of which is a mild persistent tachycardia.

Table 6-3	Signs Associated with Types of Shock			
Signs	**Hypovolemic**	**Neurogenic**	**Septic**	**Cardiogenic**
Skin temperature	Cool, clammy	Warm, dry	Cool, clammy	Cool, clammy
Skin color	Pale, cyanotic	Pink	Pale, mottled	Pale, cyanotic
Blood pressure	Drops	Drops	Drops	Drops
Level of consciousness	Altered	Lucid	Altered	Altered
Capillary refilling time	Slowed	Normal	Slowed	Slowed

- *Valvular disruption.* A sudden, forceful compressing blow to the abdomen (see Chapter 2) may damage the valves of the heart. Severe valvular injury results in acute regurgitation, where a significant amount of blood leaks back into the chamber out of which it was just pumped. These patients often rapidly develop congestive heart failure manifested by pulmonary edema and cardiogenic shock. The presence of a new heart murmur is an important clue in making this diagnosis.

Extrinsic Causes

- *Pericardial tamponade.* Fluid in the pericardial sac will prevent the heart from refilling completely during the diastolic (relaxation) phase. According to Starling's law, inadequate filling results in a diminished strength of cardiac contraction. In the case of penetrating cardiac trauma, more blood may enter the pericardial sac with each contraction, further compromising the cardiac output. Severe shock and death may rapidly follow.
- *Tension pneumothorax.* A tension pneumothorax shifts the mediastinum away from the injury. Compression and kinking of the superior and inferior venae cavae and increased pulmonary vascular resistance because of increased intrathoracic pressure drastically impede venous return to the heart, producing a significant drop in preload. Because of its impaired filling, the heart loses its efficiency as a pump and shock rapidly ensues.

Complications of Shock

Several complications may result in patients with persistent or inadequately resuscitated shock, which is why early recognition and aggressive management of shock is essential. Many prehospital care providers fail to realize that the quality of care delivered in the prehospital setting can alter a patient's hospital course and outcome. *Failure to recognize shock and initiate proper treatment in the prehospital setting may extend the patient's hospital length of stay.* Although the following complications of shock are often not seen in the prehospital setting, a prehospital care provider may encounter them while transferring patients between facilities.

ACUTE RESPIRATORY DISTRESS SYNDROME

Acute respiratory distress syndrome (ARDS) is the result of damage to the lining of the capillaries in the lung, leading to the leakage of fluid into the interstitial spaces and alveoli of the lungs. This makes it much more difficult for oxygen to diffuse across the alveolar walls and into the capillaries and bind with the RBCs. Although these patients do have pulmonary edema, it is not the result of impaired cardiac function as is the case in congestive heart failure (cardiogenic pulmonary edema). ARDS represents noncardiogenic pulmonary edema, and patients generally do not improve with diuretic therapy. Many factors have been associated with the development of ARDS, including shock, massive blood transfusions, aspiration, and severe infection. ARDS is associated with a mortality rate of about 40%, and the patients who survive may require mechanical ventilation for up to several months.

ACUTE RENAL FAILURE

Impaired circulation to the kidneys, resulting from inappropriate care of shock leading to prolonged shock, can lead to temporary or permanent renal failure. The cells that comprise the renal tubules are most sensitive to ischemia and may die if their oxygen delivery is impaired for more than 45 to 60 minutes. This acute tubular necrosis (ATN) may cause the kidneys to shut down. Because the kidneys are no longer functioning, excess fluid is not excreted and volume overload may result. Also, the kidneys lose their ability to excrete metabolic acids and electrolytes, leading to a metabolic acidosis and hyperkalemia (increased blood potassium). These patients often require dialysis for a period of several weeks to months. Most patients who develop ATN resulting from shock will eventually recover normal renal function, provided they survive.

HEMATOLOGIC FAILURE

The term *coagulopathy* refers to impairment in the normal blood-clotting capabilities. This may result from either hypothermia (decreased body temperature), reduced energy production to these cells, or depletion of the clotting substances as they are used in an effort to control bleeding (consumptive coagulopathy). The normal blood-clotting cascade involves several enzymes and eventually results in the creation of fibrin molecules that serve as a matrix to trap platelets and RBCs and form a plug in a vessel wall. These enzymes function best in a narrow temperature range (i.e., at normal body temperature). As the core temperature of the body falls, this dramatically slows down blood clotting, leading to continued hemorrhage. The blood-clotting factors may also be used up as they form blood clots in an effort to slow and control hemorrhage. Another manifestation of hematologic failure is a marked decrease in the number of WBCs, predisposing the shock patient to infection. The decreased body temperature worsens the clotting problems, which makes hemorrhage worse, which reduces the body temperature even more. Thus with inadequate resuscitation this becomes an ever worsening cycle.

HEPATIC FAILURE

Severe damage to the liver is a less common result of prolonged shock, but it may occur. Liver failure is manifested by persistent hypoglycemia (low blood sugar), a persistent lactic acidosis, and jaundice (impaired metabolism of breakdown products of old RBCs). Because the liver produces many of the clotting factors necessary for hemostasis, a coagulopathy may accompany liver failure.

MULTIPLE ORGAN FAILURE

Failure of one major body system (such as the lungs, kidneys, blood-clotting cascade, or liver) is associated with a mortality rate of about 40%. As an organ system fails, the shock state is further worsened. By the time four organ systems fail, the mortality rate is essentially 100%. Cardiovascular failure, in the form of cardiogenic and septic shock, can only occasionally be reversed.

Assessment

Shock was defined previously in this chapter as widespread inadequate tissue perfusion resulting in anaerobic metabolism and loss of energy production. Assessing a patient for shock requires checking individual systems or organs to identify the presence of shock. The question that the prehospital care provider should always ask is whether energy production is normal in a particular organ. Specifically identifying anaerobic metabolism is extremely difficult in the prehospital setting; therefore the prehospital care provider must use indirect methods, such as ventilatory rate, pulse location, cerebral function, cardiac rate, capillary refilling time, urinary output, hypothermia, and measurement of the body's total acid level. The primary survey is a gross qualitative estimation of as many organs and organ systems as possible. The goal is to find any abnormalities that might suggest the presence of anaerobic metabolism, or shock.

Simultaneous evaluation is an important part of patient assessment. This evaluation may not be done at a conscious level, but the prehospital care provider's brain nonetheless continues to gather and process information. If the prehospital care provider finds that all systems are functioning normally, no alarm is set off.

Each patient condition that should be evaluated (status of airway, ventilation, perfusion, skin color and temperature, capillary refilling time, and blood pressure) is presented separately in the next section. They are presented in the context of both the primary survey (initial assessment) and the secondary survey (focused history and physical examination).

Primary and Secondary Surveys

The following signs identify the need for continued suspicion of life-threatening conditions:

- Mild anxiety, progressing to confusion or altered LOC
- Mild tachypnea, leading to rapid, labored ventilations
- Mild tachycardia, progressing to a marked tachycardia
- Weakened radial pulse, progressing to an absent radial pulse
- Pale or cyanotic skin color
- Capillary refilling time greater than two seconds

The prehospital care provider immediately manages any compromise or failure of the airway, breathing, or circulatory system before proceeding. The following steps are described in an ordered series. However, when the prehospital care provider carries them out in the field, he or she does them all more or less simultaneously.

AIRWAY

Assessment should include evaluation of the airway to ensure its patency (see Chapter 4).

BREATHING

As noted in the pathophysiology section of this chapter, the anaerobic metabolism associated with decreased cellular oxygenation will produce an increase in lactic acid. The hydrogen (H^+) ions from the acidosis and hypoxia lead to stimulation of the respiratory center to increase the rate and depth of ventilation. Thus tachypnea is frequently one of the earliest signs of shock. A rate of 20 to 30 breaths/min indicates a borderline abnormal rate and the need for supplemental oxygen. A rate greater than 30 breaths/min indicates a late stage of shock and the need for assisted ventilation because it is generally associated with a decreased tidal volume. Both of these rates indicate the need to look for the potential sources of impaired perfusion. A patient who tries to remove an oxygen mask, particularly when such action is associated with anxiety and belligerence, is displaying another sign of cerebral ischemia. This patient has "air hunger" and feels the need for more ventilation. The presence of a mask over the nose and mouth creates a psychological feeling of ventilatory restriction. This action should be a clue that the patient is not getting enough oxygen and is hypoxic. A decreased pulse oximeter reading will confirm this suspicion.

CIRCULATION

The two components of circulation are ongoing hemorrhage and perfusion (delivery of oxygenated blood to the tissue cells). Assessment of circulation should begin with a rapid scan for significant external hemorrhage. No efforts at restoring perfusion will be effective in the face of ongoing hemorrhage. The patient can lose significant amounts of blood from scalp lacerations because of the high concentration of blood vessels and from penetrating wounds that damage major blood vessels (subclavian, axillary, brachial, radial, ulnar, carotid, femoral, or popliteal). Next the patient's LOC can be assessed. An anxious, belligerent patient should be assumed to have cerebral ischemia and anaerobic metabolism until another cause is identified. Drug and alcohol overdose and cerebral contusion are conditions that cannot be treated rapidly, but cerebral ischemia can. Therefore all patients in whom cerebral ischemia might be present should be managed as if it is present.

The next important assessment point for perfusion is the pulse. Initial evaluation of the pulse determines whether it is palpable at the artery being examined. In general, loss of a radial pulse indicates severe hypovolemia or vascular damage to the arm, especially when a central pulse, such as in the carotid or femoral artery, is weak, thready, and extremely fast. If the pulse is palpable, its character and strength should be noted:

- Is the rate strong or weak and thready?
- Is the rate normal, too fast, or too slow?
- Is the rate regular or irregular?

The prehospital care provider can check these conditions rapidly and assimilate the data to make a quick initial determination of the patient's condition.

In the secondary survey, the pulse rate is determined more precisely. The normal pulse range for an adult is 60 to 100 pulsations/min. With rates below this, except in extremely athletic individuals, an ischemic heart or a pathologic condition such as complete heart block should be considered. A pulse in the range of 100 to 120 pulsations/min identifies a patient who has early shock, with an initial cardiac response toward tachycardia. A pulse above 120 pulsations/min is a definite sign of shock unless it is due to pain or fear, and one over 140 pulsations/min is considered extremely critical and near-death.

Skin Color.   Pink skin color generally indicates a well-oxygenated patient without anaerobic metabolism. Blue (cyanotic) or mottled skin indicates unoxygenated he-moglobin and a lack of adequate oxygenation to the periphery. Pale, mottled, or cyanotic skin has inadequate blood flow resulting from one of three causes:

1. Peripheral vasoconstriction (most often associated with hypovolemia)
2. Decreased supply of RBCs (acute anemia)
3. Interruption of blood supply to that portion of the body, such as might be found with a fracture

Pale skin in one area of the body may not represent the entire body. The implications of inconsistent skin color indicate that other findings, such as tachycardia, should be used to resolve these differences and to determine if the pale skin is a localized, regional, or systemic condition. Also, cyanosis may not develop in hypoxic patients who have lost a significant number of their RBCs from hemorrhage.

Skin Temperature.   As the body shunts blood away from the skin to more important parts of the body, skin temperature decreases. A skin temperature that is cool to the touch indicates decreased cutaneous perfusion and/or decreased energy production and therefore shock. Because a significant amount of heat can be lost during the assessment phase, steps should be taken to preserve the patient's body temperature.

Capillary Refilling Time.   The ability of the cardiovascular system to refill the capillaries after the blood has been "removed" represents an important support system. Analyzing this support system's level of function by compressing the capillaries to remove all the blood and then measuring the refilling time may provide insight into the perfusion of the capillary bed being assessed. Generally, the body shuts down circulation in the most distal parts of the body first and restores this circulation last. Evaluation of the nail bed of the big toe or thumb provides the earliest possible indication that hypoperfusion is developing. Additionally, it provides a strong indication when resuscitation is complete. However, like many other signs that a patient may exhibit, several conditions, both environmental and physiologic, can alter the results. A test of the capillary refilling time is a measurement of the time required to reperfuse the skin and therefore an indirect measurement of the actual perfusion of that part of the body. It is not a diagnostic test of any specific disease process or injury. An absent pulse can result from many of the same conditions as slow capillary refilling time.

Capillary refilling time has recently been described as a poor test of shock. However, it is not a test of shock, but rather a test of perfusion of the capillary bed being analyzed. Arterial interruption from a fracture, a gunshot wound of the vessel, hypothermia, and even arteriosclerosis are conditions that produce poor perfusion, and the capillary refilling time can be decreased. Another cause of poor capillary refilling is decreased cardiac output because of hypovolemia. It is a helpful diagnostic sign and can help the prehospital care provider analyze resuscitation.

One of the better signs of adequate resuscitation may be a warm, dry, pink toe. The environmental conditions in which the patient is found when performing this test can affect the results.

Blood Pressure. Blood pressure is one of the least sensitive signs of shock. Blood pressure does not begin to drop until a patient is profoundly hypovolemic (from either true fluid loss or container-enlarged relative hypovolemia). In otherwise healthy patients, blood loss must exceed 30% of blood volume before the patient's compensatory mechanisms fail and systolic blood pressure drops below 90 mm Hg. For this reason, ventilatory rate, pulse rate and character, capillary refilling time, and LOC are more sensitive indicators of hypovolemia than is the blood pressure.

When the patient's pressure has begun to drop, an extremely critical situation exists and rapid intervention is required. In the prehospital environment, a patient who is found to be hypotensive has already lost a significant amount of blood. The presence of a hypotensive patient means that the prehospital care provider may have overlooked the early signs of shock.

The severity of the situation and the appropriate type of intervention vary based on the cause of the condition. For example, low blood pressure associated with neurogenic shock is not nearly as critical as low blood pressure with hypovolemic shock. The signs used to assess compensated and decompensated hypovolemic shock are presented in Table 6-4.

One important pitfall to avoid involves equating systolic blood pressure with cardiac output and tissue perfusion. As has been emphasized in this chapter, significant blood loss is typically required before the patient becomes hypotensive (Class III hemorrhage). Thus patients will have decreased cardiac output and impaired tissue oxygenation when they have lost 15% to 30% of their blood volume despite having a normal systolic pressure.

When assessing patients with multiple trauma, the prehospital care provider should remember that brain injuries do not cause hypotension until the cerebellum begins to herniate through the incisura and foramen magnum. Therefore if a patient with a brain injury is hypotensive, the prehospital care provider should assume that this condition is due to hypovolemia (usually blood loss) from other injuries and not from the brain injury. Young infants are the exception to this rule because they may bleed into hypovolemic shock inside their head as a result of open sutures and fontanelles.

DISABILITY

One body system that can be readily evaluated in the field is brain function. At least five conditions can produce an altered LOC or change in behavior (combativeness or belligerence) in trauma patients:

1. Hypoxia
2. Shock with impaired cerebral perfusion
3. Traumatic brain injury
4. Intoxication with alcohol or drugs
5. Metabolic processes such as diabetes, seizures, or eclampsia

Of these five, the easiest to treat—and the one that will kill the patient the most quickly if not treated—is hypoxia. Any patient with an altered LOC should be

Table 6-4	Shock Assessment in Compensated and Decompensated Hypovolemic Shock	
	Compensated	**Decompensated**
Pulse	Increased; tachycardia	Markedly increased; marked tachycardia that can progress to bradycardia
Skin	White, cool, moist	White, cold, waxy
Blood pressure range	Normal	Decreased
Level of consciousness	Unaltered	Altered, ranging from disoriented to coma

treated as if decreased cerebral oxygenation is the cause. An altered LOC is usually one of the first visible signs of shock.

The brain's function decreases as perfusion and oxygenation drop and ischemia develops. This decreased function evolves through various stages as different areas of the brain become affected. Anxiety and belligerent behavior are usually the first signs, followed by a slowing of the thought processes and a decrease of the body's motor and sensory functions. The level of cerebral function is an important and measurable prehospital sign of shock. A belligerent, combative, anxious patient or one with a decreased LOC should be assumed to have a hypoxic, hypoperfused brain until another cause can be identified. Hypoperfusion and cerebral hypoxia frequently accompany brain injury and make the long-term result even worse. Even brief episodes of hypoxia and shock may worsen the original brain injury and result in poorer outcomes.

MUSCULOSKELETAL INJURIES

Significant internal hemorrhage can occur with fractures (Table 6-5). Of greatest concern are fractures to the femur and pelvis. A single femoral fracture may be associated with up to 2 to 4 units (1000 to 2000 mL) of blood loss into a thigh. This injury alone could potentially result in the loss of 30% to 40% of an adult's blood volume, resulting in decompensated hypovolemic shock. Pelvic fractures, especially those resulting from significant falls or crushing mechanisms, can be associated with massive internal hemorrhage into the retroperitoneal space. Occasionally a victim of blunt trauma will encounter multiple fractures and Class III

Table 6-5	Approximate Internal Blood Loss Associated with Fractures	
Bone	**Approximate internal blood loss (mL)**
Rib	125
Radius or ulna	250-500
Humerus	500-750
Tibia or fibula	500-1000
Femur	1000-2000
Pelvis	1000-massive

or IV shock but no evidence of external blood loss, hemothoraces, intraabdominal bleeding, or pelvic fracture. For example, an adult pedestrian struck by a vehicle and sustaining four rib fractures, a humerus fracture, a femur fracture, and bilateral tibia/fibula fractures may experience internal bleeding of between 3000 to 5500 mL of blood. This potential blood loss is enough for the patient to die from shock if it is unrecognized and insufficiently treated.

CONFOUNDING FACTORS

Numerous factors can add confusion to the assessment of the patient for signs of shock.

Age. Patients at the extremes of life, namely the very young (neonates) and the elderly, have diminished capability to compensate for acute blood loss and other shock states. Thus a relatively minor injury may produce decompensated shock in these individuals. On the other hand, children and young adults have a tremendous ability to compensate for blood loss and may appear relatively normal on a quick scan. A closer look may reveal subtle signs of shock such as mild tachycardia and tachypnea, pallid skin with delayed capillary refilling time, and anxiety. Because of their powerful compensatory mechanisms, children found in decompensated shock represent dire emergencies. Elderly individuals may be more prone to certain complications of prolonged shock, such as acute renal failure.

Athletic Status. Well-conditioned athletes often have enhanced compensatory capabilities. Many have resting heart rates in the range of 40 to 50 beats/min. Thus a heart rate of 100 to 110 beats/min or hypotension in a well-conditioned athlete may be warning signs that indicate significant hemorrhage.

Pregnancy. During pregnancy, a woman's blood volume may increase by up to 48%. Heart rate and cardiac output during pregnancy are also increased. Because of this, a pregnant female may not demonstrate signs of shock until her blood loss exceeds 30% to 35% of her blood volume. During the third trimester, the gravid uterus may compress the inferior vena cava, greatly diminishing venous return to the heart and resulting in hypotension. Elevation of the patient's right side once she has been immobilized to a long backboard may alleviate this. Hypotension in a pregnant female that persists after performing this maneuver typically represents life-threatening blood loss.

Preexisting Medical Conditions. Patients with serious preexisting medical conditions, such as coronary artery disease and chronic obstructive pulmonary disease, are typically less able to compensate for hemorrhage and shock. These patients may experience angina as their heart rate increases in an effort to maintain their blood pressure. Patients with an implanted pacemaker are typically unable to develop the compensatory tachycardia necessary to maintain blood pressure.

Medications. Numerous medications may interfere with the body's compensatory mechanisms. Beta-blocking agents and calcium-channel–blocking agents used to treat hypertension may prevent an individual from developing a compensatory tachycardia that may maintain his or her blood pressure. Additionally, the use of nonsteroidal antiinflammatory medications, used in the treatment of arthritis and musculoskeletal pain, may impair platelet activity and blood clotting, resulting in increased hemorrhage.

Time Between Injury and Treatment. In situations where the EMS response time has been brief, patients may be encountered with life-threatening internal hemorrhage but have not yet lost enough blood to manifest severe shock (Class III or IV hemorrhage). Even patients with penetrating wounds to their aorta, venae cavae, or iliac vessels may arrive at the receiving facility with a normal systolic blood pressure if the EMS response, scene, and transport times are brief. The prehospital care provider should never assume that patients are not bleeding internally just because they "look good." Patients should be thoroughly assessed for even the most subtle signs of shock, and internal hemorrhage should be assumed to be present until it is definitively ruled out. This is one reason why continued reassessment of trauma patients is essential.

Management

Management of a patient in shock is directed toward changing the anaerobic metabolism back to aerobic metabolism. To prevent serious complications and death, time is of the essence while trying to improve oxygen delivery to the ischemic cells of the body. Resuscitation in the prehospital setting includes the following:

- Improve oxygenation of the RBCs in the lungs through appropriate airway management.
- Provide ventilatory support with a bag-valve-mask (BVM) and deliver a high concentration of oxygen.

- Improve circulation to better deliver the oxygenated RBCs to the systemic tissues and improve oxygenation at the cellular level.
- Reach definitive care as soon as possible for hemorrhage control and replacement of lost RBCs.

If the prehospital care provider does not take appropriate measures, a patient will continue to deteriorate rapidly until he or she reaches the ultimate stable condition—death.

Four questions should be asked when deciding what treatment to provide for a patient in shock:

1. What is the cause of the patient's shock?
2. What is the definitive care for the patient's shock?
3. Where can the patient best receive this definitive care?
4. What interim steps can be taken to manage the patient's condition while he or she is being transported to definitive care?

Although the first question may be difficult to answer with a high degree of diagnostic accuracy, having some idea of what is occurring can help identify which facility is best qualified to meet a patient's needs and to decide which steps to take during transport to improve the patient's condition.

Airway

The airway should be evaluated initially in all patients. Patients in need of immediate management of their airway include the following in order of importance:

1. Those who are not breathing
2. Those who have obvious airway compromise
3. Those who have ventilatory rates in excess of 20 breaths/min
4. Those who have noisy sounds of ventilation

Specific techniques of airway management are discussed in Chapter 4.

Breathing

Once a patent airway is ensured, patients in shock or those at risk for developing shock (almost all trauma patients) should initially receive an oxygen concentration as close to 100% (Fio_2 of 1.0) as possible. This kind of oxygenation can only be achieved with a device that has a reservoir attached to a concentration of oxygen, not a nasal cannula or a simple facemask. *Pulse oximetry should be monitored in virtually all trauma patients.* Once the prehospital care provider has addressed the patient's acute problems and stabilized the patient's condition, he or she may titrate the oxygen downward while maintaining an SpO_2 reading of at least 95%.

If the patient is not breathing or is not breathing with an adequate depth and/or rate, the prehospital care provider should begin ventilatory assistance using a BVM unit immediately. End-tidal CO_2 monitoring may be useful to maintain the patient in a eucapneic state (normal blood CO_2 level).

Circulation

HEMORRHAGE CONTROL

Controlling external hemorrhage is the next priority after establishing the patient's airway. Early recognition and control of external bleeding in the trauma patient helps preserve the patient's blood volume and RBCs and helps ensure continued perfusion of tissues. Hemorrhage control should proceed in a step-wise fashion:

1. *Apply direct pressure over the bleeding site with a sterile dressing if available.* This technique will control most external hemorrhage. However, in a wound with an impaled object, pressure should be applied on both sides of the object rather than over the bleeding site. If hands are required to perform other life-saving tasks, a compression dressing using gauze pads and an elastic roller bandage or an inflated blood pressure cuff can be created.
2. *Continue direct pressure with elevation if an extremity is involved and no fracture is present.*
3. *Apply direct pressure with elevation and use of a pressure point.*
4. *Apply a tourniquet.* This is used only in the direst circumstances or in some combat situations to control external hemorrhage from the extremities.

Applying direct pressure to exsanguinating hemorrhage takes precedence over insertion of intravenous lines and fluid resuscitation. For example, the prehospital care provider would make a serious error to deliver a nicely packaged shooting victim to the receiving facility who has two IV lines inserted and neatly taped in place but is hemorrhaging to death from a gunshot wound to the femoral artery and has only trauma dressings taped in place and no direct pressure being applied.

If external hemorrhage cannot be readily controlled, the patient will most likely need emergent surgery. The prehospital care provider should immediately initiate transportation to the closest appropriate facility.

Internal hemorrhage from fracture sites should also be considered. Rough handling of an injured extremity may not only convert a closed fracture to an open one, but it may also significantly increase internal bleeding from bone ends, adjacent muscle tissue, or damaged vessels. All suspected extremity fractures should be immobilized in an effort to minimize this hemorrhage. Time may be taken to individually splint several fractures if the patient has no evidence of life-threatening conditions. However, if the primary survey identifies threats to the patient's life, the patient should be immobilized rapidly to a long backboard, thereby immobilizing all the extremities in an anatomic fashion, and transported to a medical facility.

PATIENT POSITIONING

In general, trauma patients who are in shock should be transported in a supine position, immobilized to a long backboard. Special positioning, such as the Trendelenburg position (placed on an incline with the feet elevated above the head) or the "shock" position (head and torso supine with legs elevated), is no longer recommended. The Trendelenburg position may aggravate already impaired ventilatory function by placing the weight of the abdominal organs on the diaphragm and may increase intracranial pressure in patients with traumatic brain injury. More importantly, patients who are in severe hypovolemic shock are generally maximally vasoconstricted. Thus the use of the Trendelenburg position is no longer believed to result in a significant autotransfusion of blood to the vital organs from the lower extremities. Both the Trendelenburg and shock positions are contraindicated in patients with a suspected spine injury.

Expose/Environment

Maintaining the patient's body temperature within a normal range is important. Hypothermia introduces myocardial dysfunction, coagulopathy, hyperkalemia, vasoconstriction, and a host of other problems that negatively affect a patient's chance of survival. Although cold temperatures preserve tissue for a short time, the temperature drop must be very rapid and very low for preservation to occur. Such a rapid change is unacceptable for the patient in shock.

In the prehospital setting, increasing the core temperature once hypothermia has developed can be difficult; therefore all steps that can be taken in the field to preserve normal body temperature should be initiated. A patient's temperature decreases as a result of reduced energy production and loss of heat to the surrounding environment. Once the patient is exposed and examined, he or she must be protected from the environment and his or her body temperature must be maintained. Any wet clothing, including that saturated with blood, should be removed from the patient because wet clothing increases heat loss. The patient should be convered with warm blankets. An alternative involves covering the patient with plastic sheets, such as heavy, thick garbage bags. They are inexpensive, easily stored, disposable, and effective devices for heat retention. Heated, humidified oxygen, if available, may help preserve body heat, especially in intubated patients.

Once the shock patient is assessed and packaged, he or she should be moved into the warmed patient compartment of the ambulance. Ideally, the patient compartment of an ambulance is kept at 85° F (29° C) or more when transporting a severely injured trauma patient. The patient's rate of heat loss into a cold compartment is very high. The conditions must be ideal for the patient, not for the providers, because the patient is the most important person in any emergency.

Any intravenous fluids given to a shock patient should be warm, not room temperature or cold. The ideal temperature for such fluids is 102° F (39° C). Most ambulances do not have conventional rapid fluid warmers, but other steps can keep fluids at an adequate temperature. A convenient storage area for fluids is in a box in the engine compartment. Wrapping heat packs around the bag can also warm fluid. Commercially available fluid warmer units for the patient care compartment provide an easy and reliable means to keep fluids at the correct temperature; however, these units are costly.

Patient Transport

The two things that a patient in severe hemorrhagic shock needs are blood transfusions and a surgeon with an available OR. Since neither is routinely carried on an ambulance, rapid transportation to a facility that is capable of managing the patient's injuries is extremely important. Rapid transportation does not mean disregarding or neglecting the treatment modalities that are important in patient care (doing the old fashioned "scoop and run"). However, it does indicate that the prehospital care provider should quickly employ key, potentially life-saving modalities such as airway management, ventilatory support, and hemorrhage control. Time must not be wasted on an inappropriate assessment or with unnecessary immobilization maneuvers. When caring for a critically injured patient, many steps, such as warming the patient, starting intravenous therapy, and even performing the secondary survey, are accomplished in the ambulance while en route.

Pneumatic Antishock Garment

The PASG remains one of the most controversial devices ever introduced to prehospital care. One large study from the Houston EMS system failed to demonstrate a benefit of the device in hypotensive trauma patients in an urban setting with brief transport times to trauma centers with in-house trauma surgeons. A similar study run in the same institution also demonstrated the same outcome when IV fluids were used for resuscitation. Both studies should be read when developing protocols for the use of either IV fluids or the PASG. The PASG is mainly a device for controlling blood loss and not for resuscitation except in a few situations of extreme hypotension. Although the PASG has not been adequately studied in suburban and rural settings, many EMS services have removed it from their units. This approach overlooks some patients in shock who may benefit from the use of the PASG.

PHYSIOLOGY

Pressure applied by the PASG to the legs and abdomen is transmitted directly through the skin, fat, muscle, and other soft tissues to the blood vessels themselves. As the vessels are compressed, their diameters are reduced in size. The primary physiologic result is that the vascular container in body areas beneath the device is made smaller, increasing the SVR and thereby raising the systolic and diastolic blood pressures. Virtually every study of PASG application in both experimental animals and humans has documented a rise in the systolic blood pressure with the application of this device for hemorrhagic shock. The MAP is also increased, which is probably beneficial to improving tissue perfusion. In addition to the increase in SVR, a small amount of blood is shifted from the veins in the lower extremities to the central organs. Venous return is increased with inflation of the PASG, resulting in improved cardiac output. The clinical significance of this "autotransfusion" has been questioned because research has shown the amount of blood shifted to be in the range of only several hundred milliliters.

USE OF THE PASG IN HEMORRHAGIC SHOCK

In the following four situations, the PASG may have significant benefit in patients with shock from blood loss:

1. *Suspected pelvic fractures with hypotension (systolic blood pressure <90 mm Hg).* Pelvic fractures that result from anterior and posterior compression and those that result from falls may result in severe hemorrhage into the pelvic soft tissues and retroperitoneal space. Inflation of the entire PASG may decrease the volume of the pelvis and result in tamponade of the associated hemorrhage. If a PASG is not available, consideration should be given to wrapping a sheet tightly around the pelvis and tying it as a sling. This should be accomplished so that the lower extremities are maintained in an adducted and internally rotated position.
2. *Profound hypotension.* Some data suggest that patients with severe hypotension (systolic blood pressures below 50 to 60 mm Hg) may have an improved outcome when the PASG is used. The increased perfusion of the brain and heart that results from PASG inflation may contribute to the improved survival.
3. *Suspected intraperitoneal hemorrhage with hypotension.* Inflation of the entire PASG compresses intraperitoneal organs. This may result in a slowing or cessation of hemorrhage (tamponade) from the solid organs, such as the liver and spleen, and the mesenteric vessels. Several studies have demonstrated improved survival in animals receiving the PASG in models of uncontrolled intraabdominal hemorrhage.
4. *Suspected retroperitoneal hemorrhage with hypotension.* Inflation of the entire device compresses the retroperitoneal organs. Because of the increased pressure, the device may tamponade bleeding from the kidneys, aorta, and venae cavae.

The PASG is probably significantly *less effective* than direct pressure or a pressure dressing with gauze and an elastic bandage for control of external hemorrhage from the lower extremities. The prehospital care provider should only use a PASG in this manner when direct pressure cannot be applied because of manpower limitations.

CONTRAINDICATIONS FOR PASG USE

- *Penetrating thoracic trauma.* Application and inflation of the PASG increases the rate of hemorrhage from damaged blood vessels in the upper half of the body (outside the confines of the device) as the patient's blood pressure significantly increases. In the Houston PASG study, hypotensive patients with penetrating thoracic trauma clearly had a higher mortality rate when the PASG was used.
- *Splinting of lower extremity fractures.* The PASG could be thought of as a large air splint and has been suggested to immobilize fractures of the femur, tibia, and fibula. A traction splint is a much better immobilization device for fractures of the midshaft femur because it reduces the bone ends back into anatomic alignment and treats pain by combating the severe muscle spasm that develops in the thigh. Use of the PASG has been associated with the development of compartment syndromes of the calf, especially when fractures present. Use of the PASG solely as a splint for isolated lower extremity fractures where shock is not present is not recommended.
- *Evisceration of abdominal organs*
- *Impaled objects in the abdomen*
- *Pregnancy*
- *Traumatic cardiopulmonary arrest*

APPLICATION OF THE PASG

The PASG should be applied to a patient as quickly as possible once indication for its use is identified. The PASG is positioned under the patient in one of several ways. In many cases, it may be easiest to logroll the patient onto the device after spreading it out on a long backboard. Another alternative involves one prehospital care provider placing each arm into the foot ends of each of the patient's trouser legs. As one provider grabs the patient's ankles and lifts up on his or her legs, a second provider slides the PASG onto the patient's legs. The patient's pelvis is then gently lifted to complete proper placement of the garment beneath the patient. The top of the garment should come up to the lower rib margin laterally.

The straps of the PASG are securely fastened and the device is inflated, typically beginning with the legs followed by the abdomen. All three compartments may be inflated simultaneously; however, the abdominal compartment should never be inflated before the leg compartments. When the Velcro straps begin to crackle, the pressure inside the PASG is generally between 60 and 80 mm Hg. A well-trained crew can apply the device rapidly, and several studies have failed to demonstrate an increase in scene time when a PASG was used.

DEFLATION OF THE PASG

Prehospital deflation of the PASG should *not* be done except in extreme circumstances, such as evidence of a ruptured diaphragm. In such a patient, the blunt trauma ruptured the diaphragm and application and inflation of the device results in herniation of abdominal organs into the thoracic cavity. This leads to marked respiratory distress. This may mimic the development of a tension pneumothorax; however, patient deterioration will occur almost immediately after inflation of the device.

The decision to deflate the device should be made in consultation with online medical direction. Except in the unusual circumstances in which inflation of the device resulted in rapid deterioration of the patient's condition, the device should not be deflated unless the patient's vital signs are within normal limits. Even when vital signs are within normal ranges, the patient's blood volume might still be significantly depleted. The inflated PASG may have reduced the size of the patient's container (vessels) to match the available blood volume. As the PASG is deflated, the patient's container size will increase. Unless a sufficient amount of fluid is infused, cardiac preload and SVR may drop dramatically, resulting in severe hypotension and profound shock.

Volume Resuscitation

VASCULAR ACCESS

The prehospital care provider routinely obtains intravenous access in a trauma patient who has known or suspected serious injuries so that he or she can initiate volume resuscitation. Except in unusual circumstances where a patient is undergoing extrication from a vehicle or prehospital care providers are awaiting the arrival of an aeromedical helicopter, intravenous access should be obtained after the patient has been placed in the ambulance and transportation has been initiated to the closest appropriate facility. Although volume resuscitation of a trauma patient in shock makes empiric sense, no research has ever demonstrated improved survival of critically injured trauma patients when intravenous fluid therapy has been administered in the prehospital setting. Therefore *transport of the trauma patient should never be delayed to initiate IV lines.*

For patients in shock or those having potential serious injuries, two large-bore (14- or 16-gauge), short (about 1-inch long) intravenous catheters should be inserted by percutaneous puncture. The rate of fluid administration is directly proportional to the fourth power of the radius of the catheter and inversely proportional to its length (i.e., more fluid will rapidly flow through a short, large-diameter catheter than through a longer, smaller-diameter catheter). The preferred site for percu-

taneous access is a vein of the forearm. Alternative sites for intravenous access are the veins of the antecubital fossa, the hand, and the upper arm (cephalic vein). If two attempts at percutaneous access are unsuccessful in a child, inserting an intraosseous line can be considered. Central venous lines or venous cut-downs are not generally considered appropriate venous access in the prehospital setting and are rarely needed.

INTRAVENOUS SOLUTIONS

Because of its ability to transport oxygen, blood remains the fluid of choice for the resuscitation of a patient in severe hemorrhagic shock. Unfortunately blood is impractical for use in the prehospital setting because of issues related to blood typing and the fact that it is perishable when not refrigerated. Alternative solutions for volume resuscitation fall into one of four categories: (1) isotonic crystalloids, (2) hypertonic crystalloids, (3) synthetic (artificial) colloids, and (4) blood substitutes.

Isotonic Crystalloid Solutions.   Isotonic crystalloids are balanced salt solutions comprised of electrolytes (substances that separate into charged ions when dissolved in solutions). They act as effective volume expanders for a short period of time, but they possess no oxygen-carrying capacity. Immediately after infusion, crystalloids fill the vascular space that was depleted by blood loss, improving preload and cardiac output. Lactated Ringer's solution remains the isotonic crystalloid solution of choice for the management of shock because its composition is most similar to the electrolyte composition of blood plasma. It contains specific amounts of sodium, potassium, calcium, chloride, and lactate ions. Normal saline (0.9% sodium chloride solution) remains an acceptable alternative, although hyperchloremia (a marked increase in the blood chloride level) may occur with massive volume resuscitation with normal saline administration. Solutions of dextrose in water, such as D_5W, are not effective volume expanders and have no place in the resuscitation of trauma patients.

One hour after administration of a crystalloid solution, only about one third remains in the cardiovascular system. The rest has shifted into the interstitial space because both the water and the electrolytes in the solution can freely cross the capillary membranes. A rule of thumb (the 3:1 rule) is that most patients with hemorrhagic shock generally only achieve adequate resuscitation when about 300 mL of crystalloid solution has been infused for every 100 mL of blood volume that has been lost. If possible, intravenous fluids should be warmed to about 102° F (39° C) before infusion. Infusion of large amounts of room temperature or cold intravenous fluid contributes to hypothermia and increased hemorrhage.

Hypertonic Crystalloid Solutions.
Hypertonic crystalloid solutions have markedly high concentrations of electrolytes compared with blood plasma. The most common of these is hypertonic saline, which is a 7.5% solution of sodium chloride, which is more than eight times the concentration of sodium chloride found in normal saline. This is an effective plasma expander, especially in that a small 250 mL infusion often produces the same effect as infusing 2 to 3 liters of isotonic crystalloid solution. Although these solutions are somewhat more costly than isotonic crystalloids, they are considered advantageous in military situations where medics are limited in the amount of intravenous fluid they can carry. An analysis of several studies of hypertonic saline failed to demonstrate improved survival rates over the use of isotonic crystalloids.

Synthetic Colloid Solutions.
Proteins are large molecules produced by the body and are composed of amino acids. They have countless functions; however, one type of protein found in the blood, albumin, helps maintain fluid in the intravascular space. Administration of human albumin is costly and has been associated with the transmission of infectious diseases, such as hepatitis. When administered to a patient in hemorrhagic shock, synthetic colloid solutions draw fluid from the interstitial and intracellular spaces into the intravascular space, thereby producing expansion of the blood volume. Like crystalloids, colloid plasma expanders do not transport oxygen.

Gelofusine is a 4% gelatin solution produced from bovine protein and is occasionally used in Europe and Australia for fluid resuscitation. It is moderately expensive and carries a risk of severe allergic reactions. A small infusion of gelofusine produces expansion of the intravascular volume for several hours.

Hetastarch (Hespan) and dextran (Gentran) are synthetic colloids that have been created by linking numerous starch (amylopectin) or dextrose molecules together until it is similar in size to an albumin molecule. These solutions are also moderately expensive compared with crystalloids and have been associated with allergic reactions and impairment of blood typing.

Virtually no research exists involving the use of these synthetic colloid solutions in the prehospital setting and no data exist from their use in the hospital that shows them to be superior to crystalloid solutions. These products are not recommended for the prehospital management of shock.

Blood Substitutes.
Blood has several undesirable qualities, including the need to type and crossmatch, a short shelf life, perishability when not refrigerated, a potential of transmission of infectious disease, and an increasing shortage of donated units. This has led to intense research in blood substitutes in the last two decades. The military has played a central role in this research because a blood substitute that would not need refrigeration and did not require blood typing could be carried to a wounded soldier on the battlefield and infused rapidly to combat shock.

Perfluorocarbons (PFCs) are synthetic compounds that have been found to have high oxygen solubility. These inert materials can dissolve approximately 50 times more oxygen than can blood plasma. They contain no hemoglobin or protein, they are completely free of biological materials (thereby greatly reducing the threat of infectious agents being found in them), and oxygen is transported by being dissolved in the plasma portion. First-generation PFCs experienced limited usefulness because of numerous problems, including a short half-life and the need for a concurrent high Fio_2 administration. Newer PFCs have fewer of these disadvantages, but their role as oxygen carriers remains undetermined.

Most hemoglobin-based oxygen carriers (HBOCs) use the same oxygen-carrying molecule (hemoglobin) found in human blood cells; however, one under investigation uses bovine hemoglobin. The major difference between HBOCs and human blood is that the hemoglobin in HBOCs is not contained within a cell membrane. This removes the need for conducting type and crossmatch studies because the antigen-antibody risk is removed. Additionally, many of these HBOCs can be stored for long periods of time, making them the ideal solution for mass casualty incidents. Early problems with hemoglobin-based oxygen-carrying solutions included toxicity from hemoglobin. Of the several HBOCs currently involved in clinical trials, most cause vasoconstriction and gastrointestinal symptoms. Although some look promising for use in the hospital, only the product made from bovine hemoglobin does not require refrigeration, thus their applicability in the prehospital setting is limited.

DECISION-MAKING IN RESUSCITATION

Adult patients who present in Class II, III, or IV shock should receive an initial rapid bolus of 1 to 2 liters of warmed crystalloid solution, preferably lactated Ringer's. Pediatric patients should receive a bolus of 20 mL/kg of warmed crystalloid solution. As noted previously, this should virtually always occur during transport to the closest appropriate facility. Vital signs, including pulse and ventilatory rates and blood pressure, should be monitored to assess the patient's response to the initial fluid therapy. In most urban settings, the patient will be delivered to the receiving facility before the initial fluid bolus is completed.

The initial fluid bolus elicits three possible responses:

1. *Rapid response.* The vital signs return to and remain normal. This typically indicates that the patient had lost less than 20% of his or her blood volume but that the hemorrhage has stopped. Surgical intervention may still be required in these patients.

2. *Transient response.* The vital signs initially improve (pulse slows and blood pressure increases); however, during continued assessment these patients show deterioration with recurrent signs of shock. These patients have generally lost between 20% and 40% of their blood volume and have ongoing hemorrhage. Rapid surgical intervention will be required to control the bleeding.

3. *Minimal or no response.* These patients show virtually no change in the profound signs of shock after a rapid 1- to 2-liter fluid bolus. These patients typically have massive exsanguinating internal hemorrhage and are in need of immediate surgical intervention to save their lives.

In suburban and rural settings with longer transport times, fluid management of the trauma patient in shock is a more challenging and controversial issue. Theoretically, aggressive volume resuscitation could return the blood pressure to normal. This in turn may dislodge blood clots that had formed at bleeding sites in the peritoneal cavity or elsewhere and result in renewed hemorrhage that cannot be controlled until the patient reaches the OR. On the other hand, withholding intravenous fluid from a patient in profound shock only leads to further tissue hypoxia and failure of energy production. If the prehospital care provider does not provide fluid therapy, the patient may slip from decompensated shock into irreversible shock.

During prolonged transport, the prehospital care provider must attempt to maintain perfusion to the vital organs. Maintaining the systolic blood pressure in the range of 80 to 90 mm Hg, or the MAP in the range of 60 to 65 mm Hg, can usually accomplish this with less risk of renewing internal hemorrhage. Researchers are aggressively seeking the exact end point of resuscitation (Box 6-1). Although the end point has not yet been determined at the time of publication of this text, it is most likely in the range of 80 to 90 mm Hg.

During prolonged transports, the primary survey and vital signs should be reassessed frequently. Monitoring urinary output is another tool that can help guide decisions regarding the need for additional fluid therapy. Insertion of a urinary catheter should be considered so that urinary output can be monitored. Adequate urinary outputs include the following: 0.5 mL/kg/hr for an adult, 1 mL/kg/hr for a pediatric patient, and 2 mL/kg/hr for infants younger than 1 year of age. Urinary outputs of less than these amounts may be a key indicator that the patient requires further volume infusion. If time permits, placement of a nasogastric (NG) catheter should be considered for all intubated patients unless there are suspected fractures of the patient's midface. In this case, placement of an orogastric (OG) catheter should be considered. Gastric distention may cause unexplained hypotension and dysrhythmias, especially in children. Placement of an NG or OG tube may also decrease the risk of vomiting and aspiration.

Box 6-1

End-Points of Resuscitation

As noted in the text of this chapter, significant controversy surrounds prehospital fluid administration for a trauma patient who is in shock. When prehospital advanced life support was first introduced in the United States, prehospital care providers adopted the approach used by emergency physicians and surgeons in most hospitals and trauma centers—administer an intravenous crystalloid solution until the vital signs had been returned to normal (typically a pulse <100 beats/min and a systolic blood pressure >100 mm Hg).

A major contribution of PHTLS over the past two decades has been bringing about the conceptual change that, in the critically injured trauma patient, transportation should never be delayed while IV lines are placed and fluid is infused. These actions can be performed in the back of the ambulance en route to the closest appropriate facility. The critically injured trauma patient who is in shock generally requires blood and surgical intervention to control internal hemorrhage—neither of which can be accomplished in the field.

Continued

Box 6-1

End-Points of Resuscitation—cont'd

When sufficient crystalloid solution is infused to restore vital signs to normal, the patient's perfusion should be improved. Experts believed that such rapid intervention would clear lactic acid and restore energy production in the cells of the body, and also decrease the risk of developing irreversible shock and kidney failure. However, no study of trauma patients in the prehospital setting has shown that the administration of intravenous fluid decreases complications and death.

Recent research, primarily in experimental models of shock, has shown that intravenous volume resuscitation may have detrimental side effects when administered before surgical control of the source of hemorrhage. In experimental animals, internal hemorrhage often continues until the animal is hypotensive, at which point bleeding slows and a blood clot (thrombus) typically forms at the site of injury. In one sense this hypotension is protective in that it is associated with a dramatic slowing or cessation of internal hemorrhage.

When aggressive IV fluids were administered to the animals in an attempt to restore perfusion, internal hemorrhage again started and the thrombus was disrupted. In addition, crystalloid infusions may also dilute coagulation factors. These animals often had a worse outcome compared with animals that re-ceived resuscitation *after* surgical control of the injury site. A single clinical study conducted in an urban prehospital setting demonstrated a significantly worse outcome in trauma patients who received crystalloid solutions before control of internal hemorrhage (mortality rate of 62% vs. 70% in the delayed treatment group).

The findings of this single study have not been replicated in other prehospital systems, nor can the findings be generalized to rural EMS systems or patients with certain conditions, such as traumatic brain injuries. Until additional research is available, PHTLS recommends a "middle of the road" approach; especially for situations involving prolonged or delayed transport. In general, sufficient crystalloid solution should be administered intravenously to maintain a systolic blood pressure in the range of 80 to 90 mm Hg, or the mean arterial pressure (MAP) in the range of 60 to 65 mm Hg. This should maintain adequate perfusion to the kidneys with less risk of worsening internal hemorrhage compared with restoring a blood pressure to the normal range (systolic blood pressure of 100 to 120 mm Hg). Prehospital care providers should follow the recommendations of their medical control. Refer to the PHTLS MERLIN site for current information on the end-points of resuscitation controversy.

Summary

Adequate perfusion of the tissues with oxygenated blood is necessary for survival. Hemorrhagic shock is a condition in which tissue perfusion is inadequate because of loss of intravascular volume and RBCs. Without an adequate number of RBCs, a sufficient amount of oxygen cannot be carried to the cells, even when vascular volume is normal. Without adequate circulating volume, perfusion pressure is insufficient to deliver blood to the tissues for gas exchange.

Prehospital care providers direct management of the patient in shock toward optimizing circulating volume and oxygenation. These goals are achieved through aggressive management of the patient's airway, ventilation, and oxygenation and prevention of the loss of additional RBCs and blood volume through hemorrhage control. Additionally, the patient's mean arterial pressure must be maintained at a level sufficient for perfusion of the vital organs without risking renewed or increased bleeding.

In all cases, early recognition of shock and recognition of the limitations of the field management of shock are critical. The prehospital care provider must transport patients in shock without delay to the nearest facility equipped to provide definitive treatment of hemorrhage.

SHOCK MANAGEMENT ALGORITHM

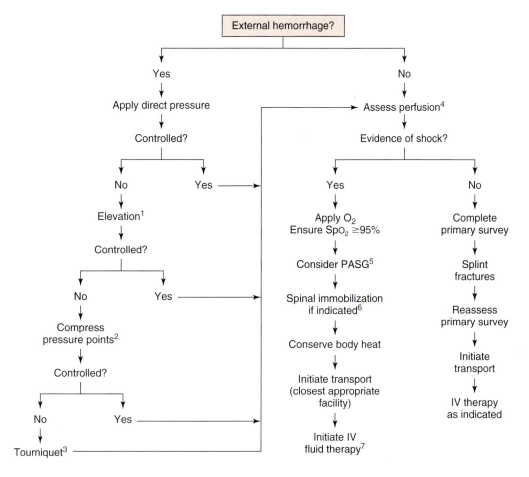

Notes:

[1]Elevation should be considered unless contraindicated by fractures or inability to elevate a specific body part.

[2]Compression should be applied proximal to the bleeding site in one of the following locations: axillary artery, brachial artery, femoral artery, or popliteal artery.

[3]A wide material such as a cravat, belt, or blood pressure cuff should be used; a tourniquet should not be placed distal to the elbow or knee.

[4]Assessment of perfusion includes, presence, quality, and location of pulses; skin color, temperature, and moisture; and capillary refilling time.

[5]PASG should be considered for decompensated shock (SBP <90 mm Hg), and suspected pelvic, intraperitoneal, or retroperitoneal hemorrhage, and in patients with profound hypotension (SBP <60 mm Hg). PASG is contraindicated in penetrating thoracic trauma, abdominal evisceration, pregnancy, impaled object in the abdomen, and traumatic cardiopulmonary arrest, or for splinting the lower extremity fractures.

[6]See Indications for Spinal Immobilization algorithm.

[7]Initiate two large-bore (14- or 16-guage) IV catheters. An initial bolus of 1 to 2 liters of warmed (102° F) lactated Ringer's solution or normal saline should be given rapidly. For pediatric patients, the initial fluid bolus should be 20 mL/kg.

Scenario Solution

The amount of kinetic energy involved and the direction of forces applied in this crash should create a high index of suspicion for intraabdominal injury and hemorrhage, even before you observe the physical findings exhibited by the patient. The primary survey confirms that the patient is in shock and in need of rapid extrication with spinal stabilization. This patient needs high-concentration oxygen immediately. Because of the distance from the nearest trauma center, you should initiate transport expediently with ongoing assessment and additional management en route.

Further management includes the initiation of two large-bore IVs for fluid replacement. Because of the presence of intraabdominal injury, you may consider use of a PASG if the patient further deteriorates. Without timely surgical intervention to achieve control of bleeding, the patient may progress through the stages of shock, causing irreversible tissue damage, resulting in immediate death or delayed death as a result of multiple organ system dysfunction.

Review Questions

Answers are provided on p. 414.

1. Which of the following best describes the term *shock* as used in this chapter?
   a. A lack of blood flow in the body that leads to aerobic metabolism
   b. A lack of adequate tissue oxygenation that leads to anaerobic metabolism
   c. A lack of adequate oxygen in the lungs as a result of airway compromise
   d. A measurement of the flow of blood in the tissues under stress

2. Hypovolemia is the medical term used to describe a condition in which:
   a. The blood volume of a given patient is considered to be within normal limits
   b. The blood volume of a given patient is above normal limits
   c. The blood volume of a given patient is less than normal
   d. The patient's systolic blood pressure is less than 90 mm Hg

3. The pneumatic antishock garment (PASG) is most appropriately used in which of the following conditions?
   a. A patient with bilateral open femur fractures who is demonstrating signs and symptoms of shock
   b. A female patient with blunt abdominal trauma who is demonstrating signs and symptoms of shock and is 20 weeks pregnant
   c. A patient with blunt abdominal and penetrating chest trauma who is demonstrating signs and symptoms of shock
   d. A patient with multiple system trauma of the abdomen and pelvis who is demonstrating signs and symptoms of shock

4. All of the following statements are true regarding the pneumatic antishock garment (PASG) except:
   a. Increased vascular resistance in the lower extremities and abdomen is beneficial to patients with systolic blood pressure between 50 and 60 mm Hg
   b. Anterior compartment syndrome is a complication associated with prolonged use of the PASG
   c. The PASG should be inflated until the patient's systolic blood pressure reaches 120 mm Hg
   d. PASG deflation in the field should only be done with online medical direction

5. In the management of shock, isotonic crystalloid solutions, such as lactated Ringer's, are preferred because:
   a. The protein molecules in crystalloid solutions act as volume expanders
   b. These solutions draw interstitial fluid into the vascular space to enhance volume
   c. These solutions will stay in the vascular space longer than water solutions, such as D_5W
   d. Their pH enhances oxygen delivery to the tissues

6. The ultimate goal of prehospital management of the trauma patient who is demonstrating signs and symptoms of shock or in which the prehospital care provider has a high index of suspicion of life-threatening injury is rapid transport to a facility that can provide surgical intervention to control hemorrhage and replacement of lost blood.
   a. True
   b. False

7. Which of the following is NOT a component of the Fick principle?
   a. Oxygen must be on-loaded to RBCs in the lung
   b. Carbon dioxide must be off-loaded from RBCs in the lung
   c. RBCs must circulate to the tissues
   d. Oxygen must be off-loaded from RBCs to tissue cells

8. Which of the following is NOT a mechanism related to failure of tissue perfusion?
   a. Skeletal muscle relaxation
   b. Relaxation of vascular smooth muscle
   c. Failure of cardiac muscle
   d. Loss of fluid volume

9. Which of the following presentations represent early shock?
   a. Tachypnea, tachycardia, diaphoresis
   b. Hypotension, tachycardia, bradypnea
   c. Altered mental status, tachycardia, hypotension
   d. Bradypnea, hypotension, altered mental status

10. Which of the following best describes mean arterial pressure (MAP)?
   a. Systolic blood pressure minus diastolic blood pressure
   b. Pulse pressure plus ½ the diastolic pressure
   c. ¼ the systolic pressure minus ⅓ the heart rate
   d. ⅓ the pulse pressure plus the diastolic pressure

REFERENCES

American College of Surgeons Committee on Trauma: *Advanced trauma life support*, Chicago, 2002, Author.

Bickell WH, Wall MJ, Pepe PE et al: Immediate versus delayed fluid resuscitation for hypotensive patients with penetrating torso injuries, *N Engl J Med* 331:1105, 1994.

Glaeser PW, Hellmich TR, Szewczuga D et al: Five-year experience in prehospital intraosseous infusions in children and adults, *Ann Emerg Med* 22:1119, 1993.

Gross SD: *A system of surgery: pathological, diagnostic, therapeutic, and operative*, Philadelphia, 1859, Blanchard and Lea.

Ketcham EM, Cairns CB: Hemoglobin-based oxygen carriers: development and clinical potential, *Ann Emerg Med* 33:326, 1999.

Marino PL: *The ICU book*, ed 2, Baltimore, 1998, Williams and Wilkins.

Mattox KL, Bickell WH, Pepe PE et al: Prospective MAST study in 911 patients, *J Trauma* 29:1104, 1989.

McSwain NE Jr: Pneumatic anti-shock garment: state of the art 1988, *Ann Emerg Med* 17:506, 1988.

O'Connor RE, Domeier R: Use of the pneumatic antishock garment (PASG), *Prehosp Emerg Care* 1:36, 1997.

Wade CE, Kramer GC, Grady JJ: Efficacy of hypertonic 7.5% saline and 6% dextran in treating trauma: a metaanalysis of controlled clinical trials, *Surgery* 122:609, 1997.

SUGGESTED READING

Allison KP, Gosling P, Jones S et al: Randomized trial of hydroxyethyl starch versus gelatine for trauma resuscitation, *J Trauma* 47:1114, 1999.

Demetriades D, Chan L, Cornwell E et al: Paramedic vs private transport of trauma patients: effect on outcome, *Arch Surg* 131:133, 1996.

Lewis FR: Prehospital intravenous fluid therapy: physiologic computer modeling, *J Trauma* 26:804, 1986.

O'Gorman M, Trabulsy P, Pilcher DB: Zero-time prehospital IV, *J Trauma* 29:84, 1989.

Trunkey DD: Prehospital fluid resuscitation of the trauma patient: an analysis and review, *Emerg Med Serv* 30(5):93, 2001.

Vassar MJ, Perry CA, Holcroft JW: Prehospital resuscitation of hypotensive trauma patients with 7.5% NaCl versus 7.5% NaCl with added detran: a controlled trial, *J Trauma* 34:622, 1993.

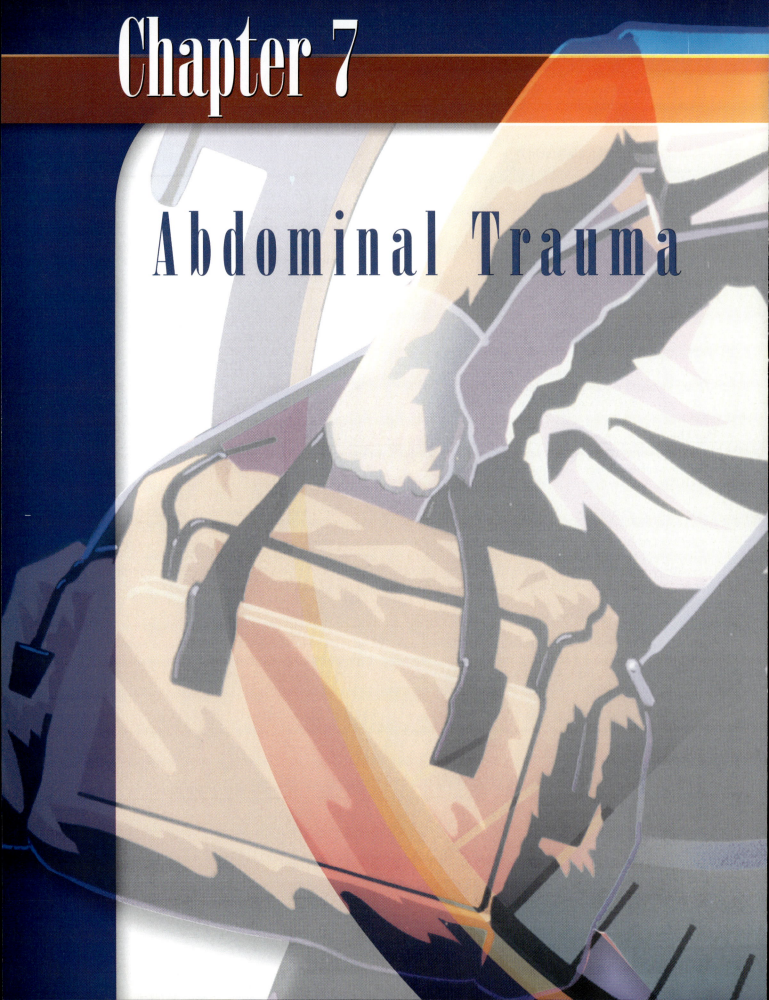

Chapter 7

Abdominal Trauma

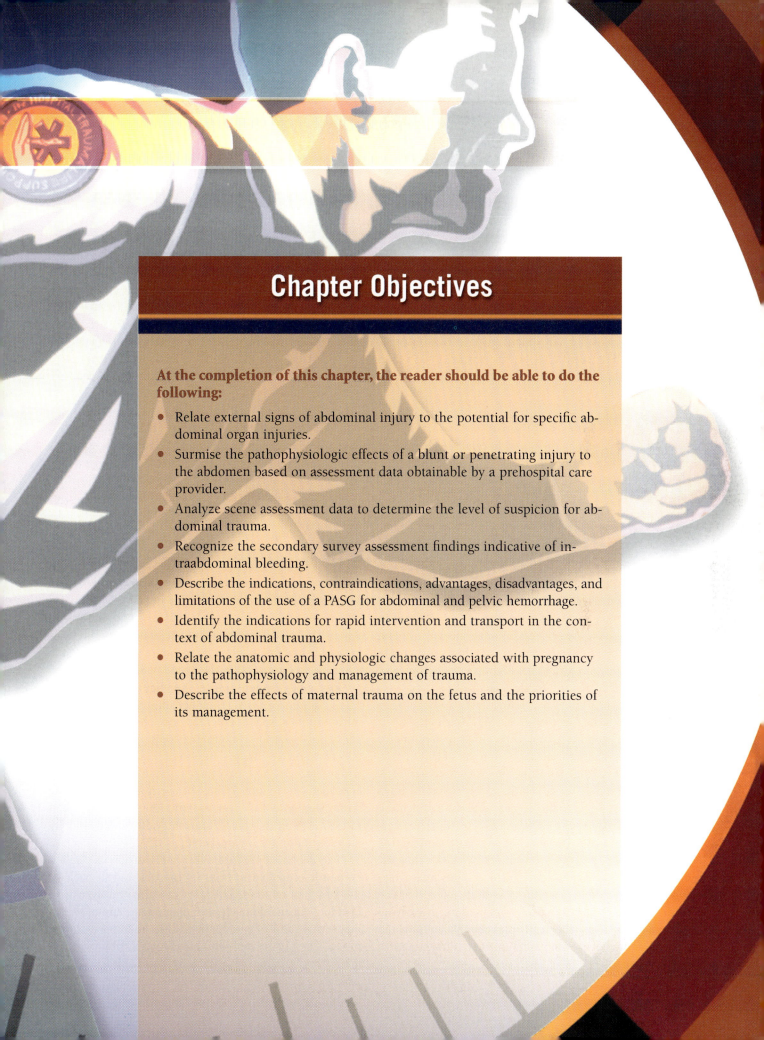

Chapter Objectives

At the completion of this chapter, the reader should be able to do the following:

- Relate external signs of abdominal injury to the potential for specific abdominal organ injuries.
- Surmise the pathophysiologic effects of a blunt or penetrating injury to the abdomen based on assessment data obtainable by a prehospital care provider.
- Analyze scene assessment data to determine the level of suspicion for abdominal trauma.
- Recognize the secondary survey assessment findings indicative of intraabdominal bleeding.
- Describe the indications, contraindications, advantages, disadvantages, and limitations of the use of a PASG for abdominal and pelvic hemorrhage.
- Identify the indications for rapid intervention and transport in the context of abdominal trauma.
- Relate the anatomic and physiologic changes associated with pregnancy to the pathophysiology and management of trauma.
- Describe the effects of maternal trauma on the fetus and the priorities of its management.

Scenario

You have been dispatched to a residence for "an injured person." En route to the scene, dispatch advises that the patient is a pregnant woman who has been assaulted and that law enforcement is en route. On arrival you are met by an anxious young woman who states that her sister is pregnant and has been beaten by her boyfriend. You find a 19-year-old female on the floor lying on her side with her knees drawn up. You observe obvious signs of a struggle in the residence. The patient has a moderate amount of blood in her hair and on her face. Her eyes are closed, but as you kneel down next to her and speak, she opens her eyes. In response to your question, the patient states that she "hit her head." She is unable to give you the details of her pregnancy or the incident. Her sister states that the patient is "about six and a half months" pregnant but has not seen a doctor.

In your assessment you find that the patient has a patent airway, a ventilatory rate of 24 breaths/min, a heart rate of 100 beats/min, and a blood pressure of 100/68 mm Hg. The patient has a scalp laceration; her pupils are equal, round, and reactive to light; her skin is pale but dry; palpation of her abdomen elicits tenderness of the lower left quadrant; and she has an obvious deformity of the right forearm.

What are the priorities in the care of this patient? What modifications to patient management are necessary because of her pregnancy? What additional information is pertinent to the care of this patient? What are the effects of the patient's condition on the fetus? Are the priorities for care of the mother different because of the pregnancy? How is the interpretation of assessment findings affected by the anatomic and physiologic changes associated with pregnancy?

The abdomen is the region of the body in which it is most difficult to correctly diagnose trauma injuries that require surgical repair. When unrecognized, abdominal injury is one of the major causes of death in the trauma patient. Because abdominal injury is difficult to correctly diagnose, the correct method of management is to transport patients with suspected abdominal injuries to the closest appropriate facility.

The extent of abdominal trauma can also be difficult to determine in the prehospital setting. Death may occur from massive blood loss caused by either penetrating or blunt injuries. Late complications and possible death occur from colon, small intestine, stomach, or pancreatic injuries that go undetected. However, blunt trauma often poses a greater threat to life because it is more difficult to diagnose than penetrating trauma. A prehospital care provider should not be as concerned with pinpointing the exact extent of abdominal trauma as with treating the clinical findings. The absence of local signs and symptoms does not rule out the possibility of abdominal trauma. A high index of suspicion based on the mechanism of injury should alert the prehospital care provider to the potential of abdominal trauma and intraabdominal hemorrhage.

Anatomy

The abdomen contains the major organs of the digestive, endocrine, and urogenital systems and major vessels of the circulatory system. The abdominal cavity is located below the diaphragm; its boundaries include the anterior abdominal wall, the pelvic bones, the vertebral column, and the muscles of the abdomen and flanks. The abdominal cavity is divided into two spaces. The retroperitoneal space (potential space behind the "true" abdominal cavity) contains the kidneys, ureters, bladder, reproductive organs, inferior vena cava, abdominal aorta, pancreas, and a portion of the duodenum, colon, and rectum (Figure 7-1). The peritoneal space (the "true" abdominal cavity) contains the large and small intestines, spleen, liver, stomach, gallbladder, and female reproductive organs (Figure 7-2).

The cephalad (toward the head) portion of the abdomen is protected in front by the ribs and in back by the vertebral column. This area contains the liver, gallbladder, spleen, stomach, and diaphragm, any of which may sustain injury as a result of a rib fracture or sternal injury. The organs most commonly injured by the same forces that fracture ribs are the liver and spleen.

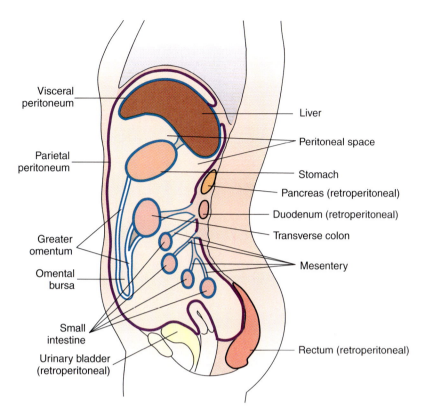

Figure 7-1 The abdomen is divided into two spaces—the peritoneal space and the retroperitoneal space. The retroperitoneal space includes the portion of the abdomen behind the peritoneum. The organs are not in contact with the peritoneal cavity. Injury to organs in this area does not necessarily produce peritonitis.

The caudad (toward the tail) portion of the abdomen is protected on all sides by the pelvis. This area contains the rectum, much of the intestine (especially when the patient is upright), the urinary bladder and ureters, and in the female, the reproductive organs. Retroperitoneal hemorrhage associated with a fractured pelvis is a major concern in this portion of the abdominal cavity. The abdomen above the pelvis and below the ribs has some soft protection by the abdominal muscles anteriorly and laterally. Posteriorly, the lumbar vertebrae provide protection with the thick, strong paraspinal and psoas muscles (Figure 7-3).

For purposes of patient assessment, the surface of the abdomen is divided into four quadrants. These quadrants are formed by drawing two lines—one in the middle from the tip of the xiphoid to the symphysis pubis and one perpendicular to this midline at the level of the umbilicus (Figure 7-4). Knowledge of anatomic landmarks is important because of the high correlation of organ location to pain response. The right upper quadrant (RUQ) includes the liver and gallbladder, the left upper quadrant (LUQ) contains the spleen and stomach, and the right lower quadrant (RLQ) and left lower quadrant (LLQ) contain primarily the intestines. A portion of the intestinal tract exists in all four quadrants. The urinary bladder is midline between the lower quadrants.

Increased intraabdominal pressure produced by compression, such as being forced against a steering column, can rupture the abdominal cavity upward through the diaphragm, much like the compression of a paper bag (see Chapters 2 and 5). Rupture to the left of the diaphragm is the injury most likely to produce problems in the early care (prehospital phase) of a patient. The intraabdominal contents forced into the chest cavity can compromise lung expansion (Figure 7-5).

Dividing the abdominal organs into hollow, solid, and vascular groups helps provide a basic physiologic understanding of them. When injured, solid and vascular organs (liver, spleen, aorta, vena cava) bleed, whereas hollow ones (intestine, gallbladder, urinary bladder) primarily spill their contents into the peritoneal cavity or retroperitoneal space. This spilling results in peritonitis (inflammation of the peritoneum or the lining of the abdominal cavity), sepsis (massive infection), and intraabdominal bleeding. Prehospital treatment involves the rapid initiation of shock management and control of hemorrhage.

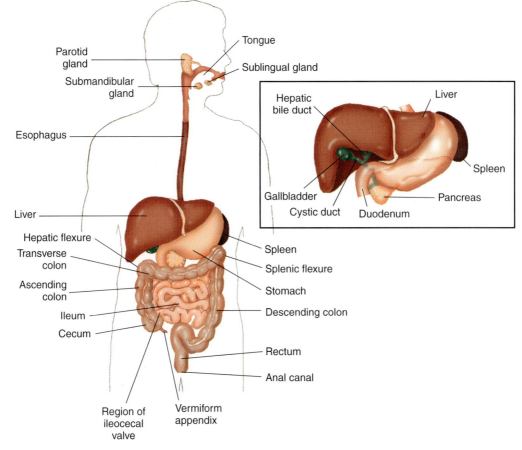

Parotid gland
Tongue
Submandibular gland
Sublingual gland
Esophagus
Hepatic bile duct
Liver
Liver
Spleen
Hepatic flexure
Spleen
Transverse colon
Splenic flexure
Gallbladder
Pancreas
Ascending colon
Stomach
Cystic duct
Duodenum
Ileum
Descending colon
Cecum
Rectum
Anal canal
Region of ileocecal valve
Vermiform appendix

Figure 7-2   The organs inside the peritoneal cavity frequently produce peritonitis when injured. Organs in the peritoneal cavity include solid organs (spleen and liver), hollow organs of the gastrointestinal tract (stomach, small intestine, and colon), and the reproductive organs.

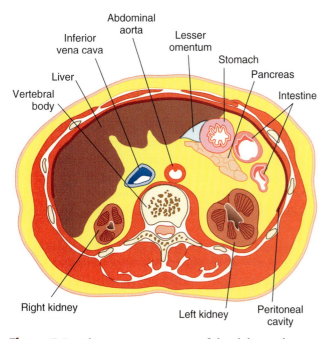

Abdominal aorta
Inferior vena cava
Lesser omentum
Stomach
Liver
Pancreas
Vertebral body
Intestine
Right kidney
Left kidney
Peritoneal cavity

Figure 7-3   This transverse section of the abdominal cavity gives an appreciation of the organs' positions in the antero-posterior direction.

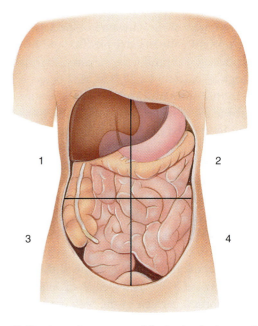

1 2 3 4

Figure 7-4   As with any part of the body, the better the description of pain, tenderness, guarding, etc., the more accurate the diagnosis. The most common system of identification divides the abdomen into four quadrants—left upper, right upper, left lower, and right lower.

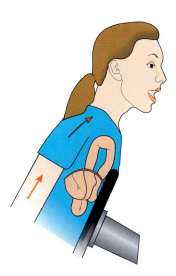

Figure 7-5   With increased pressure inside the abdomen, the diaphragm can rupture.

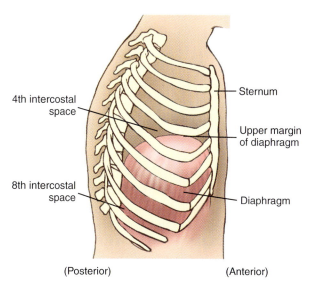

Figure 7-6   Lateral view of diaphragm position.

Pathophysiology

Injuries to the abdomen can be caused by either penetrating or blunt trauma. Penetrating trauma, such as a gunshot or stab wound, is more readily visible than blunt trauma. Multiple organ damage can occur in penetrating trauma, although it is less likely with a stab wound than with a gunshot wound. A mental visualization of the trajectory of a missile, such as a bullet or the path of a knife blade, can help identify possible injured organs.

The diaphragm extends cephalad to the fourth intercostal space anteriorly, the sixth intercostal space laterally, and the eighth intercostal space posteriorly during maximum expiration (Figure 7-6). Patients with penetrating injury to the thorax below this line may also have an abdominal injury. Penetrating wounds of the flanks and buttocks may involve organs in the abdominal cavity as well. These penetrating injuries may cause bleeding from a major vessel or solid organ and perforation of a segment of the intestine, the most frequently injured organ in penetrating trauma.

Blunt injuries to intraabdominal organs are generally the result of compression or shear forces. In compression incidents, the organs of the abdomen are crushed between solid objects, such as between the steering wheel and spinal column. Shear forces create rupture of the solid organs or rupture of blood vessels in the cavity because of the tearing forces exerted against their stabilizing ligaments and vessels. The liver and spleen can shear and bleed easily, and blood loss can occur at a rapid rate. Pelvic fractures may be associated with the loss of large volumes of blood caused by the tearing of major vessels that lie adjacent to the pelvis. Urinary bladder and urethral injuries are also a complication of pelvic fractures.

The peritoneum is sensitive to being stretched. This stretching can be caused by inflammation or distention from bleeding after trauma. In later stages of pregnancy, this irritation may go undetected because of the gradual stretching that has already taken place.

Loss of blood into the abdominal cavity, regardless of its source, can contribute to or be the primary cause of the development of shock. The release of acids, enzymes, or bacteria from the gastrointestinal tract into the peritoneal cavity will result in additional organ damage and peritonitis.

Assessment

The index of suspicion for injury should be based on the mechanism of injury and physical findings, such as ecchymosis or marks of collision. Intraabdominal bleeding should be suspected when the patient has external bruising or distention. Although these signs and symptoms indicate intraabdominal bleeding, patients with substantial intraabdominal hemorrhage often do not display them. The prehospital care provider should be alert for more subtle signs such as anxiety, agitation, and dyspnea.

The most reliable indicator of intraabdominal bleeding is the presence of shock from an unexplained source. This is why recognition of early signs is imperative. Response to the physical examination of the abdomen in the conscious patient may or may not be reliable. Pelvic or lower rib fractures can produce pain that will not necessarily be associated with intraabdominal injury. Alcohol or drugs may mask symptoms. Pediatric patients are often more unreliable, and geriatric patients may have an impaired pain response. If the patient has distracting pain from injuries, such as extremity or spinal fractures, abdominal pain may not be elicited upon palpation. Also, fresh blood in the abdomen is not an irritant to the peritoneum and, in most cases, will not cause any signs of peritonitis. The adult abdominal cavity can hold up to 1.5 liters of fluid before showing any signs of distention. Therefore a patient's physical examination can be normal, yet significant amounts of blood may be present in the abdomen. An unconscious patient or a patient who has sustained traumatic brain injury may be unable to provide any appropriate verbal response. Therefore immediate impressions from a variety of other sources of information, including kinematics, bystanders' input, and/or physical evidence, should be considered. With all of this in mind, the assessment of abdominal injury can be difficult. The following are reliable indicators for establishing the index of suspicion for abdominal injury:

- Mechanism of injury or damage to the passenger compartment (bent steering wheel)
- Outward signs of trauma
- Shock with unexplained cause
- Level of shock greater than explained by other injuries
- Presence of abdominal rigidity, guarding, or distension (a rare finding)

The assessment of a patient with suspected abdominal trauma should always include the following:

- *Inspection.* The abdomen should be exposed and observed for distension, contusions, abrasions, penetration, evisceration, impaled objects, and/or obvious bleeding. These signs can all indicate underlying injury.
- *Palpation.* Palpation of the abdomen can reveal abdominal wall defects or elicit pain in the area palpated. Voluntary or involuntary guarding, rigidity, and/or rebound tenderness may indicate bruising, inflammation, or hemorrhage. However, deep palpation of an obviously injured abdomen should be avoided because palpation can increase an existing

hemorrhage and worsen other injuries. Pelvic instability is assessed by gently applying pressure to the pelvic girdle.

Auscultation of bowel sounds is not a helpful prehospital assessment tool. Time should not be wasted trying to determine their presence or absence because this diagnostic sign will not alter the prehospital treatment of the patient.

All of these assessment tools are necessary to determine the existence of a potentially life-threatening injury.

Management

The management of abdominal trauma is simply to treat what is identified during assessment and is the same regardless of the specific organ injured. Management of a patient with abdominal injury should include the following:

1. Rapidly evaluate the scene and the patient. After ensuring scene safety, attend to any threats to life identified in the primary survey.
2. Initiate treatment for shock, including high-concentration oxygen administration.
3. Apply a pneumatic antishock garment (PASG) to reduce suspected intraperitoneal or retroperitoneal hemorrhage in patients with decompensated shock and, if indicated, to counter profound shock. The major benefit of PASG application to the injured patient is the reduction of intraabdominal hemorrhage. Evidence suggests that PASG application may be effective for controlling hemorrhage associated with pelvic fractures in patients with decompensated shock. Follow local PASG protocols and consult medical control. (See Chapter 6.)
4. Rapidly package and transport the patient to the nearest appropriate facility.
5. Initiate crystalloid intravenous fluid replacement en route to the receiving facility.

Surgical intervention remains a key need; time should not be wasted in attempts to determine the exact details of injury. In many instances, identification of specific organ injury will not be revealed until the abdomen is surgically explored.

Transporting a patient with intraabdominal injuries to a facility that does not have an operating room and a surgical team immediately available defeats the purpose of rapid transportation. The receiving facility should be chosen for its ability to provide rapid surgical management.

In addition to the general management of all abdominal injuries, unique situations will require special consideration. The following is a discussion of the management of three unique circumstances—impaled objects, evisceration, and pregnancy.

Impaled Objects

Because removal of an impaled object may cause severe additional trauma and because the object's distal end may be controlling bleeding, removal of an impaled object in the prehospital environment is contraindicated (Figure 7-7). The prehospital care provider should neither move nor remove an object impaled in a patient's abdomen. In the hospital these objects are not removed until their shape and location have been identified by radiograph evaluation and until blood replacement and a surgical team are present and ready. A prehospital care provider should stabilize the impaled object and immobilize it, either manually or mechanically, to prevent its further movement in the field and during transport. If bleeding occurs around it, direct pressure should be applied around the object to the wound with the flat of the hand. Psychological support of the patient is crucial, especially if the impaled object is visible to the patient.

The abdomen should not be palpated in these cases because palpation may produce additional tearing or intrusion by the distal end of the object. Further examination is unnecessary because the presence of impaled objects indicates the need for surgical exploration.

Evisceration

In an abdominal evisceration, a section of intestine or other abdominal organ is displaced through an open wound and protrudes externally outside the abdominal cavity (Figure 7-8). The tissue most often visualized is the fatty ommentum that lies over the intestines. Protecting the protruding section of intestine or other organ from further damage presents a special problem. Attempts should not be made to replace the protruding tissue back into the abdominal cavity. The viscera should be left on the surface of the abdomen or protruding as found. Most of the abdominal contents require a moist environment. If the intestine or some of the other abdominal organs become dry, cell death will occur. Therefore the eviscerated abdominal contents should be covered with sterile pads that are moistened with sterile saline (normal saline intravenous fluid can be used). These dressings should be periodically remoistened with sterile saline to prevent them from drying out. Wet dressing may be covered with a large dry dressing to keep the patient warm.

Pregnancy

Pregnancy causes both anatomic and physiologic changes to the body's systems. These changes affect the potential patterns of injuries and can make the assessment of a patient especially challenging. The prehospital care provider is dealing with two or more patients and must be alert to changes that have occurred throughout the pregnancy.

The uterus continues to enlarge through the thirty-eighth week of pregnancy. This anatomic change makes the uterus and its contents more susceptible to injury,

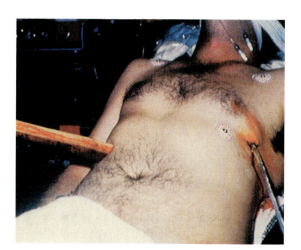

Figure 7-7 A shaft of wood entered the right side of the abdomen, pierced the diaphragm, and tore the spleen, stomach, and liver. This patient made a good recovery. (*From London PS: A colour atlas of diagnosis after recent injury, London, 1990, Wolfe.*)

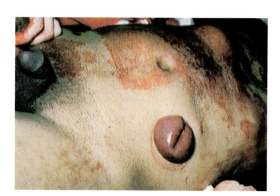

Figure 7-8 Abdominal evisceration. (*From McSwain NE Jr, Paturas JL: The basic EMT: comprehensive prehospital patient care, ed 2, St Louis, 2001, Mosby.*)

including rupture, penetration, abruptio placentae (when a portion of the placenta is pulled away from the uterine wall), and premature rupture of the membranes. The placenta and gravid uterus are highly vascular, which can result in profound hemorrhage. The hemorrhage can also be concealed inside the uterus.

The mother's heart rate increases throughout pregnancy, rising between 15 to 20 beats/min above normal by the third trimester. This makes the interpretation of tachycardia more difficult. Systolic and diastolic blood pressures drop 5 to 15 mm Hg during the second trimester but are often normal at term. Some women may have significant hypotension when supine. This condition, supine hypotension, is caused by the compression of the vena cava by the uterus and is usually relieved by placing the woman on her left side (left lateral decubitus position). If spinal immobilization is indicated, 4 to 6 inches of padding should be placed under the right side of the longboard. With the patient in this position, gravity helps to pull the uterus off of the vena cava, therefore restoring venous return to the heart. If the patient cannot be rotated, the patient's right leg should be elevated to displace the uterus to the left. These maneuvers reduce compression of the vena cava, increase venous return to the heart, and therefore increase cardiac output.

After the tenth week of pregnancy, cardiac output is increased by 1 to 1.5 L/min. The patient has a 48% increase in blood volume by term. *Because of this significant increase, 30% to 35% of the blood volume can be lost before signs and symptoms of hypovolemia become apparent.*

Although a marked protuberance of the abdomen is obvious in late pregnancy, abdominal organs remain essentially unchanged, with the exception of the uterus. Intestine that is displaced superiorly is shielded by the uterus in the last two trimesters of pregnancy. The increased size of the uterus, as well as its high blood flow, make it susceptible to both blunt and penetrating injury (Figure 7-9). The increased size and weight of the uterus alter the patient's center of gravity and increase the risk of falls. The gravid abdomen is often injured in a fall.

During the third trimester, the diaphragm is elevated and may cause mild dyspnea, especially when the patient is supine. Eclampsia, which is a late complication of pregnancy, may mimic a brain injury. A careful neurologic assessment and the discovery of any pertinent medical history are important.

Peristalsis (the propulsive, muscular movements of the intestines) is slow during pregnancy, so food may remain in the stomach many hours after eating. Therefore the pregnant patient may be at greater risk for vomiting and subsequent aspiration. As with the nonpregnant patient, auscultation of the abdomen to assess for bowel sounds is nonproductive. Searching for fetal heart tones at the scene is also nonproductive because their presence will not alter prehospital care. Rapid transport to an appropriate facility is the correct management.

Blood loss from abdominal injury can be indicated from minimal signs and symptoms up to signs of severe shock. The presence of significant amounts of blood in the peritoneal cavity usually causes pain by stretching the peritoneum. The peritoneum of the pregnant patient's abdomen is already stretching; therefore the patient may perceive less pain. The condition of the fetus often depends on the condition of the mother. However, the fetus may be in jeopardy while the mother's condition and vital signs appear stable. The goals of shock management are essentially the same as for any patient and include increased attention to providing a high concentration of oxygen to meet the needs of both the mother and the fetus.

Vigorous fluid replacement should start during transport to help combat shock in the mother and fe-

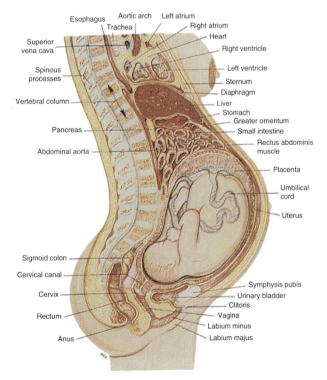

Figure 7-9 In the pregnant patient, as the uterus and fetus enlarge above the symphysis pubis, the fetus becomes more susceptible to both blunt and penetrating trauma.

tus. Any evidence of vaginal bleeding or a rigid board-like abdomen with external bleeding in the last trimester of pregnancy indicates possible abruptio placentae or a ruptured uterus. Exsanguination may occur rapidly.

Transport of the pregnant trauma patient should not be delayed. Every pregnant trauma patient should be rapidly transported—even those who appear to have only minor injuries—to the closest appropriate facility (ideally one with perinatal resources). A physician should evaluate any trauma to the abdomen of a pregnant patient. Adequate resuscitation of the mother is the key to survival of the mother and fetus.

Summary

The potential threat to life from intraabdominal injuries is extremely high. No other area of the body is more susceptible to major hemorrhage without apparent physical evidence of injury. A patient with an abdominal injury can deteriorate rapidly and without warning. Maintaining a high index of suspicion for abdominal injury is therefore crucial.

The extent of specific abdominal organ injury is seldom identifiable in the prehospital setting. Management of the patient with abdominal trauma includes rapid evaluation and preparation for transport, oxygenation, hemorrhage control, and support of circulation. A PASG is useful in the management of shock caused by abdominal and pelvic trauma as long as no contraindications to its use exist. The prehospital care provider can only achieve definitive care of the patient with abdominal trauma by transporting the patient to a facility with the ability to perform rapid surgical intervention.

Although the priorities for treatment are the same, some instances of abdominal trauma require special considerations. The anatomic and physiologic changes of pregnancy have implications for the pattern of injury, presentation of signs and symptoms of trauma, and management of the trauma patient. Management of potential fetal compromise caused by trauma in the prehospital setting is accomplished only through effective management of maternal perfusion. The patient with an abdominal impalement or evisceration also requires special handling to prevent further injury and complications. The key to optimal care of the patient with abdominal trauma is to maintain a high index of suspicion based on the mechanism of injury and shock in the absence of an obvious cause.

Scenario Solution

The patient's vital signs may be accounted for by the physiologic changes of pregnancy or may be subtle indications of shock, but combined with the known mechanism of injury and the other assessment findings, you will maintain a high index of suspicion for internal hemorrhage. The patient's scalp laceration and disorientation to the event warrant spinal immobilization, which you must modify to prevent compression of the vena cava. Because fetal oxygenation depends on maternal cardiorespiratory function, the administration of oxygen and circulatory support of the mother are the best treatment of the fetus. Additional information about the exact mechanisms of injury and information about the patient's obstetric history are pertinent to the patient's care. Because of the potential for placental abruption, transport to a trauma center with perinatal resources is ideal.

Review Questions

Answers are provided on p. 414.

1. Your patient is a 77-year-old woman who was the unrestrained driver of a vehicle that left the street and struck a utility pole head-on. The patient is awake but confused and unable to give a specific complaint. The patient has a heart rate of 72 beats/min with an irregular rhythm, a blood pressure of 82/42 mm Hg, and a ventilatory rate of 28 breaths/min. Of the various possibilities that could account for the situation and the patient's presentation, which of the following is the priority for patient care decisions?
   a. Underlying cardiac disease
   b. Abdominal hemorrhage
   c. Medication side effects
   d. Stroke

2. Which of the following injuries should create the suspicion of abdominal organ injury?
   a. Stab wound just below the right nipple
   b. Gunshot wound to the left buttock
   c. Lap belt contusion
   d. All of the above

3. Of the following, which is of highest priority in the prehospital care of the patient with a suspected abdominal injury?
   a. Crystalloid fluids en route to the receiving facility
   b. Auscultation of bowel sounds
   c. Determination of the specific organs involved
   d. Checking for peritoneal signs

4. Which of the following is NOT true regarding trauma in pregnancy?
   a. The patient is at greater risk of the aspiration of gastric contents
   b. The interpretation of vital signs is confounded by the physiologic changes of pregnancy
   c. Manual displacement of the uterus to the left in the supine patient is helpful in hypotension
   d. The priorities of care depend on the fetal heart rate

5. Which of the following is the most reliable indicator of abdominal organ injury?
   a. Otherwise unexplained hypotension
   b. Guarding on palpation of the abdomen
   c. Vomiting
   d. Absence of bowel sounds

REFERENCES

American College of Surgeons: *Abdominal trauma: advanced trauma life support*, Chicago, 2002, Author.

Berry MJ, McMurry RG, Katz VL: Pulmonary and ventilatory responses to pregnancy, immersion and exercise, *J Appl Physiol* 66(2):857, 1989.

Esposito TJ: Trauma during pregnancy, *Emerg Med Clin North Am* 12:167, 1994.

Frame SB, Timberlake GA, Rosh DS et al: Penetrating injuries of the abdominal aorta, *Am Surg* 56(10):651, 1990.

Hill DA, Delaney LM, Duflou J: A population-based study of outcome after injury to car occupants and to pedestrians, *J Trauma* 40(3):351, 1996.

Pearlman MD, Tintinalli JE, Lorenz RP: Blunt trauma during pregnancy, *N Engl J Med* 323:1606, 1991.

Schoenfeld A, Ziv E, Stein L et al: Seat belts in pregnancy and the obstetrician, *Obstet Gynecol Surv* 42(5): 275, 1987.

Timberlake GA, McSwain NE Jr: Trauma in pregnancy: a 10-year perspective, *Am Surg* 55(3):151, 1989.

Tso EL, Beaver BL, Haller JA Jr: Abdominal injuries in restrained pediatric passengers, *J Pediatr Surg* 28(7):915, 1993.

Chapter 8

Head Trauma

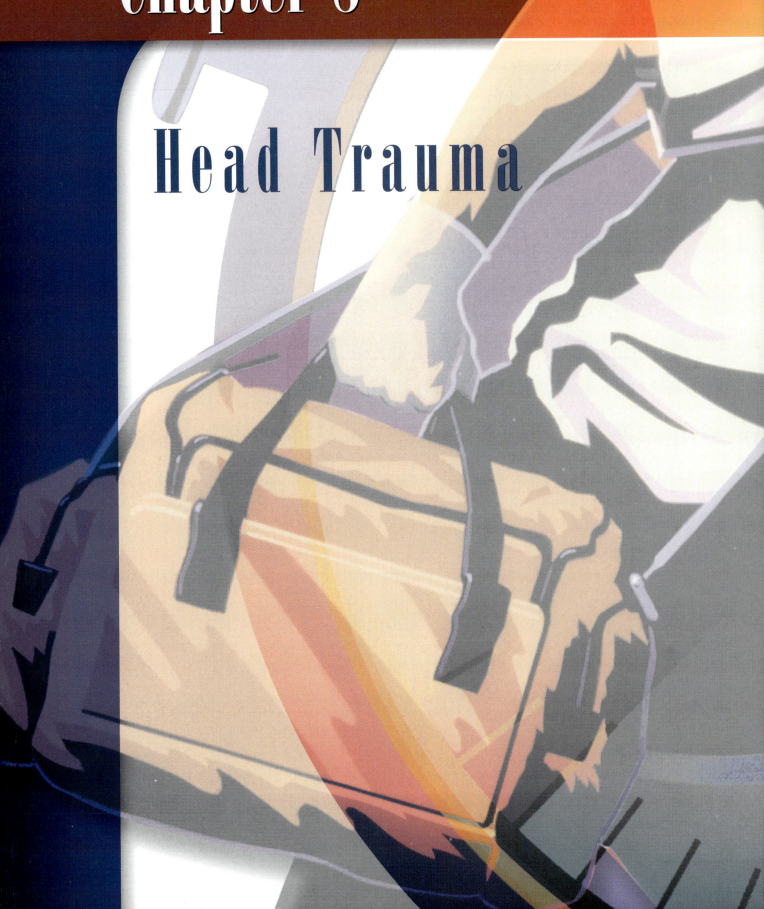

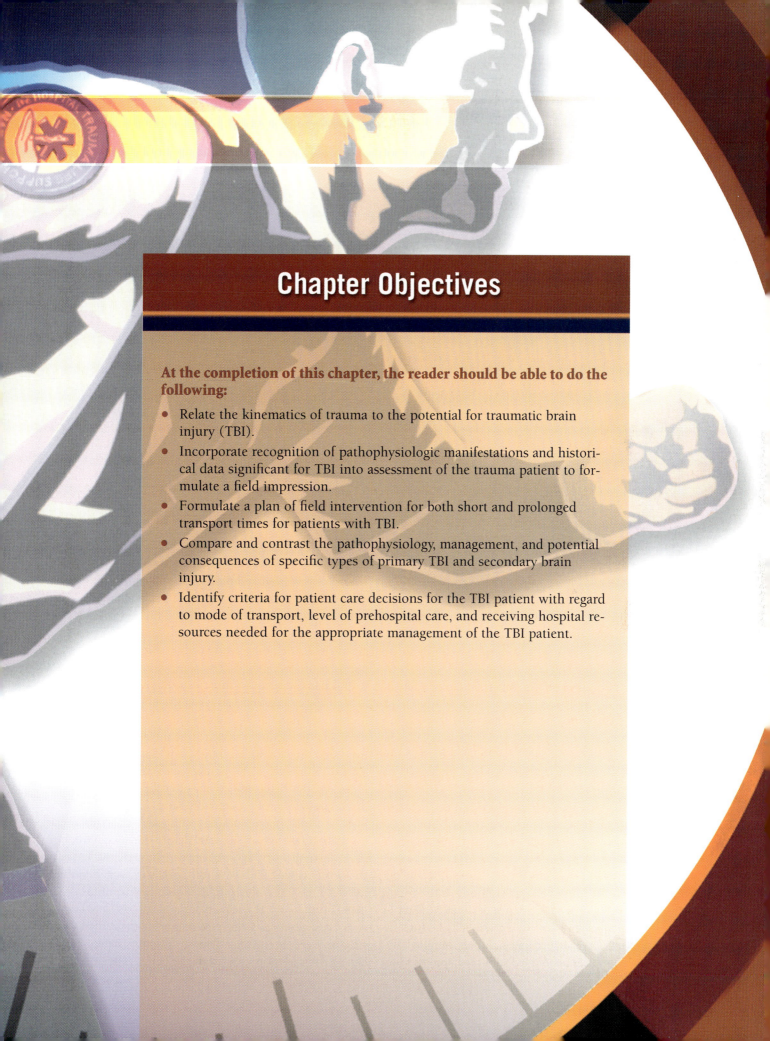

Chapter Objectives

At the completion of this chapter, the reader should be able to do the following:

- Relate the kinematics of trauma to the potential for traumatic brain injury (TBI).
- Incorporate recognition of pathophysiologic manifestations and historical data significant for TBI into assessment of the trauma patient to formulate a field impression.
- Formulate a plan of field intervention for both short and prolonged transport times for patients with TBI.
- Compare and contrast the pathophysiology, management, and potential consequences of specific types of primary TBI and secondary brain injury.
- Identify criteria for patient care decisions for the TBI patient with regard to mode of transport, level of prehospital care, and receiving hospital resources needed for the appropriate management of the TBI patient.

Scenario

You and your partner are dispatched to a construction site where a 30-year-old male ironworker lost his balance and fell about 25 feet (8 m) to a concrete floor. Bystanders state that he was unconscious for about 10 minutes but has now awakened. The scene is safe. The primary survey reveals that the patient is maintaining his airway and breathing normally. An 8 cm laceration on the right side of his scalp is bleeding copiously but is readily controlled with direct pressure and a pressure dressing. His pulse rate is 116 beats/min and his skin is warm, pink, and well perfused. He opens his eyes spontaneously and follows commands; however, he does not recall the events leading up to his fall. He exhibits some confusion as he attempts to answer questions (GCS 14). You apply oxygen via a nonrebreather mask. During spinal immobilization, he speaks incomprehensible words and now only opens his eyes and withdraws his extremities to painful stimuli (GCS 9).

How should you alter your care based on the decrease in the patient's level of consciousness? What injury is most likely present given the patient's presenting signs? What are your management priorities at this point? What actions may you need to take to combat increased intracranial pressure and maintain cerebral perfusion during a prolonged transport?

Approximately 1.6 million emergency department visits for head injury occur each year. About 500,000 of these sustain traumatic brain injury (TBI). While 80% of these patients are categorized as having only mild injuries, about 50,000 patients with TBI are pronounced dead upon arrival in the emergency department. TBI contributes significantly to the death of about half of all trauma victims. Moderate to severe brain injuries are identified in about 100,000 trauma patients annually. Mortality rates for moderate and severe brain injuries are about 10% and 30%, respectively. Of those who survive moderate and severe brain injuries, between 50% and 99% have some degree of permanent neurologic disability.

Motor vehicle crashes (MVCs) remain the leading cause of TBI in those under 65 years of age, and falls are the leading cause of TBI in the elderly. The head is the most frequently injured part of the body in patients with multisystem injuries. The incidence of gunshot wounds to the brain has increased in recent years in urban areas, and up to 60% of these victims die from their injury.

Patients with TBI represent some of the most challenging trauma patients to treat. They may be combative, and attempts to intubate can be extremely difficult because of clenched jaw muscles and vomiting. Intoxication with drugs or alcohol or the presence of shock from other injuries can hamper assessment. Occasionally, serious intracranial injuries can be present with only minimal evidence of external trauma. Skilled care in the prehospital setting, focused on maintaining vital functions, can decrease the mortality rate from TBI and may also translate into a decrease in permanent neurologic disability.

Anatomy

Knowledge of head and brain anatomy is essential to understand the pathophysiology of TBIs. The scalp is the outermost covering of the head and offers some protection to the skull and brain. The scalp is composed of several layers, including skin, connective tissue, and the periosteum of the skull. The aging process and balding may cause the scalp to thin, resulting in decreased protection. The scalp and soft tissues overlying the face are highly vascular, and seemingly minor wounds can produce significant hemorrhage. Uncontrolled hemorrhage from a complex scalp laceration can lead to hypovolemic shock. Although scalp injuries may result in copious bleeding, the hemorrhage can often be controlled with direct pressure or a pressure dressing.

The skull or cranium is composed of a number of bones that fuse into a single structure during childhood. Several small openings (foramina) through the base of the skull provide pathways for blood vessels and cranial nerves. One large opening, the foramen magnum, is located on the posterior aspect of the skull base and serves as a passageway for the brain stem to the spinal cord (Figure 8-1). In infancy, two "soft spots" (fontanelles) can often be identified between the bones. The infant has

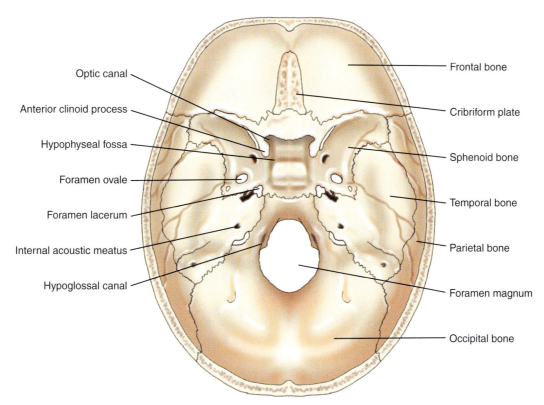

Figure 8-1   Internal view of the base of the skull.

Optic canal
Anterior clinoid process
Hypophyseal fossa
Foramen ovale
Foramen lacerum
Internal acoustic meatus
Hypoglossal canal

Frontal bone
Cribriform plate
Sphenoid bone
Temporal bone
Parietal bone
Foramen magnum
Occipital bone

no bony protection over these portions of the brain until the bones fuse, typically by 2 years of age.

Although most of the bones forming the cranium are thick and strong, the skull is especially thin in the temporal and ethmoid regions, which are more prone to fracture. The cranium provides significant protection to the brain, but the interior surface of the skull base is rough and irregular. When exposed to a blunt force, the brain may slide across these irregularities, producing cerebral contusions or lacerations.

Three separate membranes, the meninges, cover the brain (Figure 8-2). The outermost layer, the dura mater, is composed of tough fibrous tissue and lines the cranial vault (the skull or cranium). The middle meningeal arteries are located between the lateral cranium (temporal bones) and the dura mater in the epidural space. Normally the dura mater closely adheres to the inner surface of the cranial vault; however, a blow to this area of thin bone may produce a skull fracture that damages the artery, allowing blood to collect in this potential space. This injury is known as an *epidural hematoma.*

The pia mater is a thin layer that closely adheres to the cortex of the brain. Between the dura mater and pia mater lies the arachnoid membrane, which has the appearance of a spider web. Below this middle layer of the meninges is the subarachnoid space, which is filled with cerebrospinal fluid (CSF). CSF, produced in the ventricular system of the brain, surrounds the brain and spinal cord and is believed to help cushion the brain. Blunt trauma to the head that damages some of the veins between the brain and sagittal sinuses can lead to a subdural hematoma (a collection of blood between the dura mater and the arachnoid) or a subarachnoid hemorrhage (bleeding into the CSF-filled space).

The brain occupies about 80% of the cranial vault and is divided into three main regions—the cerebrum, the cerebellum, and the brain stem. The cerebrum consists of two hemispheres—the right and left—that can be subdivided into several lobes. The cerebrum houses sensory functions, motor functions, and higher intellectual functions such as intelligence and memory. The cerebellum is located in the posterior fossa of the cranium, between the brainstem and the cerebrum, and coordinates movement (Box 8-1).

The brainstem contains the medulla, an area that controls many vital functions, including breathing and heart rate. Much of the reticular activating system (RAS), the portion of the brain responsible for consciousness, is also found in the brainstem. Blunt trauma can impair the RAS, leading to a transient loss of consciousness. This occurs in a patient who sustains a concussion. The tentorium cerebelli, a portion of the dura mater, lies between

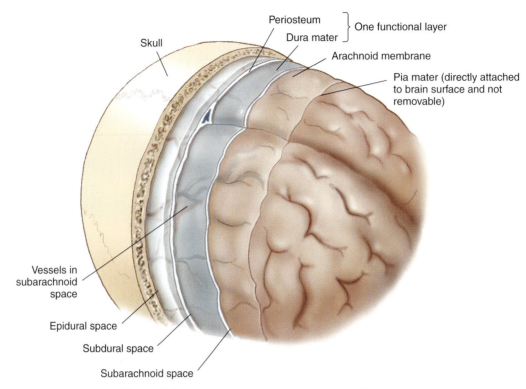

Figure 8-2 Meninges. Meningeal coverings of the brain.

the cerebrum and the cerebellum and contains an opening, the tentorial incisura, at the level of the midbrain.

The twelve cranial nerves originate from the brain and brainstem (Figure 8-3). The oculomotor nerve, cranial nerve III, controls pupillary constriction and provides an important tool in the assessment of a patient with a suspected brain injury.

Physiology

The brain has the ability to autoregulate the amount of blood flow it receives when physiologic stresses are encountered. Cerebral blood flow (CBF) remains remarkably constant with modest alterations in blood pressure; however, it begins to decrease when the mean arterial pressure (MAP) falls below 60 mm Hg. MAP can be calculated as follows:

MAP = Diastolic pressure + 1/3 Pulse pressure

The pulse pressure is calculated as the difference between the systolic pressure and the diastolic pressure. For example, the MAP of a patient with a blood pressure of 120/80 mm Hg can be calculated as follows:

MAP = 80 + 1/3 (120 − 80)
MAP = 93 mm Hg

Another important physiologic parameter is the cerebral perfusion pressure (CPP), which is the difference between the MAP and the intracranial pressure (ICP):

CPP = MAP − ICP

Normal MAP ranges from about 85 to 95 mm Hg, and ICP is normally below 20 mm Hg. Therefore CPP is normally about 70 to 80 mm Hg.

The partial pressure of carbon dioxide in arterial blood (Pa_{CO_2}) also affects CBF. An elevation of Pa_{CO_2} beyond the normal range of 35 to 45 mm Hg leads to dilation of cerebral arterioles (increasing CBF), whereas a decrease in the Pa_{CO_2} produces cerebral vasoconstriction (decreasing CBF).

Pathophysiology

TBI can be divided into two categories:

1. *Primary brain injury* (direct trauma to the brain and associated vascular injuries) represents the nerve cells (neurons) that sustain severe damage as a direct result of the initial insult, regardless of the mechanism of injury. If damaged extensively, these neurons may die. Neurons are believed to be incapable of regeneration. Depending on the location,

Box 8-1

The Brain

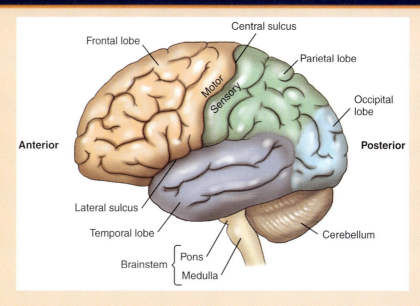

Frontal lobe
Central sulcus
Parietal lobe
Motor
Sensory
Occipital lobe
Anterior
Posterior
Lateral sulcus
Temporal lobe
Brainstem { Pons / Medulla
Cerebellum

CEREBRUM

The cerebrum is composed of the right and left cerebral hemispheres. The dominant hemisphere is the one that contains the language center. This is the left hemisphere in virtually all right-handed individuals and about 85% of left-handed individuals. The cerebrum is composed of several lobes:

- *Frontal.* Contains emotions, motor function, and expression of speech on the dominant side
- *Parietal.* Contains sensory function and spatial orientation
- *Temporal.* Regulates certain memory functions; contains the area for speech reception and integration in all right-handed and the majority of left-handed individuals
- *Occipital.* Contains vision

BRAINSTEM

- *Midbrain and upper pons.* Contain the reticular activating system, which is responsible for consciousness
- *Medulla.* Contains the cardiorespiratory centers

CEREBELLUM

Controls coordination and balance

---

function, and number of the damaged neurons, permanent neurologic damage may result if the patient survives.

2. *Secondary brain injury* refers to an extension of the magnitude of the primary brain injury by factors that result in a larger, more permanent neurologic deficit. Rapid identification and management of these conditions serve to minimize the extent of neurologic impairment. Causes of secondary brain injury can be further separated into systemic and intracranial insults.
   a. Systemic factors that may lead to secondary brain injury can often be identified and treated in the prehospital setting. These include hypoxia, hypercapnia, hypocapnia, anemia, hypotension, hyperglycemia, and hypoglycemia.
   b. With the exception of seizures, intracranial causes of secondary brain injury can only be suspected and cannot be identified in the field. Examples of intracranial insults that are diagnosed in the hospital are cerebral edema and intracranial hematomas, both of which may cause increased ICP (termed *intracranial hypertension*).

Systemic Causes

HYPOXIA, HYPOCAPNIA, AND HYPERCAPNIA

In a multisystem trauma patient, hypoxia can result from several causes, including airway obstruction, aspiration of blood or gastric contents, pulmonary contusions, and pneumothoraces. Unlike skeletal muscle that can func-

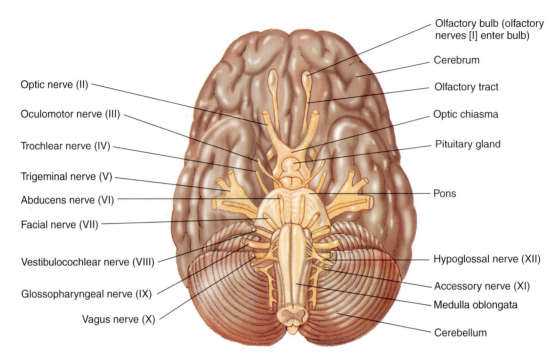

Figure 8-3   Inferior surface of the brain showing the origins of the cranial nerves.

tion in an anaerobic environment, the neurons of the central nervous system depend on a constant supply of oxygen. Confusion is often the earliest warning signal that cerebral oxygen delivery is impaired.

Ischemic brain tissue may subsequently die if even brief periods of hypoxia complicate the primary injury. Irreversible brain damage ("brain death") can occur with only 4 to 6 minutes of cerebral anoxia.

Both hypocapnia (decreased $PaCO_2$) and hypercapnia (increased $PaCO_2$) can worsen brain injury. When cerebral blood vessels constrict, as results from significant hypocapnia, CBF is compromised, leading to a decrease in oxygen delivery to the brain. Hypercapnia can result from hypoventilation from drug or alcohol intoxication or one of many abnormal ventilation patterns seen in patients with increased ICP. Hypercapnia causes cerebral vasodilation that can further increase ICP.

ANEMIA AND HYPOTENSION

Patients with severe brain injury may sustain external and internal hemorrhage from accompanying injuries. If significant blood loss occurs, the resultant anemia can dramatically impair systemic oxygen delivery and may irreversibly damage ischemic brain tissue.

After significant head trauma, the brain often loses its ability to autoregulate its CBF and it often falls to about 50% of normal within a few hours. As noted previously, the two determinants of cerebral perfusion are MAP and ICP. A fall in the MAP, as occurs in hypo-

volemic shock, can result in decreased cerebral oxygen delivery, even when ICP is normal. Hypotension may be a direct result of severe brain injury and almost always occurs shortly before death. Thus when hypotension is identified in a patient with a severe TBI, etiologies other than the brain injury, including significant internal or external hemorrhage and neurogenic shock, should be considered.

HYPOGLYCEMIA AND HYPERGLYCEMIA

Both elevations (hyperglycemia) and decreases (hypoglycemia) in blood sugar can jeopardize ischemic brain tissue. Neurons are unable to store sugar and require a continual supply of glucose to carry out cellular metabolism. In the absence of glucose, ischemic neurons can be permanently damaged. Elevated blood glucose levels in patients with TBI have also been associated with poor neurologic outcome.

Intracranial Causes

SEIZURES

A patient with acute TBI is at risk for seizures for several reasons. Hypoxia from either airway or breathing problems can induce generalized seizure activity, as can hypoglycemia and electrolyte abnormalities. Ischemic or damaged brain tissue can serve as an irritable focus to produce grand mal seizures or status epilepticus. Seizures, in turn, can aggravate preexisting hypoxia caused by impairment

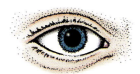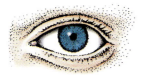

Figure 8-4 Suspect injury to the brain whenever a patient's pupils are unequal in size.

of respiratory function. Additionally, the massive neuronal activity associated with generalized seizures rapidly depletes oxygen and glucose levels, further worsening cerebral ischemia.

CEREBRAL EDEMA AND INTRACRANIAL HEMATOMAS

Cerebral edema (brain swelling) often occurs at the site of a primary brain injury. Intracellular fluid can collect within damaged neurons, and the injury can lead to the release of inflammatory substances that allow fluid to leak though capillary walls, increasing the interstitial fluid in the brain tissue. As cerebral edema develops, a dangerous cycle may be established in which the swelling further impairs oxygen delivery and compromises surrounding ischemic tissue, resulting in more edema.

Intracranial hematomas, described in detail later, are potentially life-threatening because they occupy precious space within the skull. The surrounding brain tissue can be compressed, aggravating cerebral ischemia or leading to herniation. Both cerebral edema and intracranial hematomas can result in dangerous rises in ICP.

In addition to alterations in consciousness, these problems may produce changes in pupillary function. Cerebral edema or an intracranial hematoma may force a portion of the temporal lobe (the uncus) of the cerebrum though the tentorium cerebelli in a process called *uncal herniation*. A dilated, slowly reactive ("sluggish") pupil typically indicates compression on the third cranial nerve as it crosses the tentorial incisura, wheras a dilated, nonreactive ("blown") pupil suggests uncal herniation on the same side as the abnormal pupil (Figure 8-4).

Once the fontanelles have closed, the cranial vault, in the absence of skull fractures, is essentially a rigid box with the only significant opening at its base. Thus both cerebral edema and an intracranial hematoma can compress the brainstem inferiorly through the foramen magnum in a process known as *central herniation*. Like uncal herniation, this unfortunate occurrence results in brain death (Figure 8-5).

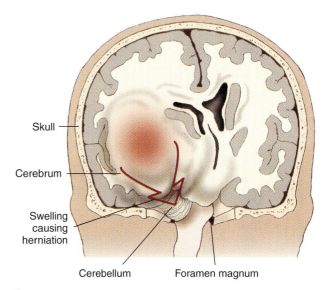

Figure 8-5 The skull is a large bony structure that contains the brain. The brain cannot escape the skull if it expands because of edema or if there is hemorrhage in the skull that presses on the brain.

Intracranial Hypertension

Increased ICP (intracranial hypertension) significantly impairs cerebral perfusion. The Monro-Kellie doctrine states that the skull, essentially a rigid box with its only large opening at the foramen magnum, contains only three elements—the brain, CSF, and blood (Figure 8-6). As the volume of one of these components increases, as occurs with brain swelling, the volume of the other two must decrease because of the fixed volume of the skull. CBF falls, and CSF is forced from the cranium down along the spinal cord. The resultant hypoxia of the brain tissue produces further cerebral edema, and the cycle repeats.

As tissue hypoxia develops in the brain, reflexes are activated in an effort to maintain cerebral oxygen delivery. To overcome rising ICP, the autonomic nervous system is activated to increase systemic blood pressure, and therefore the MAP, to maintain a normal CPP. Systolic pressures can reach up to 250 mm Hg. However, as the baroreceptors in the carotid arteries and aortic arch sense a markedly increased blood pressure, messages are sent to the brainstem to activate the parasympathetic nervous system. A signal then travels via the tenth cranial nerve, the vagus nerve, to slow the heart rate. *Cushing's phenomenon* refers to this ominous combination of markedly increased arterial blood pressure and the resultant bradycardia that can occur with severely increased ICP.

Oxygen delivery to the brain is most adversely affected when a fall in MAP occurs in a patient who also

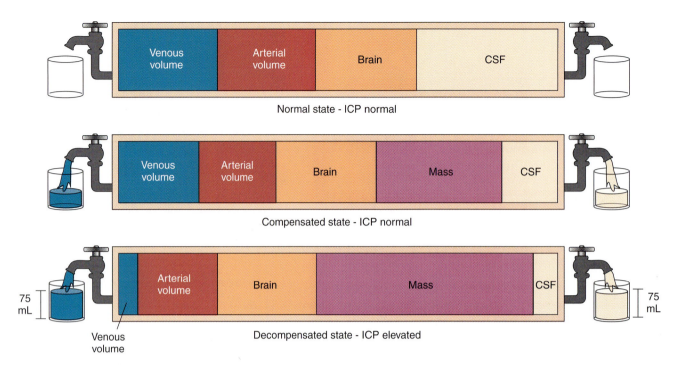

Figure 8-6   Monro-Kellie doctrine: Intracranial compensation for expanding mass. The volume of the intracranial contents remains constant. If the addition of a mass such as a hematoma results in the squeezing out of an equal volume of cerebrospinal fluid (CSF) and venous blood, the intracranial pressure (ICP) remains normal. However, when this compensatory mechanism is exhausted, an exponential increase occurs in ICP for even a small additional increase in the volume of the hematoma. (*From McSwain NE Jr, Paturas JL: The basic EMT: comprehensive prehospital patient care, ed 2, St Louis, 2001, Mosby.*)

has increased ICP. As the CPP falls toward zero, so does CBF and oxygen delivery. Unless this dire situation is rapidly corrected, permanent brain damage occurs and brain death results.

Intracranial hypertension often produces abnormal ventilatory patterns or apnea that further worsen hypoxia and significantly alter blood carbon dioxide levels. *Cheyne-Stokes ventilations* are a repeating cycle of slow, shallow breaths that become deeper and more rapid and then return to slow, shallow breaths. Brief periods of apnea may occur between cycles. *Central neurogenic hyperventilation* refers to consistently rapid, deep breaths, and *ataxic breathing* refers to erratic ventilatory efforts that lack any discernable pattern. Spontaneous respiratory function ceases with herniation and brain death.

Abnormal motor posturing typically accompanies increased ICP. Decorticate posturing involves flexion of the upper extremities and rigidity and extension of the lower extremities. A more ominous finding is decerebrate posturing wherein all extremities are extended and arching of the spine may occur. After herniation, the extremities become flaccid and motor activity is absent.

Assessment

A quick survey of the kinematics of the injury, combined with a rapid primary survey, will help identify potential life-threatening problems in a patient with a suspected TBI.

Kinematics

As with all trauma patients, assessment must include consideration of the mechanism of injury. Because many patients with severe TBI have an altered level of consciousness (LOC), key data about the kinematics must come from observation of the scene or from bystanders. The windshield of the patient's vehicle may have a "spider-web" pattern, suggesting an impact with the patient's head, or a bloody object may be present that was used as a weapon during an assault. This important information should be reported to personnel at the receiving facility because it may be essential for proper diagnosis and management of the patient.

Airway

The patency of the patient's airway should be examined. In unconscious individuals, the tongue may completely occlude the airway. Noisy ventilations indicate partial obstruction by either the tongue or foreign material. Emesis, hemorrhage, and swelling from facial trauma commonly compromise the airway of patients with TBI.

Breathing

Evaluation of respiratory function must include an assessment of the rate, depth, and adequacy of breathing. As noted previously, several different breathing patterns can result from severe brain injury. In multisystem trauma patients, thoracic injuries can impair both oxygenation and ventilation. Cervical spine fractures occur in about 2% to 5% of patients with TBI and may significantly interfere with ventilation. Pulse oximetry and end-tidal CO_2 monitors, if available, should be applied during transport because they may provide valuable information to guide further assessment and management.

Circulation

The prehospital care provider should note and quantify evidence of external bleeding, if possible. In the absence of significant external blood loss, a weak, rapid pulse in a victim of blunt trauma suggests life-threatening internal hemorrhage in the pleural spaces, peritoneum, retroperitoneum, or soft tissues surrounding long bone fractures. In an infant with open fontanelles, sufficient blood loss can occur inside the cranium to produce hypovolemic shock. A slow, forceful pulse may result from intracranial hypertension and indicate impending herniation (Cushing's phenomenon). In a patient with potentially life-threatening injuries, transport should not be delayed to measure blood pressure but should be performed en route as time permits.

Disability

During the primary survey and after the initiation of appropriate measures to treat problems identified in the airway, breathing, and circulation assessments, a baseline Glasgow Coma Scale (GCS) score should be calculated to accurately assess the patient's LOC (Table 8-1). As previously described in Chapter 3, the GCS score is calculated by using the best response noted while evaluating the patient's eyes, verbal response, and motor response. If a patient lacks spontaneous eye opening, a verbal command (e.g., "Open your eyes!") should be used. If the patient does not respond to a verbal stimulus, a painful stimulus, such as nail bed pressure with a pen or squeezing of anterior axillary tissue, should be applied.

Table 8-1 Glasgow Coma Scale	
	Points
EYE OPENING	
Spontaneous eye opening	4
Eye opening on command	3
Eye opening to painful stimulus	2
No eye opening	1
BEST VERBAL RESPONSE	
Answers appropriately (oriented)	5
Gives confused answers	4
Inappropriate response	3
Makes unintelligible noises	2
Makes no verbal response	1
BEST MOTOR RESPONSE	
Follows command	6
Localizes painful stimuli	5
Withdrawal to pain	4
Responds with abnormal flexion to painful stimuli (decorticate)	3
Responds with abnormal extension to pain (decerebrate)	2
Gives no motor response	1

Note that the lowest possible score is 3 and the highest possible score is 15.

The patient's verbal response can be examined using a question such as, "What happened to you?" If fully oriented, the patient will supply a coherent answer. Otherwise, the patient's verbal response is scored as confused, inappropriate, unintelligible, or absent. If the patient is intubated, the score is calculated from only the eye and motor scales and a "T" is added to note the inability to assess the verbal response, such as "8T."

The last component of the GCS is the motor score. A simple, unambiguous command should be given to the patient, such as, "Hold up two fingers!" or "Show me a hitchhiker's sign!" A patient who squeezes the finger of a prehospital care provider may simply be demonstrating a grasping reflex as opposed to purposefully following a command. A painful stimulus should be used if the patient fails to follow a command and the patient's *best* motor response scored. A patient who attempts to push away a painful stimulus is considered to be localizing. Other possible responses to pain include withdrawal from the stimulus, abnormal flexion (decorticate) or extension (decerebrate) of the upper extremities, or absence of a motor function.

If a depressed LOC is noted in the primary survey, the pupils should be examined quickly for symmetry and response to light. A difference of greater than 1 mm in pupil size is considered abnormal. A small percentage of the population has anisocoria, inequality of pupil size that is either congenital or acquired as the result of ophthalmic trauma. However, when anisocoria is present, both pupils will react equally.

Expose/Environment

Patients who have sustained a TBI frequently have other injuries, so the entire body should be examined for other potential life-threatening problems.

Secondary Survey (Focused History and Physical Examination)

Once life-threatening injuries have been identified and managed, a thorough secondary survey should be completed if time permits. The patient's head and face should be palpated carefully for wounds, depressions, and crepitus. Any drainage of clear fluid from the nose or ear canals may be CSF. When placed on a gauze pad or cloth, CSF may diffuse out from blood, producing a characteristic yellowish "halo." The pupillary size and response should be rechecked at this time. Because of the incidence of cervical spine fractures in patients with TBI noted previously, the neck should be examined for tenderness and bony deformities.

In a cooperative patient, a more thorough neurologic examination, assessing sensory and motor function in all extremities, should also be performed. Neurologic deficits, such as hemiparesis (weakness) or hemiplegia (paralysis), may be present on only one side of the body. These "lateralizing signs" tend to be indicative of TBI, whereas bilateral neurologic deficits, such as paraplegia, are more consistent with a spinal cord injury.

History

The prehospital care provider should obtain an AMPLE history from the patient, family members, or bystanders. Diabetes mellitus, seizure disorders, and drug or alcohol intoxication can mimic TBI. Any evidence of drug use or overdose should be noted. The patient may have a history of prior head injury and may complain of persistent or recurring headache, visual disturbances, nausea and vomiting, or difficulty speaking.

Serial Examinations

About 3% of patients with mild brain injury (GCS 14-15) may experience an unexpected deterioration in their mentation. During transport, the primary survey and assessment of the GCS should be repeated at frequent intervals. Patients with serious brain injuries can rapidly deteriorate, so trends in the GCS or vital signs should be reported to the receiving facility and documented on the patient care report. Responses to management should also be recorded.

Specific Head Trauma Conditions

Cerebral Concussion

A cerebral concussion can be thought of as a "shaking up" of the brain. The diagnosis of a concussion is made when an injured patient shows an alteration in neurologic function, most commonly a loss of consciousness, and no intracranial abnormality is identified when a computed tomography (CT) scan of the brain is performed. Other neurologic findings include memory deficits, retrograde amnesia (the inability to remember events before the injury), and antegrade amnesia (problems remembering details after regaining consciousness). This short-term memory loss often provokes anxiety and results in the patient asking questions of a repetitive nature. Severe headache, dizziness, and nausea and vomiting frequently accompany a concussion. Although most of these findings only last between several hours to a couple of days, some patients experience a postconcussive syndrome with headaches, dizziness, and difficulty concentrating for weeks and up to months after a severe concussion.

Skull Fractures

Fractures of the skull can result from either blunt or penetrating trauma. Linear fractures account for about 80% of skull fractures; however, a powerful impact may produce a depressed skull fracture, where fragments of bone are driven toward or into the underlying brain tissue (Figure 8-7). Although simple linear fractures can be diagnosed only with a radiographic study, depressed skull fractures can often be palpated during a careful physical examination. A closed, nondepressed skull fracture by itself is of little clinical significance, but its presence dramatically increases the risk of an intracranial hematoma. Open skull fractures can result from a particularly severe impact or from a gunshot wound and serve as an entry site for bacteria, predisposing the patient to meningitis. If the dura mater is torn, brain tissue or CSF may leak from an open skull fracture.

Basilar skull fractures (fractures to the floor of the cranium) should be suspected if CSF is draining from the nostrils or ear canals. Periorbital ecchymosis, often referred to as "raccoon eyes," and Battle's sign, in which ecchymosis is noted over the mastoid area behind the ears, often occur with basilar skull fractures, although they may take several hours after injury to become apparent.

Intracranial Hematoma

Intracranial hematomas are divided into three general types—epidural, subdural, and intracerebral. Because the signs and symptoms of these have significant overlap, specific diagnosis in the prehospital setting is almost impossible, although the prehospital care provider may suspect an epidural hematoma based on the characteristic clinical presentation. Even so, a definitive diagnosis can only be made after a CT scan performed at the receiving facility. Because these hematomas occupy space inside the rigid skull, they may produce rapid increases in ICP, especially if they are sizable.

EPIDURAL HEMATOMA

Epidural hematomas account for about 2% of TBIs that require hospitalization and have a mortality rate of about 20%. These hematomas often result from a low-velocity blow to the temporal bone, like the impact from a punch or baseball. A fracture of this thin bone damages the middle meningeal artery, resulting in arterial bleeding that collects between the skull and dura mater (Figure 8-8). The classic history for an epidural hematoma is that the patient experienced a brief loss of consciousness, then regained consciousness, and then experienced a rapid decline in consciousness. During the period of consciousness, the lucid interval, the patient may be oriented or lethargic and may complain of a headache.

As a patient's LOC worsens, examination can reveal a dilated and sluggish or nonreactive pupil on the side of the impact (ipsilateral side). Because motor nerves cross over in the spinal cord, hemiparesis or hemiplegia typically occurs on the side opposite the impact (contralateral side). If the hematoma is recognized early and the patient undergoes prompt neurosurgical intervention, the prognosis is generally excellent because the patient usually does not have serious underlying brain injury.

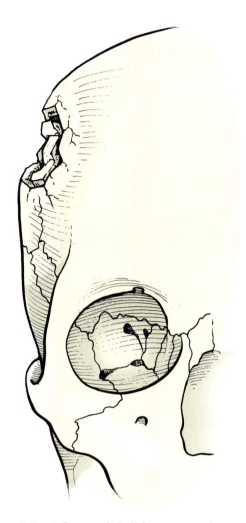

Figure 8-7   A depressed skull fracture may force particles of bone into the brain tissue.

SUBDURAL HEMATOMA

Subdural hematomas account for about 30% of severe brain injuries. In addition to being more common than epidural hematomas, they also differ in etiology, location, and prognosis. As opposed to the arterial hemorrhage, which produces an epidural hematoma, a subdural hematoma generally results from a venous bleed from bridging veins that are torn during a violent blow to the head. In this injury, the blood collects in the subdural space, between the dura mater and the arachnoid (Figure 8-9). Focal neurologic deficits may be present immediately after the trauma, or the signs may be delayed for days to months. Subdural hematomas are classified into three types depending on how quickly neurologic findings present:

1. In an *acute subdural hematoma*, neurologic deficits can be identified within 72 hours of the injury and usually sooner. The patient usually has a history of a

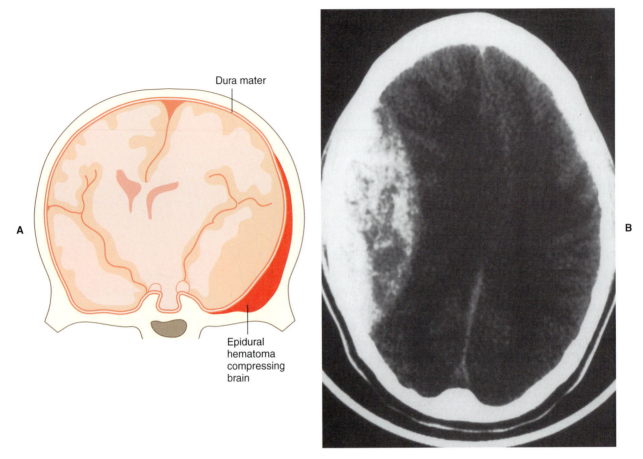

Figure 8-8 **A**, Epidural hematoma. **B**, Computed tomography (CT) of an epidural hematoma. (*B from Cruz J:* Neurologic and neurosurgical emergencies, *Philadelphia, 1998, WB Saunders.*)

high-velocity mechanism of injury such as an MVC or an assault with a rigid object. Because significant underlying brain injury is often associated with this condition, the mortality rate ranges from 50% to 60%, even with prompt diagnosis and early surgical drainage.

2. *Subacute subdural hematomas* develop more gradually as signs and symptoms develop over 3 to 21 days. Because of the slower accumulation of blood and less-extensive brain injury, subacute subdural hematomas have a mortality rate of about 25%.

3. *Chronic subdural hematomas* may present with neurologic findings months after a seemingly minor head injury. This condition commonly occurs in patients with chronic alcoholism who are prone to frequent falls and has a mortality rate of about 50%.

In addition to alterations in consciousness, specific neurologic findings may vary depending on the location of the hematoma; however, the patient or family members may complain of headache, visual disturbances, personality changes, difficulty speaking (dysarthria), and hemiparesis or hemiplegia.

INTRACEREBRAL HEMATOMA

Damage to blood vessels within the brain itself may produce an intracerebral hematoma or cerebral contusion. These occur fairly commonly, accounting for about 20% to 30% of severe brain injuries. Although these injuries are typically the result of blunt trauma, they may also occur from penetrating trauma such as a gunshot wound to the brain. In blunt trauma, cerebral contusions may be numerous. One hematoma generally occurs at the point of impact as the brain collides with the inside of the skull (the "coup" injury), and a second lesion may occur directly opposite from the point of impact as the brain tears away from the cranium (the "contracoup" injury). These hematomas may enlarge after the injury and produce seizures and marked increases in ICP. The specific neurologic findings depend on the location and size of the hematoma.

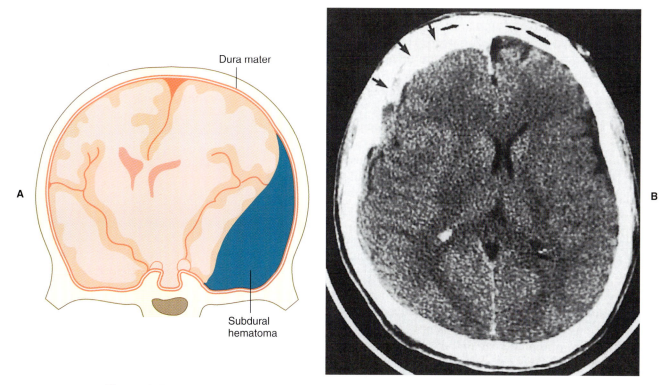

Figure 8-9   **A**, Subdural hematoma. **B**, Computed tomography (CT) of a subdural hematoma. (*B from Cruz J:* Neurologic and neurosurgical emergencies, *Philadelphia, 1998, WB Saunders.*)

Management

Effective management of a patient with TBI begins with orderly interventions focused on treating any life-threatening problems identified in the primary survey. Once these problems are addressed, the patient should be rapidly packaged and transported to the nearest facility capable of caring for TBI.

Airway

Patients with depressed LOCs may be unable to protect their airway. A retrospective study has documented an improved mortality rate in patients with TBI who received prehospital endotracheal intubation. Thus all patients with a severe TBI (GCS 8 or less) should be considered for intubation, although this can be extremely challenging because of the patient's combativeness, clenched jaw muscles (trismus), vomiting, and the need to maintain inline cervical spine stabilization on the patient. The use of neuromuscular blocking agents as part of a rapid sequence intubation protocol may facilitate successful intubation. Based on animal studies, an intravenous dose of lidocaine (1 mg/kg) may blunt an increase in ICP during intubation. Blind nasotracheal in-

tubation can serve as an alternative technique, but the presence of midface trauma is a relative contraindication for this procedure. Suction equipment should be readily available. If initial attempts at intubation are unsuccessful, prolonged laryngoscopy should be avoided, especially if there is a short transport time. An oropharyngeal airway with bag-valve-mask (BVM) ventilation or percutaneous transtracheal ventilation are reasonable alternatives.

Breathing

All patients with suspected TBI should receive supplemental oxygen. The use of pulse oximetry is strongly recommended because hypoxia can worsen neurologic outcome. Oxygen concentration can be titrated when using pulse oximetry; however, the oxygen saturation (SpO_2) should be maintained at 95% or higher. If pulse oximetry is not available, oxygen should be provided via a nonrebreather facemask for a spontaneously breathing patient. For intubated patients, an oxygen concentration of 100% (FiO_2 of 1.0) should be maintained with a BVM device. If hypoxia persists despite oxygen therapy, the provider should attempt to identify and treat all likely etiologies, including aspiration and tension pneumothoraces. Use of positive end-expiratory pressure (PEEP) valves may be considered to improve oxygenation; however, levels of PEEP greater than 15 cm H_2O may increase ICP.

Because both hypocapnia and hypercapnia can aggravate brain injury, end-tidal CO_2 monitoring ($ETCO_2$ or capnography) may be considered, with an acceptable $ETCO_2$ range being 30 to 35 mm Hg. If capnography is not available, the provider should use normal ventilatory rates when assisting ventilation in patients with TBI—10 breaths/min for adults, 20 breaths/min for children, and 25 breaths/min for infants. Overly aggressive hyperventilation produces cerebral vasoconstriction that in turn leads to a decrease in cerebral oxygen delivery. Routine *prophylactic* hyperventilation has been shown to worsen neurologic outcome and should not be used.

Circulation

Both anemia and hypotension are important causes of secondary brain injury, so efforts should be taken to prevent or treat these conditions. Control of hemorrhage is essential. Direct pressure or pressure dressings should be applied to any external hemorrhage. Complex scalp wounds can produce significant external blood loss. Several gauze pads held in place by an elastic roller bandage creates an effective pressure dressing to control bleeding; however, this should not be applied to a depressed or open skull fracture unless significant hemorrhage is present because it may aggravate brain injury and lead to an increase in ICP. Direct gentle pressure may also limit the size of extracranial (scalp) hematomas. Gentle handling and immobilization to a long backboard in anatomic alignment can minimize interstitial blood loss around fractures.

Because hypotension further worsens brain ischemia, standard measures should be employed to combat shock. In patients with traumatic brain injury, the combination of hypoxia and hypotension is associated with a mortality rate of about 75%. If shock is present and major internal hemorrhage is suspected, prompt transport to a trauma center takes priority over brain injuries. Hypovolemic and neurogenic shock are aggressively treated by resuscitation with isotonic crystalloid solutions; however, transport should not be delayed to establish intravenous access. Although assessing blood volume is extremely difficult in the prehospital setting, the provider should return the patient to a state of normal circulating blood volume (euvolemia). To preserve cerebral perfusion, attempts should be made to maintain a systolic blood pressure of at least 90 to 100 mm Hg;

however, excessive volume resuscitation may lead to uncontrolled internal hemorrhage, increased cerebral edema, and increased ICP. For adult TBI patients with normal vital signs and no other suspected injuries, intravenous fluid at a rate of no more than 125 mL/hr should be administered and adjusted if signs of shock develop. If indicated by the patient's injuries, such as suspicion of a severe pelvic fracture, a PASG may be applied and inflated.

Disability

Neurosurgical interventions to insert devices to monitor ICP or evacuate intracranial hematomas are not performed in the field. As has been emphasized, prehospital management of TBI primarily consists of measures aimed at reversing and preventing factors that cause secondary brain injury. Prolonged or multiple grand mal seizures can be treated with intravenous administration of a benzodiazepine, such as diazepam, lorazepam, or midazolam. These drugs should be cautiously titrated because hypotension and ventilatory depression may occur.

Because of the significant incidence of cervical spine fractures, patients with suspected TBI should be placed in spinal immobilization. Some degree of caution must be exercised when applying a cervical collar to a patient with TBI. Some evidence suggests that a tightly fitted cervical collar can impede venous drainage of the head, thereby increasing ICP. Application of a cervical collar is not mandatory as long as the head and neck are sufficiently immobilized.

Transportation

To achieve the best possible outcome, patients with moderate and severe TBI should be transported directly to a trauma center that has the ability to perform a CT scan and provide prompt neurosurgical intervention. If such a facility is not available, aeromedical transport from the scene to an appropriate trauma center should be considered.

The patient's pulse rate, blood pressure, SpO_2, and GCS should be reassessed and documented every 5 to 10 minutes during transport. PEEP valves may be used cautiously if persistent hypoxia exists because levels of PEEP greater than 15 cm H_2O may increase ICP. The patient's body heat should be preserved during transport.

Controversy exists regarding the optimal position for a patient with TBI. In general, patients with TBI should be transported in a supine position because of the presence of other injuries. Although elevating the head of the ambulance stretcher or long backboard (reverse Trendelenburg position) may decrease ICP, cerebral perfusion pressure may also be jeopardized, especially if the head is elevated higher than 30 degrees.

The receiving facility should be notified as early as possible so that they can make appropriate preparations before the patient's arrival. The radio report should include information regarding the mechanism of injury, initial GCS score and vital signs, other serious injuries, and the response to management.

Prolonged or Delayed Transport

When there is a delay in transport or a prolonged transport time to an appropriate facility, the prehospital care provider may consider additional management options. For patients with an abnormal GCS score, the blood glucose level should be checked. If the patient is hypoglycemic, a 50% dextrose solution can be administered until the blood sugar is restored to a normal level.

Appropriate management of increased ICP in the prehospital setting is extremely challenging because the ICP is not monitored in the field unless the patient is undergoing interfacility transfer and an ICP monitor or ventriculostomy has been placed at the referring center. Although a declining GCS score may well represent increasing ICP, it may also be the result of worsening cerebral perfusion from hypovolemic shock. Warning signs of possible increased ICP and herniation include the following:

- Decline in GCS score of two points or more
- Development of a sluggish or nonreactive pupil
- Development of hemiplegia or hemiparesis
- Cushing's phenomenon

The decision to intervene and manage increased ICP should be based on written protocol or made in consultation with medical control at the receiving facility. Possible temporizing management options include sedation, chemical paralysis, osmotherapy (the use of osmotically active agents that may assist in the treatment of intracranial hypertension), and controlled hyperventilation. Small doses of benzodiazepine sedatives should be titrated cautiously because of the potential side effects of hypotension and ventilatory depression. Use of a long-acting neuromuscular blocking agent, such as vecuronium, may be considered if the patient is intubated. If the cervical collar is believed to be too tight, it may be loosened slightly or removed, provided that the head and neck are adequately immobilized with other measures.

Osmotherapy with mannitol (0.25 to 1 g/kg) can be given intravenously. However, aggressive diuresis may produce hypovolemia that can further worsen cerebral perfusion. Furosemide may be administered, in doses of 0.3 to 0.5 mg/kg, with mannitol for severely increased ICP. If an osmotic agent is used, the patient should be maintained in a euvolemic state.

Controlled mild therapeutic hyperventilation may be considered for obvious signs of herniation. If capnography is available, hyperventilation to an $ETCO_2$ of 25 to 30 mm Hg is acceptable. Otherwise the provider should use the following ventilatory rates: 20 breaths/min for adults, 30 breaths/min for children, and 35 breaths/min for infants. Steroids have not been shown to improve the outcome of patients with TBI and should not be administered. *Prophylactic hyperventilation has no role in TBI, and therapeutic hyperventilation, if instituted, should be stopped if signs of intracranial hypertension resolve.*

Brain Death and Organ Donation

The diagnosis of "brain death" is made when no reasonable hope exists for recovery of brain function. For a patient to qualify as "brain dead," the following four criteria must be met: a Glasgow Coma Scale score of 3, nonreactive pupils, no spontaneous ventilatory activity, and absence of brainstem reflexes, such as the corneal reflex or the oculocephalic reflex. Some additional tests that may be useful in determining brain death include absence of activity on an electroencephalogram (EEG), no evidence of cerebral blood flow (CBF) on CBF study, and ICP exceeding MAP for more than 1 hour. To document brain death, these findings must be identified in the absence of hypothermia and drug or alcohol intoxication.

Victims of traumatic brain injury that progresses to brain death provide an important source of organs for transplantation. In 1999, TBI was the cause of brain death for more than 40% of individuals from whom organs were procured, with the majority of organs coming from those between 18 and 49 years of age. Despite the presence of a fatal brain injury, an individual's heart, lungs, liver, kidneys, pancreas, and corneas may benefit others with chronic illnesses.

MANAGEMENT OF SUSPECTED TRAUMATIC BRAIN INJURY

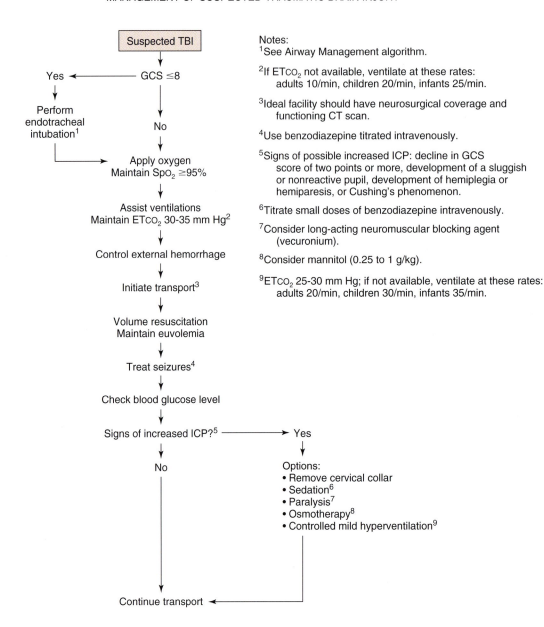

Notes:
[1]See Airway Management algorithm.

[2]If ETCO$_2$ not available, ventilate at these rates:
adults 10/min, children 20/min, infants 25/min.

[3]Ideal facility should have neurosurgical coverage and functioning CT scan.

[4]Use benzodiazepine titrated intravenously.

[5]Signs of possible increased ICP: decline in GCS score of two points or more, development of a sluggish or nonreactive pupil, development of hemiplegia or hemiparesis, or Cushing's phenomenon.

[6]Titrate small doses of benzodiazepine intravenously.

[7]Consider long-acting neuromuscular blocking agent (vecuronium).

[8]Consider mannitol (0.25 to 1 g/kg).

[9]ETCO$_2$ 25-30 mm Hg; if not available, ventilate at these rates: adults 20/min, children 30/min, infants 35/min.

The following appears within the flowchart image:

Suspected TBI

GCS ≤8 — Yes → Perform endotracheal intubation[1]

No

Apply oxygen
Maintain SpO$_2$ ≥95%

Assist ventilations
Maintain ETCO$_2$ 30-35 mm Hg[2]

Control external hemorrhage

Initiate transport[3]

Volume resuscitation
Maintain euvolemia

Treat seizures[4]

Check blood glucose level

Signs of increased ICP?[5] → Yes

No

Options:
• Remove cervical collar
• Sedation[6]
• Paralysis[7]
• Osmotherapy[8]
• Controlled mild hyperventilation[9]

Continue transport

Summary

Head injury is a common reason for emergency department visits. A large proportion of these patients have TBI. Of these, the severity of the primary injury is incompatible with resuscitation 10% of the time. For the remainder of patients with TBI, aggressive management to maintain cerebral perfusion and prevent secondary brain injury can make a difference in morbidity and mortality from TBI. Two of the most important goals in the early treatment of TBI are the management of ventilation and maintenance of cerebral perfusion pressure, which can both be addressed to some degree in the prehospital setting en route to definitive care. Therefore the role of the prehospital care provider in caring for the patient with TBI is significant.

The severity of TBI may not be immediately apparent; therefore the prehospital care provider must maintain a high index of suspicion based on mechanism of injury and must perform serial neurologic evaluations of the patient, including Glasgow Coma Scale scores and pupillary response. Not infrequently, TBI is concomitant with multisystem trauma, so the prehospital care provider must attend to all problems in their appropriate priority. Not only are airway, breathing, and circulation always the priorities of patient care, but they are specifically important in the management of TBI in preventing secondary brain injury.

The prehospital care provider accomplishes the goals of immediate prehospital management of the TBI patient in the short term by controlling hemorrhage from other injuries, maintaining a systolic blood pressure of at least 90 to 100 mm Hg, providing oxygenation to maintain an SpO_2 of at least 95%, and providing well-managed ventilation to maintain an $ETCO_2$ of 30 to 35 mm Hg. When transport to an appropriate facility is prolonged, the prehospital care provider pursues these goals more aggressively with sedation, chemical paralysis, osmotherapy, and controlled hyperventilation. The prehospital care provider not only has an important role in the prehospital care of the TBI patient; he or she also has a significant influence on in-hospital care by selecting the appropriate facility to which to transport the patient. At least equally important to patient treatment and transport decisions is the need for prehospital care providers to play a high-profile role in TBI prevention through patient and public education efforts.

Scenario Solution

The rapid decrease in this patient's GCS score is extremely worrisome, so you should transport the patient to a facility with neurosurgical coverage immediately upon completion of spinal immobilization. Given the lucid interval demonstrated by this patient, suspect the presence of an epidural hematoma. Examination of the eyes may reveal an enlarged, sluggishly reactive pupil on the right side, and weakness or paralysis may develop on the left side of his body. A CT scan at the receiving trauma center can confirm the diagnosis.

Once en route, you should reevaluate the patient's airway and breathing and apply a pulse oximeter. If his SpO_2 is less than 95%, you should apply supplemental oxygen and assist ventilations with a bag-valve-mask device. Additionally, given the mechanism of injury, you should consider a pneumothorax. If the GCS score further deteriorates, you must consider intubating this patient, preferably using a rapid sequence technique. You should reassess the scalp wound to ensure that hemorrhage is adequately controlled and start two large-bore IV lines. You should measure the patient's vital signs and take a blood pressure reading. The mild tachycardia may be suggestive of compensated shock from intraabdominal hemorrhage from the liver or spleen or retroperitoneal hemorrhage from a pelvic fracture. You should perform a complete secondary survey to rule out additional injuries and determine a blood glucose level. During transport, you should frequently assess the patency of the patient's airway, measure his vital signs, and check his GCS score and pupillary response. You should notify the receiving facility of the patient's condition and update it if any significant changes occur.

If transport to an appropriate facility is prolonged and the patient's neurologic status continues to deteriorate, you may take further measures. After endotracheal intubation, you may titrate a benzodiazepine sedative intravenously. You may consider a dose of mannitol, as well as modest, controlled hyperventilation. When combined with appropriate neurosurgical intervention, aggressive prehospital care should improve the outcome of patients with moderate to severe TBI.

Review Questions

Answers are provided on p. 414.

1. Which of the following factors would have the greatest adverse effect on a patient with moderate to severe traumatic brain injury (TBI)?
   a. Mean arterial pressure (MAP) less than 60 mm Hg
   b. $PaCO_2$ between 35 and 45 mm Hg
   c. PaO_2 above 98 mm Hg
   d. Systolic blood pressure above 120 mm Hg

2. A patient who withdraws from painful stimuli, opens eyes on verbal command, and cannot speak because of intubation has a Glasgow Coma Scale score of which of the following?
   a. 8
   b. 8T
   c. 7
   d. 7T

3. A sharp blow to the temporal area of the skull is most highly associated with which of the following injuries?
   a. Chronic subdural hematoma
   b. Basilar skull fracture
   c. LaForte III fracture
   d. Epidural hematoma

4. Which of the following is the most frequent cause of TBI in the elderly?
   a. Motor vehicle crashes
   b. Falls
   c. Stroke
   d. Assault

5. The presence of cerebrospinal fluid in blood can be detected by absorbing the blood onto a 4-inch by 4-inch piece of gauze and observing which of the following?
   a. Horizontal bands of pinkish staining
   b. Immediate clot formation
   c. Glossy black striations
   d. A yellowish halo

6. Which of the following is a manifestation of Cushing's phenomenon?
   a. Bradycardia
   b. Hypotension

c. Hypoglycemia
d. Hypercapnia

7. Your patient is a 23-year-old male who was the driver of a small vehicle that sustained a significant side impact from another vehicle. The patient is immobilized, and you are en route to the hospital. The patient is confused, asking repetitive questions, and becoming increasingly agitated. He has made repeated attempts to remove the cervical collar you placed on him, stating that it is too tight despite the fact that you have explained its necessity to him. Which of the following actions should you undertake next?
   a. Loosen the cervical collar (provided spinal immobilization is maintained) to improve venous return
   b. Restrain the patient's hands with soft restraints

c. Sedate the patient with benzodiazepines
d. Explain to the patient that this is the way the cervical collar is supposed to fit

8. Your patient is a 70-year-old female who was the driver of a vehicle that collided head-on with a semi. She has a large hematoma on her forehead; is unresponsive with cool, pale, moist skin; and has a ventilatory rate of 30 breaths/min, a heart rate of 124 beats/min, and a blood pressure of 88/52 mm Hg. These findings indicate suspicion for which of the following?
   a. Basilar skull fracture
   b. Cervical spine injury
   c. Hypovolemic shock
   d. Brain stem herniation

REFERENCES

American College of Surgeons: Head trauma. In Committee on Trauma, American College of Surgeons: *Advanced trauma life support*, Chicago, 2002, Author.

Brain Trauma Foundation: *Guidelines for prehospital management of traumatic brain injury*, New York, 2000, Brain Trauma Foundation.

Chestnut RM, Prough DS: Critical care of severe head injury, *New Horizons* 3:365, 1995.

Cooper KR, Boswell PA, Choi SC: Safe use of PEEP in patients with severe brain injury, *J Neurosurg* 63:552, 1985.

Davies G, Deakin C, Wilson A: The effect of a rigid collar on intracranial pressure, *Injury* 27:647, 1996.

Feldman Z, Kanter MJ, Robertson CS et al: Effect of head elevation on intracranial pressure, cerebral perfusion pressure and cerebral blood flow in head-injured patients, *J Neurosurg* 76:207, 1992

Kolb JC, Summer RL, Galli RL: Cervical collar-induced changes in intracranial pressure, *Amer J Emerg Med* 17:135,1999.

McGuire G, Crossley D, Richards J, Wong D: Effects of varying levels of positive end-expiratory pressure on intracranial pressure and cerebral perfusion pressure, *Crit Care Med* 25:1059, 1997.

Rosner MJ, Coley IB: Cerebral perfusion pressure, intracranial pressure and head elevation, *J Neurosurg* 65:636, 1986.

Winchell RJ, Hoyt DB: Endotracheal intubation in the field improves survival in patients with severe head injury, *Arch Surg* 132:592, 1997.

SUGGESTED READING

Muizelaar JP, Marmarou A, Ward JD et al: Adverse effects of prolonged hyperventilation in patients with severe brain injury: a randomized clinical trial, *J Neurosurg* 75:731, 1991.

Teasdale G, Jennett B: Assessment of coma and impaired consciousness: a practical scale, *Lancet* 2:81,1974.

Valadka AB: Injury to the cranium. In Mattox KL, Feliciano DV, Moore EE: *Trauma*, ed 4, Norwalk, Conn, 2000, Appleton and Lange.

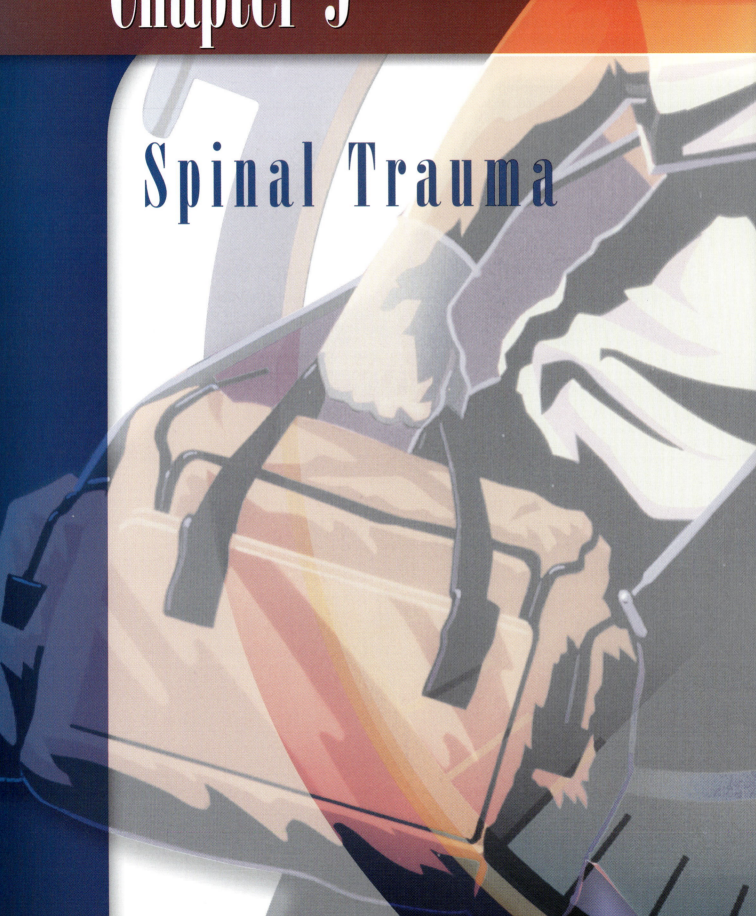

Chapter 9

Spinal Trauma

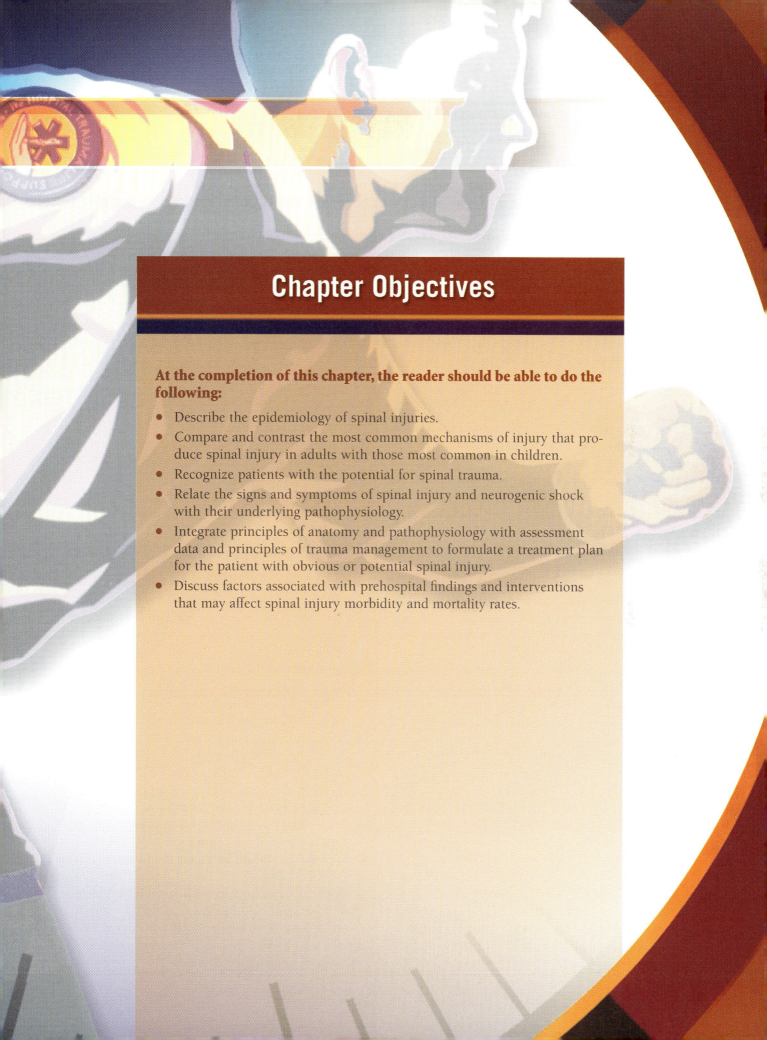

Chapter Objectives

At the completion of this chapter, the reader should be able to do the following:

- Describe the epidemiology of spinal injuries.
- Compare and contrast the most common mechanisms of injury that produce spinal injury in adults with those most common in children.
- Recognize patients with the potential for spinal trauma.
- Relate the signs and symptoms of spinal injury and neurogenic shock with their underlying pathophysiology.
- Integrate principles of anatomy and pathophysiology with assessment data and principles of trauma management to formulate a treatment plan for the patient with obvious or potential spinal injury.
- Discuss factors associated with prehospital findings and interventions that may affect spinal injury morbidity and mortality rates.

Scenario

You have been dispatched to a residence for an unknown problem. Upon arrival, you find a male, approximately 45 years of age, lying supine in the front yard of a house. The scene is safe, and you hear the siren from the fire department first response vehicle approaching. Police are already on the scene.

As you begin your primary survey, you find an unresponsive male patient who apparently fell from a second story window. He has abrasions and an obvious hematoma on his right temple. His airway is open, and he is breathing, although it does not appear to be regular. The patient has weak radial and carotid pulses. He shows no obvious signs of external blood loss. His skin appears normal and warm in the lower extremities. His upper extremities are pale, cool, and clammy.

What pathological processes explain the patient's presentation? What intermediate interventions and further assessments are needed? What are the management goals for this patient?

Spinal trauma, if not recognized and properly managed in the field, can result in irreparable damage and leave a patient paralyzed for life. Some patients sustain immediate spinal cord damage as a result of trauma. Others sustain an injury to the spinal column that does not initially damage the cord; cord damage may result later with movement of the spine. Because the central nervous system is incapable of regeneration, a severed cord cannot be repaired. The consequences of inappropriately moving a patient with a spinal column injury, or allowing the patient to move, can be devastating. Failure to properly immobilize a fractured spine may produce a much worse outcome than, for example, failure to properly immobilize a fractured femur.

Spinal cord injury can have profound effects on human physiology, lifestyle, and financial circumstances. Human physiology is affected because the use of extremities or other areas is severely limited as a result of cord damage. Lifestyle is affected because spinal cord injury usually results in changes to daily activity levels and independence. Spinal cord injury also alters financial circumstances. A patient with this injury requires both acute and long-term care. The lifetime cost of this care is estimated at approximately $1.25 million for a permanent spinal cord injury.

About 15,000 to 20,000 spinal cord injuries occur annually. Spinal cord injury can occur at any age; however, it commonly occurs in those 16 to 35 years of age because this age group is involved in the most violent and high-risk activities. Most trauma patients are between 16 and 20 years of age. The second largest group of patients is between 21 and 25 years of age, and the third largest group is between 26 and 35 years of age. Common causes are motor vehicle crashes (MVCs; 48%), falls (21%), penetrating injuries (15%), sports injuries (14%), and other injuries (2%).

Sudden violent forces acting on the body can move the spine beyond its normal range of motion by either impacting on the head or neck or by driving the torso out from under the head. Four concepts make the possible effect on the spine clearer when evaluating the potential for injury:

1. The head is like a bowling ball perched on top of the neck, and its mass often moves in a different direction from the torso, resulting in strong forces being applied to the neck (cervical spine and/or spinal cord).
2. Objects in motion tend to stay in motion, and objects at rest tend to stay at rest.
3. Sudden or violent movement of the upper legs displaces the pelvis, resulting in forceful movement of the lower spine. Because of the weight and inertia of the head and torso, force in an opposite (contra) direction is applied to the upper spine.
4. Lack of neurologic deficit *does not* rule out bone or ligament injury to the spine or conditions that have stressed the spinal cord to the limit of its tolerance.

Some trauma patients with neurologic deficit will have a temporary or permanent spinal cord injury. Other patients have neurologic deficit caused by either a peripheral nerve injury or an extremity injury not associated with spinal cord injury. The prehospital care provider should assume that any patient who has sustained any of the following injuries has a potential spinal injury:

- Any mechanism that produced a violent impact on the head, neck, torso, or pelvis
- Incidents that produce sudden acceleration, deceleration, or lateral bending forces to the neck or torso
- Any fall, especially in the elderly
- Ejection or a fall from any motorized or otherwise powered transportation device
- Any victim of a shallow-water incident

Any such patient should be manually stabilized in a neutral inline position (unless contraindicated) before being moved even slightly and until the need for spinal immobilization has been assessed.

Spinal cord injuries can result from improper handling. Therefore the potential consequences of a mishandled spinal column or spinal cord injury require that the prehospital care provider err on the side of caution when the mechanism of injury suggests a possible spinal cord injury. The lack of findings suggesting a spinal cord injury discovered during an examination are not sufficient cause to completely rule out the possibility. The prehospital care provider should fully assess any patient who may have sustained spinal trauma and protect the entire spine.

Anatomy and Physiology

Vertebral Anatomy

The spinal column is composed of 33 bones called *vertebrae*, which are stacked on top of one another. Except for the first (C1) and second (C2) vertebrae at the top of the spine and the fused sacral and coccygeal vertebrae at the lower spine, all of the vertebrae are nearly alike in form, structure, and motion (Figure 9-1). The largest part of each vertebra is the anterior part called the *body*. Each vertebral body bears most of the weight of the vertebral column and torso superior to it. Two curved sides called the *neural arches* are formed by the pedicle and posteriorly by the lamina. The posterior part of the vertebra is a tail-like structure called the *spinous process*. In the lower five cervical vertebrae this posterior process points directly posterior, whereas in the thoracic and lumbar vertebrae it points slightly downward in a caudad (toward the feet) direction.

Most vertebrae also have similarly styled protuberances called *transverse processes* at each side near their

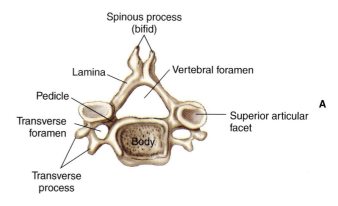

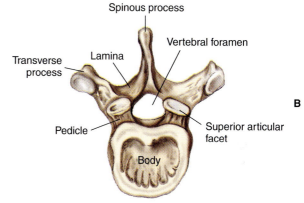

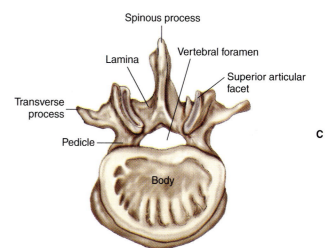

Figure 9-1   Except for the fused sacral and coccygeal vertebrae, each vertebra has the same parts as the others. The body (anterior portion) of each vertebra gets larger and stronger because it must support more weight nearing the pelvis. A, Fifth cervical vertebra. B, Thoracic vertebra. C, Lumbar vertebra.

anterior lateral margins. The transverse and spinous processes serve as points for muscle attachment and are therefore fulcrums for movement. The neural arches and the posterior part of each vertebral body form a near-circular shape with an opening in the center called the *vertebral foramen*. The spinal cord passes through this

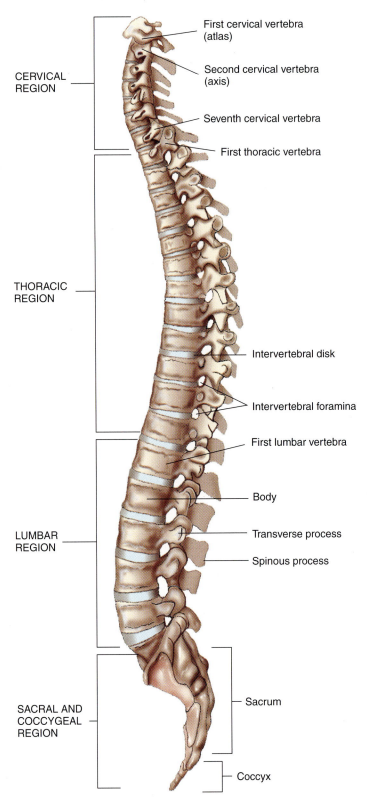

CERVICAL REGION

First cervical vertebra (atlas)

Second cervical vertebra (axis)

Seventh cervical vertebra

First thoracic vertebra

THORACIC REGION

Intervertebral disk

Intervertebral foramina

First lumbar vertebra

Body

LUMBAR REGION

Transverse process

Spinous process

SACRAL AND COCCYGEAL REGION

Sacrum

Coccyx

Figure 9-2   The vertebral column is not a straight rod, but a series of blocks that are stacked to allow for several bends or curves. At each of the curves, the spine is more vulnerable to fractures, thus the origin of the term "breaking the S in a fall."

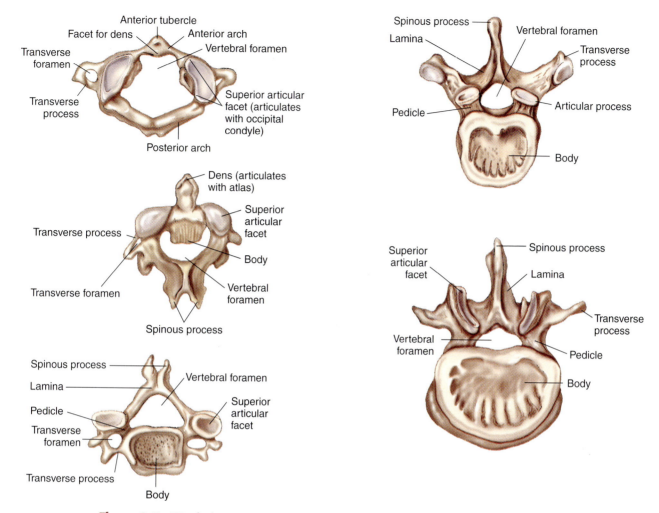

Figure 9-3   Weight bearing increases on the lower vertebral bodies, which are thick and stronger to carry this load.

opening. The cord is protected somewhat from injury by the bony vertebrae surrounding it. Each vertebral foramen lines up with that of the vertebrae above and the vertebrae below to form the hollow spinal canal through which the spinal cord passes.

Vertebral Column

As previously mentioned, the individual vertebrae are stacked on top of one another in an S-like shape (Figure 9-2). This organization allows extensive multidirectional movement while imparting maximum strength. The spinal column is divided into five individual regions for reference. Beginning at the top of the spinal column and descending downward, these regions are the cervical, thoracic, lumbar, sacral, and coccygeal regions. Vertebrae are identified by the first letter of the region in which they are found and their sequence from the top of

that region. The first cervical vertebra is called C1, the third thoracic vertebra T3, the fifth lumbar vertebra L5, and so on throughout the entire spinal column. Each vertebra supports increasing body weight as the vertebrae progress down the spinal column. Appropriately, the vertebrae from C3 to L5 become progressively larger to accommodate the increased weight and workload (Figure 9-3).

Located at the top end of the spinal column are the seven cervical vertebrae that support the head. The cervical region is flexible to allow for total movement of the head. Next are twelve thoracic vertebrae. Each pair of ribs connects posteriorly to one of the thoracic vertebrae. Unlike the cervical spine, the thoracic spine is relatively rigid with little movement. Below the thoracic vertebrae are the five lumbar vertebrae. These are the most massive of all the vertebrae. The lumbar area is also flexible,

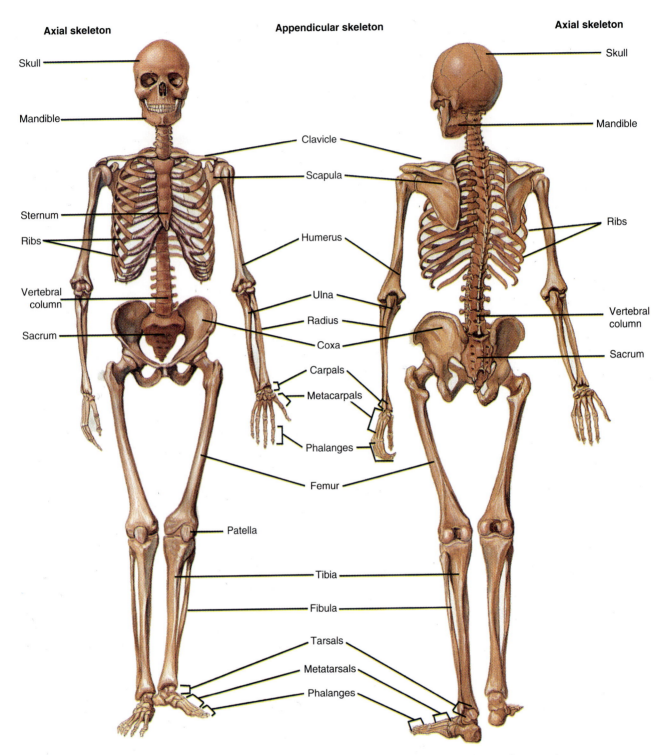

Axial skeleton   **Appendicular skeleton**   **Axial skeleton**

Skull

Mandible

Sternum

Ribs

Vertebral
column

Sacrum

Clavicle

Scapula

Humerus

Ulna

Radius

Coxa

Carpals

Metacarpals

Phalanges

Femur

Patella

Tibia

Fibula

Tarsals

Metatarsals

Phalanges

Skull

Mandible

Ribs

Vertebral
column

Sacrum

Figure 9-4   The spine is attached to the legs by attachments to the pelvis at the sacroil-
iac joints. The head is like a bowling ball that balances on top of the spine.

allowing for movement in several directions. The five
sacral vertebrae are fused, forming a single structure
known as the *sacrum*. The four coccygeal vertebrae are
also fused, forming the *coccyx* (tailbone). Approximately
55% of spinal injuries occur in the cervical region, 15%

in the thoracic region, 15% at the thoracolumbar junction, and 15% in the lumbosacral area.

   Ligaments and muscles tether the spine from the base
of the skull to the pelvis. These ligaments and muscles
form a web that sheathes the entire bony part of the

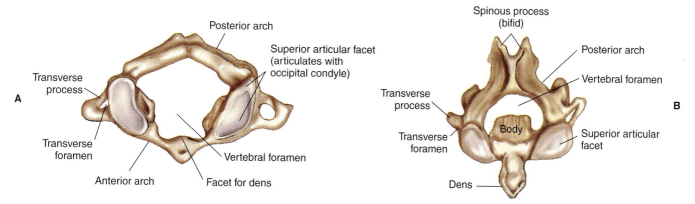

Figure 9-5 The first (A) and second (B) cervical vertebrae are shaped differently than the rest of the vertebrae of the spine. Their function is to support the skull and allow rotation and anterior-posterior motion of the head.

spinal column, holding it in normal alignment and allowing for movement. If these ligaments and muscles are torn, excessive movement of one vertebra in relation to another occurs. In the presence of torn spinal ligaments, this excessive movement may result in dislocation of the vertebrae, which can compromise the space inside the spinal canal and thus damage the spinal cord.

The anterior and posterior longitudinal ligaments connect the vertebral bodies anteriorly and inside the canal. Ligaments between the spinous processes provide support for flexion-extension (forward and backward) movement, and those between the lamina provide support during lateral flexion (side bending).

The head balances on top of the spine, and the spine is supported by the pelvis (Figure 9-4). The skull perches on the ring-shaped first cervical vertebra (C1) referred to as the *atlas*. The *axis*, C2, is also basically ring shaped but has a spur (the odontoid process) that protrudes like a tooth into the anterior arch of the atlas. The axis allows the head an approximately 180-degree range of rotation (Figure 9-5).

The human head weighs between 16 and 22 lb (7 to 10 kg), approximately the same weight as an average bowling ball. The weight and position of the head atop the thin and flexible neck, the forces that act upon the head, the small size of the supporting muscle, and the lack of ribs or other bones help make the cervical spine particularly susceptible to injury. At the level of C3, the spinal cord occupies approximately 95% of the spinal canal (the spinal cord occupies approximately 65% of the spinal canal area at its end in the lumbar region), and only 3 mm of clearance exists between the cord and the canal wall. Even a minor dislocation at this point can produce compression of the spinal cord. The posterior

neck muscles are strong, permitting up to 60% of the range of flexion and 70% of the range of extension of the head without any stretching of the cord. However, when sudden violent acceleration, deceleration, or lateral force is applied to the body, the significant weight of the head on the narrow cervical spine can amplify the effects of sudden movement.

The sacrum is the base of the spinal column, the platform upon which the spinal column rests. Between 70% and 80% of the body's total weight rests on the sacrum. The sacrum is a part of both the spinal column and the pelvic girdle, and it is joined to the rest of the pelvis by immovable joints.

Spinal Cord Anatomy

The spinal cord is continuous with the brain and starts from the base of the brain stem, passing through the foramen magnum (the hole at the base of the skull) and through each vertebra to the level of the second lumbar (L2) vertebra. Blood is supplied to the spinal cord by the vertebral and spinal arteries.

The spinal cord itself consists of gray matter and white matter. The white matter contains the anatomic spinal tracts. Spinal tracts are divided into two types:

1. *Ascending nerve tracts* carry sensory impulses from body parts through the cord up to the brain. Ascending nerve tracts can be further divided into tracts that carry the different sensations of pain and temperature; touch and pressure; and sensory impulses of motion, vibration, position, and light touch. The nerve tracts that carry pain and temperature sensation cross over in the body, meaning that the nerve root with that information from

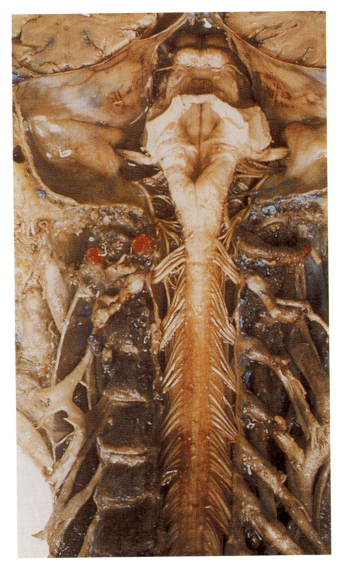

Figure 9-6 The spinal nerves branch from each side of the spinal cord to provide motor and sensory innervation to the torso and extremities.

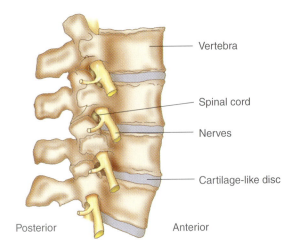

Figure 9-7 The cartilage between each vertebral body is called the *intervertebral disc*. These discs act as shock absorbers. If damaged, the cartilage may protrude into the spinal canal, compressing the cord or the nerves that come through the intervertebral foramina.

the right side of the body crosses over to the left side of the spinal cord and then goes up to the brain. In contrast, the nerve tract that carries the sensory information for position, vibration, and light touch does not cross over in the spinal cord. Thus this sensory information is carried up to the brain on the same side of the spinal cord as the nerve roots.

2. *Descending nerve tracts* are responsible for carrying motor impulses from the brain through the cord down to the body, and they control all muscle movement and muscle tone. These descending tracts also do not cross over in the spinal cord. Therefore the

motor tract on the right side of the cord controls motor function on the right side of the body. These motor tracts do cross over in the brain stem, so the left side of the brain controls motor function on the right side of the body and vice versa.

As the spinal cord continues to descend, pairs of nerves branch off from the cord at each vertebra and extend to the various parts of the body (Figure 9-6). The spinal cord has 31 pairs of spinal nerves, named according to the level from which they arise. Each nerve has two roots on each side. The dorsal root is for sensory impulses and the ventral root is for motor impulses. Neurologic stimuli pass between the brain and each part of the body through the cord and particular pairs of these nerves. As they branch from the spinal cord, these nerves pass through a notch in the inferior lateral side of the vertebra, posterior to the vertebral body, called the *intervertebral foramen*. Cartilage-like intervertebral discs lie between the body of each vertebra and act as shock absorbers (Figure 9-7).

These nerve branches have multiple control functions, and their level in the spinal cord is represented by dermatomes. A dermatome is the sensory area on the body for which a nerve root is responsible. Collectively, dermatomes allow the body areas to be mapped out for each spinal level (Figure 9-8). Dermatomes help determine the level of a spinal cord injury. Two landmarks that the prehospital care provider should keep in mind are the nipple level, which is the

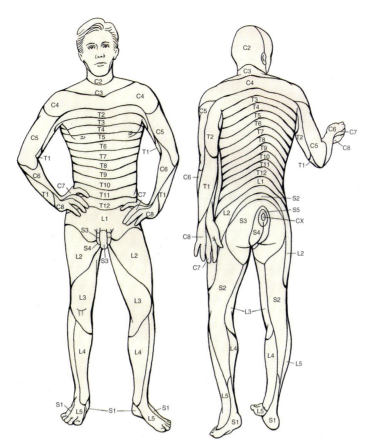

Figure 9-8 A dermatome map shows the relationship between areas of touch sensation on the skin and the spinal nerves that correspond to that area of sensation. Loss of sensation in that area may indicate injury to the spinal nerve.

T4 dermatome, and the umbilicus level, which is the T10 dermatome.

For example, in adults the process of inhalation and exhalation requires both chest excursion and proper changes in the shape of the diaphragm. The diaphragm is innervated by the phrenic nerves, which branch from the nerves arising from the cord between levels C2 and C5. If the cord above the level of C2 or the phrenic nerves are cut or the nerve impulses are otherwise disrupted, a patient will lose the ability to breathe spontaneously. Therefore this patient will need positive-pressure ventilation.

The spinal cord is surrounded by cerebrospinal fluid (CSF) and is encased in a dural sheath. This dural sheath covers the brain and continues down to the second sacral vertebra, where a saclike reservoir (the great cistern) exists. CSF produced by the brain passes around the cord and is absorbed in this cistern. CSF performs the same function for the cord as for the brain—as a cushion against injury during rapid and severe movement.

Pathophysiology

The bony spine can normally withstand forces of up to 1000 foot-pounds (1360 Joules) of energy. High-speed travel and contact sports can routinely exert forces well in excess of this amount on the spine. Even in a low- to moderate-speed vehicle crash, the body of an unrestrained 150 lb (68 kg) person can easily place 3000 to 4000 foot-pounds (4080 to 5440 Joules) of force against the spine as the head is suddenly stopped by the windshield or roof. Similar force can occur when a motorcyclist is thrown over the front of the motorcycle or when a high-speed skier collides with a tree.

Skeletal Injuries

Various types of injuries can occur to the spine, including the following:

- Compression fractures of a vertebra that can produce total body flattening of the vertebra or wedge compression

- Fractures that produce small fragments of bone that may lie in the spinal canal near the cord
- Subluxation, which is a partial dislocation of a vertebra from its normal alignment in the spinal column
- Overstretching or tearing of the ligaments and muscles, producing an unstable relationship between the vertebrae

Any of these skeletal injuries may immediately result in the irreversible cutting of the cord, or they may compress or stretch the cord. However, in some patients, damage to the vertebrae results in an unstable spinal column but does not produce an immediate cord injury. In addition, patients who have cervical spine injuries also have a 10% chance of having another spine fracture. Therefore the entire spine must be immobilized in every patient suspected of having a spinal column injury.

A lack of neurologic deficit does not rule out a bony fracture or an unstable spine. Although the presence of good motor and sensory responses in the extremities indicates that the cord is currently intact, it does not indicate the absence of injured vertebrae or associated bony or soft tissue structures. A significant percentage of patients with an unstable bony spine have no neurologic deficit. A full assessment is still required.

Specific Mechanisms of Injury that Cause Spinal Trauma

The specific mechanisms of injury that cause spinal trauma are as follows:

- *Axial loading* can occur in several ways. Most commonly, this compression of the spine occurs when the head strikes an object and the weight of the still-moving body bears against the stopped head, such as when the head of an unrestrained occupant strikes the windshield or when the head strikes an object in a shallow-water diving incident. Compression and axial loading also occur when a patient sustains a fall from a substantial height and lands in a standing position. This drives the weight of the head and thorax down against the lumbar spine while the sacral spine remains stationary. About 20% of falls from a height greater than 15 feet involve an associated lumbar spine fracture. During such an extreme energy exchange, the spinal column tends to exaggerate its normal curves, and fractures and compressions occur at such areas. The spine is S-shaped; therefore it can be said that the compressive forces tend to break the

patient's S. These forces compress the concave side and open the convex side of the spine.
- *Excessive flexion (hyperflexion), excessive extension (hyperextension),* and *excessive rotation (hyperrotation)* can cause bone damage and tearing of muscles and ligaments, resulting in impingement on or a stretching of the spinal cord.
- *Sudden or excessive lateral bending* requires much less movement than flexion or extension before injury occurs. During lateral impact, the torso and the thoracic spine are moved laterally. The head tends to remain in place until it is pulled along by the cervical attachments. The center of gravity of the head is above and anterior to its seat and attachment to the cervical spine; therefore the head will tend to roll sideways. This movement often results in dislocations and bony fractures.
- *Distraction* (overelongation of the spine) occurs when one part of the spine is stable and the rest is in longitudinal motion. This pulling apart of the spine can easily cause stretching and tearing of the cord. Distraction injury is a common mechanism of injury in children's playground injuries and in hangings.

Although any one of these types of violent movements may be the dominant cause of spinal injury in a given patient, one or more of the others will usually also be involved.

Spinal Cord Injuries

Primary injury occurs at the time of impact or force application and may cause cord compression, direct cord injury (usually from sharp or unstable bony fragments), and/or interruption of the cord's blood supply. Secondary injury occurs after the initial insult and can include swelling, ischemia, or movement of bony fragments. Cord concussion results from the temporary disruption of the spinal cord functions distal to the injury. Cord contusion involves bruising or bleeding into the spinal cord's tissues, which may also result in a temporary loss of cord functions distal to the injury (spinal "shock"). Spinal shock is a neurologic phenomenon that occurs for an unpredictable variable period of time after spinal cord injury, resulting in loss of all sensory and motor function, flaccidity and paralysis, and loss of reflexes below the level of the spinal cord injury. Cord contusion is usually caused by a penetrating type of injury or movement of bony fragments. The severity of injury resulting from the contusion is related to the amount of bleeding into the tissue. Damage to or disruption of the spinal blood supply can result in local cord tissue ischemia. Cord compression is pres-

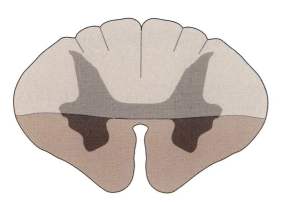

Figure 9-9   Anterior cord syndrome.

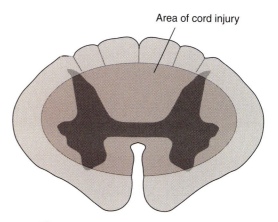

Figure 9-10   Central cord syndrome.

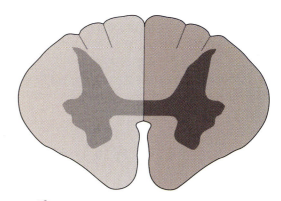

Figure 9-11   Brown-Séquard syndrome.

sure on the spinal cord caused by swelling, which may result in tissue ischemia and in some cases may require decompression to prevent a permanent loss of function. Cord laceration occurs when cord tissue is torn or cut. Neurologic deficits may be reversed if the cord has sustained only slight damage; however, it usually results in permanent disability if all spinal tracts are disrupted.

Spinal cord transection can be categorized as complete or incomplete. In complete cord transection, all spinal tracts are interrupted and all cord functions distal to the site are lost. Because of the effects of swelling, determination of loss of function may not be accurate until 24 hours after the injury. Most complete cord transections result in either paraplegia or quadriplegia depending on the level of the injury. In incomplete cord transection, some tracts and motor/sensory functions remain intact. Prognosis for recovery is greater than with complete transections. Types of incomplete cord injuries include the following:

- *Anterior cord syndrome* (Figure 9-9) is a result of bony fragments or pressure on spinal arteries. Symptoms include loss of motor function and pain, temperature, and light touch sensations. However, some light touch, motion, position, and vibration sensations are spared.
- *Central cord syndrome* (Figure 9-10) usually occurs with hyperextension of the cervical area. Symptoms include weakness or paresthesia in the upper extremities but normal strength in the lower extremities. This syndrome causes varying degrees of bladder dysfunction.
- *Brown-Séquard syndrome* (Figure 9-11) is caused by penetrating injury and involves hemitransection of the cord involving only one side of the cord. Symptoms include complete cord damage and loss of

function on the affected side (motor, vibration, motion, and position) with loss of pain and temperature sensation on the side opposite the injury.

Neurogenic "shock" secondary to spinal cord injury represents a significant additional finding. Neurogenic shock from spinal cord injury is caused by different mechanisms that result from the neurologic deficits produced by injury to the spinal cord. Injury to the vasoregulatory fibers produces loss of sympathetic tone to the vessels or vasodilation. The skin will be warm and dry and the pulse rate will be slow, but the blood pressure will be low. When the cord is disrupted, the body's sympathetic compensatory mechanism cannot maintain control of the muscles in the walls of the blood vessels below the point of disruption. These arteries and arterioles dilate, enlarging the size of the vascular container and producing relative hypovolemia and partial loss of systemic vascular resistance (SVR). Instead of the tachycardia commonly associated with hypovolemic shock, this type of injury is associated with a normal heart rate or a slight bradycardia. Neurogenic shock results from vasodilation, which may cause hypoperfusion (see p. 174).

Assessment

Spinal injury, as with other conditions, should be assessed in the context of other injuries and conditions present. The primary survey is the first priority. However, often the patient first needs to be moved. Therefore a rapid scene assessment and history of the event should determine if the possibility of a spinal injury exists. If a spinal injury might exist because of a concerning mechanism, it can only be confirmed by use of appropriate radiographic studies. This supposition also holds true for nonconcerning mechanisms until completion of the critical criteria. Therefore the patient's spine must be manually protected. The patient's head is brought into a neutral inline position, unless contraindicated (see p. 241). The head is maintained in that position until the manual stabilization is replaced with a spine immobilization device such as a half-spine board, longboard, or vest-type device. Any necessary movement done by hospital personnel involved in assessing and managing the patient should include continuous manual protection of the spine.

Using Mechanism of Injury to Assess Spinal Cord Injury

Traditionally, prehospital care providers have been taught that injury is based solely on the mechanism of injury and that spinal immobilization is required for any patient with a motion injury. This generalization has caused a lack of clear clinical guidelines for assessment of spine injuries. However, assessment for spinal immobilization should also include assessment of the motor and sensory function, presence of pain or tenderness, and patient reliability as predictors of spinal cord injury. In addition, the patient may not complain of pain in the spinal column because of pain associated with a more distracting injury, such as a fractured femur. Alcohol or drugs that the patient may have ingested may also blunt the patient's perception of pain and mask serious injury.

The primary focus of a prehospital care provider should be to recognize the indications for spinal immobilization rather than to attempt to clear the spine clinically. In most EMS runs, a delay in the field to do an in-depth neurologic motor and sensory examination in trauma patients is not a useful expenditure of time. Rather, the prehospital care provider should assume that the spine is injured, immobilize the patient on a backboard, and transport the patient to an appropriate facility where a complete examination can be accomplished. A complete neurologic examination is a time-consuming process. The field is not the environment for this to take place.

Blunt Trauma

The major causes of spinal injury in adult patients, in order of frequency, are as follows:

1. MVCs
2. Shallow water incidents
3. Motorcycle crashes
4. All other injuries and falls

The major causes of spinal injury in pediatric patients, in order of frequency, are as follows:

1. Falls from heights (generally two to three times the patient's height)
2. Falls from a tricycle or bicycle
3. Being struck by a motor vehicle

As a guideline, the prehospital care provider should assume the presence of spinal injury and an unstable spine with the following situations:

- Any mechanism that produced a violent impact on the head, neck, torso, or pelvis (e.g., assault, entrapment in a structural collapse)
- Incidents that produce sudden acceleration, deceleration, or lateral bending forces to the neck or torso (e.g., moderate- to high-speed MVCs, pedestrians struck by a vehicle, involvement in an explosion)
- Any fall, especially in the elderly
- Ejection or a fall from any motorized or otherwise powered transportation device (e.g., scooters, skateboards, bicycles, motor vehicles, motorcycles, recreational vehicles)
- Any victim of a shallow-water incident (e.g., diving or body surfing)

Other situations that are commonly associated with spinal damage include the following:

- Head injuries with any alteration in LOC
- Significant helmet damage
- Significant blunt injury to the torso or above the clavicles
- Impacted or other deceleration fractures of the legs or hips
- Significant localized injuries to the area of the spinal column

The wearing of proper seat belt restraints has proved to save lives and reduce head, face, and thoracic injuries. However, the use of proper restraints does not rule out the possibility of spinal injury. In significant frontal impact collisions when sudden severe deceleration occurs, the restrained torso stops suddenly but the unrestrained head attempts to continue its forward movement. Held by the strong posterior neck muscles, the head can only move forward slightly. If the force of deceleration is strong enough, the head then rotates down until the chin strikes the chest wall, frequently rotating across the diagonal strap of the shoulder restraint (Figure 9-12). Such rapid forceful hyperflexion and rotation of the neck can result in compression fractures of the cervical vertebrae, jumped and locked facets (dislocation of the articular processes), and stretching of the spinal cord. Different mechanisms can also cause spinal trauma in restrained victims of rear or lateral collisions. The amount of damage to the vehicle and the patient's other injuries are the key factors in determining if a patient needs to be immobilized.

The patient's ability to walk *should not* be a factor in determining whether a patient needs to be treated for spinal injury. A significant number of patients who required surgical repair of unstable spinal injuries were found "walking around" at the scene or walked into the emergency department at the hospital. An unstable spine can only be ruled out by use of radiographic examination or by a lack of any positive mechanism.

Penetrating Trauma

Penetrating injury represents a special consideration regarding the potential for spinal trauma. In general, if a patient did not sustain definite neurologic injury at the moment that the trauma occurred, there is little concern for a spinal injury. This is because of the mechanism of injury and the kinematics associated with the force involved. Penetrating objects generally do not produce unstable spinal fractures as does blunt force injury because penetrating trauma produces little risk of unstable ligamentous or bony injury. A penetrating object causes injury along the path of penetration. If the object did not directly injure the spinal cord as it penetrated, the patient will not likely develop a spinal cord injury.

Indications for Spinal Immobilization

The mechanism of injury can be used as an aid to determine indications for spinal immobilization. Figure 9-13 provides an algorithm for indications of spinal immobilization. The key point always is that a prehospital care provider should use good clinical judgment and, *if in doubt, immobilize.*

Patients who have sustained penetrating injury such as gunshot or stab wounds should be considered to have a concerning mechanism of injury when they complain of

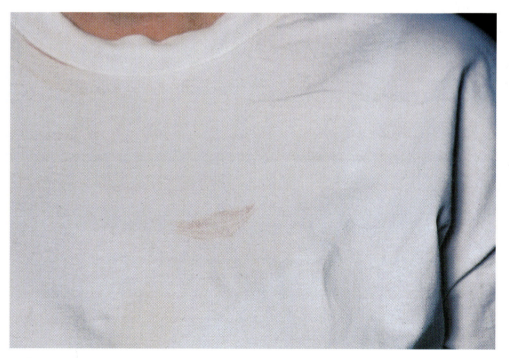

Figure 9-12 The lipstick mark on this patient's left chest indicates that the lips touched the anterior chest during impact. The severe flexion and moderate rotation resulted from head motion around the diagonal shoulder strap. The resultant injury to the patient was a locked facet at C5 and C6. The patient was correctly immobilized as a result of recognition of this sign and the proper interpretation of the information.

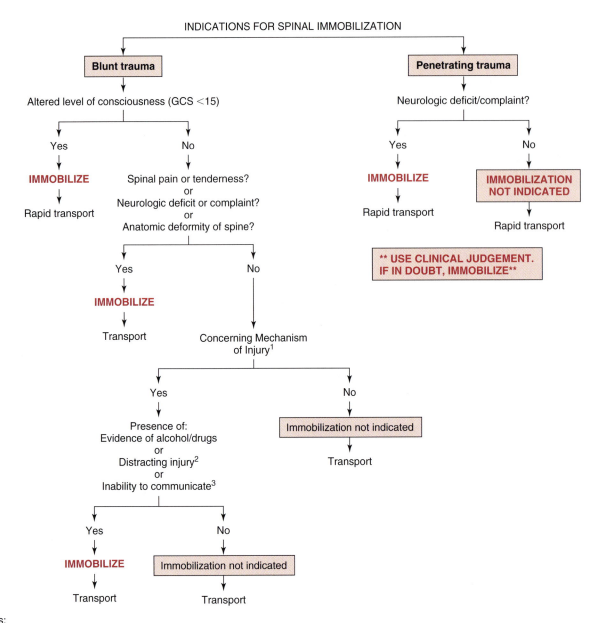

INDICATIONS FOR SPINAL IMMOBILIZATION

Blunt trauma

Altered level of consciousness (GCS <15)

Yes → **IMMOBILIZE** → Rapid transport

No → Spinal pain or tenderness?
or
Neurologic deficit or complaint?
or
Anatomic deformity of spine?

Yes → **IMMOBILIZE** → Transport

No → Concerning Mechanism of Injury[1]

Yes → Presence of:
Evidence of alcohol/drugs
or
Distracting injury[2]
or
Inability to communicate[3]

Yes → **IMMOBILIZE** → Transport

No → Immobilization not indicated → Transport

No → Immobilization not indicated → Transport

Penetrating trauma

Neurologic deficit/complaint?

Yes → **IMMOBILIZE** → Rapid transport

No → **IMMOBILIZATION NOT INDICATED** → Rapid transport

** USE CLINICAL JUDGEMENT. IF IN DOUBT, IMMOBILIZE**

Notes:
[1]Concerning Mechanisms of Injury
• Any mechanism that produced a violent impact to the head, neck, torso, or pelvis (e.g., assault, entrapment in structural collapse, etc.)
• Incidents producing sudden acceleration, deceleration, or lateral bending forces to the neck or torso (e.g., moderate- to high-speed MVC, pedestrian struck, involvement in an explosion, etc.)
• Any fall, especially in the elderly
• Ejection or fall from any motorized or human-powered transportation device (e.g., scooters, skateboards, bicycles, motor vehicles, motorcycles or recreational vehicles)
• Victim of shallow-water diving incident

[2]Distracting Injury
Any injury that may have the potential to impair the patient's ability to appreciate other injuries. Examples of distracting injuries include a) long bone fracture; b) a visceral injury requiring surgical consultation; c) a large laceration, degloving injury, or crush injury; d) large burns, or e) any other injury producing acute functional impairment.
(Adapted from Hoffman JR, Wolfson AB, Todd K. Mower WR: Selective cervical spine radiography in blunt trauma: methodology of the National Emergency X-Radiography Utilization Study [NEXUS], *Ann Emerg Med* 461, 1998.)

[3]Inability to communicate. Any patient who, for reasons not specified above, cannot clearly communicate so as to actively participate in their assessment. Examples: speech or hearing impaired, those who only speak a foreign language, and small children.

Figure 9-13   Indications for spinal immobilization.

neurologic symptoms or have findings such as numbness, tingling, or loss of motor or sensory function or actual loss of consciousness. If no neurologic complaints or findings in patients with penetrating injury exist, then the spine does not need to be immobilized (although the backboard may still be used for lifting and transport purposes).

In the setting of blunt trauma, certain conditions should mandate spinal immobolization:

1. *Altered LOC (GCS <15)*. This includes the following:
   - *Acute stress reactions (ASRs)*. ASRs are temporary responses of the autonomic nervous system. A sympathetic ASR is the "fight-or-flight" response in which bodily functions increase and pain masking occurs. A parasympathetic ASR slows bodily functions and may result in syncope. If signs of a sympathetic ASR are present, the patient is considered unreliable.
   - *Traumatic brain injury (TBI)*. TBI may involve temporary loss of consciousness and necessitate spinal immobilization of the patient. In some instances, belligerence and uncooperative behavior may be the only signs of injury.
   - *Altered mental status (AMS)*. Patients with AMS include psychiatric patients, patients with Alzheimer's disease, or patients with AMS caused by trauma. These patients should be immobilized.
2. *Spinal pain or tenderness*. This includes pain or pain on movement, point tenderness, and deformity and guarding of the spinal area.
3. *Neurologic deficit or complaint*. These include bilateral paralysis, partial paralysis, paresis (weakness), numbness, prickling or tingling, and neurogenic spinal shock below the level of the injury. In males, a continuing erection of the penis, called *priapism*, may be an additional indication of spinal cord injury.
4. *Anatomic deformity of the spine*. This includes any deformity noted upon physical examination of the patient.

However, the absence of these signs does not rule out bony spinal injury (Box 9-1).

When a patient has a concerning mechanism of injury in the absence of the conditions just listed, the prehospital care provider must consider the patient's reliability. A reliable patient is calm, cooperative, and sober. An unreliable patient may exhibit any of the following:

- *Intoxication*. Patients who are under the influence of drugs or alcohol are immobilized and managed as if they had spinal injury until they are calm, cooperative, and sober.

Box 9-1

Signs and Symptoms of Spinal Trauma

- Pain to the neck or back
- Pain on movement of the neck or back
- Pain on palpation of the posterior neck or midline of the back
- Deformity of the spinal column
- Guarding or splinting of the muscles of the neck or back
- Paralysis, paresis, numbness, or tingling in the legs or arms at any time after the incident
- Signs and symptoms of neurogenic shock
- Priapism (in males)

- *Distracting injuries*. Distracting injuries are severely painful or bloody injuries that may prevent the patient from giving reliable responses during the assessment. Examples of distracting injuries include a fractured femur or a large burn (see Figure 9-13).
- *Communication barriers*. Communication problems include language barriers, deafness, very young patients, or patients who for any reason cannot communicate effectively.

The prehospital care provider should continually recheck patient reliability at all phases of an assessment. If at any time the patient exhibits these signs or symptoms, it should be assumed that the patient has a spinal injury and full immobilization management techniques should be implemented.

In most situations the prehospital care provider may feel that the mechanism of injury is not indicative of neck injury (e.g., falling on an outstretched hand and producing a Colles' fracture). In such situations, in the presence of a normal examination and proper assessment, spinal immobilization is not indicated.

Management

The management for a suspected unstable spine is to immobilize the patient in a supine position on a rigid longboard in a neutral inline position. The head, neck, torso, and pelvis should each be immobilized in a neutral inline position to prevent any further movement of the unstable spine that could result in damage to the spinal cord. Spinal immobilization follows the common principle of fracture management (i.e., immobilizing the joint above and the joint below an injury). Because of the anatomy of the spinal column and the interaction caused by forces that affect any part of the spine, this principle simply needs to be extended to spinal immobilization. The joint above the spine means the head, and the joint below means the pelvis.

Moderate anterior flexion or extension of the arms will not cause significant movement of the shoulder girdle. Any movement or angulation of the pelvis results in movement of the sacrum and of the vertebrae attached to it. For example, lateral movement of both legs together can result in angulation of the pelvis and lateral bending of the spine.

The body is considerably wider at the hips than at the ankles. When the prehospital care provider rolls a patient to the side and allows the lower legs to remain on the ground, the patient moves out of lateral alignment, which may angulate the pelvis and result in moving the lower and midspine. Therefore in patients with suspected spine injury, the legs need to be maintained in a midline neutral position that is in line with the rest of the body. Logrolling methods that call for elevating an arm over the head when the patient is rolled on his or her side are not recommended because they can cause movement of the spine. The ankles may be elevated off the ground.

Fractures of one area of the spine are commonly associated with fractures of other areas of the spine. Therefore the entire weight-bearing spine (cervical, thoracic, lumbar, and sacral) should be considered as one entity and the entire spine immobilized and supported to achieve proper immobilization. The supine position is the most stable position to ensure continued support during handling, carrying, and transporting a patient. It also provides the best access for further examination and additional resuscitation and management of a patient. When the patient is supine, the airway, mouth and nose, eyes, chest, and abdomen can be accessed simultaneously.

Patients usually present in one of four general postures—sitting, semiprone, supine, or standing. The prehospital care provider must protect and immobilize the patient's spine immediately and continuously from the time he or she discovers the patient until he or she mechanically secures the patient to a longboard. Techniques and equipment, such as manual stabilization, half-spine boards, immobilization vests, scoop litters, proper logroll methods, or rapid extrication with full manual stabilization, are interim techniques that are used to protect a patient's spine. These techniques allow for safe movement of a patient from the position in which he or she was found until full supine immobilization on a rigid longboard can be implemented.

Prehospital care providers often focus too much on particular immobilization devices without an understanding of the principles of immobilization and how to modify these principles to meet individual patient needs. Specific devices and immobilization methods can only be safely used with an understanding of the anatomic principles that are generic to all methods and equipment. Any inflexible detailed method for using a device will not meet the varying conditions found in the field. Regardless of the specific equipment or method used, the management of any patient with an unstable spine should follow the general steps described in the next section.

General Method

When the possibility of an unstable spine exists, the prehospital care provider should do the following:

1. Move the patient's head into a proper neutral inline position (unless contraindicated) (see p. 241). Continue manual support and inline stabilization without interruption.
2. Evaluate the patient in the primary survey, and provide any immediately required intervention.
3. Check the patient's motor ability, sensory response, and circulation in all four extremities if the patient's condition allows.
4. Examine the patient's neck, and measure and apply a properly fitting, effective cervical collar.
5. Position the device, such as a shortboard or vest-type device, on the patient, or place the patient on the device, such as a long backboard.
6. Immobilize the patient's torso to the device so that it cannot move up, down, left, or right.
7. Evaluate and pad behind the patient's head or chest as needed.
8. Immobilize the patient's head to the device, maintaining a neutral inline position.
9. Once the patient is on the long backboard, immobilize his or her legs so that they cannot move anteriorly or laterally.
10. Fasten the patient's arms to the backboard.
11. Reevaluate the primary survey, and reassess the patient's motor ability, sensory response, and circulation in all four extremities if the patient's condition allows.

Manual Inline Stabilization of the Head

Once the prehospital care provider has determined from the mechanism of injury that an unstable spine exists, the first step is to provide manual inline stabilization. The patient's head is grasped and carefully moved into a neutral inline position unless contraindicated (see below). A proper neutral inline position is maintained without any significant traction. Only enough pull should be exerted on a sitting or standing patient to cause axial unweighting (taking the weight of the head off the axis and the rest of the cervical spine). The head should be constantly maintained in the manually stabilized neutral inline position until the completion of mechanical immobilization of the torso and head. In this way, the patient's head and neck are immediately immobilized and remain so until after examination at the hospital. Moving the head into a neutral inline position presents less risk than if the patient were carried and transported with the head left in an angulated position. In addition, both immobilization and transport of the patient are much simpler with the patient in a neutral position.

Movement of the patient's head into a neutral inline position is *contraindicated* in a few cases. If careful movement of the head and neck into a neutral inline position results in any of the following, the movement must be STOPPED:

- Neck muscle spasm
- Increased pain
- Commencement or increase of a neurologic deficit such as numbness, tingling, or loss of motor ability
- Compromise of the airway or ventilation

Neutral inline movement should not be attempted if a patient's injuries are so severe that the head presents with such misalignment that it no longer appears to extend from the midline of the shoulders. In these situations, the patient's head must be immobilized in the position in which it was initially found. Fortunately, such cases are rare.

Rigid Cervical Collars

Rigid cervical collars alone do not adequately immobilize; they simply aid in supporting the neck and promote a lack of movement. Rigid cervical collars limit flexion by about 90% and limit extension, lateral bending, and rotation by about 50%. A rigid cervical collar is an important adjunct to immobilization but *must always be used with manual stabilization or mechanical immobilization* provided by a suitable spine immobilization device. A soft cervical collar is of no use as an adjunct to spinal immobilization.

The unique primary purpose of a cervical collar is to protect the cervical spine from compression. Prehospital methods of immobilization (using a vest, shortboard, or a longboard device) still allow some slight movement because these devices only fasten externally to the patient, and the skin and muscle tissue move slightly on the skeletal frame even when the patient is extremely well mobilized. Most rescue situations involve movement when carrying and loading the patient. This type of movement also occurs when an ambulance accelerates and decelerates in normal driving conditions.

An effective cervical collar sits on the chest, posterior thoracic spine and clavicle, and trapezius muscles, where the tissue movement is at a minimum. This still allows movement at vertebrae C6, C7, and T1 but prevents compression of these vertebrae. The head is immobilized under the angle of the mandible and at the occiput of the skull. The rigid collar allows the unavoidable loading between the head and the torso to be transferred from the cervical spine to the collar, eliminating or minimizing the cervical compression that could otherwise result.

Even though it does not immobilize, a cervical collar aids in limiting head movement. The rigid anterior portion of the collar also provides a safe pathway for the lower head strap across the neck.

The collar must be the correct size for the patient. A collar that is too short will not be effective and will allow significant flexion. A collar that is too large will cause hyperextension or full motion if the chin is inside of it. A collar must be applied properly. A collar that is too loose will be ineffective in helping to limit head movement and can accidentally cover the anterior chin, mouth, and nose, obstructing the patient's airway. A collar that is too tight can compromise the veins of the neck.

A collar should be applied after bringing the patient's head into a neutral inline position. If the head is not in a neutral inline position, use of any collar is difficult and should not be considered. A collar that does not allow the mandible to move down and the mouth to open without motion of the spine will produce aspiration of gastric contents into the lungs if the patient vomits and therefore should not be used. Alternative methods to immobilize a patient when a collar cannot be used may include use of such items as blankets, towels, and tape. A prehospital care provider may need to be creative when presented with these types of patients. Whatever method is used, the basic concepts of immobilization should be followed.

Rigid Cervical Collars

- Do not immobilize by themselves
- Must be properly sized for each patient
- Must not inhibit a patient's ability to open his or her mouth or the prehospital care provider's ability to open the patient's mouth if vomiting occurs
- Should not obstruct or hinder ventilation in any way

Immobilization of the Torso to the Device

Regardless of the specific device that the prehospital care provider uses, he or she must immobilize the patient's torso to the device so that the torso cannot move up, down, left, or right. The rigid device is strapped to the torso and the torso to the device. The device is secured to the patient's torso so that the head and neck will be supported and immobilized when affixed to it. The patient's torso and pelvis are immobilized to the device so that the thoracic, lumbar, and sacral sections of the spine are supported and cannot move. The torso should be immobilized to the device before the head is secured. In this way, any movement of the device that may occur when fastening the torso straps is prevented from angulating the cervical spine.

Many different specific methods for immobilizing the device to the torso exist. Protection against movement in any direction—up, down, left, or right—should be achieved at both the upper torso (shoulders or chest) and the lower torso (pelvis) to avoid compression and lateral movement of the vertebrae of the torso. Immobilization of the upper torso can be achieved with several specific

methods. The prehospital care provider must understand the basic anatomic principles common to each method. Cephalad movement of the upper torso is prohibited by use of a strap on each side, fastened to the board inferior to the upper margin of each shoulder, which then passes over the shoulder and is fastened at a lower point. Caudad movement of the torso can be prohibited by use of straps that pass snugly around the pelvis.

In one method, two straps (one going from each side of the board over the shoulder, then across the upper chest and through the opposite armpit to fasten to the board on the armpit side) produce an X, which stops any upward, downward, left, or right movement of the upper torso. The same immobilization can be achieved by fastening one strap to the board and passing it through one armpit, then across the upper chest and through the opposite armpit to fasten to the second side of the board. Then a strap or cravat is added to each side and passed over the shoulder to fasten it to the armpit strap (like a pair of suspenders).

The prehospital care provider can achieve immobilization of the upper torso of a patient with a fractured clavicle by placing backpack-type loops around each shoulder through the armpit and fastening the ends of each loop in the same handhole. The straps remain near the lateral edges of the upper torso and do not cross the clavicles. With any of these methods the straps are over the upper third of the chest and can be fastened tightly without producing the ventilatory embarrassment that is commonly produced by tight straps placed lower on the thorax.

Immobilization of the lower torso can be achieved by use of a single strap fastened tightly over the pelvis at the iliac crests. If the longboard will have to be upended or

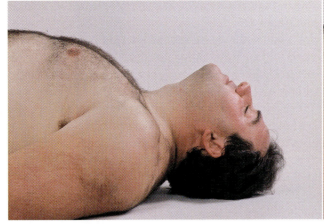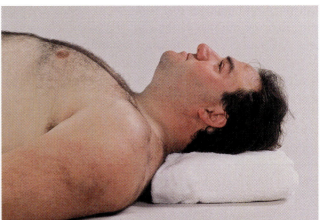

Figure 9-14   **A**, In some patients, pulling the skull back to the level of the backboard can produce severe hyperextension. **B**, Padding is needed between the back of the head and the backboard to prevent such hyperextension.

carried on stairs or over a distance, a pair of groin loops will provide stronger immobilization than the single strap across the iliac crests.

Lateral movement or anterior movement away from the rigid device at the midtorso can be prevented by use of an additional strap around the midtorso. Any strap that surrounds the torso between the upper thorax and the iliac crests should be snug but not so tight that it inhibits chest excursion or causes a significant increase in intraabdominal pressure.

Maintenance of Neutral Inline Position of the Head

In many patients, when the head is placed in a neutral inline position, the outer measurement of the occipital region at the back of the head is between ½ and 3½ inches anterior of the posterior thoracic wall (Figure 9-14, *A*). Therefore in most adults a space exists between the back of the head and the device when the head is in a neutral inline position, so suitable padding should be added before securing the head to the device (Figure 9-14, *B*). To be effective, this padding must be made of a material that does not readily compress. Firm semirigid pads designed for this purpose or folded towels can be used. The amount of padding needed must be individualized for each patient. A few individuals require none. If too little padding is inserted or if the padding is of an unsuitable spongy material, the head will be hyperextended when head straps are applied. If too much padding is inserted, the head will be moved into a flexed position. Both hyperextension and flexion of the head can increase spinal cord damage and are contraindicated.

The same anatomic relationship between the head and back is true when most people are supine—whether on the ground or on a backboard. When most adults are supine, the head falls back into a hyperextended position. Upon arrival, the prehospital care provider should move the head into a neutral inline position and manually maintain it in that position, which in many adults will require holding the head up off the ground. Once the patient is placed on the longboard and the head is about to be fastened to the board, proper padding (as described) should be inserted between the back of the head and the board to maintain the neutral position.

In small children (generally those with a body size of a 7 year old or younger), the size of the head is much larger relative to the rest of the body than it is in adults, and the muscles of the back are less developed. When a small child's head is in a neutral inline position, the back of the head usually extends between 1 and 2 inches (2.5 to 5 cm) beyond the posterior plane of the back. Therefore if a small child is placed directly on a rigid surface, the head will be moved into a position of flexion (Figure 9-15, *A*).

Placing small children on a standard longboard results in unwanted flexion. The longboard needs to be modified by either creating a recess in the board or inserting padding under the torso to maintain the head in a neutral position (Figure 9-15, *B*). The padding placed under the torso should be of the appropriate thickness so that the head lies on the board in a neutral position; too much will result in extension, too little in flexion. The padding under the torso must also be firm and evenly shaped. Use of irregularly shaped or insufficient padding, or plac-

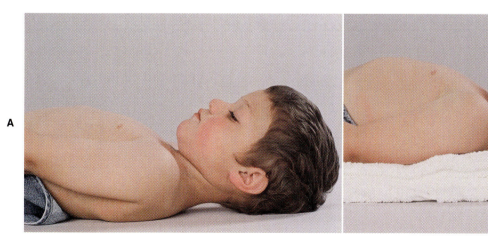

A, **B**

Figure 9-15 **A**, The larger size of a child's head relative to body size, combined with the reduced development of the posterior thoracic muscles, produces hyperflexion of the head when a child is placed on a backboard. **B**, Padding beneath the shoulders and torso will prevent this hyperflexion.

ing it under only the shoulders, can result in movement and misalignment of the spine.

Completing Immobilization

HEAD

Once the patient's torso has been immobilized to the rigid device and appropriate padding inserted behind the head as needed, the head should be secured to the device (only after securing the torso). Because of the rounded shape of the head, it cannot be stabilized on a flat surface with only straps or tape. Use of these alone will still allow the head to rotate and move laterally. Also, because of the angle of the forehead and the slippery nature of moist skin and hair, a simple strap over the forehead is unreliable and can easily slide off. Although the human head weighs about the same as a bowling ball, it has a significantly different shape. The head is ovoid, being longer than it is wide and having almost completely flat lateral sides, like a bowling ball that has had about 2 inches (5 cm) cut off its left and right sides. Adequate external immobilization of the head, regardless of method or device, can only be achieved by placing pads or rolled blankets on these flat sides and securing them with straps or tape. In the case of vest-type devices, this is accomplished with hinged side flaps that are part of the vest.

The side pieces, whether they are preshaped foam blocks or rolled blankets, are placed on the flat lateral planes of the head. The side pieces should extend to an area at least as wide as the opening of the patient's ears or beyond and stack at least as high as the level of the patient's eyes. Two straps or pieces of tape surrounding these head pieces draw the sides together. When it is packaged between the blocks or blankets, the head now has a flat posterior surface that can be realistically fixed to a flat board. The upper forehead strap is placed tightly across the front of the lower forehead (across the supraorbital ridge) to help prevent anterior movement of the head. This strap should be pulled tightly enough to indent the blocks or blankets and rest firmly on the forehead.

The use of chin cups or straps encircling the chin prevents opening of the mouth to vomit, so these devices should not be used. The device that holds the head—regardless of type—also requires a lower strap to help keep the side pieces firmly pressed against the lower sides of the head and to further anchor the device and prevent anterior movement of the lower head and neck. The lower strap passes around the side pieces and across the anterior rigid portion of the cervical collar. The prehospital care provider must ensure that this strap does not place too much pressure on the front of the collar, which could produce an airway or venous return problem at the neck. Use of sandbags secured to the longboard on the sides of the head and neck represents a dangerous practice. Regardless of how well they are secured, these heavy objects can shift and move. Should the need arise to rotate the patient and board to the side, the combined weight of the sandbags can produce localized lateral pressure against the cervical spine. Raising or lowering the head of the board when moving and loading the patient, or any sudden acceleration or deceleration of the ambulance, can also produce shifting of the bags and movement of the head and neck.

LEGS

Significant outward rotation of the legs may result in anterior movement of the pelvis and movement of the lower spine. Tying the feet together eliminates this possibility.

The patient's legs are immobilized to the board with two or more straps—one strap proximal to the knees at about midthigh and one strap distal to the knees.

The average adult measures between 14 and 20 inches (35 to 50 cm) from one side to the other at the hips and only 6 to 9 inches (15 to 23 cm) from one side to the other at the ankles. When the feet are placed together, a V shape is formed from the hips to the ankles. Because the ankles are considerably narrower than the board, a strap placed across the lower legs can prevent anterior movement but will not prevent the legs from moving laterally from one edge of the board to the other. If the board is angled or rotated, the legs will fall to the lower edge of the board, which can angulate the pelvis and produce movement of the spinal column.

One way to effectively hold the patient's lower legs in place is to encircle them several times with the strap before attaching it to the board. The legs can be kept in the middle of the board by placing blanket rolls between each leg and the edges of the board before strapping.

ARMS

For safety, the patient's arms should be secured to the board or across the torso before moving the patient. One way to achieve this is with the arms placed at the sides on the board with the palms in, secured by a strap across the forearms and torso. This strap should be snug but not so tight as to compromise the circulation in the hands.

The patient's arms should not be included in either the strap at the iliac crests or in the groin loops. If the straps are tight enough to provide adequate immobilization of the lower torso, they can compromise the circulation in the hands. If the straps are loose, they will not provide adequate immobilization of the torso or arms. Use of an additional strap exclusively to hold the arms makes it possible to open the strap for taking a blood pressure measurement or starting an intravenous line once the patient is in the ambulance without compromising the immobilization. If the arm strap is also a torso strap, loosening it to free just an arm has the side effect of loosening the torso immobilization as well.

Most Common Mistakes

The following are the three most common immobilization errors:

1. *Inadequate immobilization.* Either the device can move significantly up or down on the torso or the head can still move excessively.

2. *Immobilization with the head hyperextended.* The most common cause is a lack of appropriate padding behind the head.

3. *Readjusting the torso straps after the head has been secured.* This causes movement of the device on the torso, which results in movement of the head and cervical spine.

Complete spine immobilization is generally not a comfortable experience for the patient. As the degree and quality of the immobilization increases, the patient's comfort decreases. Spine immobilization is a balance between the need to completely protect and immobilize the spine and the need to make it tolerable for the patient.

Criteria for Evaluating Immobilization Skills

The prehospital care provider needs to practice immobilization skills in hands-on sessions using mock patients before use with real patients. When practicing or when evaluating new methods or equipment, the following generic criteria will serve as good tools for measuring how effectively the "patient" has been immobilized:

- Was manual inline stabilization initiated immediately, and was it maintained until it was replaced mechanically?
- Was an effective, properly sized cervical collar applied appropriately?
- Was the torso secured before the head?
- Can the device move up or down the torso?
- Can the device move left or right at the upper torso?
- Can the device move left or right at the lower torso?
- Can any part of the torso move anteriorly off the rigid device?
- Does any tie crossing the chest inhibit chest excursion, resulting in ventilatory compromise?
- Is the head effectively immobilized so that it cannot move in any direction, including rotation?

- Was padding behind the head used if necessary?
- Is the head in a neutral inline position?
- Does anything inhibit or prevent the mouth from being opened?
- Are the legs immobilized so that they cannot move anteriorly, rotate, or move from side to side, even if the board and patient are rotated to the side?
- Are the pelvis and legs in a neutral inline position?
- Are the arms appropriately secured to the board or torso?
- Have any ties or straps compromised distal circulation in any limb?
- Was the patient bumped, jostled, or in any way moved in a manner that could compromise an unstable spine while the device was being applied?
- Was the procedure completed within an appropriate time frame?

Many methods and variations can meet these objectives. The prehospital care provider should base selection of a specific method and specific equipment on the situation, the patient's condition, and available resources.

Summary

The vertebral column is composed of 33 separate vertebrae stacked on top of one another. Their major functions are to support the weight of the body and allow movement. The spinal cord is enclosed within the vertebral column and is vulnerable to injury from abnormal movement and positioning.

When support for the vertebral column has been lost as a result of injury to the vertebrae or to the muscles and ligaments that help hold the spinal column in place, injury to the spinal cord can occur. Because the cord does not regenerate, permanent injury, often involving paralysis, can result.

The presence of spinal trauma and the need to immobilize the patient can be indicated either by the mechanism of injury, the presence of other injuries that could only occur with sudden violent forces acting on the body, or specific signs and symptoms of vertebral or spinal cord injury. Damage to the bones of the spinal column is not always evident. If an initial injury to the cord has not occurred, a neurologic deficit may not be present even though the spinal column is unstable. The presence of any one of these indications, regardless of the absence of any of the others, should cause the prehospital care provider to assume that an unstable spine exists and to manage it accordingly.

Immobilization of spinal fractures, as with other fractures, requires immobilization of the joint above and the joint below the injury. For the spine, the joints above are the head and neck and the joints below are the torso and pelvis.

The device that the prehospital care provider uses should immobilize the head, chest, and pelvis areas in a neutral inline position without causing or allowing movement. Interim methods and devices to protect the spine can be used until the patient is immobilized in a supine position on a longboard.

Scenario Solution

This patient is exhibiting signs of head trauma and classic signs of neurogenic shock. Unopposed parasympathetic influence on the vascular system below the point of spinal injury results in an increased size of the vascular container and imposes a relative hypovolemia. The body's response to decreased tissue perfusion is normal above the point of spinal cord injury, resulting in typical signs of shock caused by sympathetic nervous system response. Patients with neurogenic shock, however, are bradycardic as opposed to tachycardic.

The first priorities of care are to continue to maintain a patent airway and oxygenation and assist ventilation to ensure an adequate minute volume while concurrently providing manual stabilization of the cervical spine. You must immobilize the patient effectively and efficiently on a long backboard and transport the patient without delay to a trauma center. You may manage hypotension caused by neurogenic shock with intravenous fluids en route to the trauma center.

The goals of prehospital management for this patient are to prevent additional spinal cord trauma, maintain tissue perfusion to prevent secondary brain injury and anaerobic metabolism, and transport without delay to a trauma center for definitive care.

Review Questions

Answers are provided on p. 414.

1. The largest percentage of spinal cord injuries are due to which of the following mechanisms?
   a. Sports injuries
   b. Motor vehicle crashes
   c. Falls
   d. Penetrating trauma

2. Which of the following is the anatomic location of most spinal injuries?
   a. Lumbar spine
   b. Thoracic spine
   c. Coccygeal spine
   d. Cervical spine

3. A spinal cord injury at which of the following levels is most likely to interfere with the patient's ventilatory effort?
   a. C5
   b. C7
   c. T2
   d. T10

4. Which of the following types of musculoskeletal injury may result in spinal cord damage?
   a. Subluxation
   b. Compression fractures
   c. Torn ligaments
   d. All of the above

5. When stabilizing the cervical spine of a patient for whom a well-fitted cervical collar is not available, it is best to do which of the following?
   a. Use a collar that is shorter than needed
   b. Use a collar that is taller than needed
   c. Use an alternative material, such as a towel
   d. Not attempt cervical spine stabilization

REFERENCES

Chan D, Goldberg R, Tascone A et al: The effect of spinal immobilization on healthy volunteers, *Ann Emerg Med* 23:48, 1994.

Cooper C, Dunham CM, Rodriguez A: Falls and major injuries are risk factors for thoracolumbar fractures: cognitive impairment and multiple injuries impede the detection of back pain and tenderness, *J Trauma* 38:692, 1995.

Cordell WH, Hollingsworth JC, Olinger ML et al: Pain and tissue-interface pressures during spine-board immobilization, *Ann Emerg Med* 26:31, 1995.

Cornwell EE III, Chang DC, Bonar JP et al: Thoracolumbar immobilization for trauma patients with torso gunshot wounds: is it necessary? *Arch Surg* 136(3):324, 2001.

Domeier RM, Evans RW, Swor RA et al: Prehospital clinical findings associated with spinal injury, *Prehosp Emerg Care* 1:11, 1997.

Domeier RM, National Association of EMS Physicians Standards and Practice Committee: Indications for prehospital spinal immobilization, *Prehosp Emerg Care* 3:251, 1997.

Marion DW, Pryzybylski G: Injury to the vertebrae and spinal cord. In Mattox KL, Feliciano DV, Moore EE, editors: *Trauma*, New York, 2000, McGraw-Hill.

Meldon SW, Moettus LN: Thoracolumbar spine fractures: clinical presentation and the effect of altered sensorium and major injury, *J Trauma* 38:1110, 1995.

Pennardt AM, Zehner WJ: Paramedic documentation of indicators for cervical spine injury, *Prehosp Disaster Med* 9:40, 1994.

Ross SE, O'Malley KF, DeLong WG et al: Clinical predictors of unstable cervical spine injury in multiply injured patients, *Injury* 23:317, 1992.

Tator CH: Spinal cord syndromes: physiologic and anatomic correlations. In Menezes AH, Sonntag VKH, editors: *Principles of spinal surgery*, New York, 1995, McGraw-Hill.

Tator CH, Fehlings MG: Review of the secondary injury theory of acute spinal cord trauma with special emphasis on vascular mechanisms, *J Neurosurg* 75:15, 1991.

Specific Skills

Spine Management

Manual Inline Stabilization

Principle: To maintain the cervical spine in a neutral inline position until the patient is completely immobilized.

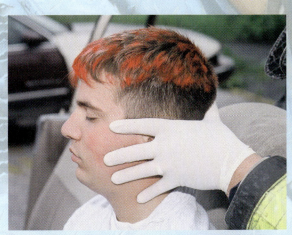

Behind

From behind the patient, the prehospital care provider places his or her hands over the patient's ears without moving the patient's head. The thumbs are placed against the posterior aspect of the patient's skull. The little fingers are placed just under the angle of the mandible. The remaining fingers are spread on the flat lateral planes of the patient's head. Pressure is applied in such a manner as to maintain the head in a stable position. If the head is not in a neutral inline position, the provider slowly moves the head until it is, unless contraindicated. The provider brings his or her arms in and rests them against the seat, headrest, or torso for additional support.

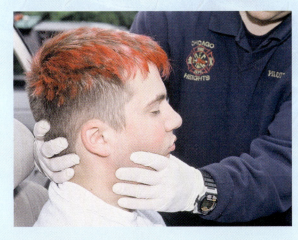

Side

Standing at the side of the patient, the prehospital care provider passes his or her arm over the patient's shoulder closest to the provider and cups the back of the patient's head with his or her hand being careful not to move the patient's head. The thumb and first finger of one hand are placed on either side of the patient's face. The thumb and finger should rest in the notch formed where the patient's teeth and maxilla join. Enough pressure is supplied to support and stabilize the patient's head. If the patient's head is not in a neutral inline position, the provider slowly moves the head until it is, unless contraindicated. The provider braces his or her elbows on the patient's torso for additional support.

Specific Skills

Front

Standing directly in front of the patient, the prehospital care provider places his or her hands on both sides of the patient's head as shown. The little fingers are placed at the posterior aspect of the patient's skull. One thumb is placed in the notch between the patient's upper teeth and the maxilla on each cheek. The remaining fingers are spread on the flat lateral planes of the patient's head. Pressure is applied in such a manner as to maintain the head in a stable position. If the patient's head is not in a neutral inline position, the provider slowly moves the head until it is, unless contraindicated. The provider brings his or her arms in and braces the elbows against the patient's torso for additional support.

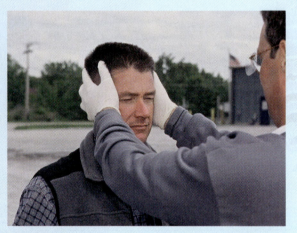

Note: The provider can also use this method when kneeling alongside the thorax of a supine patient and facing toward his or her head.

Supine Patient

The prehospital care provider positions himself or herself above the supine patient's head, either kneeling or lying. The hands are placed on either side of the patient's head, covering the patient's ears with the palms. The fingers are spread in a fashion to stabilize the patient's head with the fingers pointing toward the patient's feet (caudal). The fourth and fifth digits of each hand should wrap around the posterior portion of the patient's skull. The elbows and forearms can be rested on either the ground or the provider's knees for additional support.

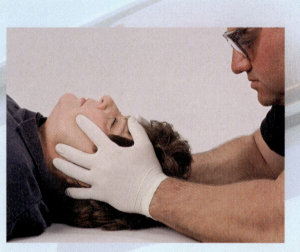

Logroll

Principle: To turn a patient while maintaining manual stabilization with minimal movement of the spine. The logroll is indicated for (1) positioning a patient onto a longboard or other device to facilitate movement of the patient and (2) turning a patient with suspected spinal trauma to examine the back.

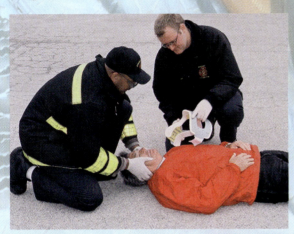

Supine Patient

While one prehospital care provider maintains neutral in-line stabilization at the patient's head, a second provider applies a properly sized cervical collar.

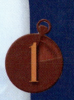

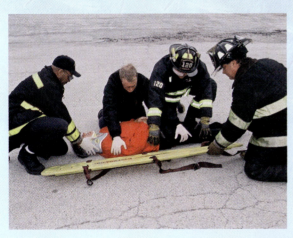

While one provider maintains neutral inline stabilization, a second provider kneels at the patient's midthorax and a third provider kneels at the level of the patient's knees. The patient's arms are straightened and placed palms-in next to the torso while the patient's legs are brought into neutral alignment. The patient is grasped at the shoulder and hips in such a fashion as to maintain a neutral inline position of the lower extremities. The patient is "logrolled" slightly onto his or her side. The long backboard is placed with the foot end of the board positioned between the patient's knees and ankles (the head of the long backboard will extend beyond the patient's head).

Specific Skills

The long backboard is held at an angle against the patient's back. The patient is logrolled onto the long backboard, and the board is lowered to the ground with the patient.

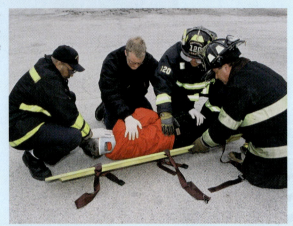

Once on the ground, the patient is grasped firmly by the shoulders, the pelvis, and the lower extremities.

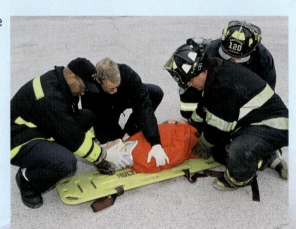

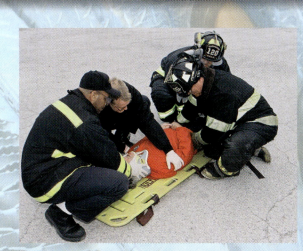

The patient is moved upward and laterally onto the long backboard. Neutral inline stabilization is maintained without pulling on the patient's head and neck.

The patient is positioned onto the long backboard with his or her head at the top of the board and his or her body centered.

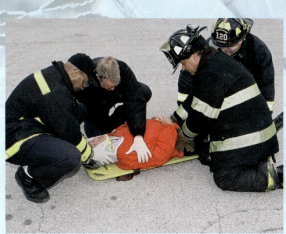

Specific Skills

Semiprone Patient

When a patient presents in a semiprone position, a stabilization method similar to that used for the supine patient can be used. The method incorporates the same initial alignment of the patient's limbs, the same positioning and hand placement of the prehospital care providers, and the same responsibilities for maintaining alignment.

The patient's arms are positioned in anticipation of the full rotation that will occur. *With the semiprone logroll method, a cervical collar can only be safely applied once the patient is in an inline position and supine on the longboard, not before.*

Whenever possible, the patient should always be rolled away from the direction in which the patient's face initially points. One provider establishes inline manual stabilization of the patient's head and neck. Another provider kneels at the patient's midthorax and grasps the patient's opposite shoulder and wrist and pelvis area. A third provider kneels at the patient's knees and grasps the patient's wrist and pelvis area and lower extremities. The long backboard is placed on the lateral edge with the foot of the board between the patient's knees and ankles.

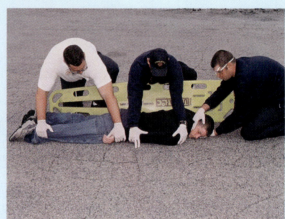

The patient is logrolled onto his or her side. The patient's head rotates less than the torso, so by the time the patient is on his or her side (perpendicular to the ground), the head and torso have come into proper alignment.

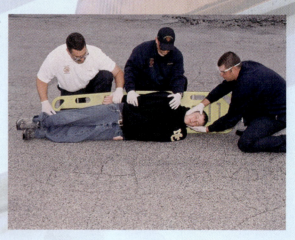

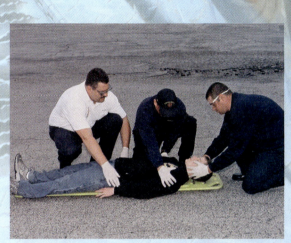

Once the patient is supine on the long backboard, the patient is moved upward and toward the center of the board. The prehospital care providers should take care not to pull the patient but to maintain neutral inline stabilization. Once the patient is positioned properly on the long backboard, a properly sized cervical collar can be applied and the patient can be secured to the backboard.

Longboard Immobilization

Principle: To fully immobilize a supine patient to a longboard while maintaining the head and neck in a neutral position and minimizing the risk of additional injuries.

Longboard immobilization is indicated when spinal immobilization is indicated (see Figure 9-13). This is not to be confused with transporting a trauma patient strapped to a longboard for ease of movement when immobilization is NOT indicated.

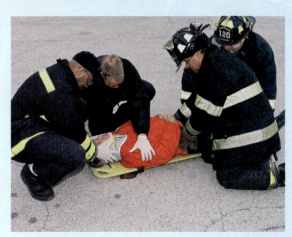

Adult Patient

The patient's head and neck are moved into a neutral inline position (unless contraindicated) (see p. 241), manual inline stabilization is maintained, and a properly sized cervical collar is applied. With an acceptable method, the patient is positioned on the long backboard.

Specific Skills

While maintaining manual stabilization, the patient's upper torso is first secured to the backboard. The lower torso (pelvis) is then secured. The patient's body must be secured in such a fashion as not to allow any movement up, down, or laterally. Padding is inserted under the patient's head as needed to maintain a neutral inline position, and pads or rolled towels are placed on each side of the patient's head.

Note: When immobilizing the patient's head to the backboard, a strap is fastened tightly over the pads and the lower forehead. A second strap is placed over the pads and the rigid cervical collar and fastened snugly to the board.

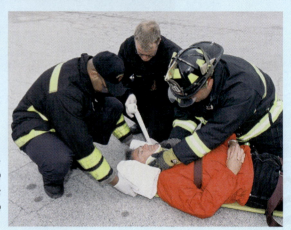

The final step in immobilizing the patient to the board is to secure the lower extremities. Padding is placed between the patient's legs and on the outside of the legs to help prevent movement. The straps are placed distal to the patient's knees and just above the knees, and the patient's lower legs are secured with the toes pointing straight up.

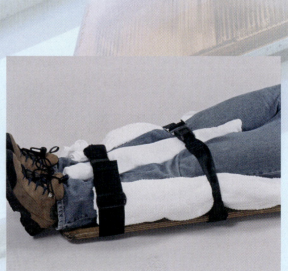

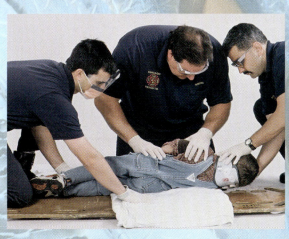

Pediatric Patient

Two major adjustments from the adult method are necessary when immobilizing a small child to a long backboard. Because of the relatively large size of the child's head in comparison to his or her body, padding is needed under the torso to elevate it and maintain the spine in a neutral alignment. The accompanying photo shows prehospital care providers preparing a child for immobilization to a long backboard. Note that the padding extends from the patient's shoulders down to the top of the pelvis and to the lateral sides of the board.

Note: Small children are usually narrower than an adult-sized backboard. Padding should be placed between the child's sides and the sides of the board to prevent lateral movement. Pediatric-sized devices take these differences into account and are preferable if available.

Standing Long Backboard Application

Principle: To fully immobilize a standing patient to a longboard while maintaining the head and neck in a neutral position and minimizing the risk of additional injury.

This application is indicated for spinal immobilization of a trauma patient who is ambulatory but is found to have an indication for spinal immobilization (see Figure 9-13).

Two general methods exist for immobilizing a standing patient to a long backboard. The first method involves securing the standing patient's torso and head to the board before lowering the board to the ground. This method causes some discomfort to the patient and may not allow the patient to be lowered to the ground without movement. The second method involves manual stabilization of the patient to the board while lowering the board and patient to the ground and then securing the patient to the board. This second method is the preferred method and can be accomplished with three rescuers.

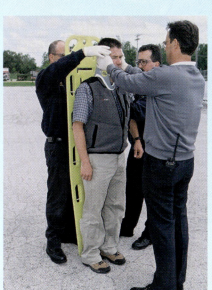

Three or More Providers

Prehospital care providers can apply manual inline stabilization from either behind the patient or in front of the patient. Once manual inline stabilization is applied, a properly sized rigid cervical collar can be applied. A long backboard is placed behind the patient from the side and pressed against the patient. Once the board is in place, manual inline stabilization is maintained until the patient is secured to the long backboard.

Specific Skills

One prehospital care provider stands on either side of the patient (turned slightly toward the patient) and inserts the hand that is closest to the patient under the patient's armpit and grasps the nearest handhold of the backboard without moving the patient's shoulders. The other hand grasps a higher handhold on the board. While manual inline stabilization is maintained, the patient and backboard are lowered to the ground.

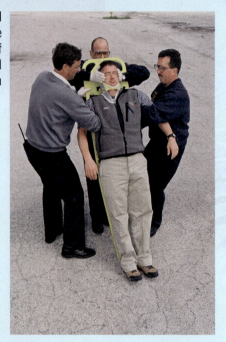

As the patient is lowered to the ground, manual stabilization is maintained through rotation of the hands. Once the patient and board are on the ground, the patient is secured to the long backboard.

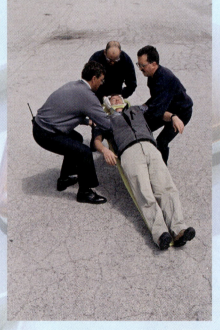

Two Providers

When three or more prehospital care providers are not available, two providers can achieve immobilization. The two providers stand on each side of the patient, turned slightly toward the patient. Each provider places his or her hand that is closest to the patient under the patient's armpit and grasps the nearest handhold on the backboard. The other hand is placed with the palm surface (finger extended) against the lateral sides of the patient's head and pressed inward toward each other to maintain manual stabilization.

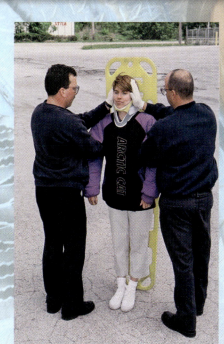

The patient is lowered, along with the backboard, to the ground. The prehospital care providers must work together during this move to ensure maximum manual stabilization. Once the patient and backboard are on the ground, manual inline stabilization is maintained while a properly sized cervical collar is applied and the patient is secured to the long backboard.

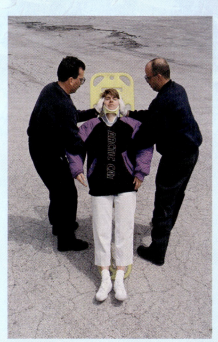

Specific Skills

Sitting Immobilization (Vest-Type Extrication Device)

Principle: To immobilize a trauma patient without critical injuries before moving him or her from a sitting position.

This type of immobilization is used when spinal stabilization is indicated for a sitting trauma patient with no life-threatening conditions.

Several brands of vest-type extrication devices are available. Each model is slightly different in design, but any one can serve as a general example. The KED is used in this demonstration. The details (but not the general sequence) are modified when using a different model or brand of extrication device. Also during this demonstration the roof and windshield of the vehicle have been removed for clarification purposes.

1 Once manual inline stabilization is initiated and a properly sized cervical collar is applied, the patient is positioned in an upright seated position with an adequate amount of space between the patient's back and the vehicle seat.

Note: Before placing the vest-type device behind the patient, the two long straps (groin straps) are unfastened and placed behind the vest device. After placing the vest device behind the patient, the side flaps are placed around the patient and moved until the side flaps are touching the patient's armpits.

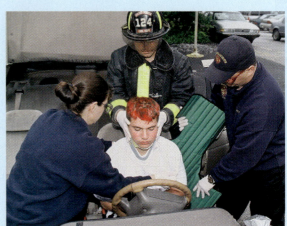

2 The torso straps are positioned and fastened, starting with the middle chest strap followed by the lower chest strap. Each strap is tightened after attachment. Use of the upper chest strap at this time is optional. If the upper chest strap is used, then the provider should ensure that it is not so tight that it impedes the patient's ventilations. The upper chest strap should be tightened just before moving the patient.

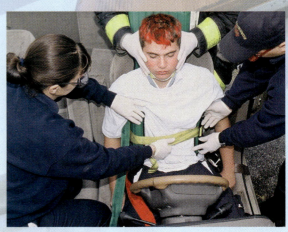

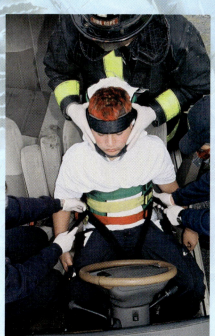

Each groin strap is positioned and fastened. Each groin strap is placed under the patient's leg and attached to the vest on the same side as the strap's origin. Using a back-and-forth motion, the strap is worked under the patient's thigh and buttock until it is in a straight line in the inter-gluteal fold from front to back. Once the groin strap is in place, each strap is tightened. The patient's genitalia should not be placed under the straps but to the side of each strap.

Note: The torso straps should be evaluated and readjusted as needed. Pads should be placed behind the patient's head as needed to maintain a neutral inline position. The head flaps will need to be positioned, which will involve careful changing of the hands supporting the patient's head. The patient's head is secured to the head flaps of the vest device. The provider should be careful not to seat the patient's mandible or obstruct his or her airway. All straps should be rechecked before moving the patient. If the upper chest strap has not been secured, it should be attached and tightened.

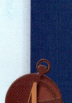

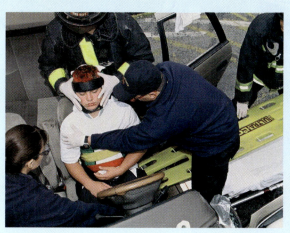

If possible, the ambulance cot with a long backboard should be brought to the opening of the vehicle door. The long backboard is placed under the patient's buttocks so that one end is securely supported on the vehicle seat and the other end on the ambulance cot. If the ambulance cot is not available or the terrain will not allow the placement of the cot, other prehospital care providers can hold the long backboard while the patient is rotated and lifted out of the vehicle.

Specific Skills

While rotating the patient, the patient's lower extremities must be elevated onto the seat. If the vehicle has a center console, the patient's legs should be moved over the console one at a time.

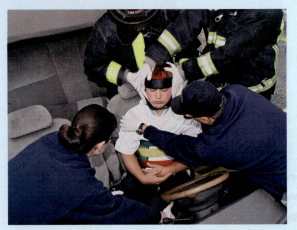

Once the patient is rotated with his or her back to the center of the long backboard, the patient is lowered to the board while keeping the legs elevated. After placing the patient onto the long backboard, the two groin straps are released and the patient's legs are lowered. The patient is positioned by moving him or her up on the board with the vest device in place. The provider should consider releasing the upper chest strap at this time.

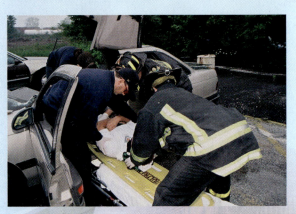

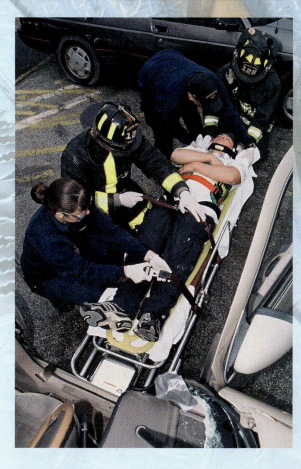

Once the patient is positioned on the long backboard, the vest device is left secured in place to continue to immobilize the patient's head, neck, and torso. The patient and vest device are secured to the long backboard. The patient's lower extremities are immobilized to the board, and the long backboard is secured to the ambulance cot.

Rapid Extrication

Principle: To manually stabilize a patient with critical injuries before and during movement from a sitting position.

Three or More Providers

Sitting patients with life-threatening conditions and indications for spinal immobilization (see Figure 9-13) can be rapidly extricated. Immobilization to an interim device before moving the patient provides more stable immobilization than when using only the manual (rapid extrication) method. However, it requires an additional 4 to 8 minutes to complete. The prehospital care provider should use the vest or halfboard methods in the following situations:

• When the scene and patient's condition are stable and time is not a primary concern

or

• When a special rescue situation involving substantial lifting or technical rescue hoisting exists, and significant movement or carrying of the patient is involved before it is practical to complete the supine immobilization to a longboard

Rapid extrication is indicated in the following situations:
• When the patient has life-threatening conditions identified during the primary survey
• When the scene is unsafe and clear danger to the prehospital care provider and patient exists, necessitating rapid removal to a safe location
• When the patient needs to be moved quickly to access other more seriously injured patients

Note: Rapid extrication is only selected when life-threatening conditions are present and not on the basis of personal preference.

Specific Skills

1 Once the decision is made to rapidly extricate a patient, manual inline stabilization of the patient's head and neck in a neutral position is initiated. This is best accomplished from behind the patient. If a provider is unable to get behind the patient, manual stabilization can be accomplished from the side. Whether from behind the patient or the side, the patient's head and neck are brought into a neutral alignment, a rapid assessment of the patient is performed, and a properly sized cervical collar is applied. An ambulance cot with a long backboard should be placed next to the open vehicle door.

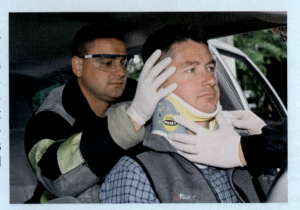

2 While manual stabilization is maintained, the patient's upper torso and lower torso and legs are controlled. The patient is rotated in a series of short, controlled movements until control of manual stabilization can no longer be maintained.

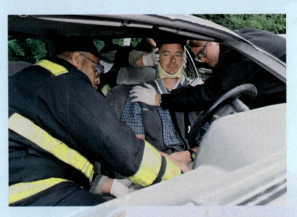

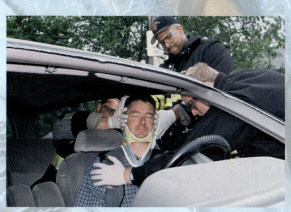

A second prehospital care provider goes outside the vehicle and takes control of the manual stabilization. The provider in the back seat moves and takes control of the patient's lower torso and legs.

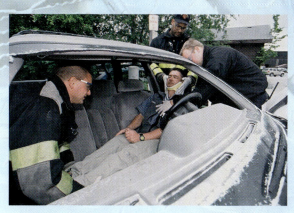

The rotation of the patient is continued until the patient can be lowered out of the vehicle door opening and onto the long backboard. The long backboard is placed with the foot end of the board onto the vehicle seat and the head end on the ambulance cot. If the cot cannot be placed next to the vehicle, other prehospital care providers can hold the long backboard while the patient is lowered onto the backboard.

Specific Skills

Once the patient's torso is down on the board, the weight of the patient's chest is controlled while the patient's pelvis and lower legs are controlled. The patient is moved upward onto the long backboard. The prehospital care provider who is maintaining manual stabilization should take caution not to pull the patient but to support the patient's head and neck.

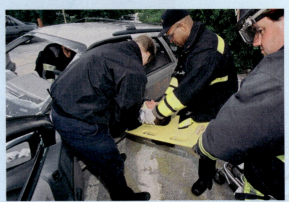

After the patient is positioned onto the long backboard, the prehospital care providers can secure the patient to the board and the board to the ambulance cot. The patient's upper torso is secured first, then the lower torso and pelvis area, then the head. The patient's legs are secured last. If the scene is unsafe, the patient should be moved to a safe area before being secured to the board or cot.

Note: This represents only one example of rapid extrication. Because very few field situations are ideal, prehospital care providers may need to modify the steps for extrication for the particular patient and/or situation. The principle of rapid extrication should remain the same regardless of the situation—maintain manual stabilization throughout the extrication process without interruption and maintain the entire spine in an inline position without unwanted movement. Any positioning of the prehospital care providers that works can be successful. However, numerous position changes and hand position takeovers should be avoided because they invite a lapse in manual stabilization.

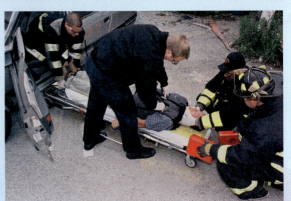

The rapid extrication technique can effectively provide manual inline stabilization of the patient's head, neck, and torso throughout a patient's removal from a vehicle. The following are three key points of rapid extrication:

1. One prehospital care provider *must* maintain stabilization of the patient's head and neck at all times, another must rotate and stabilize the patient's upper torso, and a third must move and control the patient's lower torso, pelvis, and lower extremities.
2. Maintaining manual inline stabilization of the patient's head and neck is impossible if attempting to move the patient in one continuous motion. The prehospital care providers must limit each movement, stopping to reposition and prepare for the next move. Undue haste will cause delay and may result in movement of the spine.
3. Each situation and patient may require adaptation of the principles of rapid extrication. This can only work effectively if the maneuvers are practiced. Each provider must know the actions and movements of the other providers.

Two Providers

In some situations an adequate number of providers may not be available to rapidly extricate a critical patient. In these situations a two provider technique is useful.

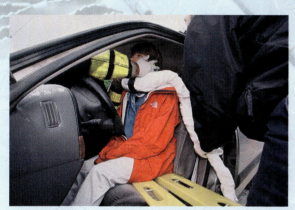

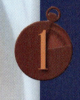

One prehospital care provider initiates and maintains manual inline stabilization of the patient's head and neck. A second provider places a properly sized cervical collar on the patient and places a prerolled blanket around the patient. The center of the blanket roll is placed at the patient's midline on the rigid cervical collar. The ends of the blanket roll are wrapped around the cervical collar and placed under the patient's arms.

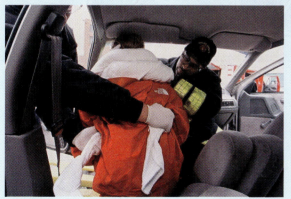

The patient is turned using the ends of the blanket roll and until the patient's back is centered on the door opening.

Specific Skills

3 The first provider takes control of the blanket ends, moving them under the patient's shoulders, and moves the patient by the blanket while the second provider moves and controls the patient's lower torso, pelvis, and legs.

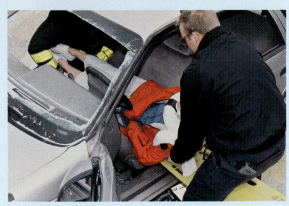

Helmet Removal

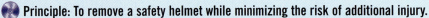
Principle: To remove a safety helmet while minimizing the risk of additional injury.

Patients who are wearing full face helmets must have the helmet removed early in the assessment process. This provides immediate access to assess and manage a patient's airway and ventilatory status. It ensures that hidden bleeding is not occurring into the posterior helmet, and allows the provider to move the head (from the flexed position caused by large helmets) into neutral alignment. It also permits complete assessment of the head and neck in the secondary survey and facilitates spinal immobilization when indicated (see Figure 9-13). The prehospital care provider should explain to the patient what is going to happen. If the patient verbalizes that the provider should not remove the helmet, the provider should explain that properly trained personnel can remove it by protecting the patient's spine. Two providers are required for this maneuver.

1 One provider takes position above the patient's head. With his or her palms pressed on the sides of the helmet and fingertips curled over the lower margin, the first provider stabilizes the helmet, head, and neck in as close to a neutral inline position as the helmet allows. A second provider kneels at the side of the patient, opens or removes the face shield if needed, and undoes or cuts the chinstrap.

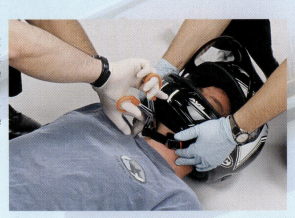

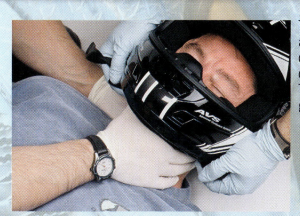

The patient's mandible is grasped between the thumb and the first two fingers at the angle of the mandible. The other hand is placed under the patient's neck on the occiput of the skull to take control of manual stabilization. The provider's forearms should be resting on the floor or ground or on his or her thighs for additional support.

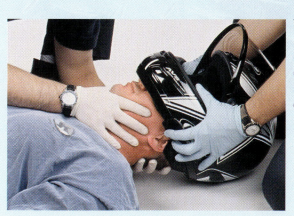

The first provider pulls the sides of the helmet slightly apart, away from the patient's head, and rotates the helmet with up-and-down rocking motions while pulling it off of the patient's head. Movement of the helmet is slow and deliberate. The provider takes care as the helmet clears the patient's nose.

Specific Skills

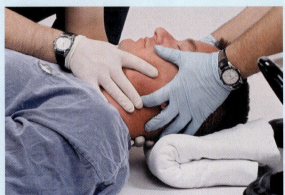

4

Once the helmet is removed, padding should be placed behind the patient's head to maintain a neutral inline position. Manual stabilization is maintained, and a properly sized cervical collar is placed on the patient.

Note: Two key elements are involved in helmet removal:
1. *While one provider maintains manual stabilization of the patient's head and neck, the other provider moves. At no time should both providers be moving their hands.*
2. *The provider must rotate the helmet in different directions, first to clear the patient's nose and then to clear the back of the patient's head.*

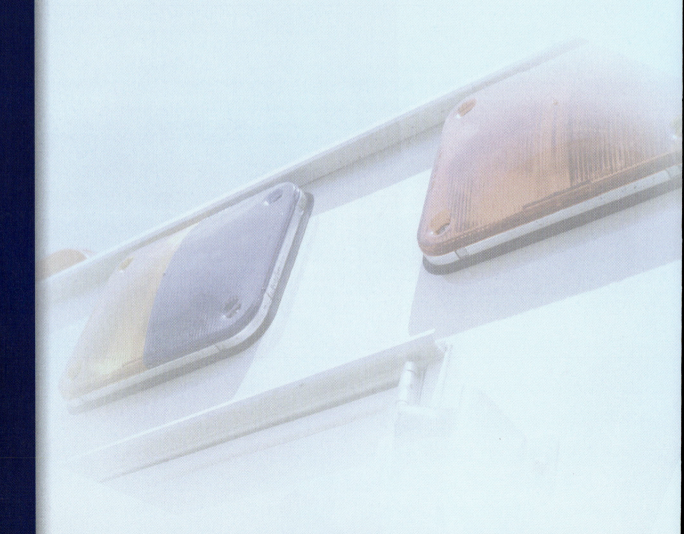

Padding to Maintain a Neutral Inline Position

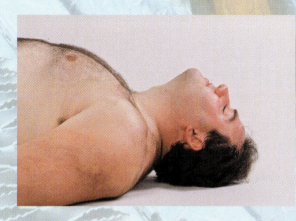

Failure to properly pad behind the patient's head can result in either hyperextension or hyperflexion of the patient's neck. This may result in excessive movement of the spine and or compromise the airway.

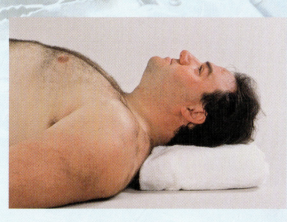

Proper padding behind the head will place the head and neck in a neutral inline position. Each patient will require different amounts of padding based on his or her body type. Proper alignment will have the opening of the patient's ear in line with the point of his or her shoulder, with his or her face centered on the midline.

Padding to Secure the Patient to the Long Backboard

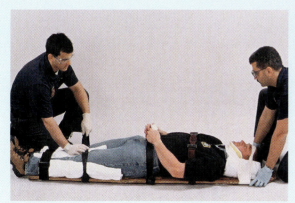

When securing a patient to a long backboard, the provider must fill all voids between the sides of the patient and the sides of the long backboard with padding. Filling the side voids with proper strapping will help prevent the patient from moving laterally on the board.

Chapter 10

Musculoskeletal Trauma

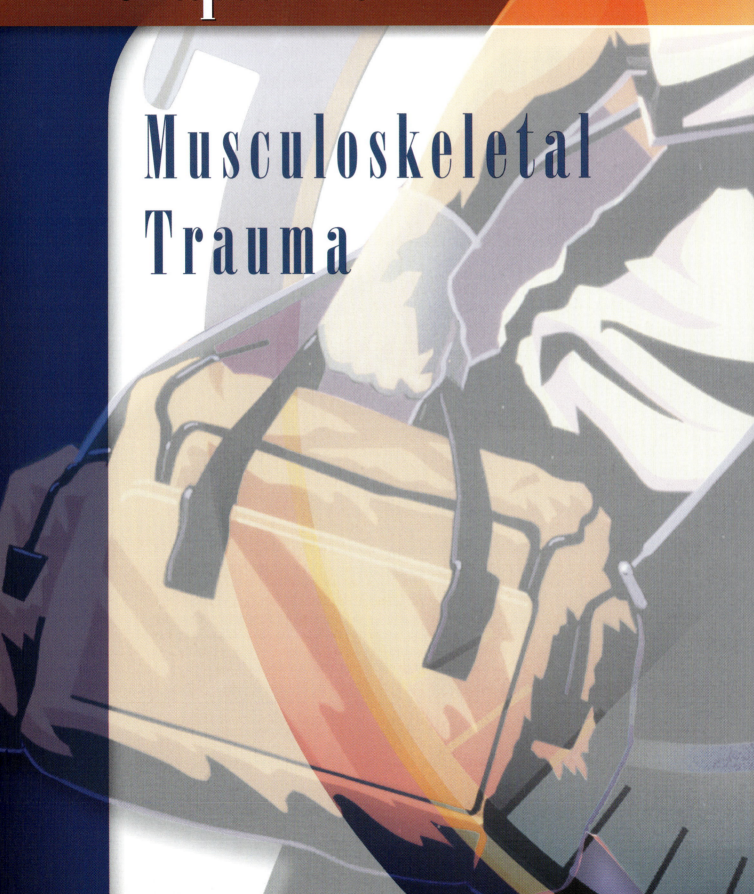

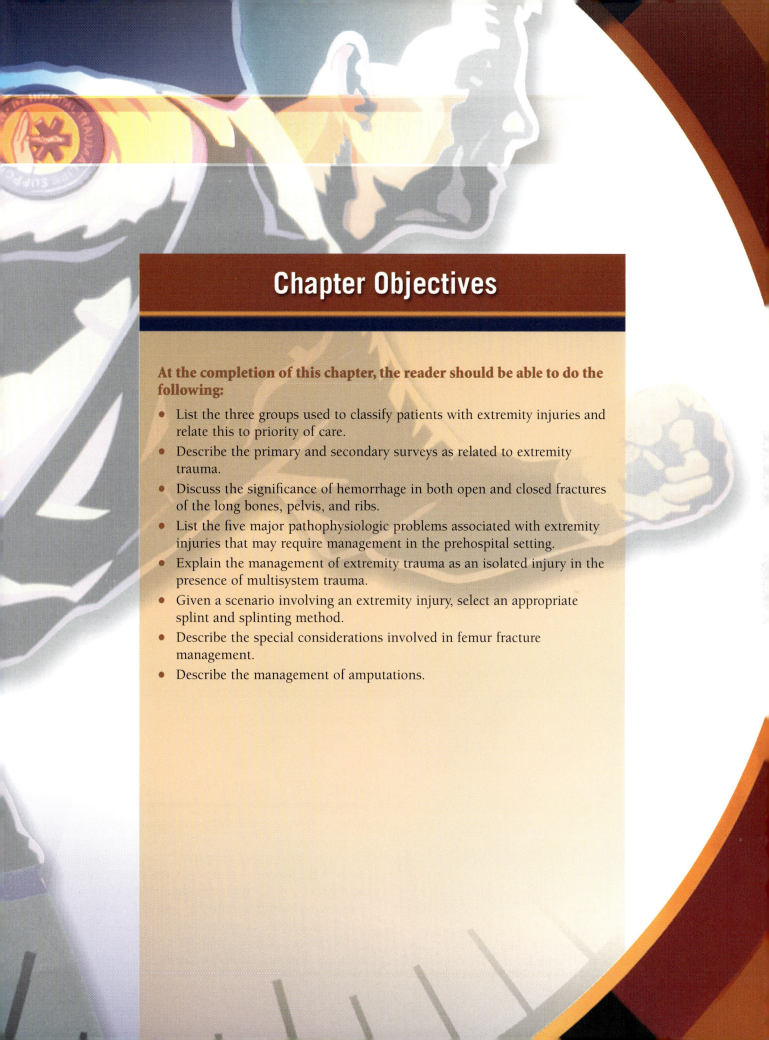

Chapter Objectives

At the completion of this chapter, the reader should be able to do the following:

- List the three groups used to classify patients with extremity injuries and relate this to priority of care.
- Describe the primary and secondary surveys as related to extremity trauma.
- Discuss the significance of hemorrhage in both open and closed fractures of the long bones, pelvis, and ribs.
- List the five major pathophysiologic problems associated with extremity injuries that may require management in the prehospital setting.
- Explain the management of extremity trauma as an isolated injury in the presence of multisystem trauma.
- Given a scenario involving an extremity injury, select an appropriate splint and splinting method.
- Describe the special considerations involved in femur fracture management.
- Describe the management of amputations.

Scenario

You and your partner are called to the scene of a single vehicle versus utility pole collision. On arrival at the scene you find a vehicle resting on all four tires, partially wrapped around a utility pole on the driver's side. The extrication crew informs you that the vehicle is safe for entry and disentanglement will take no more than 4 minutes. Upon gaining access to your patient, you find an alert 23-year-old male complaining of severe upper left arm pain and who appears short of breath. The patient's skin color is pale, he is tachycardic and tachypneic, and his skin is warm.

How would you complete the assessment on this patient? What injuries would you expect to find? How does the mechanism of injury lead you to these expectations? What is your first priority in the care of this patient? What is your second priority in the care of this patient? On what body systems should you focus your treatment of this patient?

Extremity injury, although common in trauma patients, rarely poses an immediate life-threatening condition. Extremity trauma can be life-threatening when it produces severe blood loss (hemorrhage), either externally or from internal bleeding into the extremity.

When caring for a critical trauma patient, there are two primary considerations with regard to extremity injuries:

1. Do not overlook a life-threatening condition in the extremities or a life-threatening condition caused by an extremity injury.
2. The presence of horrible looking but noncritical extremity injuries must not distract from caring for life-threatening injuries to other areas of the body (Figure 10-1).

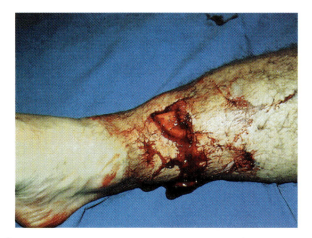

Figure 10-1   An open injury of the lower leg with protruding bone ends. (*From Vallotton J:* Color atlas of mountain medicine, *St Louis, 1991, Mosby.*)

If a life-threatening or potentially life-threatening condition is discovered anywhere in the body during the primary survey (initial assessment), the secondary survey (focused history and physical examination) should not be started. Any deficiencies found during the primary survey should be corrected before moving to the secondary survey. This may mean delaying the secondary survey until the patient is en route or even until arrival at the emergency department.

Each critical trauma patient is secured to a longboard in a supine position, with as much normal anatomic positioning as possible, to allow for resuscitation. This positioning is called *anatomic splinting*. Securing the patient to the longboard can effectively support and splint every bone and joint. If this can be done in an efficient manner, it will not detract from focusing on critical conditions. The prehospital care provider is not responsible for differentiating among the types of musculoskeletal injuries, but for identifying and treating life-threatening injuries and, if time permits, identifying and stabilizing extremity injuries.

Anatomy and Physiology

Understanding the gross anatomy and physiology of the human body is an important piece of the prehospital care provider's fund of knowledge. Anatomy and physiology is the foundation on which assessment and management are based. Without a good grasp of the structures of the bones and muscles, one will not be able to relate mechanism of injury (MOI) and superficial injuries to injuries that are internal. Although this textbook does not discuss all of the anatomy and physiology of the musculoskeletal system, it reviews some of the basics.

The mature human body has approximately 206 bones separated into categories by shape—long, short, flat, sutural, and sesamoid. Long bones have a greater length than width (e.g., femur, humerus, and radius). Short bones are nearly equal in length and width (e.g.,

metacarpals and metatarsals). Flat bones are usually thin and compact (e.g., sternum, ribs, and scapulae). Sutural bones are part of the skull and are located between the joints of certain cranial bones. Sesamoid bones are bones located within tendons over a bony surface. The patella is the largest sesamoid bone (Figure 10-2).

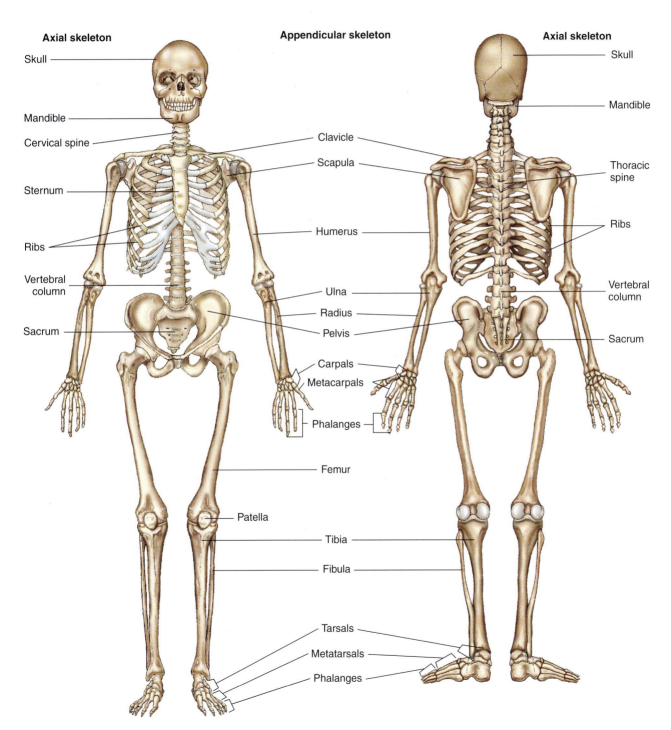

Figure 10-2   Appendicular skeleton.

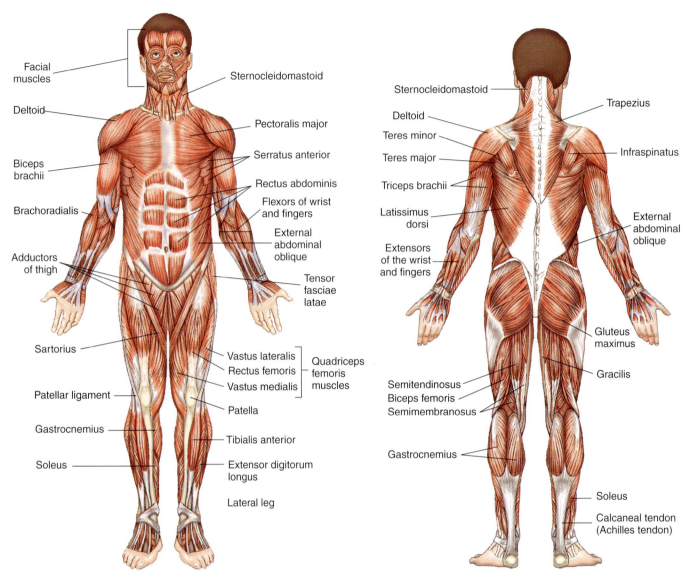

Figure 10-3   Muscular system.

The human body has over 700 individual muscles, which are categorized by function. The muscles that are specific to this chapter are the voluntary or skeletal muscles. They are termed *skeletal* because they move the skeletal system. Muscles in this category voluntarily move the structures of the body (Figure 10-3).

Other important structures discussed in this chapter are *tendons* and *ligaments*. A tendon is a band of tough, inelastic, fibrous tissue that connects a muscle to bone. It is the white part at the end of a muscle that directly attaches a muscle to the bone that it will move. A ligament is a band of tough, fibrous tissue connecting bone to bone. It is strong, and its function is to hold joints together.

Pathophysiology

Injuries to the extremities result in five major problems that require prehospital management:

1. Hemorrhage
2. Instability (fractures and dislocations)
3. Soft tissue injury (strains and sprains)
4. Loss of tissue (amputation)
5. Compartment syndrome.

The first four are discussed in this chapter. Compartment syndrome is discussed in the Appendix.

Hemorrhage

Hemorrhage is the loss of blood from the vessels of the vascular system. The torn vessels can be large or small. The ability of the body to respond to and control these tears is a function of the size of the vessel, the pressure within the vessel, the presence of clotting factors, and the ability of the vessel to go into spasm. This means that the rate of blood loss is directly related to the size of the hole in the blood vessel and the transmural pressure. Imagine the blood vessels as plumbing inside a home and the water inside the pipes as blood. If the plumbing has a leak, the amount of water lost is directly related to the size of the hole and the transmural pressure inside the pipe. For example, if the hole in the pipe is 1 inch (2.54 cm) in diameter and the pressure inside the plumbing is 100 psi, more water will leak out than if the hole is 1 inch (2.54 cm) in diameter and the pressure inside the plumbing is 50 psi. This was first described by Bernoulli, a Swiss mathematician, with the following equation. The specifics of the equation are just nice to know, but the principle itself is important. The equation explains how the size of the hole and the transmural pressure are directly related to the amount of blood that will escape thorough the hole:

$$Q = \frac{AP + 2V}{E}$$

where Q is the rate of leakage, A is the area of laceration, P is the transmural pressure (intraluminal pressure minus extraluminal pressure), E is the density of fluid media, and V is the velocity of fluid flow (inside the vessel).

The blood flow or rate of leakage out of a laceration in a vessel is proportional to the difference between the size of the hole in the vessel wall and the intraluminal and extraluminal pressures. The first step in the management of hemorrhage should be to increase the extramural pressure (pressure on skin or over laceration) by applying external pressure on the area overlying the injury. As opposed to the pipes inside a home, blood vessels are compressible. Compression of the blood vessels will decrease the amount of blood loss. Increasing external pressure (applying direct pressure to the injury) serves two purposes:

1. It reduces the transmural pressure, thus reducing blood loss.
2. It compresses the sides of the torn vessel, reducing the area of the opening and reducing blood flow out of the vessel. For example, if a garden hose has a

hole in it while the water is running, one can decrease the amount of water lost by applying pressure to the outside of the hose. This maneuver reduces transmural pressure and makes the defect smaller, changing two parts of the Bernoulli equation. The outcome is reduced water loss.

Although the body has other mechanisms of hemorrhage control, such as clotting factors and vessel spasm, the prehospital care provider has the most control over the mechanical measures (direct pressure).

Instability of the Bone or Joint

Tears of the supporting structures of a joint, fracture of a bone, or major muscle or tendon injury affect the capability of an extremity to support itself. The two divisions of instability to the bone or joint are fractures and dislocations.

FRACTURES

If a bone is fractured, immobilizing it will reduce the potential for further injury and pain to the patient. Movement of the sharp ends of the bone inside the muscle and in the vicinity of vessels and nerves can produce significant additional injuries.

The two general types of fractures are open fractures and closed fractures. Fractures are further defined as greenstick, comminuted, etc. This text does not discuss all of the types of fractures because it does not alter field management.

Closed fractures are fractures in which the bone has been broken but the patient has no loss of skin integrity (i.e., the skin is intact) (Figure 10-4). Closed fractures can range in seriousness from a hairline fracture (a crack along the shaft of the bone) to a comminuted fracture (splintering or crushing of a bone).

Closed fractures may produce an additional source for major internal hemorrhage into tissue compartments. An example is a closed femur fracture. Closed fractures can result in significant internal blood loss. A femur may be broken in several places, or the fracture may be comminuted. Each site has the potential for large amounts of blood loss by laceration of the vessels or the vascular muscles near the fracture site. A total blood loss of 1000 to 2000 mL per thigh can occur. Because of the natural tamponade effect of the surrounding tissue, muscles, and skin, smaller quantities of hemorrhage are more common.

Another example of a fracture that may result in a large volume of blood loss is a pelvic fracture. As a blood-manufacturing center of the body, the pelvis has a large blood supply. Multiple vascular plexuses lie

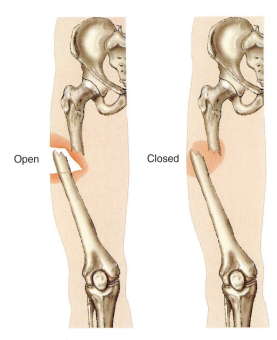

Figure 10-4 Open versus closed fracture.

adjacent to the pelvis, especially on the inner surface. An unstable pelvis associated with a rapidly distending abdomen is an indication of a large volume of blood loss; proper immobilization and rapid transport are required. As with other fractures, compression and fracture stabilization are important to control hemorrhage. A pneumatic antishock garment (PASG) is helpful in controlling pelvic hemorrhage; in this situation the PASG is not controversial and it works well (see Chapter 6).

Open fractures are those in which the integrity of the skin has been interrupted. They are usually caused by bone ends perforating the skin from the inside or the crushing or laceration of the skin by an object at the time of the injury. A laceration caused by bone ends is common and may or may not cause a gross hemorrhage. The prehospital care provider should not try to replace the bones; however, the bones occasionally return to a near-normal position when realigned or by the muscle spasms that usually occur with fractures. Complications of open fractures include external hemorrhage, further damage to the muscles and nerves, and bone infection.

DISLOCATIONS

Joints are held together by ligaments between the bones. The bones are attached to muscles by tendons. Joint movement is accomplished by muscles contracting (shortening). Reduction of muscle length pulls the tendons that are attached to a bone and moves the extremity. A dislocation is a separation of two bones at the joint (whereas a fracture is a separation of two pieces of broken bone). A

dislocation produces an area of instability that the prehospital care provider must secure. Dislocations can produce a great deal of pain and can be difficult to distinguish from a fracture. Individuals with prior dislocations have a more lax supporting structure and can have frequent dislocations. These patients usually know what the problem is and can help in assessment and stabilization.

Soft Tissue Injury

Injuries to muscles and ligaments are more common than injuries to bones. Soft tissue injuries occur when a joint or muscle is torn or stretched beyond its normal limits. Strains and sprains are two types of these injuries. Differentiation between these two injuries is very difficult without radiographic study.

A *strain* is a soft tissue injury that involves the tearing of muscle fibers that can occur anywhere in the musculature. Strains are characterized by pain with movement, with little or no swelling.

A *sprain* is an injury in which ligaments are stretched or partially torn. Sprains are characterized by extreme pain, swelling, and possible hematoma. Externally, they may look like a fracture. Sprains are caused by a sudden twisting of the joint beyond its normal range of motion. Definitive differentiation between a sprain and a fracture is available only through a radiographic study.

Loss of Tissue

When tissue has been totally separated from an extremity, the tissue is completely without nutrition and oxygenation. This type of injury is termed *amputation* or *avulsion*. An amputation is the loss of part or all of a limb, and an *avulsion* involves the tearing away of soft tissue. Initially bleeding may be severe with these injuries; however, the body's defense mechanism will cause the vessels at the injured site to constrict, and the blood loss may diminish. Local trauma can break apart the clots or interrupt the spasm, and bleeding can reoccur.

The longer the amputated portion is without oxygen, the less likely that it can be replaced successfully. Cooling the amputated body part—without freezing it—will reduce the metabolic rate and prolong this critical time.

Assessment

Within the scope of triage, musculoskeletal trauma can be categorized into three main types:

1. Isolated non–life-threatening musculoskeletal trauma (isolated limb fractures)

2. Non–life-threatening musculoskeletal trauma, but with multisystem life-threatening trauma (life-threatening injuries and limb fractures)
3. Definite musculoskeletal life-threatening injuries (pelvic and femur fractures with life-threatening blood loss)

The purpose of the primary survey is to identify and treat life-threatening injuries. The presence of a non–life-threatening musculoskeletal injury can be an indicator of a possible multisystem trauma. The prehospital care provider should ask the following questions in this situation:

- If enough lateral force was delivered to fracture a humerus, a bone covered by thick muscle, can there also be damage to the lungs?
- Could a potential life-threatening injury exist to the thoracic region or the organs of the upper abdomen with a simple rib fracture?
- Could a potential life-threatening injury occur with multiple lacerations to the face and fractures to the underlying bony structures of the maxilla, mandible, and frontal bones of the face?

The answer to all of these questions is yes. Although the prehospital care provider must not be distracted by the presence of musculoskeletal trauma, he or she must recognize the injuries as possible indicators of the presence of life-threatening injuries. This action may delay or even prevent a potential life-threatening injury from becoming life-threatening.

Mechanism of Injury

Determining the MOI is one of the most important functions that a prehospital care provider performs to adequately begin the management of a trauma patient. Rapidly determining the MOI and low- versus high-energy transference (e.g., falling from a bike versus being thrown from a motorcycle) will lead the prehospital care provider to the recognition of most critical injuries. Optimally, the best source for the MOI is directly from the patient. If the patient is unresponsive, details of the injury mechanism can be obtained from witnesses. Often a "best guess" approach to the events based on injuries can be used if no one was present at the time of the incident. This information should be reported to the receiving facility and documented on the run report.

Based on the history of the MOI obtained, the prehospital care provider should already have a high index of suspicion as to the injuries that a patient sustained. Primary injuries are the most obvious based on the MOI; however, from a musculoskeletal aspect, barring blood loss, these injuries are not life-threatening and can be treated with splints. Secondary injuries are not as obvious but are on the "path of injury." The following examples further illustrate the difference between primary and secondary injuries:

- If a patient jumps out of a window feet first, the primary injury suspicion would be fractures to the calcaneus, tibia, fibula, femur, pelvis, and spine and aortic stress injuries. However, secondary injuries might include abdominal injury or head injury from tumbling forward after hitting the ground.
- If a patient is involved in a motorcycle collision with a telephone pole and hits his or her head on the pole, primary injuries will be head, cervical spine, and thoracic injury. A secondary injury might include a femur fracture from "catching" the femur on the handlebars.
- Another example is a patient who is riding in the passenger side of a vehicle that is involved in a side impact collision. As discussed in Chapter 2, Newton's first law of motion states that a body in motion will stay in motion until acted upon by an equal but opposite force. The vehicle is the moving object until acted upon by the other vehicle. For example, the door of the target vehicle is pushed against the upper arm, which can then push into the chest wall, producing rib fractures, lung contusion, and possibly a fractured humerus. Primary extremity suspicion would include humerus, pelvis, and femur fractures. Secondary injury suspicion would include rib fractures, chest wall muscle injury, and lung and heart injuries. One secondary injury to be investigated is an abrasion from a deployed air bag. Another possible secondary injury from a side impact collision results from an unrestrained passenger becoming a missile (object) inside the vehicle. The other vehicle striking the passenger side sets the passenger in motion until he or she is stopped by another object, such as the driver. However, near-side injuries are more severe than far-side injuries. In this case the MOI for the driver is the unrestrained passenger's body.

Musculoskeletal injuries in and of themselves are usually not life-threatening, but the injuries can alert the prehospital care provider to a more serious injury. Appropriately visualizing the incident from the first object set in motion until the last possible object that could be set in motion is the crux of truly understanding MOI and its importance.

Primary and Secondary Surveys

The first step of any assessment is scene safety and situation. Once the scene is safe, the prehospital care team can continue. The primary survey addresses the most life-threatening conditions that can be identified and managed. If the patient has no life-threatening injuries, the prehospital care provider proceeds to the secondary survey.

In the secondary survey, the prehospital care provider should do the following:

- Visually assess the patient for swelling, lacerations, abrasions, hematomas, color, movement, capillary refilling time, and deformity.
- Feel for pulses, temperature, crepitation, and movement.
- If the patient is conscious, question the patient about sensation, pain, and MOI and ask the patient to describe how the pain feels.
- Note that voluntary movement of the extremities tests for neurologic and muscular involvement.

Lacerations may bleed a little or a lot. As noted previously, direct pressure is the best initial method to control bleeding. Hemorrhage contained within the soft tissue will produce swelling and ecchymosis (bruising). Hematomas and deformity may indicate a closed fracture. Pain indicates potential serious injury unless the patient has loss of sensation to that area as a result of nerve injury.

Pulses, movement, and sensation are an important part of assessments. Lack of pulses, movement, and/or sensation may indicate a lack of blood flow or neurologic defects in conjunction with other signs. The primary survey is performed to establish a baseline and identify initial injury. Reassessment of the patient on multiple occasions is to identify changes.

Crepitus is the feeling that the bones can make when the fractured ends rub against one another. Crepitus can be elicited by palpating the site of injury and by motion of the bones. This sounds like a snap, crackle, and pop. Another analogy is the popping of bubble packing. Although the prehospital care provider frequently notes this feeling of bones grating against one another during the assessment of a patient, it can produce further injury. Therefore once the crepitus is noted, additional or repetitive steps to produce it should not be taken. Crepitus is a distinct feeling that is not easily forgotten.

The prehospital care provider can almost never rule out a fracture by physical examination in the field, regardless of his or her skill level. Many fractures can be asymptomatic, especially immediately after the injury when the muscles may contract and hold the bone ends together. Many times sprains or strains can present signs and symptoms identical to those of a fracture. In addition, the patient may be distracted from the presence of a fracture by the presence of other injuries, or the patient may be unconscious and unable to verbalize the extent of the pain or injuries. The presence of a fracture can only be ruled out by appropriate radiographic evaluation of the injured part. Therefore if in doubt, the injury should be treated as a fracture.

Hemorrhage

External arterial bleeding should be identified during the primary survey and controlled after the patient's airway

Table 10-1	Approximate Internal Blood Loss Associated with Fractures	
Bone	**Approximate internal blood loss (mL)**
Rib	125
Radius or ulna	250-500
Humerus	500-750
Tibia or fibula	500-1000
Femur	1000-2000
Pelvis	1000-massive

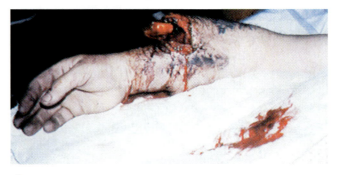

Figure 10-5 Open fracture. (*From London PS: A colour atlas of diagnosis after recent injury, London, 1990, Wolfe.*)

and breathing are managed. Generally this type of bleeding is assessed easily, but assessment can be difficult when blood is hidden under a patient or in heavy or dark clothing. Therefore all of the patient's clothing should be removed.

Estimation of blood loss is extremely difficult. The patient may have been moved from the site of injury or blood may be concealed by waterproof or dark-colored clothing, absorbed through the surface that the patient is lying on or into the clothes, or washed away in water or by rain. Overt signs of external blood loss may not always be apparent.

The prehospital care provider should rapidly assess the potential blood loss caused by extremity trauma. This will help evaluate the potential of blood loss that will lead to decreased perfusion and shock. Such advanced knowledge will prepare the prehospital care provider for the possibility of systemic deterioration and indicates the initial steps to prevent its occurrence. Life-threatening hemorrhage and shock should be immediately identified, regardless of the source, and managed as part of the primary survey. Continued swelling of an extremity or a cold, pale, pulseless extremity is potentially a hematoma and indicates internal arterial hemorrhage. Significant internal blood loss can be associated with fractures (Table 10-1).

Open and Closed Fractures

Open fractures may be easy to locate on a trauma patient (Figure 10-5). Bone ends may or may not be visible. The prehospital care provider should consider any open wound near a possible fracture to be an open fracture and treat it as such. Pulses, movement, sensation, and color should be assessed initially and reassessed continuously as with any fracture.

Closed fractures are usually accompanied with swelling and hematomas. Crepitus may or may not be present. Pulses, movement, sensation, and color should be assessed and then reassessed continuously for changes.

Strains and sprains may appear like a closed fracture. Because these injuries can only be differentiated by radiography, strains and sprains should be treated as if they are closed fractures.

Femur fractures present with an additional problem compared with the rest of the skeletal structure—hemorrhage. Because of the amount of space in the pelvic cavity, hemorrhage may occur with few external signs of difficulty. Likewise, because the femur is covered with large thick muscle tissue, excessive bleeding into that tissue may cause an excessive blood loss with only minimal external swelling. The first indication of difficulty may be shock. Patients who present with possible femur fractures should be closely monitored for any changes that may result from the blood loss.

Dislocations

Dislocations are easy bone injuries to discover during physical examination (Figures 10-6 and 10-7). This injury usually involves a great deal of pain to the patient. Pain and deformity usually are the initial findings. Gentle examination will identify that the bones on either side of the joint are out of position. Attempted motion of the joint will usually produce pain and may not be possible because the bones are locked by the

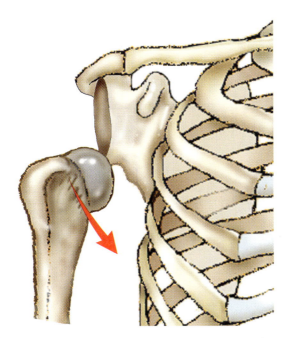

Figure 10-6 A dislocation is a separation of a bone from a joint. (*From McSwain NE Jr, Paturas JL: The basic EMT: comprehensive prehospital patient care, ed 2, St Louis, 2001, Mosby.*)

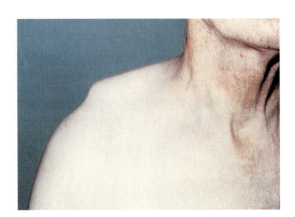

Figure 10-7 Dislocation of the acromioclavicular joint. (*From London PS: A colour atlas of diagnosis after recent injury, London, 1990, Wolfe.*)

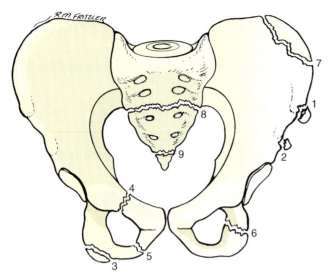

Figure 10-8   Fractures of individual pelvic bones. *1,* Avulsion of anterosuperior iliac spine. *2,* Avulsion of anteroinferior iliac spine. *3,* Avulsion of ischial tuberosity. *4,* Fracture of superior pubic ramus. *5,* Fracture of inferior pubic ramus. *6,* Fracture of ischial ramus. *7,* Fracture of iliac wing. *8,* Transverse fracture of sacrum. *9,* Fracture of coccyx.

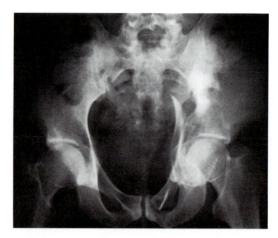

Figure 10-9   Pelvic radiograph demonstrating a complex comminuted fracture of the left hemipelvis. *(Courtesy of Riverside Methodist Hospitals, Columbus, Ohio.)*

abnormal relationship. Hematomas are not usually present with dislocations, with the exception of the knee, because the joint has only a minimal blood supply. The close proximity of the popliteal artery and the strong attachments of this vessel to the femur and the tibia make it vulnerable to damage (see Chapter 2).

Pelvic Fractures

One of the major complications with a pelvic fracture is hemorrhage (Figures 10-8 and 10-9). Because of the amount of space within the pelvic cavity, a great deal of bleeding may occur with few external signs of difficulty. Onset of shock without an obvious source may be explained by this condition. Therefore patients with pelvic fractures should be closely observed for the development of shock, and intravenous access should be obtained as soon as possible without delaying transport. Aggressive palpation or manipulation of the pelvis (pelvic rock) can increase blood loss. To assess the pelvis, gentle palpation is acceptable but should only be performed once. Gentle manual pressure anterior to posterior will illicit signs of instability.

Amputations

Amputations are evident to a prehospital care provider as he or she approaches the scene (Figure 10-10). This type of injury receives a great deal of attention from bystanders, and the patient may or may not know that

the extremity is missing. Psychologically the prehospital care provider must deal with this injury cautiously. If the patient does not know the extremity is missing, to tell him or her about the injury on scene may or may not be beneficial. The patient may not be ready to deal with the loss of a limb and should be told after being managed. The missing extremity should be located for possible reattachment. Even if it is not possible to regain complete function of the extremity, the patient may regain partial function. The primary survey should be performed before looking for a missing extremity. The look of an amputation may be horrifying, but if the patient is not breathing, the loss of the limb is secondary.

Amputations may or may not be accompanied by significant bleeding. The patient may complain of pain distal to the amputation. This *phantom pain* is the sensation that pain exists in an extremity that has been removed. The reason for phantom pain is not understood completely, but it may be because the brain does not realize that the extremity is not present.

Management

The prehospital care provider must follow the following priorities at all times when managing a patient with extremity injuries:

1. Manage any life-threatening conditions.
2. Manage any limb-threatening conditions.
3. Manage all other conditions (if time allows).

Adherence to these priorities does not imply that extremity injuries should be ignored or that injured ex-

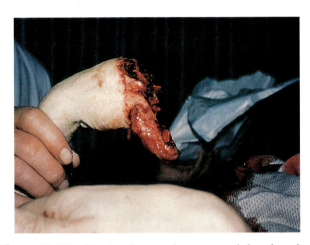

Figure 10-10   Hand with a nearly amputated thumb and amputated fingers. (*From London PS:* A colour atlas of diagnosis after recent injury, *London, 1990, Wolfe.*)

tremities should not be protected from further harm. It means that in multisystem trauma patients with extremity injuries that are not life-threatening, abbreviated general measures should be used to care for the extremity injuries. This will allow the prehospital care provider to focus on those injuries and conditions that directly threaten the patient's life. The easiest and fastest way to accomplish abbreviated care of extremity injuries is to correctly immobilize the patient onto a longboard.

The prehospital care provider must prioritize the critical injuries of patients with life-threatening conditions in addition to extremity trauma. This allows for essential lifesaving intervention where and when it will be most beneficial to the patient. This may mean abbreviating the care of specific extremity injuries so that focus can remain on those conditions that are life-threatening to the patient.

Patients with life-threatening extremity trauma (hemorrhage) but no other critical problems should be identified during the primary survey. These patients should have appropriate interventions, including initial management of shock and rapid transport to the facility that can best treat their condition. In patients without life-threatening injuries or conditions, extremity trauma can be identified and managed during the secondary survey.

If an extremity is under abnormal stress because of the patient's position or pathologic angulation, the prehospital care provider should attempt to straighten the extremity. This will mean moving the extremity back to a normal anatomic position. Having the extremity back in a normal position will help with splinting and improving circulation.

An injured extremity should be moved as little as possible. The primary objective of splinting is to prevent movement of the body part. This will help decrease the patient's pain and prevent further soft tissue damage and hemorrhage. To effectively immobilize any long bone in an extremity, the entire limb should be immobilized. To do this, the injured site should be supported manually while the joint and bone above (proximal to) and the joint and bone below (distal to) the injury site are immobilized.

The general management for suspected fractures includes the following steps:

1. Stop any bleeding and treat the patient for shock.
2. Evaluate for distal neurovascular function.
3. Support the area of injury.
4. Immobilize the injured extremity, including the joint above and the joint below the injury site.
5. Reevaluate the injured extremity after immobilization for changes in distal neurovascular function.

Three points are important to remember when applying any type of splint:

1. Pad rigid splints to help adjust for anatomic shapes and to help increase the patient's comfort.
2. Remove jewelry and watches so they will not inhibit circulation as additional swelling occurs.
3. Assess neurovascular functions distal to the injury site before and after applying any splint and periodically thereafter.

This text is written as a continuing education course; therefore dressing and bandaging is not discussed within this chapter.

Splints: Equipment and Methods

Various splints and splinting materials are available, including the following:

- *Rigid splints* cannot be changed in shape (Figure 10-11). They require that the body part be positioned to fit the splint's shape. Examples of rigid splints include board splints (wood, plastic, or metal) and inflatable "air splints." This group of splints also includes the longboard.
- *Formable splints* can be molded into various shapes and combinations to accommodate the shape of the injured extremity (Figure 10-12). Examples of formable splints include vacuum splints, pillows, blankets, cardboard splints, wire ladder splints, and foam-covered moldable metal splints.

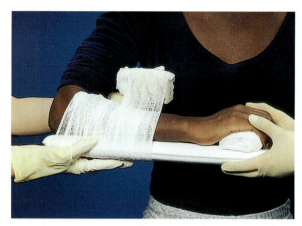

Figure 10-11   Rigid splint. (*Stoy W: Mosby's EMT-Basic textbook, St Louis, 1996, Mosby.*)

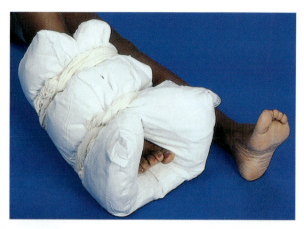

Figure 10-12   Formable splint. (*Stoy W: Mosby's EMT-Basic textbook, St Louis, 1996, Mosby.*)

- *Traction splints* are designed to maintain mechanical inline traction to help realign fractures (Figure 10-13). Traction splints are most commonly used to stabilize femur fractures.

Hemorrhage

The prehospital care provider can usually detect significant hemorrhage easily unless it is internal. In general, obvious hemorrhages are controlled by using direct pressure first, then elevation and pressure points, and as the last resort, use of a tourniquet. Direct pressure is accomplished by placing a dressing over the wound and applying pressure with the heel of the hand. For direct pressure, once a dressing is applied, it remains. If the bleeding goes through the first dressing, another dressing should be placed on top of the first one without removing it. If adequate manual pressure is not available, an Ace bandage should be applied as a pressure dressing. If a fracture is associated with gross bleeding, the extremity should be realigned and splinted while direct pressure is applied to the open wound. Hopefully this procedure will also help control the bleeding.

In the case of internal hemorrhage, direct pressure applied to the outside of the body over the area of suspected injury will help the bleeding, just as it would for an open wound.

If direct pressure does not completely control bleeding, elevation of the extremity above the level of the heart is the next step. Pressure points are used to try to impede blood flow distal to the artery in which the pressure is applied. The main pressure points used are the axillary, brachial, popliteal, and femoral. Direct pressure is placed to the closest artery above the hemorrhage site. Tourniquets are rarely used—only under

extreme circumstances (or for combat situations, see Chapter 16) and as a last resort.

Open and Closed Fractures

The first considerations in open fractures are to control hemorrhage and treat for shock. Open wounds should be covered with a sterile pressure dressing and pressure applied to further control bleeding. The limb should then be adequately immobilized. In the case of open femur fractures, the prehospital care provider should first apply a sterile dressing to the wound and then use a traction splint to straighten the extremity and stabilize the fracture. If the bone ends return into the wound, the outcome will not be altered as long as the physician who cares for the patient is informed that the bone ends initially were outside of the body. Returning the bone ends inside the body will expose it to outside contaminants and bacteria. The physician and other hospital personnel should be informed of the initial condition of the wound and any changes that occurred as a result of its management in the field. This information must also be documented on the run report.

Both open and closed fractures can be immobilized with the use of rigid or air splints. Rigid splints are easier to use because once an air splint is inflated, it cannot be deflated or inspected further. Padding should be used with a rigid splint to ensure that no movement inside the splint is allowed. If a pulse is no longer detected where it once was, the injury becomes more of a priority. Ice packs can be used to decrease pain and swelling.

The prehospital care provider should manage strains and sprains just like fractures because differentiation between these injuries is not possible in the field.

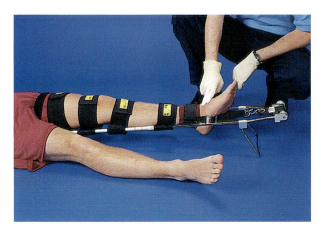

Figure 10-13   Traction splint. (*Stoy W: Mosby's EMT-Basic textbook, St Louis, 1996, Mosby.*)

Dislocations

As a general rule, suspected dislocations should be splinted in the position found. If a pulse is not detectable, the prehospital care provider may manipulate the joint to try to return blood flow. This manipulation will cause the patient a great deal of pain, so the patient should be prepared before moving the extremity. Ice packs can be used to decrease pain and swelling.

Any splint that is available should be used to splint the injury in the position in which it is found. Documentation of how the injury was found and of the presence of pulses, movement, sensation, and color before and after splinting is important.

The National Association of EMS Physicians (NAEMSP) recommends reduction of dislocations when transport time is prolonged. Their rationale is that joints are more difficult to reduce if they are left in a dislocated position for a prolonged time; therefore the prehospital care provider should attempt reduction in the field. The written local protocols should include the exact procedure for reduction.

Pelvic Fractures

Pelvic fractures, especially if hemorrhage is suspected, can be difficult to manage. Not only is bleeding a concern, but a patient with such an unstable fracture is difficult to move. If the patient is not suspected of having a hemorrhage, the best way to stabilize the fracture may be with a scoop stretcher and padding. A PASG can be very useful in maintaining the integrity of the pelvis with or without a suspected hemorrhage. If a PASG is unavailable, consideration should be given to wrapping a sheet tightly around the pelvis and tying it as a sling. This

position should maintain the lower extremities in an adducted and internally rotated position.

Amputations

Amputation presents another special problem. Principles of managing an amputated part include the following:

- Clean the amputated part by gentle rinsing with lactated Ringer's solution.
- Wrap the part in sterile gauze moistened with lactated Ringer's solution, and place it in a plastic bag or container.
- After labeling the bag or container, place it in an outer container filled with crushed ice.
- DON'T freeze the part by placing it directly on the ice or by adding another coolant such as dry ice.
- Transport the part along with the patient to the closest appropriate facility.

Transport of a patient should not be delayed to locate a missing amputated part. If the amputated part is not readily found, law enforcement officials or other responders should remain at the scene to search for it. When the amputated part is being transported in a separate vehicle from the patient, the prehospital care provider should ensure that the transporters of the amputated part understand clearly where the patient is being transported and how to deal with the part once they locate it. The receiving facility should be notified as soon as the part is located and transportation of the part should be initiated as soon as possible.

Femur Fractures

Femur fractures represent a special consideration because of the musculature of the thigh. The thigh muscles have tremendous strength and commonly cause closed femur fractures to present with overriding bone ends and obvious deformity with angulation. This can be a major contributing factor to hypovolemic shock because of the creation of a "third space" for hemorrhage.

The application of traction, both manually and by the use of a mechanical device, will help promote tamponading of internal third-space bleeding and decrease the patient's pain. Contraindications to the use of a traction splint include the following:

- Fractured pelvis
- Hip injury with gross displacement
- Any significant injury to the knee
- Avulsion or amputation of the ankle and foot

Impaired or Absent Circulation

Impaired or absent circulation at or distal to the injury site will place an extremity in jeopardy. After stabilizing all life-threatening conditions or injuries, the next priority is to correct any condition that threatens an extremity. Slight repositioning of the extremity toward a normal position will often reinstate circulation and is not time-consuming. The extremity should not be moved to the extreme range of either full extension or full flexion. If one or two attempts do not restore circulation, continued attempts will not likely prove successful. In such cases it is safer and more prudent to splint the limb as it lies and rapidly transport the patient to the nearest appropriate facility.

Pain Management

Prehospital control of pain is not usually an achievable goal; however, the prehospital care provider certainly should address pain management. Analgesics are recommended for isolated joint and limb injuries but are generally not advocated in multisystem trauma patients. Before administering pain medication, the prehospital care provider should attempt to decrease the pain by addressing the basics first. Once the fracture or dislocation is stabilized and splinted, the patient should experience a great reduction in pain. Stabilizing the effected extremity decreases the amount of movement of the area, thus decreasing the amount of discomfort. The patient should be observed for signs of alcohol or drug use if he or she does not appear to be in a great deal of pain with significant injuries.

Pain medications should be used judiciously and as tolerated by the patient. Circumstances in which analgesics should not be administered include when the patient presents or develops signs and symptoms of shock, pain is significantly relieved with stabilization and splinting, or the patient appears under the influence of drugs and/or alcohol. Medication should not be administered without understanding the potential complications.

Summary

The management of patients with extremity trauma varies based on an evaluation of the priority of the patient's extremity injuries compared with all of that patient's other injuries and conditions.

In patients with multisystem trauma, the prehospital care provider directs his or her attention toward the primary survey and the finding and management of all life-threatening injuries, including internal or external hemorrhage in the extremities. These patients should be rapidly secured to a longboard in a normal, supine, anatomic position to efficiently stabilize all injured extremities and allow for focus on meeting the patient's critical needs. The prehospital care provider often cannot provide care of individual injuries that are not life-threatening in multisystem trauma patients until the patient's systemic condition is stabilized. The prehospital care provider should not be distracted from life-threatening conditions by the gross appearance of any noncritical injuries or by the patient's request for management of them.

Patients with noncritical isolated injuries represent another category. The initial priority is to establish that the patient does not have life-threatening injuries. Only after the prehospital care provider has fully assessed the patient and found that the patient has only isolated injuries without any systemic implication can the patient be managed in the normal prescribed way. When the mechanism of injury indicates sudden violent changes in motion, multisystem trauma, or spinal trauma, the prehospital care provider must anticipate potential systemic decline and include the patient's age, physical condition, and medical history in the evaluation for potential systemic decline.

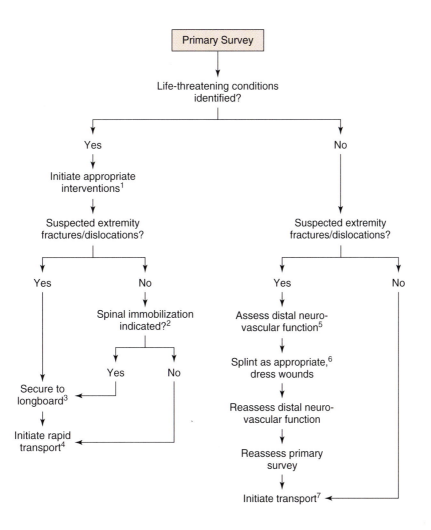

[1]Airway management, ventilatory support, shock therapy.

[2]See Indications for Spinal Immobilization algorithm (p. 238).

[3]Injured extremities are immobilized in anatomic position by securing to longboard.

[4]Transport to closest appropriate facility (trauma center, if available); assess distal neurovascular function and apply traction splint (if suspected femur fracture) as time permits.

[5]Assess perfusion (pulses and capillary refilling) and neurologic function (motor and sensory) distal to the suspected fracture or dislocation.

[6]Use appropriate splinting technique to immobilize suspected fracture or dislocation; if suspected midshaft femur fracture, apply traction splint.

[7]Transport to closest appropriate facility.

Scenario Solution

Based on the chief complaints of shortness of breath and upper left arm pain, you should listen for lung sounds. Auscultation reveals diminished lung sounds to that side, indicating the possibility of damage to the left lung. You must perform manual stabilization of the spine and administer 15 L/min of oxygen via a nonrebreather mask before rapidly extricating this patient from the vehicle. Continuous monitoring of the patient's ventilatory status is vital because of the possibility for a simple pneumothorax to progress to a tension pneumothorax. Anatomic splinting along the patient's body when he is secured to a long backboard would provide adequate immobilization during transport. If the patient's ventilatory status improves with oxygen, you can use additional splinting methods if time permits. If the patient's ventilatory status worsens, consider endotracheal intubation.

Review Questions

Answers are provided on p. 414.

1. In an adult patient, blood loss into the tissue from a fractured femur may be as much as which of the following?
   a. 250 to 500 mL
   b. 500 to 1000 mL
   c. 1000 to 2000 mL
   d. 2500 to 5000 mL

2. Which of the following is the technique of extremity fracture immobilization in which a patient who has extremity fractures in the presence of life-threatening injuries is placed on a long backboard without splinting of individual injuries?
   a. Supine splinting
   b. Anatomic splinting
   c. Physical splinting
   d. Functional splinting

3. Which of the following musculoskeletal injuries is/are NOT usually treated in the prehospital setting?
   a. Hemorrhage
   b. Amputation
   c. Compartment syndrome
   d. Infection
   e. Both c and d

4. Which of the following is an injury characterized by tearing away of tissue?
   a. Sprain
   b. Strain
   c. Incision
   d. Avulsion

5. Which of the following musculoskeletal injuries may indicate serious associated injury?
   a. Rib fracture
   b. Scapular fracture
   c. Pelvic fracture
   d. All of the above

REFERENCES

American College of Surgeons Committee on Trauma: *Advanced trauma life support*, Chicago, 2002, American College of Surgeons.

Goth P, Garnett G: Clinical guidelines for delayed or prolonged transport: II. Dislocations. Rural Affairs Committee, National Association of Emergency Medical Services Physicians, *Prehospital Disaster Med* 8(1):77, 1993.

McSwain NE Jr, Paturas JL, editors: *The basic EMT: comprehensive prehospital patient care*, ed 2, St Louis, 2001, Mosby.

Seyfer AE: *Guidelines for management of amputated parts*, Chicago, 1996, American College of Surgeons Committee on Trauma.

Chapter 11

Thermal Trauma: Injuries Produced by Heat and Cold

Chapter Objectives

At the completion of this chapter, the reader should be able to do the following:

- List the two sources of body heat.
- List four mechanisms of heat transfer into and out of the body.
- List the types of energy that create local injury.
- List criteria for assessing burn severity.
- List two life-threatening injuries that result from burns that require pre-hospital treatment.
- List five signs that indicate inhalation injury and possible respiratory complications after a burn injury.
- Apply the rule of nines for adult and pediatric patients.
- List key assessment and management elements for chemical and electrical burns.
- Differentiate between critical and noncritical hyperthermia.
- List the major elements of management of hyperthermia from different causes.
- Differentiate between superficial and deep frostbite.
- Formulate a management plan for the patient with local cold injury.
- Differentiate between primary and secondary hypothermia.
- Formulate a management plan for the patient with hypothermia.
- Differentiate between the mechanisms and management of submersion and immersion hypothermia.

Scenario

A 19-year-old male restaurant worker cooking with hot grease scalds his hand and spills the hot grease on his entire right leg, which is now blistering. *Is this a critical burn? What are the depth and body surface area involved?* Firefighters bring an unresponsive child out of a structure fire after finding her hiding under a bed. The child has no visible burns. *What is the most likely cause for the child's unresponsiveness?* An elderly male is found unresponsive in his cool New England home one February morning. His ventilations are slow and shallow, and he has a weak, slow carotid pulse. *What type of hypothermia do you suspect? How will you treat him?* A marathon runner is found wandering around off the course, confused, diaphoretic, and barely ambulatory. *What are the possible causes of his disorientation? Is this a threat to his life as a result of a thermal problem or other cause? Does the fact that he is diaphoretic make any difference in your assessment?* On a day with temperatures well below freezing, a homeless woman complains of numb lower extremities with no sensation in her feet and ankles. *Do you attempt to rewarm this injury in the field? What are the possible complications of rewarming?*

This chapter covers a wide range of possible injuries and illnesses caused by thermal trauma. Thermal trauma includes a variety of different injuries and conditions. For discussion purposes, these are divided into two main categories—*heat* and *cold.* Each of these is further divided into *localized* (cutaneous) *conditions*, such as burns or frostbite, and *systemic conditions*, such as hyperthermia or hypothermia, which produce a generalized effect on the entire body. Within the heat category are the differences between burn injuries (from both thermal and nonthermal sources), those conditions in which body temperature is elevated, and those that are prompted by heat but in which the body temperature itself is not elevated. The cold category includes frostbite, hypothermia, and immersion and submersion injuries. Some cold injuries are insidious and sneak up on patients, especially the very young and the elderly.

This chapter also includes discussion of the different priorities necessary for the management of thermal trauma patients. For example, the severely hypothermic patient requires rewarming in the hospital setting, but the patient's core temperature may need to be stabilized before he or she is transported to the hospital without causing ventricular fibrillation. The burn patient with multisystem trauma is treated first for trauma and any systemic burn-related deficits and only secondarily for the actual surface burn injuries.

Anatomy

The skin, the largest organ of the body, is composed of three tissue layers—the epidermis, dermis, and subcutaneous tissue. The *epidermis*—the outermost layer—is made up entirely of epithelial cells with no blood vessels. Underlying the epidermis is the thicker *dermis,* made up of a framework of connective tissues that contain blood vessels, nerve endings, sebaceous glands, and sweat glands. The *subcutaneous layer* is a combination of elastic and fibrous tissue as well as fatty deposits (Figure 11-1).

The skin serves many functions for the body, the most important being to form a protective barrier against the outside environment, which helps prevent infection. The skin also prevents fluid loss and helps regulate body temperature. The dermal layer contains nerve endings that convey impulses between the brain and the body. When thermal injuries occur to skin tissue, many or all of these functions are either destroyed or severely impaired. This protective layer must have adequate perfusion with red blood cells (RBCs) and other nutrients to survive. Heat, in addition to coagulating the protein, can compromise blood flow.

An understanding of the surface area of the various regions of the body will help the prehospital care provider estimate the relative size of the area that is burned. This determination will in turn help determine how much fluid replacement the patient needs. The percentage of the body's total surface area represented by each part or region of the body varies with the size of that region. This percentage also varies as the individual develops in size from an infant to a fully mature adult. An approximate estimation can be made by using the rule of nines (Figure 11-2). Although this is not completely accurate, it is close enough for determining fluid replacement needs, estimating mortality, and computing other components of burn therapy that use body surface area (BSA) as a factor.

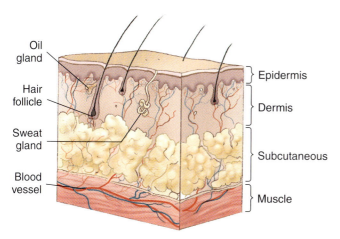

Figure 11-1   The skin is composed of three tissue layers—epidermis, dermis, and subcutaneous—and associated muscle. Some layers contain structures such as glands, hair follicles, blood vessels, and nerves. The depth of the burn determines the portion of these organs involved.

Physiology

Normally, the body functions within a narrow temperature range of about 5 degrees on either side of 98° F (37° C ± 3° C). If the internal temperature (the core temperature) falls outside this range, serious injury or death may result. This narrow range is maintained by homeostatic mechanisms regulated by the hypothalamus. The hypothalamus receives sensory input from both the core of the body and the outer regions, known as the *shell*, and initiates heat production and conservation measures or reduces heat production and increases methods of heat loss. The body gains heat primarily as a by-product of metabolism. The body can increase heat production by increasing metabolism, mostly by large muscle activity such as shivering. The body is far less efficient at gaining heat from external sources, such as standing in front of a fire or lying on a beach in the sun. The body reduces heat losses by vasoconstriction and shunting of the heat, carrying blood away from the skin. Certain medications can also interfere with thermoregulation (Box 11-1).

Heat (energy) is transferred from an area of greater concentration to an area of lower concentration by the following four methods. Since heat is transferred from greater temperature to lower temperature, the human body can both gain and lose heat by these methods. The prehospital care provider must understand how heat is transferred in order to treat a patient with either heat or cold injury.

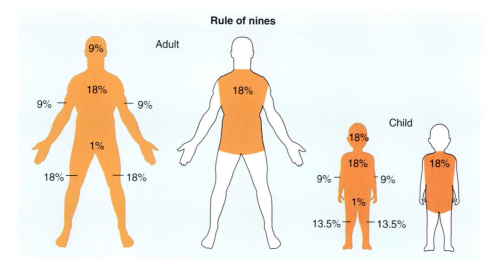

Figure 11-2   Determining the amount of burn involved is a major consideration in the resuscitation of the burn patient. The rule of nines is a fairly accurate and simple approach to this determination.

Box 11-1

Medications that Interfere with Thermoregulation

DRUGS THAT INCREASE HEAT PRODUCTION
Thyroid hormone
Amphetamines
Tricyclic antidepressants
Lysergic acid diethylamide (LSD)

DRUGS THAT DECREASE THIRST
Haloperidol

DRUGS THAT DECREASE SWEATING
Antihistimines
Anticholinergics
Phenothiazines

DRUGS THAT CHANGE THERMOREGULATION BY VASOACTIVE ABILITY
Alcohol
Nicotine

---

1. *Radiation* is the direct transfer of energy from a warm object to a cooler one by infrared radiation. This does not use an intermediary such as air or water. The sun warms the earth through space by this method of energy transfer. Heat lamps at restaurants work this way also. Some hospitals use these types of lights to keep patients warm.

2. *Conduction* is the transfer of heat between two objects in direct contact with each other. Heat "flows" from the hand to what is touched if what is touched is cooler than the hand. This is important if a patient is lying on the cold ground or the hot pavement. A patient will generally lose heat twice as fast to the ground as to the air. Therefore the prehospital care provider should get the patient off the ground rather than just covering the patient with a blanket. A patient will lose heat significantly faster in water than in air of the same temperature, so it is also important to keep the patient dry.

3. *Convection* is the heating of water or air in contact with a body, removal of that air (such as with wind) or water, and then the heating of the new air or water that replaces what is left. A scuba diver's wetsuit guards against convection. This is also the primary mechanism of wind chill (Table 11-1).

4. *Evaporation* of water from liquid to a vapor is an extremely effective method of heat loss. A basal level

of both water and accompanying heat loss from exhaled air, skin, and mucus membranes is called *insensible loss* and is caused by evaporation. This insensible loss is normally about 10% of basal heat production, but when the body temperature rises, this process becomes more active (sensible) and sweat is produced. The amount of water produced can be up to almost 4 liters per hour. The resulting heat loss can be 30 times the normal insensible loss.

Several medical and iatrogenic conditions, including medications, may lead to impairment of thermoregulation and therefore predispose patients to heat and cold injury and illness. Hyperthermia and hypothermia caused by these conditions are called *secondary illnesses*.

Heat-Related Conditions and Injuries

Human skin shows no apparent damage when exposed to higher-than-normal temperatures (up to 104° F [40° C]), even for relatively long periods of time. However, when exposed to much higher temperatures for shorter lengths of time or only moderately higher temperatures for longer periods of time, tissue destruction occurs. The same temperature/time principle is true for exposure to varying degrees of cold.

Thermal injuries also differ with regard to location, extent, and depth. Heat injury to the hands, feet, genitalia, or face and burns that completely encircle body areas are high priority injuries. Other key factors for the prehospital care provider to consider in burn patients are inhalation injuries, length of exposure, core body temperature, and the patient's age, general health, other injuries, and medical history.

Burn injury is the fourth leading cause of trauma deaths, preceded only by motor vehicle crashes (MVCs), penetrating trauma, and falls. Millions of people each year seek the care of a physician for treatment of burns. Approximately 75,000 require hospitalization, and approximately 6000 die every year. Prevention efforts, such as public education about smoke detectors, are responsible for a significant decrease in burn-related deaths. However, long-term morbidity is still a significant problem associated with burns. The types of burns vary depending on the age group involved. For instance, scalds from hot liquids are found more often in toddlers, whereas flame burns are most frequently seen in older children. Industrial burns from liquids or caustic agents are most common in adults.

Table 11-1   Windchill

Estimated wind speed (in mph)	Actual thermometer reading (° F)											
	50	40	30	20	10	0	−10	−20	−30	−40	−50	−60
	Equivalent chill temperature (° F)											
Calm	50	40	30	20	10	0	−10	−20	−30	−40	−50	−60
5	48	37	27	16	6	−5	−15	−26	−36	−47	−57	−68
10	40	28	16	4	−9	−24	−33	−46	−58	−70	−83	−95
15	36	22	9	−5	−18	−32	−45	−58	−72	−85	−99	−112
20	32	18	4	−10	−25	−39	−53	−67	−82	−96	−110	−124
25	30	16	0	−15	−29	−44	−59	−74	−88	−104	−118	−133
30	28	13	−2	−18	−33	−48	−63	−79	−94	−109	−125	−140
35	27	11	−4	−21	−35	−51	−62	−82	−98	−113	−129	−145
40	26	10	−6	−21	−37	−53	−69	−85	−100	−116	−132	−148

(Wind speeds greater than 40 mph have little additional effect.)	Little danger. In <5 hr with dry skin. Maximum danger of false sense of security.	Increasing danger. Danger from freezing of exposed flesh within 1 minute.	Great danger. Flesh may freeze within 30 seconds.

Trenchfoot and immersion foot may occur at any point on this chart.

From Sanders M: *Mosby's paramedic textbook*, ed 2, St Louis, 2001, Mosby.

Instructions: *Measure* local temperature and wind speed if possible. If not, *estimate*. Enter table at closest 10° F interval along the top with appropriate wind speed along left side. Intersection gives approximate equivalent chill temperature (that is, the temperature that would cause the same rate of cooling under calm conditions). Note that regardless of cooling rate, you do not cool below the actual air temperature unless wet.

Associated injuries account for a significant part of morbidity and mortality caused by thermal injuries. Inhalation injuries are a cause of death. Chemical injury to the lung tissue and toxic by-products of combustion are both prime contributors to pulmonary pathology. Injury to the tracheobronchial tree is generally due to superheated gases. Injury to the lung is usually due to chemicals.

Cutaneous Heat Injuries (Burns)

Heat coagulates protein. This is how an egg cooks. This is also the primary mechanism of injury with burns. Low levels of heat for a long period of time or high heat for a short time that have equal energy exchange produce the same result.

The priorities of care for burn victims follow the same principles and priorities as for any trauma patient:

1. Stop the burning process (thermal or chemical).

2. Use the primary survey for assessment and management.
3. Provide specific care for individual wounds (burns).

Many patients die as a result of thermal injuries because they have inhaled the carbonaceous by-products of combustion, inhaled toxic gases, or been in a hypoxic environment for a sustained period of time—not from their actual burn injuries. Often these effects may not present with alarming signs and symptoms immediately after the injury. The probability of such associated conditions should be recognized, a high concentration of oxygen provided, and ventilations assisted as necessary.

A victim of a fire who has been in a confined area for any length of time must be considered to have carbon monoxide in his or her blood as well as potential pulmonary and systemic problems caused by toxic inhalation. Such a patient should be considered unstable, regardless of contradictory findings during the primary and secondary surveys, and should be transported to an appropriate facility without delay. Oxygen should be administered in a concentration of at least 85% (FiO$_2$ of 0.85). Pulse oximetry may be inaccurately high with these patients because carbon monoxide fools a pulse oximeter into giving a normal reading when the patient may actually be hypoxic.

Burn trauma often includes other nonthermal injuries resulting from falls, jumping, or being struck by objects. In some cases these related injuries can be more serious and present a greater risk to life than the burns. The prehospital care provider should assess for the presence of associated injuries.

BURN ASSESSMENT

Scene Assessment.
Upon arrival at the scene of an incident, the prehospital care provider must assess the situation rapidly and thoroughly. Potential safety threats to the patient and crew should be identified and addressed immediately. If the fire department has arrived, the chief fire officer can make this determination. Prehospital care providers should *not* attempt rescues for which they do not have specific training, experience, and equipment.

Once the patient is in a safe place, the burning process must be stopped to eliminate further injury and tissue damage.

Primary Survey (Initial Assessment).
During the primary survey, close attention should be paid to the patient's airway, including a search for signs of inhalation injury. These include burns of the face and upper torso, singed facial and nasal hairs, carbonaceous sputum, hoarseness, stridor, or burns around the mouth and nose. Smoke poisoning, carbon monoxide poisoning, and respiratory injuries should be considered when the exposure has occurred in a confined space. Once the airway is secure, assessment should include the pulse rate, ventilatory effort, skin color, and level of consciousness (LOC).

Secondary Survey (Focused History and Physical Examination).
With critical patients in a potentially unstable environment, performing a secondary survey is inappropriate until both the patient and the environment have been secured from danger. In many cases the only way to ensure a secure environment is to move the patient. The prehospital care provider should pay attention to critical injuries and to stabilizing the spine. When no critical conditions require attention and the environment is safe, a thorough head-to-toe examination, evaluating the burns and other injuries, pertinent medical history, and allergies (when this information is available) should be performed rapidly. During this time, sites for placement of intravenous lines can be located.

BURN MANAGEMENT

Airway and Breathing.
Because of the high possibility of inadequate oxygenation and impaired circulation, any patient, conscious or unconscious, who has sustained a thermal injury should be treated with high-concentration supplemental oxygen and the airway and breathing monitored for adequacy. Carbon monoxide and cyanide respond to an oxygen concentration as close to 100% (FiO$_2$ of 1.0) as possible. The provider should use this during transport whenever the potential of either exists. A stable patient with an intact gag reflex and airway should be given oxygen and monitored. An endotracheal tube should be placed as required. Burns that lead to laryngeal problems early include edema from steam or chemical injury. Although management using an endotracheal tube may be required, edema of the laryngeal structures may allow only one attempt. The most experienced person on the scene should perform this attempt. The potential for laryngospasm is high in patients with a heat-injured larynx.

In the apneic or hypoxic patient, endotracheal intubation should be accomplished early to allow positive-pressure ventilation and prevent aspiration. If the hypoxic patient has a gag reflex, rapid sequence intubation (RSI) should be considered. Blind nasotracheal intubation may be required if RSI is not part of the training of the providers on the scene. Laryngospasm may result from contact of the device with the cords. If the airway becomes obstructed, percutaneous transtracheal jet ventilation is appropriate if local protocols allow.

In patients with charred burns surrounding the entire chest, expansion of the thoracic cavity may be extremely limited. Restricted chest excursion, caused by lack of elasticity of the burned tissue, results in inadequate tidal and minute volumes. A few of these patients may need to have incisions (escharotomies) made in the burned tissue to allow for better chest excursion. Appropriately trained personnel may need to do this in the field. The decision to perform this procedure should be made in conjunction with the receiving burn surgeon. If trained personnel are not available, the patient should be intubated, have ventilation supported with a bag-valve-mask (BVM) and high-concentration of oxygen, and be rapidly transported to the nearest facility capable of resuscitating a severely burned patient.

Circulation.   Associated injuries in a burn patient can lead to a decrease in circulatory blood volume, diminishing transport of oxygen to the body organs. The decrease in blood volume commonly associated with burns does *not* happen immediately after the burn injury. Usually 6 to 8 hours pass before this type of shock occurs. Shock at the scene is most often due to other causes. Management of hypovolemia should include the following measures:

- Assessment for associated injuries should be performed.
- Administration of intravenous lactated Ringer's solution or normal saline with large-bore catheters and tubing at a desired rate should be performed en route to the receiving facility, unless other conditions contraindicate fluids.

An unburned arm should be used for intravenous access unless both upper extremities are affected. In this case, the intravenous line should be placed through the burned area using a slightly longer catheter to prevent the catheter from being dislodged by associated edema that may develop later.

Although many formulas for fluid replacement exist, the Parkland formula serves as a good acute prehospital care guideline because it does not depend on laboratory findings. This formula indicates that the patient should receive 4 mL of fluid in the first 24 hours for every 1% of BSA with second- and third-degree burns (see p. 299) per kilogram of the patient's weight. One half of this total amount is to be given in the first 8 hours.

🔵 **Fluid replacement in first 24 hours =**
4 mL × Percentage of BSA × Weight (kg)

The following example using this method illustrates the need for early intravenous fluid administration. A 70 kg patient has partial-thickness burns on 50% of his BSA. The fluid replacement required in the first 8 hours can be calculates as follows:

Fluid replacement
in first 24 hours = 4 mL × 50% BSA × 70 kg
$$= 14{,}000 \text{ mL, or } 14 \text{ L}$$
$$\frac{14 \text{ L}}{2} = 7 \text{ L in first 8 hours}$$

The following formula can be used to figure drops per minute using a 10-drop administration set:

$$\textbf{Drops per minute} = \frac{\textbf{Amount to be infused} \times \textbf{Drip set}}{\textbf{Time (min)}}$$
$$= \frac{\textbf{7000 mL} \times \textbf{10 gtt set}}{\textbf{480 min}}$$
= **145 drops/min through one line or 72 drops/min each through two lines**

The 8-hour total can be used as the basis for calculating the drip rate that begins in the field. However, the patient's hemodynamic status and other injuries should also be taken into account.

Many burn centers now use other acceptable methods of fluid replacement. Every prehospital care provider should know and use the method preferred by the treatment facility to which he or she will transport burn patients.

PAIN MANAGEMENT

The pain experienced by a burn patient is related to the severity of the burn. Third-degree (full-thickness) burns are painless because of the destruction of the nerve receptor endings; however, second-degree (partial-thickness) burns involve a great deal of pain. Because partial-thickness burns are usually associated with full-thickness burns, a patient with full-thickness burns may experience a great deal of pain.

Analgesics, such as morphine or nitrous oxide, can be used to relieve the pain. Because morphine can cause vasodilation, especially if hypovolemia is present, fluid resuscitation must be adequate. Morphine is reported to metabolize faster in the presence of burns and must be dosed accordingly. Both morphine and nitrous oxide can induce ventilatory depression, and they can be dangerous if shock or ventilatory problems are present. Fentanyl is becoming more popular because it does not have the hemodynamic and ventilatory effects of morphine. The use of all analgesics should be based on the patient's overall condition, not just the amount of pain; however, pain should be treated adequately. Any analgesics should be administered intravenously.

Another method of pain relief is cooling the wound with cool, moist, sterile pads. No evidence indicates that such therapy produces pain relief; however, the cooling sensation is sometimes of psychological benefit to the patient. Adding cool, moist pads in such cases to cool the wound and reduce the amount of tissue injury is also not based on facts. When cool, moist, sterile pads are used, they should cover only 10% of the BSA and for only 10 to 15 minutes at a time. The preferred method of dressing burns is with dry sterile dressings. In the seriously burned patient, the hypothermia brought on by the wet dressings could seriously compromise the patient. *Heat loss by conduction is significantly greater with water than with air.*

WOUND CARE

Wound care is performed in the burn patient to prevent further damage and infection. All clothing around the burn should be removed with care to not pull away any clothing that is stuck to the wound. Where active bleeding is present, pressure dressings should be applied and any associated injuries should be treated before covering the burn area. The patient should be wrapped in a clean or sterile dry sheet. Any type of dressing that shreds and leaves particles in the wound and any ointment or solutions should be avoided. All burned tissue should be covered with dry dressings. *The prehospital care provider should not attempt to open blisters* because they are a protective mechanism. Débridement should not be attempted in the field. *Rings and jewelry should be removed from patient.* Jewelry keeps in heat, and fingers that have been burned will swell; if they have not been burned, they will swell later during fluid shifts. *Time is of the essence.* Once immediate life-threatening injuries are managed and shock management is initiated, the patient should be transported to an appropriate facility.

EVALUATION OF POTENTIALLY CRITICAL BURNS

Seven factors must be considered to determine which burn patients are the most critical:

1. Depth of the burn
2. BSA involved
3. Age of the patient
4. Pulmonary injury
   a. Smoke inhalation
   b. Toxic by-product inhalation
5. Associated injuries
   a. Airway burns
   b. Other associated nonburn injuries
6. Special considerations
   a. Chemical burns
   b. Electrical burns
   c. Carbon monoxide poisoning
7. Preexisting disease

Depth of the Burn. The first step in the evaluation of the burn itself is a visual examination to determine the depth (Figure 11-3). This assessment is only an estimate because the full extent of the injury may not be apparent for several days.

- Superficial burns (first-degree burns) (Figure 11-4)
  - Injury to the epidermis only
  - Red, inflamed, and painful skin
- Partial-thickness burns (second-degree burns) (Figure 11-5)
  - Injury to both the epidermis and dermis
  - Skin with reddened areas, blisters, or open, weeping wounds

---

Injuries Requiring Burn Unit Care

Patients with serious burns should receive care at centers that have special expertise and resources. Initial transport or early transfer to a burn unit should result in a lower mortality rate and fewer complication. A burn unit may treat adults, children, or both. The Committee on Trauma of the American College of Surgeons believes that patients with burn injury who meet the following criteria should be referred to a burn unit:

1. Inhalation injury
2. Partial-thickness burns over greater than 10% of the total body surface area (TBSA)
3. Full-thickness (third-degree) burns in any age group.
4. Burns that involve the face, hands, feet, genitalia, perineum, or major joints
5. Electrical burns, including lightning injury
6. Chemical burns
7. Burn injury in patients with preexisting medical disorders that could complicate management, prolong recovery, or affect mortality
8. Any patients with burns and concomitant trauma (e.g., fractures) in which the burn injury poses the greatest risk of morbidity or mortality; if the trauma poses the greater immediate risk, the patient may be initially stabilized in a trauma center before transfer to a burn unit
9. Burned children in hospitals without qualified personnel or equipment for the care of children
10. Burn injury in patients who will require special social, emotional, or long-term rehabilitative intervention.

From American College of Surgeons Committee on Trauma: *Resources for optimal care of the injured patient: 1999*, Chicago, 1998, American College of Surgeons.

- Complaints of a great deal of pain
- Significant fluid loss, which may occur with subsequent shock
- Full-thickness burns (third-degree burns) (Figure 11-6)
  - Injury to the epidermis, dermis, and subcutaneous tissue (possibly deeper)
  - Skin that appears charred or leathery and may be bleeding
  - No pain (although associated second-degree burns will cause pain)
  - Capillary refill absent

Body Surface Area Involved.   The chart for BSA (see Figure 11-2) can be used to estimate the total area of involved skin. In figuring fluid replacement, only the areas of partial- and full-thickness (second- and third-degree) burns are used. In an adult, each arm's surface area is approximately 9% of the total BSA. The total surface area of the torso is 36%. The front of the torso is 9% for the chest to the lower border of the ribcage and 9% for the abdomen. The back of the torso is 9% for the shoulders down to the lower border of the ribcage and 9% for the lumbar back. Each leg is 18%, or 9% for the front and 9% for the back of the leg. The head is 9% and the genital area is 1%. (Note that all but the last are multiples of 9.) In a child between 3 and 9 years of age, the arms, front and back of the torso, and genitalia are all estimated to be the same percentage as in an adult. However, in a child under 3 years of age, because of the relatively larger size of the head and smaller size of the legs, the percentage for the head is increased to 18% and the percentage for each leg is decreased to 13.5%. (Compared with an adult, 4.5% is subtracted from each leg and the combined 9% is added to the head.) For smaller burns, the patient's hand (excluding the fingers) can be used as a scale (palm ≈ 1% BSA). However, the rule of nines is simply an initial

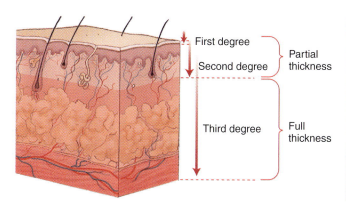

Figure 11-3   Burns are divided into superficial (first-degree), partial-thickness (second-degree), and full-thickness (third-degree) categories. Each level carries different prognostic, diagnostic, and therapeutic implications.

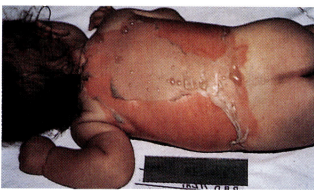

Figure 11-5   Partial-thickness burn. (*From McSwain NE Jr, Paturas JL, editors:* The basic EMT: comprehensive prehospital patient care, *ed 2, St Louis, 2001, Mosby.*)

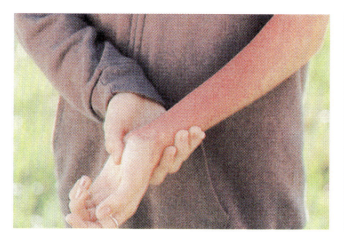

Figure 11-4   Superficial burn. (*From McSwain NE Jr, Paturas JL, editors:* The basic EMT: comprehensive prehospital patient care, *ed 2, St Louis, 2001, Mosby.*)

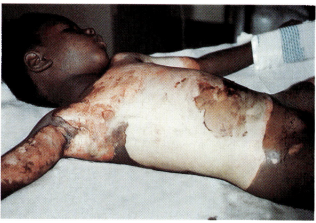

Figure 11-6   Full-thickness burn. (*From Sanders M:* Mosby's paramedic textbook, *ed 2, St Louis, 2001, Mosby.*)

estimate. Most studies show that using the rule of nines results in an underestimate of the ultimate size of the burn calculated using a weight/height nomogram in the hospital. This difference is not relevant in most prehospital situations.

Age of the Patient. A burn patient's age has a significant effect on his or her survival. The very young and the very old respond poorly to burn injury. Elderly patients may have many preexisting conditions that can complicate their care. Reduced vital organ function, decreased resistance to infection, and atherosclerotic vascular disease make age a major factor in burn management. As patients age there is a gradual increase in mortality from burns because of the body's general inability to respond to massive insult. This gradual decrease in survival can be estimated by adding the age of the patient in years to the percentage of BSA of partial- and full-thickness burns. For example, the probability of mortality of a 60-year-old patient with partial- and full-thickness burn on 30% of his body can be estimated as follows:

60 (age in years) + 30% (BSA burned) = 90% probability of mortality

Pulmonary injury and sepsis are the major components that affect a patient's overall outcome. Preexisting medical conditions, either diagnosed or undiagnosed before admission, can adversely affect both of these components. Preexisting medical conditions usually increase with advancing age and are a part of the reason that age is an important factor in determining a critical burn injury.

Pulmonary Injury
Smoke Inhalation. Smoke inhalation injuries account for over 50% of deaths each year from burns. Of the 75,000 victims hospitalized for major burns, 30% are treated for smoke poisoning and inhalation injuries.

The upper airway may be injured by direct heat. This is especially true when steam is involved. Air cannot usually conduct enough calories (heat) into the nose and mouth to produce a burn, but water (steam) can. Steam injuries are usually to the larynx and vocal cords but not any deeper.

The smoke particles that are inhaled are the main cause of pulmonary trauma. This type of injury is a form of chemical damage to the cells that line the bronchi and alveoli. If the smoke particles are filtered out and not allowed to reach the lungs, injury may not occur. Wearing some type of mask (even a wet handkerchief) in a house filled with smoke reduces such injuries significantly. A prehospital care provider should not enter a smoke-filled area without adequate training and protection.

Fluid overload after such an injury can further compromise pulmonary injury. Intravenous fluid therapy should be administered, following careful guidelines in the resuscitation of the burn injury patient.

Toxic By-product Inhalation. Much of the long-term lung damage in inhalation injuries is caused by toxic fumes or smoke. Many of these by-products are highly acidic and cause destruction of the epithelial lining of the bronchi, alveoli, and pulmonary capillaries. After exposure, initial pulmonary symptoms may not become clinically apparent for up to 12 to 36 hours. Generally speaking, the earlier symptoms present, the more severe the damage. Moreover, various toxic, volatile by-products (such as cyanide) may be released when materials such as plastics burn, resulting in inhalation poisoning.

Associated Injuries
Airway Burns. Dry heat and steam inhalation injuries are usually limited to the upper airway, whereas burns to the lower airway (including the lungs) may be caused by smoke particles. Heat, upon entering the air passages, dissipates in the nasopharynx and upper airway, causing burns and inflammation. Airway obstruction secondary to edema may occur within 24 hours. When the potential for losing the airway exists because of the progression of edema, intubation should be considered as early as possible.

Other Associated Nonburn Injuries. Falls, vehicle crashes, and electrical injuries are other possible causes of injury during a fire. Shock produced directly from and only by the burn injury appears late. Early shock is produced by hypovolemia, hypoxia, or some other cause, not the burn. *A burn patient who is displaying signs of shock soon after the injury is most probably not in shock from the burn but from associated injuries that produce hypovolemia, such as internal hemorrhage from damaged organs or broken bones, or from severe hypoxia caused by pulmonary injury.* The mechanism of injury should be reviewed, and other injuries that might cause shock should be assessed.

In burn injuries, as with all trauma, shock occurs when the patient has a deficiency of circulating blood volume with decreased tissue oxygenation. The body's response to a burn is the formation of edema. Any burn, no matter how small, will produce edema at the burn site. When the burn is as great as 20% of the BSA, the fluid shift from the vascular compartment to the tissue will be significant. This will produce a gradual decrease in circulating fluid volume that becomes detectable as hypoperfusion of the body tissues manifested by hypotension and other signs of shock. This fluid shift does not become apparent until a large amount has been lost. Such a shift usually requires several hours to become noticeable. Hypovolemic shock (and shock of any kind) in the prehospital phase is not secondary to the burn but is caused by another injury.

Evaluation of the circulating blood volume in a severely burned patient may be difficult, and the blood pressure may be unreliable. Tachycardia may be the first indication of impending shock but can also be present because of the pain associated with a partial-thickness burn. The burn patient should be managed in the same manner as any other trauma patient. Upon identification of the signs of shock, the patient should be managed as if hypovolemic shock is present. Fluid replacement, heat conservation (after the burning process has been stopped), immobilization of possible fractures, hemorrhage control, and high-concentration supplemental oxygen should be used as indicated. Adequate pain management should also be provided.

Special Considerations

Chemical Burns.   A chemical burn occurs when the skin comes in contact with various caustic agents. The prehospital care provider must be careful not to become a victim. *In most cases*, dilution and washing away of the chemical with copious amounts of water is the first step in management. The chemical continues to react until it is completely removed. This is also true for dry chemicals after brushing off any powder. The skin will contribute water to any reaction, so it is better to flush and dilute the chemical with a copious amount of water. *Flushing should begin immediately.* Neutralizing agents should not be used because they may cause further exothermic (heat) injuries from chemical reactions, producing sudden additional heat, burning, and tissue damage. The exact amount of time required for irrigation cannot be predicted. Therefore flushing should begin at the scene and continue until arrival at the receiving facility.

The prehospital care provider should notify the receiving facility in advance so that they can be ready to continue irrigation and prepare a suitable area to contain the washed-off materials. If the identity of the chemical is known, it should be relayed so the receiving facility can prepare any special antidotes before the patient's arrival. The materials safety data sheet (MSDS) for the chemical, if available, should be found and transported with the patient.

If the chemical is a dry powder, as much as possible should be brushed off before flushing to reduce the chemical concentration. While flushing is in progress, the patient's clothes should be removed. The patient's shoes must be removed early to avoid pooling water that contains high chemical concentrations. The prehospital care provider should avoid runoff or splattering onto himself or herself or his or her clothing. *The safety of the prehospital care provider is paramount. Standard precautions (gloves, gowns, and eye protection) are necessary.*

Chemical burns of the eye should be irrigated with large volumes of saline; topical anesthetic agents (such as tetracaine) may be applied if necessary to control eyelid movement. The patient's hands may need to be restrained; even the most cooperative patient may have difficulty allowing someone to irrigate his or her eyes. Irrigation should continue en route to the receiving facility. The patient should be positioned so that the runoff will not spill into the other eye. The use of a Morgan lens may be helpful. The prehospital care provider should be familiar with local protocols.

Chemicals that require special treatment are as follows:

- *Dry lime and soda ash.* Like any powder, these powders should be brushed off because contact with water will form a corrosive substance. The contaminated areas should not be irrigated unless they are already wet. Large quantities of water should be used if the burning process has already begun.
- *Phenol.* Phenol is widely used as an industrial cleaning agent. Although phenol is not water soluble, flushing with large amounts of water may be beneficial.
- *Lithium and sodium metal.* These are substances that react with water, releasing heat and toxic fumes. Any large metal chunks that remain in or around the burn should be removed and placed in oil.
- *Hydrogen fluoride and hydrofluoric acid.* Death from these types of burns have been reported with as little as 2.5% BSA involved. When transport is prolonged, calcium gluconate or calcium chloride can be mixed with lubricant jelly (a premixed product is available) and applied to the burned area, which may slow the damage.

If the prehospital care provider is unsure about treatment for a chemical burn, he or she should ask medical control to contact the nearest poison control center or CHEMTREC at 800-424-9300.

Electrical Burns. The degree of tissue damage in an electrical burn is related to the amount of current involved and the duration of the exposure. The first priority is to determine if the patient is still in contact with the electrical source. If this cannot be determined with certainty, *the patient should not be touched.* Attempts to remove the patient from contact with any electrical source should only be done by those who are trained to do so. Electrical injury burns can cause cardiac arrest. Cardiopulmonary resuscitation (CPR) may be required with such patients.

Electrical burns are actually thermal burns as the resistance of the tissues converts electrical energy into heat in direct proportion to the amperage and current of the source. The smaller the body part, the more intense the heat and the smaller the area to dissipate that heat. Therefore small body parts like fingers and toes, hands, feet, and forearms will sustain more damage than the trunk. Muscle contraction can cause fractures of lumbar vertebrae, the humerus, or even the femur and may dislocate shoulders and hips. Muscular cell damage releases myoglobin and potassium and can cause injury similar to crush syndrome. Electrical cardiac damage includes actual rupture of the heart wall or the papillary muscles. Household current in North America at 110 volts generally does little physical damage but may cause ventricular fibrillation. Alternating current is more likely to cause ventricular fibrillation than direct current.

The three types of electrical injury are as follows:

1. *Current burns.* Electrical current passes through the tissue, causing extensive areas of necrosis along the current's pathway. The skin is often charred and in some cases has exploded apart. These burns typically have entry and exit wounds. These patients should be assumed to have associated injuries to the nerves, bones, muscles, blood vessels, and other organs along the pathway between the entry and exit points.
2. *Arc (flash) burns.* Arc burns occur by arcing of electricity between two contact points close together near the skin. With these injuries the skin can be exposed to temperatures of 4500° to 5400° F (2500° to 3000° C), producing significant cutaneous burns. Such injuries are typically superficial and are recognized by the loss or singeing of hair along the arc's pathway. Deep injury may be evident, especially at flexed joints, as the electricity jumps from body part to body part, such as the forearm to the upper arm or from the arm into the chest.

3. *Contact burns.* Contact burns occur when electrical current passes through a metallic object (such as a wire or tool) and causes the metal to become superheated. The object may slice through tissue and usually results in very deep burns.

Initial management for patients of electrical burns includes an intravenous lactated Ringer's solution or normal saline running wide open. This helps prevent kidney failure by flushing myoglobin, a by-product of muscle damage, through the kidneys. Additional treatment includes administration of sodium bicarbonate. The following are key points to consider with electrical injuries:

- Do not become part of the circuit. However, patients do not store electricity and are safe to touch if they are no longer in contact with the electrical source.
- Anticipate greater tissue damage than is visible externally.
- Examine the patient for associated injuries to bones and internal organs, and immobilize as necessary.
- Administer volume replacement to protect the kidneys from tubular necrosis and subsequent shutdown.
- Monitor the patient for possible cardiac dysrhythmias.
- Transport *all* electrical burn patients to an appropriate facility.

Carbon Monoxide Poisoning. All patients who have sustained a thermal injury in an enclosed area, whether the patient presents with symptoms or not, should be suspected of having and treated for carbon monoxide poisoning. The symptoms of carbon monoxide poisoning include hypoxia with an altered mental state, neurologic deficits, and severe headache. The presence of cherry red color, although classic, is seldom seen because it is masked by cyanosis from unoxygenated hemoglobin. Reliance on cherry red skin color to determine carbon monoxide poisoning is dangerous and is a finding, like crepitus, that is helpful when present but provides no information when absent.

Carbon monoxide, a colorless, odorless, tasteless gas, has greater than 200 times the affinity for hemoglobin than for oxygen. This decreases the oxygen-carrying capacity of hemoglobin. In addition, the presence of carbon monoxide decreases the offloading of oxygen from hemoglobin, therefore decreasing oxygen delivery to the tissues. Because the half-life of carboxyhemoglobin is relatively long, all patients with symptoms suggestive of carbon monoxide poisoning should be treated with high concentrations of oxygen. This elevates the partial pressure of arterial oxygen (PaO_2), enhances displacement of carbon monoxide from the hemoglobin molecule, and improves saturation of hemoglobin with oxygen. At an oxygen concentration of 100% (Fio$_2$ of 1.0), the carboxyhemoglobin half-life will be reduced from over 4 hours to between 40 and 60 minutes. The patient should be transported to an appropriate facility. If a burn center is available within a reasonable access time, other hospitals should be bypassed. Patients with very high concentrations of carbon monoxide may require hyperbaric oxygen treatment.

Preexisting Disease. Conditions that exist before the onset of the burn injury can compromise the outcome. The conditions that occur during and after the resuscitation of a burn patient, such as sepsis, large volumes of fluid replacement, pulmonary edema, multiple operative procedures, prolonged bed confinement, decreased control of temperature regulatory mechanisms, and skin grafts, are part of the recovery from a burn. Any condition such as congestive heart failure, renal failure, hypertension, or atherosclerotic peripheral vascular disease can have a negative effect on the patient's prognosis.

Systemic Heat Injuries

Elevated body temperatures, derived externally from the environment or internally from increased metabolism, can cause illness and death by overwhelming the body's ability to dissipate heat. Normal acclimatization to changes in environmental heat occurs over about 2 weeks. The amount of sweat produced in the acclimated person increases, and the salts lost in sweat decrease. Dehydration secondary to sweating can add to susceptibility to heat illness and can cause its own problems. As little as a 4% dehydration can cause a 50% loss of muscle strength, and a 6% dehydration significantly increases the risk for heat illness. Most heat illness occurs after several days in a row of exposure to heat and humidity, especially early in the season before acclimatization. When heat buildup is greater than heat loss, internal body systems begin to malfunction. High cellular temperature causes damage in all of the body's systems and individual organs. No single target organ bears the majority of damage. Muscle, liver, kidney, cardiovascular, and central nervous system cells all sustain damage. In certain instances, only rapid intervention by prehospital personnel can alter this destructive path. Several types or stages of signs and symptoms of systemic heat injuries exist, including heat cramps, heat syncope, heat edema, heat exhaustion, and heat stroke. These terms do not describe the physiologic changes that occur; however, because of the common usage of these terms, they continue to be used. The prehospital care provider should recognize that these terms are simply names. They are not distinct conditions but represent points along a continuum of heat illness from relatively mild to life-threatening disease.

HEAT EXHAUSTION

Heat exhaustion results from excessive fluid and electrolyte loss through sweating and lack of adequate fluid replacement when the patient is exposed to high environmental temperatures for a sustained period of time, usually several days. Activity during such a period of exposure can increase fluid loss to the point of hypovolemia. The patient's signs and symptoms are those of dehydration. The management is the same as for dehydration.

Assessment. Patients with heat exhaustion may complain of headache, drowsiness, euphoria, nausea, lightheadedness, or anxiety; or display signs of fatigue and apathy. They may feel better while lying down but become light-headed when they attempt to stand or sit (orthostatic hypotension). Their skin usually feels cool and clammy. Profuse sweating is not unusual. Ventilations and pulse rates may be rapid, and the pulse may feel thready at the radial artery. Systolic blood pressure may be normal or slightly decreased, and an orthostatic test of vital signs (tilt test) will be positive. The patient's core body temperature may be either normal or slightly elevated.

Management. Management of heat exhaustion is similar to that of any hypovolemic patient, although the patient should be moved into a cool environment rather than a warm one. The patient should be kept in a supine position, and any heavy clothing should be removed. Even if the patient is alert, oral rehydration is usually not as effective because patients are often nauseous and the absorption of liquid out of the stomach is limited to about 8 ounces every 20 minutes. Preferably, lactated Ringer's solution or normal saline should be administered intravenously. Two to four liters of crystalloid infusion for an adult is not unusual. Proper temperature control and regular monitoring of vital signs during transport are essential.

HEAT CRAMPS

Heat cramps usually occur in individuals with heat exhaustion who are not acclimated to a hot environment. Heat cramps accompany heat exhaustion in up to 60% of cases. Heat cramps occur in a patient who is at rest and are often confused with exercise cramps that result from a buildup of lactic acid. Heat cramps are due to a loss of balance between electrolytes and water. The primary electrolytes lost in such cases are sodium and potassium. Water loss may also add to the onset of heat cramps, but so may overhydration with water alone. Sudden cooling of muscles has also been implicated. Between 15 and 20 grams of sodium can be lost through sweating with heavy muscular activity in hot environments.

Assessment. Patients with heat cramps typically complain of muscle cramping in the lower extremities, back, abdomen, or arms. The muscles involved are generally the larger muscle groups. The muscles feel tight and hard when palpated.

Management. Immediate management includes removal of the patient from the hot environment and gentle stretching of the muscle to alleviate the cramp. The patient should drink fluids containing an electrolyte solution. Salt tablet usage is discouraged because the osmotic fluid shift can cause vomiting and damage to the stomach lining. Rarely does a heat cramp patient need intravenous fluids. Heat exhaustion, which may coexist with heat cramps, should not be ruled out.

HEAT STROKE

Heat stroke can occur suddenly from such circumstances as a baby left in a hot vehicle, an adult transported in improperly ventilated vehicles, or exposure to confined spaces with poor ventilation, such as a boiler room or an attic. Heat stroke also can develop slowly over days, especially in the elderly. Large groups of patients often overwhelm emergency services during heat waves. The two different types of heat stroke are as follows:

1. *Classical heat stroke* is most often seen in the elderly. This usually age-related problem can be worsened by the various medications that an elderly person may be taking. Exposure to high room temperatures without benefit of air conditioning over time can lead to dehydration and is a classic presentation during the hot summer months. This is especially common in large cities where effective home ventilation is either not possible or not used. Scene assessment will provide information helpful in the identification of this condition.

2. *Exertional heat stroke* stems from a combination of high environmental temperature, high humidity, and physical activity. All of these conditions can rapidly elevate internal heat production and limit the body's ability to unload heat. The body reaches the point where it can no longer regulate heat gain or loss. Under certain conditions when the humidity reaches above 75%, the body is no longer able to lose heat by sweating. Athletes who practice in high humidity are prone to exertional heat stroke.

The combination of ambient temperature (read on a thermometer) and relative humidity is called *heat stress index* (Box 11-2). This may be a better way of predicting potential systemic heat injury than the ambient temperature alone. If the patient was working in direct sunlight, near surfaces that radiate large amounts of heat, or in heavy protective clothing, 10 degrees should be added to the figure on the table. Wearing impermeable clothing such as turnout gear or hazardous materials suits during physical activity leads to rapid heat overload and heat stroke. If the condition is not recognized and managed immediately, body temperatures above 106° to 108° F (41° to 42° C) are possible and death or permanent disability is imminent.

Assessment. Heat stroke patients typically present with hot, flushed skin. They may or may not be sweating depending on where they are found and whether they have classical or exertional heat stroke. Blood pressure may be elevated or diminished, and the pulse is usually tachycardic and thready. The patient's LOC can range from altered and confused to unconscious, and seizure activity may also be present. The key clues to separate heat stroke from one of the other heat-related conditions are the elevation in body temperature and LOC. Any patient who is warm to the touch with an altered mental status (confused, disoriented, or combative) should be suspected of having heat stroke and should be treated accordingly.

Management. Heat stroke is a true emergency. The higher the temperature and the longer a patient remains with an elevated internal temperature, the more destructive and deadly the condition becomes. High core (and thus brain) temperatures are much more destructive when combined with advancing age. Adult patients often cannot tolerate temperatures that pediatric patients can tolerate.

Management consists of rapidly cooling the patient with whatever means are available. Ice water poured directly over the patient is the fastest method of cooling. If ice is not immediately available, cool water immersion or cool water with forced evaporation by use of a fan is effective. Ice water does not cause vasoconstriction sufficient to prevent cooling. Cooling should begin before transport, with special attention given to the cooling of

Box 11-2

Heat Stress Index

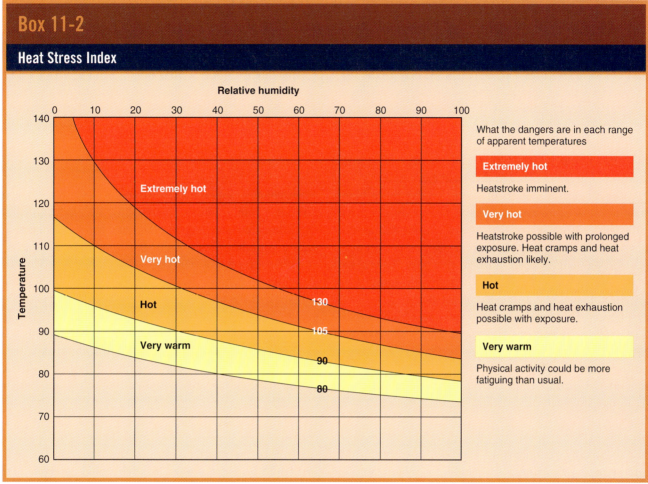

From Sanders M: *Mosby's paramedic textbook*, ed 2, St Louis, 2001, Mosby.

the head and scalp. Blood vessels are closest to the surface in the groin, axilla, and anterior lateral neck. About 40% of heat loss occurs in the head and neck. Some steps that the prehospital care provider can take include removing heavy clothing, placing the patient in an air-conditioned ambulance, and pouring bottled irrigation fluids over the patient. Fanning the patient will promote evaporation and removal of heat. Ice packs should be placed in the groin area, in the axillae, and around the neck. Seizures, which will elevate temperature, should be stopped using benzodiazepines or even paralytics.

Cold-Related Conditions and Injuries

Cold injuries differ from burn injuries, although the skin is involved in both situations. Pulmonary complications predominate with burn patients, whereas changes in core temperature and reduced circulation are the pri-

mary associated complications with cold injuries. The clinical conditions of cold injuries often are not as dramatic as with heat trauma, neither in rapidity of onset nor as immediately visible diagnostic clues. The extent of injury to the skin may appear much more superficial with a cold-related condition than that produced by a similar degree of burn. Prolonged exposure and moisture are the usual causative factors in cold injuries.

Cutaneous Conditions of Cold

Unless injury is due to a super-cooled liquid splash, cold injuries to the skin are generally isolated to such body areas as the fingers, toes, hands, feet, face, and ears—places where a significant difference exists between the surface area and the blood volume that circulates through the body part. These body parts are more exposed and farther away from the core temperature zone of the trunk, making them more susceptible to cold injuries. The most common injury to these areas is frostbite.

FROSTBITE

Frostbite is the actual freezing of the water in the body tissue as a result of exposure to freezing or below-freezing temperatures. The body's normal response to lower-than-desirable temperatures is to reduce blood flow to the skin surface to reduce heat exchange with the environment. The body accomplishes this by vasoconstriction of peripheral blood vessels in an attempt to shunt warm blood to the body's core to maintain a normal body temperature. Reduction of this blood flow greatly reduces the amount of heat delivered to the distal extremities.

The longer the period of exposure, the more blood flow is reduced to the periphery. The body conserves core temperature at the expense of extremity and skin temperature. The heat loss from the tissue becomes greater than the heat supplied to that area. In cases of below-freezing temperatures when the extremities are left unprotected, the intracellular and extracellular fluids can freeze. This results in the formation of ice crystals. As the ice crystals form, they expand and cause damage to local tissues. Blood clots may also form, further impairing circulation to the area. Use of drugs, such as nicotine or alcohol, and wet or tight and constricting clothing can further contribute to the development of frostbite.

The assessment of any patient who has been in below-freezing temperatures without proper clothing and shelter should always include an examination of those body parts that are most susceptible to frostbite. Hydrocarbon fluids, such as gasoline, can cause immediate frostbite when spilled onto exposed skin in below-freezing temperatures because of rapid evaporation and conduction. Frostbite can also immediately result from warm, moist skin contacting extremely cold metal because of rapid conduction.

Frostbite is divided into two types:

1. *Superficial frostbite*, also called *frost nip*, is the less severe type of frostbite. The patient feels slight pain or a burning sensation in the affected extremity, which later develops into numbness. The skin of the affected area will appear grayish or yellow. When digital pressure is applied to the area, the tissue below the discolored extremity will feel soft and malleable like normal tissue.
2. *Deep frostbite* develops if a patient does not recognize or react to the numbing sensation of the extremity. If the freezing of the tissue continues, the affected area becomes more waxy-looking. When the nerve endings become frozen, the numbness and pain stop. The frozen parts are hard and are not pli-

able when the affected tissue is compressed. The longer an extremity is allowed to remain frozen and the lower the temperature of the environment, the more severe the injury will be. The severity of deep frostbite cannot be determined until the frozen body part has thawed and the body begins to repair the damage. Frostbitten extremities may continue to improve gradually over several days to several weeks. Early excision or the opening of blisters is not recommended for frostbite.

Assessment. Superficial frostbite is usually assessed through a combination of recognizing the environmental conditions; considering the patient's chief complaint of pain or numbness of a digit, hand, foot, or facial area; and observing discolored skin in the same area. The environmental conditions must be below freezing. Gentle palpation of the area can determine if the underlying tissue is compliant or hard when compressed. The patient with superficial freezing will usually complain of increased discomfort during the manipulation of the frostbitten area. In cases of deep frostbite, the frozen tissue will be hard and usually is not painful when touched or compressed.

Management. The immediate management of frostbite is to move the frostbite patient from the cold environment into a heated area. The prehospital care provider should always suspect systemic hypothermia. Patients with superficial frostbite should be placed with the affected area against a warm body surface, such as covering the patient's frostbitten ears with warm hands or placing affected fingers into the armpits. Superficial frostbite only needs to be warmed at normal body temperatures.

The prehospital care for deep frostbite should consist of appropriate shelter, supportive care, and early transport to an appropriate facility. The patient can drink something warm (and nonalcoholic) if it is available, depending on the patient's LOC and other injuries. Tobacco use (smoking, chewing, or using nicotine patches) should be discouraged because nicotine causes further vasoconstriction.

Attempts to begin rewarming of deep frostbite patients in the field can be hazardous to the patient's eventual recovery and are not recommended unless long transport times are involved. Deep frostbite should be rewarmed in a controlled setting for the following reasons:

- The rewarming of the extremity should be a rapid immersion process, using consistent water temperatures of 102° to 108° F (38.5° to 42° C).

- The rewarming process is an extremely painful event for the patient. Intravenous analgesics are usually required for pain relief.
- If rewarming attempts have been started and for some reason the extremity is allowed to refreeze, gangrene may occur and the extremity or a part of the extremity may have to be amputated.

As mentioned previously, the severity of deep frostbite injuries is determined after the thawing process is completed. Frostbite is categorized into four degrees of severity similar to the categorization of burns. Superficial frostbite is classified as first degree. The most severe, fourth degree, usually develops gangrene shortly after thawing.

If rewarming has been initiated, the affected body parts should be elevated gently to reduce swelling while maintaining the rewarming process. Individual digits should be separated carefully with cotton or gauze to reduce skin irritation and to decrease the chance of the digits sticking together. If blisters have formed on the extremity, they should be left intact and not punctured. While transporting a patient once rewarming has begun, the prehospital care provider should not allow the thawed part to refreeze. Pain relief may be necessary during transport.

Systemic Conditions of Cold

The most common systemic cold injury or condition is hypothermia. *Hypothermia* is defined as the condition in which the core body temperature is measured below 95° F (35° C) when using a rectal thermometer placed at least 15 cm (6 inches) into the rectum. Unlike frostbite, hypothermia can occur in environments with temperatures well above freezing. Hypothermia can affect healthy individuals who are placed into adverse conditions unprepared (*primary hypothermia*) or can develop secondary to the patient's existing illness or injury (*secondary hypothermia*). If unrecognized or improperly treated, hypothermia can be fatal—in some cases within 2 hours. A 50% mortality rate exists in cases of secondary hypothermia caused by complications of other injuries and in severe cases in which the core body temperature is below 90° F (32° C).

Many variables promote hypothermia. Environmental conditions can lower a patient's core body temperature to the point where his or her mental status is affected. Impairment progresses from poor judgment to initial confusion to stupor and eventually coma. In such cases the patient must rely on others to recognize the condition. If the condition is unrecognized and untreated, death may be imminent.

As the body's core temperature falls below 95° F (35° C), the heart rate, ventilatory drive, blood pressure, and cerebral and peripheral blood flow all begin to decrease. The reduced peripheral blood flow shunts warm blood to the core at the expense of the shell. This higher core blood volume causes "cold diuresis" and ultimately hypovolemia. Skeletal muscles begin to shiver in an attempt to produce heat, at first subtly and then more violently. This eventually ceases and the muscles become stiff as the core temperature drops below 90° F (32° C). Because of decreased cardiac output and increased oxygen deficit caused by shivering, peripheral cellular hypoxia develops with increased lactic acid production and eventual metabolic acidosis in the periphery. However, oxygenation and blood flow are maintained in the core. Cerebral metabolism and therefore oxygen demand decrease by 6% to 10% per degree centigrade drop in core temperature. This means that cerebral oxygenation is preserved despite bradycardia and bradypnea.

The pupils become fixed and dilated only at extremely low core temperatures. With moderate hypothermia, pupillary reflexes are normal. The PR, QRS, and QTC intervals are prolonged. ST and T wave changes and J or Osborn waves may be present and may mimic other electrocardiographic abnormalities, such as an acute myocardial infarction (AMI). Atrial fibrillation and extreme bradycardias develop and may continue between 83° F and 90° F (28° C and 32° C). When the core temperature reaches 80° to 82° F (26.7° to 28° C), any physical stimulation of the heart can cause ventricular fibrillation. The stimulation could be caused by CPR or possibly by rough handling of the patient. At these extremely low core temperatures, pulse and blood pressure are not detectable and the joints are stiff. However, a patient should not be assumed to be dead until he or she is rewarmed and still has no signs of life (ECG, pulse, ventilation, and mental function).

SEVERITY AND EXPOSURE

The severity of hypothermia is determined by the core temperature of the body at its lowest reading. Hypothermia is classified into two types: (1) mild, with a core temperature of 90° F (32° C) and above, and (2) profound, with a core temperature below 90° F (32° C). The duration of exposure that contributes to the hypothermic condition is divided into three categories:

1. *Acute.* Sudden lowering of core temperature in minutes, such as immersion in cold water
2. *Subacute.* Lowering of the core temperature over 1 hour to several days

308 PREHOSPITAL TRAUMA LIFE SUPPORT

3. *Chronic.* Lowering of the core temperature slowly over weeks (usually occurs in the elderly)

The significance of exposure time deals with the difference between the core and the peripheral body temperatures. The longer the patient is exposed, the closer the core temperature becomes to the peripheral skin temperature. With minimal exposure time before rewarming, serum glucose levels remain within normal to slightly above normal limits, permitting adequate aerobic metabolism to occur. With normal cellular metabolism, lactic acid production and acid base balance will remain within normal limits.

As exposure time lengthens, as in subacute and chronic conditions, the core temperature more closely approaches the peripheral body temperature. When this occurs, hypoglycemia and acidosis begin to develop, and continued aerobic metabolism is threatened. Although the exact length of exposure is significant, any patient can develop profound hypothermia in a short time span.

HYPOTHERMIC SITUATIONS

Prehospital personnel encounter hypothermic patients in many different settings and situations. Four broad categories describe the settings—immersion hypothermia, submersion hypothermia, field hypothermia, and urban hypothermia.

Immersion Hypothermia. Immersion hypothermia occurs when an individual is placed into a cold environment without preparation or planning. Someone who has fallen through the ice in a pond or river is immediately in danger of hypothermia. Near-drowning victims in water 70° F (21° C) or colder also fall into this category. These situations are usually acute hypothermia settings.

Submersion Hypothermia. Submersion hypothermia is a combination of hypothermia and hypoxia. Cases exist with remarkable results in resuscitating cold water near-drowning patients. Successful resuscitation without neurologic impairment has occurred in cases of cold water submersion of up to 66 minutes. The mammalian diving reflex, which involves instinctive breath holding, vital function slowing, and blood shunting to the body's core, all increase survivability. Cold water is also thought to protect the central nervous system from the otherwise damaging effects of cerebral hypoxia.

Several factors may influence the outcome of a cold water submersion patient:

- *Age.* The large number of successful infant and child resuscitations in the United States and Europe

has been well documented. The smaller mass of a child's body cools faster than an adult's body, thus permitting fewer harmful by-products of anaerobic metabolism to form and causing less irreversible damage.
- *Submersion time.* The shorter the length of submersion, the less chance the patient has for cellular damage caused by hypoxia. The prehospital care provider should obtain accurate information concerning submersion time. Immersion greater than 66 minutes is probably fatal. However, rescue and resuscitation efforts should be initiated regardless of the length of submersion.
- *Water temperature.* Water temperatures of 70° F (21° C) and below are capable of inducing hypothermia. The colder the water, the better the chance of survival. This is probably due to a decreased metabolism when the body is quickly chilled.
- *Struggle.* Submersion victims who struggle less have a better chance of being resuscitated (unless their struggling efforts are successful enough to avoid drowning). Less struggle means less muscle activity, which translates to less heat (energy) production and less vasodilation. These in turn cause decreased muscular oxygen deficits (decreased deficits mean less CO_2 and lactic acid production), and thus the rate of cooling is increased.
- *Cleanliness of the water.* Patients generally do better after resuscitation if they were submerged in clean water rather than muddy or contaminated water. Chances of survival between freshwater and salt-water submersions are the same.
- *Quality of CPR and resuscitative efforts.* Patients who receive adequate and effective CPR, combined with proper rewarming and advanced life support (ALS) measures, generally do better than patients for whom one or more of these items was substandard. Immediate initiation of CPR is a key factor for submersion hypothermia patients.
- *Associated injuries or illness.* Patients with an existing injury or illness, or who become ill or injured in combination with the submersion, do not fare as well as otherwise healthy individuals.

The preceding list of factors that appear to contribute to a submersion patient's chances of successful recovery is based on ongoing research. Every submersion patient should have full resuscitation efforts made, regardless of the presence or absence of any of these factors. A patient should be warm and dead before resuscitation is terminated.

Field Hypothermia.   Field hypothermia involves a protracted exposure to the elements, usually by healthy individuals who participate in outdoor sports and adventure activities. Skiing, backpacking, hunting, climbing, and other outdoor sports enthusiasts can become overexposed to cold temperatures and placed in danger of hypothermia.

Urban Hypothermia.   Urban hypothermia is sometimes missed because of the possibility of a more common illness or injury. Various acute and chronic medical conditions may make the patient more susceptible to hypothermia. In turn, the underlying hypothermia may hamper the effectiveness of normal treatment modalities. Hypothermia should be suspected in all of the following cases:

- Newborns and infants
- Patients with alcohol-related illness or injury
- Patients with drug use or overdose, including both recreational drug abuse and abuse of certain prescription drugs (e.g., beta blockers and sedatives)
- Patients with cocaine-induced hypothermia
- All elderly patients, regardless of obvious injury or illness
- Patients with diseases such as hypothyroidism, heart disease, and diabetes
- Burn patients
- Patients with malnutrition
- Homeless individuals who are underclothed and/or in shelters

A typical situation in which hypothermia may not be suspected is a cool, rainy day with a temperature of 60° F (15° C). The patient "sleeping off" a heavy alcohol intake, wearing wet clothing, and lying on cool pavement or a sidewalk is a perfect situation for unrecognized severe hypothermia.

ASSESSMENT

The prehospital care provider should highly suspect hypothermia even when the environmental conditions are not highly suggestive (e.g., wind, moisture, temperature). Rectal temperatures are not commonly assessed in the field nor widely used as a vital sign in most prehospital systems. Ambulances usually only carry a standard-range oral or rectal (for infants) thermometer, which only reads to 94° F (34.4° C). Electronic thermometers are also not useful in hypothermic situations. To obtain hypothermic temperatures, a low-range rectal thermometer is necessary. In colder climates, prehospital care units should carry these inexpensive thermometers.

The best assessment finding that a prehospital care provider can seek when suspecting hypothermia is muscular shivering and the patient's LOC. Mildly hypothermic patients (core temperature higher than 90° F [32° C]) will have an altered LOC and usually show signs of confusion, slurred speech, altered gait, and clumsiness. They will be slow in their actions and are usually found in a nonambulatory state—sitting or lying. They will be shivering. Law enforcement and EMS personnel may misinterpret this condition as drug or alcohol intoxication.

When the patient's core temperature falls below 90° F (32° C), profound hypothermia is present and the patient will probably not complain of feeling cold. Shivering will be absent, and the patient's LOC will be markedly decreased, possibly to the point of unconsciousness and coma. The patient's pupils will react slowly or may be dilated and fixed. The patient's palpable pulses may be diminished or absent, and his or her systolic blood pressure may be low or indeterminate. The patient's ventilations may have slowed to as few as one or two breaths per minute. An ECG may show atrial or ventricular fibrillation.

MANAGEMENT

Prehospital care of the hypothermic patient consists of prevention of further heat loss, gentle handling, initiation of rapid transport, and rewarming (in certain circumstances).

This includes moving the patient to the warm ambulance or to a warm shelter if transportation is not immediately available. Wet clothing should be removed by cutting to avoid unnecessary movement and agitation of the patient. The patient's head should be covered with warm blankets. The patient should be covered with an outer windproof layer to prevent convective and evaporative heat loss. If the patient is conscious and alert, he or she can drink warm sweet fluids. The patient should avoid alcohol and caffeine drinks. Intravenous fluids should be warmed to 104° F (40° C) and administered if an intravenous line can be started without unduly agitating the patient. *The patient should not be given cold (room temperature) fluids.* This fluid is below body temperature and will make the patient colder. These two forms of therapy are minimal at best for rewarming, and the prehospital care provider should use common sense to decide whether fluids (orally or intravenously) are worth the risks of aspiration, coughing, and painful stimuli.

Hot packs or massaging of the patient's extremities are not recommended. Rewarming of the extremities, or other methods that increase peripheral circulation before central rewarming can occur, can increase acidosis and hyperkalemia and can actually decrease the core temperature (*after drop*). This complicates resuscitation and may precipitate nonresponsive ventricular fibrillation.

The phrase "they are not dead until they are warm and dead" was coined specifically for hypothermic patients. All efforts to resuscitate the patient should continue until actual brain death is determined with the core temperature in the normal range.

In the more profoundly hypothermic patient, gentle handling is of utmost importance. If an ECG is available, cardiac monitoring should be used to assess the patient's electrical activity. In the absence of palpable pulses, this may be the only way to determine whether CPR is warranted. *If the ECG shows any kind of organized electrical cardiac rhythm, CPR should not be started regardless of the absence of a palpable pulse.* CPR usually will precipitate ventricular fibrillation in such patients. If ventricular fibrillation is present, normal CPR should be initiated and continued until the patient has been transported and rewarmed at the hospital. In contrast, submersion victims, like any other drowning victim, should be treated with immediate CPR (if the patient is apneic and pulseless) and full advanced cardiac life support procedures.

The patient with profound hypothermia may be unresponsive. In this case, airway adjuncts such as oral pharyngeal airways and endotracheal tubes should be used if needed. Oxygen administration is even more important and can be provided through a mask or BVM. The patient may benefit more if the oxygen can be warmed, even if by use of a pocket mask. Warmed oxygen administered before movement may prevent fibrillation during transport.

In the profoundly hypothermic patient, defibrillation and conventional advanced cardiac life support drug therapy may not be beneficial because of the depressed core temperature.

In the rare event that rewarming is attempted in the field because of the inability to transport a patient (se-

vere blizzard or other disaster), the patient should be placed in a bathtub or similar-sized container full of warm water (104° F [40° C]). The patient's extremities should be left out of the water so that the body's core will warm first. This will help avoid "after drop," which results when the extremities warm more quickly than the core and vasodilate, causing central hypotension and promoting ventricular fibrillation. This type of rewarming is a last-ditch effort. Central rewarming in a hospital setting is the preferred method.

Environmental Emergencies in Mass Casualty and Disasters

Heat and cold are major players in many special situations of mass care. Prevention and preparation for treatment of a large number of environmentally injured patients should be part of the planning for any mass gathering or disaster. Whether a rock concert or a county fair, the possibility of a large number of patients at almost any gathering is real, especially during summer outdoor gatherings. A hot summer day has obvious possibilities for heat stroke or exhaustion. However, a sudden or late afternoon thunderstorm can drop the temperature 20 or more degrees in as little as 5 minutes and follow with rain and wind to chill a lightly dressed crowd quickly. This means that prehospital care providers should plan for both heat and cold injury care with mist tents, adequate drinking water, blankets, and sheltered areas. A school bus that overturns one cold winter morning on a rural icy road may involve exposure of many victims for over an hour or more. Many mass casualty plans involve patient-collecting stations for triage and treatment before transport. How to protect patients from the heat or cold in such collecting stations must be part of the planning. Floods happen year round and produce a large number of wet and possibly cold people. Explosions can present a large number of burn and respiratory patients. Environmental concerns must be part of special event and mass casualty incident planning.

Summary

The prehospital care provider should consider a patient with a major burn just as he or she would consider any other multisystem trauma patient and manage him or her accordingly. Airway maintenance is of prime importance with all burn victims. Aggressive prehospital management of the acutely burned patient may reduce mortality in the two thirds of burn patients who die annually before reaching definitive care.

The following are major considerations when managing burn patients:

- Do not become a victim yourself. Address potential safety threats to the crew and patient immediately upon arrival.
- Airway management is the most important consideration for the burn patient. Have all equipment ready so that intubation, if required, proceeds smoothly.
- Provide high-concentration supplemental oxygen to all patients suspected of inhalation injuries.
- The primary cause of shock in the severely burned patient is hypovolemia. Treat shock with proper fluid replacement. If shock presents early, it is caused by other injuries; identify and manage these injuries.
- Irrigate most chemical injuries with copious amounts of water.
- Transport burn patients without delay to an appropriate facility.
- Avoid hypothermia.

The prehospital care provider can prevent deaths by use of systematic prehospital patient assessment and management, based on the pathophysiology and its etiology. In a severely injured multisystem trauma patient, *the trauma and systemic effects of the burn should be treated first, and then the burn should be treated.*

Cold and heat injuries can result from environmental conditions and underlying medical conditions. They can cause both localized and systemic complications for the patient and present situations that can threaten life and limb. Proper recognition, assessment, and management by prehospital personnel can limit the danger that cold and heat injuries may cause and lower the morbidity and mortality rates of these emergencies. In certain cases of hypothermia, basic treatment modalities in the field are more productive for the patient than aggressive ALS interventions. Proper assessment of the environmentally ill patient can make the difference in resuscitation and long-term recovery.

Scenario Solution

A 19-year-old male has full- and partial-thickness grease burns on his hands and right leg from toes to hip. This case represents a common problem—a patient presents with obvious, horrific looking injuries, and the prehospital care provider is drawn immediately to those injuries, thus failing to find other more life-threatening conditions. To properly manage this patient, you must first assess the scene. If the scene is safe, you should then stop the burning process. Next, conduct the primary survey. After the primary survey, provide specific care for the burn. In this case, burn care would involve covering of the burn with dry, sterile dressings; initiation of IV therapy, if applicable; and pain relief if the patient is hemodynamically stable. Transport the patient to a burn center if one is available.

A child hiding under a bed during a fire is a common scenario for firefighters. In this case the unresponsive child without burns is probably hypoxic. Immediate and aggressive airway control, 100% oxygen, and ventilation are necessary.

The elderly male who is unresponsive in his cool home may have a variety of problems from hypoglycemia to cerebrovascular accident. You must consider all of these, but hypoglycemia is not likely with the bradycardia; however, you still should check the patient's blood sugar level as with all patients with an altered level of consciousness (LOC). The patient's unresponsiveness may be due to cardiac dysrhythmias, such as sick sinus or a heart block. A core temperature reading would help with the diagnosis, but you should consider any elderly patient who is in a room that is not heated to at least the patient's age in degrees and who has an altered LOC to be hypothermic. The type of hypothermia is chronic hypothermia. You should give him warm, humidified oxygen and an IV started with warmed normal saline if possible. Movement should be gentle to avoid precipitating ventricular fibrillation.

The marathon runner who has wandered off course is another diagnostic dilemma. This patient may have hypoglycemia, and several environmental issues could be the cause of his disorientation. If the patient is cool to the touch or has a depressed core temperature, then he has hypothermia probably caused by a combination of a cool and/or rainy day or a low carbohydrate intake while running. You should get the patient out of any wet clothing, dry him, and wrap him to prevent further heat loss. If the patient is able to swallow, you may give him warm, sweet, nonalcoholic and noncaffeinated beverages. If the patient is warm or has an elevated core temperature, then the problem is heat stroke. In this case you must cool the patient immediately. The fact that the patient is wet or dry makes no difference. The altered LOC is a much greater concern.

The homeless woman with frostbite is a much more straightforward case. You must first rule out or treat the patient for systemic hypothermia. In most traditional situations you should not try to thaw the patient's limbs in the field because the pain control issue and the chances of refreeze are too great. Once the patient is in the hospital, thawing is best done in a water bath between 102° and 108° F (38° and 42° C).

Review Questions

Answers are provided on p. 414.

1. Which of the following is LEAST efficient as a source of heat production for the body?
   a. Drinking hot cocoa or coffee
   b. Shivering
   c. Running
   d. Walking

2. A 7-year-old child who caught his shirt on fire while on a camping trip has sustained burns to the anterior chest and abdomen. What percentage of body surface area is involved?
   a. 36%
   b. 9%
   c. 18%
   d. 24%

3. Signs of possible inhalation injury in the burn patient include all of the following EXCEPT:
   a. Purulent green sputum
   b. Stridor
   c. Singed facial hair
   d. Burns of the upper torso

4. Which of the following patients should be cared for in a burn center?
   a. A 30-year-old male with 9% partial-thickness burns of the left leg
   b. A 45-year-old female with 5% full-thickness burns of the right arm
   c. A 15-year-old male with superficial and partial-thickness burns of the upper back
   d. An otherwise healthy 65-year-old female with 9% partial-thickness burns of the chest

5. You have been dispatched to a local high school football practice field for a "person down." On your arrival you find a 17-year-old male who became disoriented during preseason practice and then had a seizure. He is flushed with warm skin, is mildly diaphoretic, responds only to painful stimulus, and has a weak, rapid radial pulse and a blood pressure of 92/60 mm Hg. Of the following, which is most likely to be the patient's problem?
   a. Heat exhaustion
   b. Classic heat stroke
   c. Exertional heat stroke
   d. Heat cramps

6. Treatment of heat stroke includes all of the following EXCEPT:
   a. Administering an oral rehydration solution containing electrolytes
   b. Pouring ice water over the patient
   c. Placing ice packs in the groin
   d. Preventing further seizure activity

7. Hypothermia develops:
   a. Rapidly, with a sudden lowering of core temperature
   b. Gradually, over hours to days
   c. Chronically, over a period of weeks
   d. All of the above

8. Which of the following factors DOES NOT influence survival from cold water submersion?
   a. Gender
   b. Age
   c. Water temperature
   d. Cleanliness of the water

9. All of the following treatments may be appropriate to the hypothermic patient EXCEPT:
   a. Use caution to prevent agitation of the patient
   b. Apply hot packs to the groin and axillae
   c. Cut away wet clothing
   d. Administer warm nonalcoholic oral fluids

REFERENCES

American College of Surgeons Committee on Trauma: *Advanced trauma life support,* Chicago, 2002, American College of Surgeons.

Auerbach PS: *Wilderness medicine: management of wilderness and environmental emergencies,* ed 3, St Louis, 1995, Mosby.

Forgey WW, editor: *Wilderness Medical Society practice guidelines for wilderness emergency care,* ed 2, Guilford, Conn, 2000, The Globe Pequot Press.

McSwain NE Jr, Paturas JL, editors: *The basic EMT: comprehensive prehospital patient care,* ed 2, St Louis, 2001, Mosby.

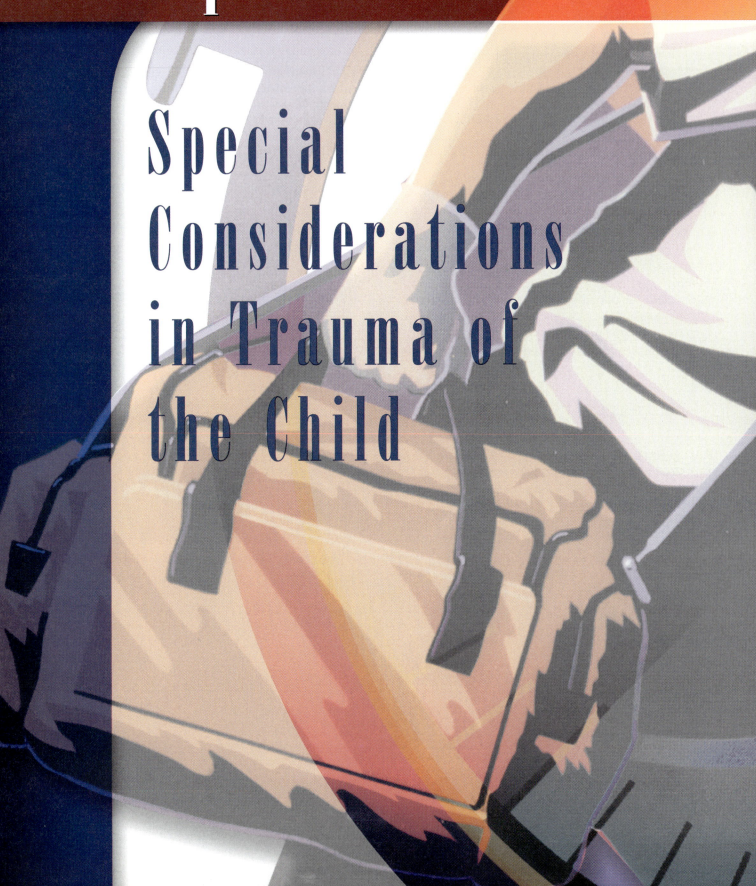

Chapter 12

Special Considerations in Trauma of the Child

Chapter Objectives

At the completion of this chapter, the reader should be able to do the following:

- Identify the unique differences in injury patterns for children.
- Demonstrate an understanding of the special importance of managing the airway and restoring adequate tissue oxygenation in pediatric patients.
- Identify the quantitative vital signs for children.
- Demonstrate an understanding of management techniques for the various injuries found in pediatric patients.
- Calculate the Pediatric Trauma Score.
- Identify the signs of pediatric trauma suggestive of child abuse.

Scenario

You are called to a pedestrian versus motor vehicle incident. A child has been struck by a sports utility vehicle (SUV) at a busy intersection that is known for its rush hour crashes. You know that the posted speed limit in this area is 45 miles per hour (72 km/hr). No weather-related factors are involved on this average spring afternoon.

Upon arrival at the scene you see that the police have secured and blocked traffic from the area around the child. As you approach the patient, you see a young boy, approximately 10 years of age, lying on his back with his left leg angulated in a dramatic outward position. You also note that the child appears calm.

Your primary and secondary surveys reveal a 12-year-old boy who tells you that his name is Scott. He has central and distal pulses at a rate of 110 beats/min, the radial pulse being weaker than the carotid; his blood pressure is 80 mm Hg by palpation; and his ventilatory rate is 20 breaths/min, slightly irregular, but without abnormal sounds. As you talk with Scott you also note that, despite having an obvious angulated left femur, he is not complaining of significant pain and he appears to be resting comfortably. As you continue to talk with him, you note that he has an altered awareness of his surroundings and what happened to him. You also note that his pupils are slightly dilated, and his skin is pale and sweaty. A woman who identifies herself as a friend of the family tells you that Scott's mother is en route and that you should wait for her.

What are the management priorities for this patient? What are the most likely injuries in this child? Where is the most appropriate destination for this child?

Injury is the most common cause of death of American children. Tragically, 20% to 40% of these deaths may be preventable. Just as with all aspects of pediatric care, proper assessment and management of an injured child requires a thorough understanding of the unique characteristics of childhood growth and development.

Good pediatric care is far more than a simple application of adult principles to a smaller person. Children have common patterns of injury, unique physiologic responses, and special needs based on their size, maturity, and psychosocial development.

This chapter first describes the special characteristics of the pediatric trauma patient and then reviews optimal trauma management and its rationale. Although the unique characteristics of pediatric injury are important for the prehospital care provider to understand, the basic life support measures using the primary and secondary surveys are the same for every patient, regardless of size.

The Child as a Trauma Patient

Demographics of Pediatric Trauma

Many unique characteristics should be addressed when considering the child as a trauma patient. The incidence of blunt (as opposed to penetrating) trauma is highest in the pediatric population. Although the National Pediatric Trauma Registry (NPTR) continues to identify blunt trauma as the most common mechanism of injury over the last 4 years, penetrating injury has increased to almost 15% of cases. The consequences of penetrating trauma are relatively predictable, but blunt trauma mechanisms have a greater potential for multisystem injury.

Falls are the most common cause of injury and occur most frequently in children younger than 14 years of age. Trauma to pedestrians struck by vehicles is the next most common mechanism. According to statistics, injury is "accidental" in 87% of cases, sports related in 4%, and the result of assault in 5%. Multisystem involvement is the rule rather than the exception; therefore all organ systems should be assumed to be injured until proven otherwise. Although minimal external evidence of injury may be present, the presence of potentially significant internal derangement of every major organ should be assumed until ruled out by definitive assessment or careful follow-up evaluation.

Kinematics of Pediatric Trauma

A child's size produces a smaller target to which linear forces from fenders, bumpers, and falls are applied. Because of diminished body fat, increased elasticity of connective tissue, and close proximity of multiple organs, these forces are not dissipated as well as in the adult and therefore disperse more energy to multiple organs. Because the skeleton of a child is incompletely calcified and contains multiple active growth centers, it is more resilient than that of an adult. However, the skeleton of a child is less able than that of an adult to absorb the kinetic forces applied during a traumatic event and may allow significant internal derangement with apparently minor external injury. For example, although rib fractures are uncommon, pulmonary contusion is common.

Thermal Homeostasis

The ratio between a child's body surface area (BSA) and body volume is highest at birth and diminishes throughout infancy and childhood. This means that relatively more surface area exists through which heat can be lost quickly. As a result, thermal energy loss becomes a significant stress factor in a smaller child. Although this may not be life-threatening by itself, it frequently provides additional stress to the child who may be hypotensive and in severe pain. Severe hypothermia will frequently initiate irreversible cardiovascular collapse.

Psychosocial Issues

The psychologic ramifications of caring for an injured child can also present a major challenge. Particularly with a very young child, regressive psychologic behavior may result when stress, pain, or other perceived threats intervene in a child's environment. A child's ability to interact with unfamiliar individuals in strange surroundings is usually limited and makes history-taking and cooperative manipulation extremely difficult. An understanding of these characteristics and a willingness to cajole and soothe an injured child is frequently the most effective means of achieving good rapport and obtaining a more comprehensive assessment of the child's physiologic state. Additionally, the child's caregivers or parents will frequently have needs and issues that need to be addressed to successfully care for the child. In many cases the caregivers need to be viewed as additional patients.

Recovery and Rehabilitation

Another problem unique to the pediatric trauma patient is the effect that injury may have on subsequent growth and development. Unlike an anatomically mature adult, a child must not only recover from the injury but must also continue the normal growing process and development. The effect of injury on this process—especially in terms of long-term disability, growth deformity, or abnormal subsequent development—cannot be overestimated. Children sustaining even minor injury may have prolonged disability either in cerebral function, psychologic adjustment, or an organ system disability. As many as 60% of children with severe multiple trauma have personality changes, and 50% are left with subtle cognitive or physical handicaps. Additionally, pediatric trauma can substantially affect siblings and parents, resulting in a high incidence of family dysfunction, including divorce. The cost of correcting these problems can be staggering and lifelong.

The effect of inadequate or inappropriate care in the immediate posttraumatic period may have consequences not only on the child's survival but also, and perhaps more importantly, on the quality of the child's life for years to come. Major organ injury may exist in the face of minimal external signs. A high index of suspicion and clinical common sense should prompt transport of the child to an appropriate facility for a more thorough evaluation when any possibility of severe injury exists.

Pathophysiology

In terms of death and disability, the ultimate result of care for the injured child is largely determined by the quality of care rendered in the first moments after injury. During these critical minutes, a systematized primary survey is the best defense against overlooking an injury that may be fatal or that may cause unnecessary morbidity. As in the adult, the three most common causes of immediate death in the child are hypoxia, massive hemorrhage, and overwhelming central nervous system (CNS) trauma. Lack of expedient triage and transport to the most appropriate center for treatment can compound any or all of these problems.

Hypoxia

The first priority in prehospital care is always the establishment of a patent airway. Confirming that a child has an open and functioning airway does not preclude the need for assisted ventilation and supplemental oxygen, especially where CNS injury or hypoperfusion may be present. Injured children can rapidly deteriorate from labored breathing and tachypnea to a state of total exhaustion and apnea. Once an airway is established, the rate and depth of ventilation should be evaluated to confirm adequate alveolar ventilation. If alveolar ventilation is not adequate, merely providing excessive concentration of oxygen will not prevent ongoing cellular hypoxia.

Adequate oxygenation is especially critical to the initial care of the patient with traumatic brain injury. A patient may be densely obtunded and yet have an excellent potential for good functional recovery if cerebral hypoxia can be avoided. If possible, patients who require advanced airway management should be preoxygenated before intubation. In many cases, this basic maneuver may be all that is necessary to begin reversal of hypoxia and improve the margin of safety when intubation is performed.

Hemorrhage

Most pediatric injuries do not cause immediate exsanguination. Unfortunately, children who sustain injuries with major blood loss die within moments or are dead on arrival at the receiving facility. Most injured children who require emergency care have multiple organ injuries with at least one component associated with blood loss. This hemorrhage may be extremely minor (such as cutaneous lacerations or contusions) or potentially life-threatening (such as a ruptured spleen, lacerated liver, or avulsed kidney).

As in adults, the injured child compensates for hemorrhage by increasing systemic vascular resistance (SVR) at the expense of peripheral perfusion. Blood pressure alone is an inadequate marker for shock. Ineffective organ perfusion is a more appropriate indication of shock and is evidenced by a decreased level of consciousness (LOC), diminished skin perfusion (decreased temperature, poor color, and delayed capillary refilling time), and decreased urine output. However, unlike in the adult, the early signs of hemorrhage in the child may be subtle and difficult to identify. Tachycardia may be caused by hypovolemia or may be the result of fear or pain. Moreover, the normal heart rate of a child varies with age. Poor peripheral perfusion may be the result of hypotension, hypothermia, or both. If the prehospital care provider misses the early subtle signs, a child may lose so much circulating blood volume that compensatory mechanisms fail. In this case, cardiac output plummets, organ perfusion disappears, and the child plunges into decompensated and usually fatal shock. Therefore the vital signs of every child who sustains blunt trauma should be carefully monitored to detect those subtle signs. Inadequate resuscitation could result in profound cardiovascular collapse at a later time.

A major reason for the rapid transition to decompensated shock is the gradual loss of red blood cell (RBC) mass. Restoration of shed blood with crystalloid solutions will provide a transient increase in blood pressure, but the solutions will dissipate as the fluid leaks across capillary membranes. The net effect is that circulating volume will be gradually replaced with an increasingly diluted RBC mass, which has virtually no oxygen-carrying capacity. The child should be assessed in light of this possibility and it should be assumed that any child who requires more than one 20 mL/kg bolus of crystalloid solution may be rapidly deteriorating.

A common error in the initial evaluation of an injured child is the tendency to overresuscitate the patient once venous access has been secured. In the face of minimal bleeding and normal vital signs, a bolus of 20 mL/kg can artificially dilute the hematocrit (a measure of the packed cell volume of RBCs in the total blood volume) and introduce a potential error in the diagnosis of hemorrhage. Given the high incidence of traumatic brain injury with associated blunt trauma and the relatively low incidence of severe hemorrhagic shock, fluid overresuscitation of a child with a traumatic brain injury may be more detrimental than effective and may actually worsen evolving cerebral edema. Careful assessment of the child's vital signs and evaluation of the effect of therapeutic intervention must be the primary consideration immediately after the injury.

Brain Injury

The pathophysiologic changes that follow trauma to the CNS begin within a matter of minutes. Early and adequate resuscitation is the key to increased survival of children with a CNS injury. Although a certain percentage of CNS injuries are overwhelmingly massive and fatal, many children present with CNS injuries that are made more severe by subsequent hypoperfusion or ischemia. Adequate oxygenation and ventilation are extremely critical in the management of traumatic brain injuries. Even densely comatose children may recover if they do not develop cerebral hypoxia.

For given degrees of injury severity as measured by the Abbreviated Injury Scale (AIS), children have a lower mortality rate and higher potential for survival than their adult counterparts. However, with the introduction of an extracranial injury in association with the cerebral injury, the child's survival curve matches that of the adult. This illustrates the potentially negative effect of associated injury on outcome from CNS trauma.

Children with traumatic brain injury frequently present with a mild degree of obtundation (sensory dullness), and they may have sustained a period of unconsciousness not recorded during initial evaluation. A history of loss of consciousness is one of the most important prognostic indicators of potential CNS injury, and the prehospital care provider should investigate and record it for every case. Likewise, complete documentation of baseline neurologic status, including the following, is important:

- Response to sensory stimulation
- Pupillary reaction
- Motor function

These are essential steps in initial pediatric trauma care. CNS injury is a pathophysiologic continuum that begins as an initial depolarization of the intracranial neurons and proceeds along a recognizable course of secondary edema and hypoperfusion. The absence of adequate baseline assessment makes ongoing follow-up and evaluation of intervention extremely imprecise and difficult.

Attention to detailed history-taking is especially important in cases of potential cervical spinal cord injury. Since a child's skeleton is incompletely calcified and has multiple active growth centers, minimal, if any, radiographic evidence may exist of a mechanism of injury that may have caused a stretch or contusion of the spinal cord. A transient neurologic deficit may be the only indicator of a potentially significant cervical spinal cord injury.

Assessment

The small and variable size of the pediatric patient (Table 12-1), the diminished caliber and size of the vascular system, and the unique anatomic characteristics of the airway frequently cause the standard procedures used in basic life support to be extremely challenging and technically difficult. The immediate availability of appropriately sized equipment is essential for successful initial management of an injured child. Attempting to place an overly large intravenous cannula or an inappropriately sized endotracheal tube can cause more harm than good. For this reason, Broselow and colleagues devised a length-based resuscitation tape. The tape allows for rapid identification of a patient's height with a correlated estimation of weight, size of equipment to be used, and appropriate dosages of potential resuscitative drugs. Effective pediatric trauma resuscitation mandates the availability of appropriately sized laryngoscope blades, endotracheal tubes, nasogastric tubes, Foley catheters, chest tubes, blood pressure cuffs, oxygen masks, bag-valve-mask (BVM) resuscitators, and other associated equipment.

Airway

As in the adult, the immediate priority and focus in the child is on airway management. The relatively large tongue and more anterior position of the airway make small children more likely to have an airway obstruction than adults. The smaller the child, the greater the disproportion between the size of the cranium and midface and the greater the propensity of the posterior pharyngeal area to "buckle" as the relatively large occiput forces passive flexion on the cervical spine. In the absence of trauma, the pediatric patient's airway is best protected by a slightly superior anterior position of the midface, known as the *sniffing position*. In the pediatric trauma patient, the neck should be kept inline to prevent the hyperflexion at C5-C6 and hyperextension at C1-C2 that occurs with the sniffing position.

The child's larynx is smaller than that of an adult, has a slightly more anterocaudad angle (forward and toward the feet), and is frequently more difficult to visualize for direct cannulation (Figure 12-1). Despite these characteristics, the most reliable means of ventilation in the child with airway compromise is direct orotracheal intubation. Nasotracheal intubation requires blind passage around a relatively acute posterior nasopharyngeal angle and can cause severe bleeding or even inadvertent penetration of the cranial vault. In the absence of appropriate intubation equipment, BVM ventilation with 100% oxygen (FiO_2 of 1.0) is an acceptable alternative. A child with craniofacial injuries that cause upper airway obstruction should be considered for immediate percutaneous transtracheal ventilation. This is only a temporary measure, and a more definitive airway should be established as soon as safely possible.

Breathing

As in all trauma patients, a significantly traumatized child typically needs an oxygen concentration of 85%

Table 12-1	Height and Weight Range for Pediatric Patients		
		Range of mean norms	
Group	Age	Average height (cm)	Average weight (kg)
Newborn	Birth-6 wk	51-63	4-5
Infant	7 wk-1 yr	56-80	4-11
Toddler	1-2 yr	77-91	11-14
Preschool	2-6 yr	91-122	14-25
School age	6-13 yr	122-165	25-63
Adolescent	13-16 yr	165-182	62-80

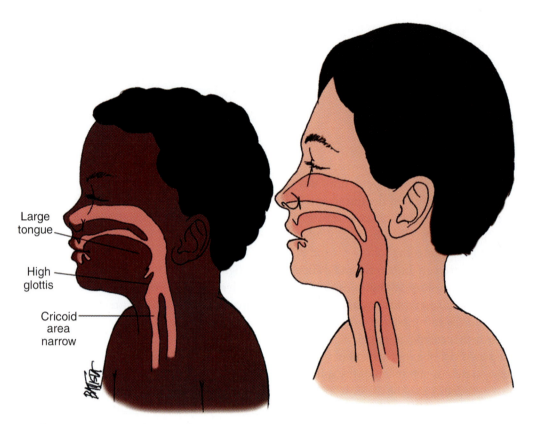

Figure 12-1 Comparison of the adult and child airways. (*Stoy W: Mosby's EMT-Basic textbook, St Louis, 1996, Mosby.*)

Large tongue

High glottis

Cricoid area narrow

to 100% (FiO_2 of 0.85 to 1.0). This is accomplished by use of supplemental oxygen and an appropriately sized pediatric mask. When hypoxia occurs in the small child, the body compensates by increasing the ventilatory rate (tachypnea) and by a strenuous increase in ventilatory effort, including increased thoracic excursion efforts and the use of accessory muscles in the neck and abdomen. This increased effort can produce severe fatigue, resulting in ventilatory failure. Ventilatory distress can rapidly progress from a compensated ventilatory effort to ventilatory failure, then respiratory arrest, and ultimately cardiac arrest secondary to the respiratory problem.

Evaluation of the child's level of ventilation with early recognition of distress and the provision of ventilatory assistance are key elements in the management of the pediatric trauma patient. The normal ventilatory rate of infants and children younger than 4 years of age is two to three times that of adults (Table 12-2).

Tachypnea with signs of increased effort or difficulty may be the first manifestation of respiratory distress and/or shock. As distress increases, additional signs and symptoms include shallow breathing with minimal chest movement. Breath sounds may be weak or infrequent,

and air exchange at the nose or mouth may be reduced or minimal. Ventilatory effort becomes more labored and may include the following:

- Head bobbing with each breath
- Gasping or grunting
- Flared nostrils
- Stridor or snoring
- Suprasternal, supraclavicular, and intercostal retractions
- Use of accessory muscles of neck and abdomen
- Distention of the abdomen when the chest falls (seesaw effect between the chest and abdomen)

The effectiveness of a child's ventilation should be evaluated using the following indicators:

- Rate and depth (minute volume) and effort confirm adequate ventilation.
- Breath sounds confirm the depth of exchange.
- Wheezing, rales, or rhonchi indicate inefficient alveolar oxygenation.
- Pink skin indicates adequate ventilation.

Table 12-2   Ventilatory Rates for Pediatric Patients

Group	Age	Ventilatory rate (breaths/min)	Ventilatory rate (breaths/min) that indicates possible decrease in minute volume and need for ventilatory assistance with BVM
Newborn	Birth-6 wk	30-50	<30 or >50
Infant	7 wk-1 yr	20-30	<20 or >30
Toddler	1-2 yr	20-30	<20 or >30
Preschool	2-6 yr	20-30	<20 or >30
School age	6-13 yr	(12-20)-30	<20 or >30
Adolescent	13-16 yr	12-20	<12 or >20

- Dusky, gray, cyanotic, or mottled skin indicates insufficient oxygen exchange.
- Anxiety, restlessness, or combativeness are possible early signs of hypoxia.
- Lethargy, lowered LOC, or unconsciousness are probable advanced signs of hypoxia.

A rapid evaluation of ventilation includes assessment of the patient's ventilatory rate (particularly tachypnea), ventilatory effort (degree of labor, nostril flaring, accessory muscle use, retraction, seesaw movement), auscultation (air exchange, bilateral symmetry, pathologic sounds), skin color, and mental status. Central (rather than peripheral) cyanosis is a fairly late and often inconsistent sign.

In the child initially presenting with tachypnea and increased ventilatory effort, a subsequently decreasing ventilatory rate and apparent lessening in effort may indicate exhaustion and further reduced ventilation. This should not be misinterpreted as always being a sign of improvement.

Ventilatory assistance should be given to children with diminished air exchange or those in acute ventilatory distress. Because the main problem is one of inspired volume rather than concentration of oxygen, assisted ventilation is best given by use of a BVM device. Use of the correct mask size is essential for obtaining a proper mask seal, providing the proper tidal volume, and ensuring that hyperinflation (resulting in gastric distention) or barotrauma does not occur.

When obtaining a mask seal in infants, caution should be exercised to avoid compressing the floor of the mouth because this pushes the tongue back into the airway and against the soft palate. Pressure on the uncalcified soft trachea should also be avoided. One or two hands can be used to obtain a mask seal. Gastric disten-

tion can result in regurgitation or prevent adequate ventilation by limiting diaphragmatic excursion.

Once the prehospital care provider has initiated ventilation, he or she should supplement the BVM with an oxygen reservoir attached to high-concentration oxygen (FiO_2 of 0.85 to 1.0). Because a child's airway is so small, initial and periodic suctioning may be necessary. In infants, who are often obligate nose breathers, the nostrils should also be suctioned.

Changes in a child's ventilatory status can be subtle, and ventilatory effort can rapidly deteriorate until ventilation is inadequate and hypoxia occurs. The patient's breathing should be evaluated as part of the primary survey and carefully rechecked periodically to ensure its continued adequacy. Pulse oximetry should be monitored, and effort should be made to keep the SpO_2 at greater than 95%.

Circulation

The survival rate from immediate exsanguinating injury is low in the pediatric population. Fortunately, the incidence of this type of injury is also low. External hemorrhage should be identified and controlled during the primary survey. Injured children usually present with at least some circulating blood volume and respond appropriately to volume replacement. As in the assessment of the airway, a single measurement of heart rate or blood pressure does not equate with physiologic stability. Close monitoring of vital signs is absolutely essential to prevent hypotension and shock. The normal ranges for pulse rate and blood pressure for different age groups are presented in Tables 12-3 and 12-4.

If the primary survey suggests severe hypotension, the most likely cause is blood loss—either through a major external wound (readily observable), an intrathoracic wound (identifiable by diminished ventilatory mechanics and auscultatory findings), or loss of blood from a major intraabdominal injury. Because blood is not a compressible medium, blood loss from a major intraabdominal injury will frequently produce abdominal distention and increasing abdominal girth.

A major consideration in the assessment of a pediatric patient is compensated shock. Because of their increased physiologic reserve, children with hemorrhagic injury frequently present with only slightly abnormal vital signs. Initial tachycardia may not only be the result of hypovolemia but also the effect of psychologic stress, pain, and fear. Moreover, a small patient may have a systolic blood pressure that, while considered alarmingly low for an adult, may be within the normal range for a healthy child. All injured children should have their blood pressure, heart rate, ventilatory rate, and overall CNS status monitored closely. A child with hemorrhagic injury can maintain adequate circulating volume by increasing his or her peripheral resistance to maintain mean arterial pressure. In the child, signs of significant hypotension develop with the loss of approximately 25% of the circulating volume. If initial resuscitation is inadequate, circulating volume will eventually diminish to a point below which increased peripheral resistance can maintain arterial pressure. The concept of evolving shock must be of prime concern in the initial management of an injured child and is a major indication for transport to an appropriate fa-

Table 12-3 Pulse Rates for Pediatric Patients

Group	Age	Pulse rate (beats/min)	Pulse rate (beats/min) that indicates a possible serious problem (bradycardia or tachycardia)
Newborn	Birth-6 wk	120-160	<100 or >150
Infant	7 wk-1 yr	80-140	<80 or >120
Toddler	1-2 yr	80-130	<60 or >110
Preschool	2-6 yr	80-120	<60 or >110
School age	6-13 yr	(60-80)-100	<60 or >100
Adolescent	13-16 yr	60-100	<60 or >100

Table 12-4 Blood Pressure for Pediatric Patients

Group	Age	Expected range for blood pressure (mm Hg)*	Lower limit of systolic blood pressure (mm Hg)
Newborn	Birth-6 wk	74-100 50-68	<70
Infant	7 wk-1 yr	84-106 56-70	<70
Toddler	1-2 yr	98-106 50-70	<70
Preschool	2-6 yr	98-112 64-70	<70
School age	6-13 yr	104-124 64-80	<80-90
Adolescent	13-16 yr	118-132 70-82	<80-90

*The top numbers represent systolic range, and the bottom numbers represent diastolic range.

cility and proper physician evaluation of even minor-appearing injuries.

Disability

After assessment of airway, breathing, and circulation, the primary survey must include an assessment of neurologic status. Although the AVPU scale (Alert, responds to Verbal stimulus, responds to Painful stimulus, Unresponsive) remains a rapid screening tool for assessment of LOC, it should be combined with a careful examination of the pupils to determine whether they are equal, round, and reactive to light. As in adults, the Glasgow Coma Scale (GCS) provides a more thorough assessment of neurologic status; however, the scoring for the verbal section for children under 4 years of age must be modified (Table 12-5). Because of limited communications skills in this age group, the child's behavior should be observed carefully.

Table 12-5 Pediatric Verbal Score

Verbal response	Verbal score
Appropriate words or social smile; fixes and follows	5
Crying but consolable	4
Persistently irritable	3
Restless, agitated	2
No response	1

The GCS score should be repeated frequently and used to document progression or improvement of neurologic status during the postinjury period (refer to Chapters 3 and 8 for a review of the GCS). A more thorough assessment of motor and sensory function should be performed in the secondary survey if time permits.

Expose/Environment

Children should be examined for other potential life-threatening injuries; however, they may be frightened at attempts to remove their clothes. Because children are more prone to developing hypothermia, once the examination to identify other injuries is complete, the patient's bare skin should be covered to preserve body heat.

Pediatric Trauma Score

The decision as to which child requires what level of care must proceed from a careful and rapid evaluation of the entire child. Overlooking potential additional organ system injury and inadequately managing the patient are the two most common problems encountered in this area. For this reason, the Pediatric Trauma Score (PTS) (Figure 12-2) has been developed to provide a reliable and simple protocol for assessment and to provide numeric quantitation that is predictive of outcome in regard to morbidity and mortality. It consists of a categorization system in which six components of pediatric injury are graded and then added together to produce a score predictive of injury severity and potential for mortality. The system is based on an analysis of pediatric injury patterns and is designed to provide a protocol

Component	+2	+1	−1
Size	Child/adolescent >20 kg	Toddler 11-20 kg	Infant <10 kg
Airway	Normal	Assisted: O$_2$ mask, cannula	Intubated: ETT, cricothyroidotomy
Consciousness	Awake	Obtunded, lost consciousness	Coma, unresponsive
Systolic blood pressure	90 mm Hg Good peripheral pulses, perfusion	51-90 mm Hg Carotid, femoral pulse palpable	<50 mm Hg Weak or no pulses
Fracture	None seen or suspected	Single closed fracture anywhere	Open or multiple fractures
Cutaneous	No visible injury	Contusion, abrasion, laceration <7 cm not through fascia	Tissue loss, any gun shot wound or stab through fascia

Figure 12-2 The Pediatric Trauma Score is primarily designed to function as a checklist. Each component can be assessed by basic physical examination. Airway evaluation is designed to reflect intervention required for effective care. An open fracture is graded −1 for fracture and −1 for cutaneous injury. As clinical observation and diagnostic evaluation continue, further definition and reassessment will establish a trend that predicts severity of injury and potential outcome.

checklist to ensure that all the major factors relative to outcome from pediatric injury are considered in the initial evaluation of the child. The PTS is different than the Revised Trauma Score (RTS), which only considers the blood pressure, ventilatory rate, and GCS score. The PTS is intentionally designed as a checklist that addresses the six factors critical to outcome from injury in the pediatric patient.

Size is the first component because it is readily observed and is a major consideration in the infant/toddler group, which has the highest mortality rate from injury. The airway is assessed next. The functional status and the type of care required to provide adequate ventilation and oxygenation are considered.

The most important factor in initial assessment of the CNS is LOC. Because children frequently sustain transient loss of consciousness during an injury, the obtunded grade (+1) is applied to any child with loss of consciousness—no matter how fleeting. This grade identifies the patient as likely to develop potentially fatal yet frequently treatable intracranial injuries secondary to brain injury.

Systolic blood pressure assessment is arranged primarily to identify those children in whom evolving preventable shock may occur (51 to 90 mm Hg systolic blood pressure; +1). Regardless of size, a child whose systolic blood pressure is below 50 mm Hg (−1) is in obvious jeopardy. On the other hand, a child whose systolic blood pressure exceeds 90 mm Hg (+2) probably falls into a better outcome category than a child with even a slight degree of hypotension. If the appropriately sized blood pressure cuff is not available, the systolic pressure is assessed as +2 if the radial or pedal pulse is palpable, +1 if only the carotid or femoral pulse is palpable, and −1 if no pulse is palpable.

Because of the high incidence of skeletal injury in the pediatric population and its potential contribution to mortality and disability, the presence of a fracture is included in the PTS as a component.

Finally, the skin is assessed for open or visible wounds and penetrating injury.

By nature of its design, the PTS serves as a straightforward checklist that ensures that all components necessary to identify a critically injured child are considered.

Vital Signs and Quantitative Norms

The term *pediatric* or *child* includes a vast range of physical development, emotional maturity, and body sizes. The approach to the patient and the implications of many injuries vary greatly between an infant and an adolescent.

In most anatomic and therapeutic dosage considerations, a child's weight (or specific height or length) serves as a more accurate indicator than does exact chronologic age. Table 12-1 describes the average height and weight for healthy children of varying ages.

The acceptable ranges of quantitative vital signs vary for the different ages within the pediatric population. The prehospital care provider cannot use adult norms as guidelines in smaller children. An adult ventilatory rate of 30 breaths/min is tachypneic, and an adult heart rate of 120 beats/min is tachycardic. Both are considered alarmingly high in an adult and are significant pathologic findings. However, the same findings in an infant may be well within the normal ranges.

Studies in the pediatric literature and lists in various pediatric texts may not be consistent, displaying the normal ranges for different age groupings. As an additional complication, in a child who has been injured and has no previous history of normal vital signs, a conservative approach dictates viewing borderline signs as if they are pathologic—even though in that individual child they may be physiologically acceptable. The

guidelines in Tables 12-2, 12-3, and 12-4 can aid in evaluating vital signs. These tables represent ranges into which the findings of most children in these age groups will fall. They do not define the limits of good health but only describe the ranges that are statistically common.

Several commercially available items serve as rapid references for pediatric vital signs and equipment size. These include the length-based resuscitation tape (Broselow tape) and several slide-rule–type plastic scales. The following guideline formulas can also be used to estimate the expected finding for any age:

> **Weight (kg) = 8 + (2 × child's age in years)**
> **Systolic blood pressure (mm Hg) =**
> **80 + (2 × child's age in years)**
> **Total vascular blood volume (mL) =**
> **80 mL × child's weight in kg**

As in adults, quantitative vital signs in children, though important, are only an additional piece of information in making an assessment. One must remember how rapidly a child can deteriorate into either critical ventilatory difficulty or decompensated shock. Vital signs should be considered along with mechanism of injury and other clinical findings.

As a predictor of injury, the PTS has a statistically significant inverse linear relationship with patient mortality. There is a threshold score of 8, below which injured children should be taken to an appropriate pediatric trauma center. These are the children in whom the potential for preventable mortality and morbidity is greatest.

Secondary Survey (Focused History and Physical Examination)

The secondary survey of the child should follow the primary survey only after life-threatening conditions have been identified and managed. The thorax should be evaluated for potential cardiac or pulmonary contusions, both of which may be worsened by overly aggressive fluid resuscitation. Because the increased resiliency of a child's ribs may have allowed transmission of significantly greater energy to underlying thoracic organs, the patient may have an extensive pulmonary contusion with no external signs. Trauma patients frequently have full stomachs; therefore the possibility of aspiration exists. This is especially true for children who are obtunded or who have posttraumatic seizure activity.

Although rib fractures are rare in childhood, they are associated with a high risk of death. Even if a rib fracture is an isolated injury, it should be viewed as an indicator of severe trauma. The risk of mortality increases with the number of ribs fractured.

Examination of the abdomen should focus on distention, tenderness, discoloration, or presence of a mass. Careful palpation of the iliac crests may suggest an unstable pelvic fracture and increase suspicion for possible retroperitoneal or urogenital injury.

Each extremity should be palpated to rule out deformity, diminished vascular supply, or neurologic deficit. A child's incompletely calcified skeleton with its multiple growth centers increases the possibility of epiphyseal (growth plate) disruption. Accordingly, any area of edema, pain, tenderness, or diminished range of motion should be carefully evaluated and suspected as being fractured until ruled out by radiographic examination. In adults and children alike, a missed orthopedic injury in an extremity has little effect on mortality, but it may have a major long-term effect on deformity and disability.

Management

The keys to pediatric trauma survival are rapid assessment, appropriate aggressive management, and transport to a facility capable of managing pediatric trauma.

Airway

The primary goal of the initial resuscitation of an injured child is restoration of adequate tissue oxygenation as quickly as possible. Oxygenation and circulation are as essential to an injured child as they are to an adult. The first priority of assessment and resuscitation is the establishment of a patent airway.

A patent airway should be ensured and maintained with suctioning, manual maneuvers, and airway adjuncts along with proper spinal protection throughout. As in the adult, initial management may include cervical spine stabilization. When elevating a child's chin, compressing the soft tissues of the neck and trachea should be avoided. Once manual control of the airway is achieved, an oropharyngeal airway can be placed if no gag reflex is present. The device should be inserted carefully and gently, parallel to the course of the tongue rather than turned 90 or 180 degrees in the posterior oropharynx as in the adult. Use of a tongue blade to depress the tongue is helpful. Visualized orotracheal intubation is the preferred method of definitive airway control.

Careful attention to airway maintenance and immobilization are especially important in the obtunded child whose LOC is altered. Moreover, in providing initial cervical spine stabilization of the child, the size disproportion of the occiput should be considered. Adequate padding should be placed under the patient's torso so that the cervical spine is maintained in a straight line rather than forced into slight flexion because of the occiput (Figure 12-3).

Breathing

The patient's minute volume and ventilatory effort should be evaluated carefully. Because of the potential for rapid deterioration from hypoxia to ventilatory arrest,

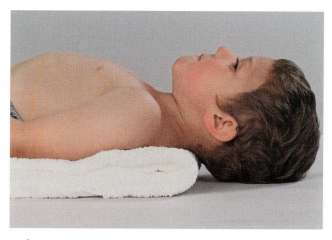

Figure 12-3 Provide adequate padding under the torso.

Pediatric Endotracheal Intubation

As in the adult, endotracheal intubation of a child should include careful attention to the cervical spine. One person should maintain the patient's head in a neutral position while another person intubates. The narrowest portion of the pediatric airway is the cricoid ring, so uncuffed endotracheal tubes should always be used in infants and toddlers. The appropriately sized endotracheal tube can be estimated by evaluating the diameter of the child's fifth finger or the diameter of the patient's external nares. A slight amount of cricoid pressure frequently brings the anterior structures of the child's larynx into better view and will passively obstruct the esophagus, thus diminishing gastric insufflation. Pharmacologically assisted intubation should include the use of atropine sulfate to prevent bradycardia. Heart rate is a major determinant of perfusion in pediatric patients.

A common error that occurs during intubation of children under emergency circumstances is an overly aggressive insertion of the endotracheal tube that causes right mainstem bronchial intubation. The chest should always be auscultated directly after the endotracheal tube is placed for bilateral breath sounds. Placement of the tube should also be frequently reassessed, especially after any movement of the patient. In addition to confirming endotracheal tube placement, auscultation may rule out the possibility of other pulmonary injury. The child with a compromised airway and a pulmonary injury who has been successfully intubated may be in greater jeopardy for the development of a tension pneumothorax as a result of more efficient delivery of tidal volume to the lungs.

PASG in Children

Currently, use of a pneumatic antishock garment (PASG) in children is limited to patients who can be properly fitted into either a pediatric or adult garment. In most cases, this latter group could be considered "almost adult-sized" children, and PASG use follows the same indications and contraindications as for adults (see Chapter 6).

The most frequently cited caution regarding the use of a PASG on pediatric patients is the possibility of the abdominal section overlapping the lower ribs. When the abdominal section is inflated in such cases, this invariably provokes ventilatory compromise and significant respiratory distress.

No present studies indicate any benefit from PASG use on children. In the absence of specific studies, the prehospital care provider should assume that the use of the garment on a child smaller than the general size for which the garment has been designed (pediatric or adult size) is potentially dangerous and should not attempt it. Alternatively, the use of a PASG should not be withheld on a patient whose body size is large enough simply because the patient is chronologically still a child.

ventilation should be assisted if dyspnea and increased ventilatory effort are observed. A properly sized BVM with a reservoir and high-flow oxygen to provide an oxygen concentration of between 85% and 100% (FiO_2 of 0.85 to 1.0) should be used. Continuous pulse oximetry serves as an adjunct for ongoing assessment of airway and breathing. The SpO_2 should be kept at greater than 95%.

Circulation

Once the patient's external hemorrhage is controlled, perfusion should be evaluated. The pediatric vascular system is commonly able to maintain a normal blood pressure until severe collapse occurs, at which point it is often unresponsive to resuscitation. Therefore fluid resuscitation should be started whenever signs of compensated hypovolemic shock are present, especially in those patients who present with decompensated shock. Lactated Ringer's solution or normal saline in 20 mL/kg boluses should be used. Transportation should not be delayed to start IV therapy.

For pediatric trauma patients who display any signs of hemorrhagic shock or hypovolemia, key factors to survival are blood replacement and rapid initiation of transport to a suitable facility.

VASCULAR ACCESS

Fluid replacement in a child with severe hypotension or signs of shock must deliver adequate fluid volume to the right atrium as directly as possible to avoid further reducing cardiac preload. The most appropriate initial site for intravenous access is above the diaphragm. Intravenous access should first be attempted at the antecubital fossa. In the absence of adequate venous access at this location, the saphenous vein at the ankle should be considered. The saphenous vein is a distal point below the diaphragm; however, the availability of this vessel usually ensures reliable vascular access.

In the unstable or potentially unstable patient, attempts at peripheral access should be limited to two in 90 seconds. If access is unsuccessful, central access via intraosseous infusion should be considered in the child.

Percutaneous cannulation of the external jugular or saphenous cutdown are other possibilities if the prehospital care provider is properly trained and credentialed. Cannulation of the femoral vein is associated with the risk of thrombosis and circulatory compromise of the leg. Placement of a subclavian catheter in an injured child should be performed only under the most controlled circumstances within the hospital; this should not be attempted in the prehospital setting.

Vascular access should be obtained in any child who needs fluid replacement. However, the establishment of a "to keep open" (TKO) intravenous "lifeline" in anticipation of the potential need for fluid replacement represents a prehospital problem without an easy answer. In adults, an intravenous line is established if any chance of its need exists. Because of the possibility of evolving shock and a child's potential to decompensate rapidly, a greater indication for TKO intravenous lines in children appears to be warranted. However, starting an intravenous line in children can be extremely difficult and time-consuming and may add to the child's psychologic trauma.

The determination of which pediatric patients should have an IV access line started depends on transport times and other factors. If the prehospital care provider is unsure as to which patients need IV access or if fluid replacement has become indicated during transport, he or she should contact medical direction.

FLUID THERAPY

As in the adult, lactated Ringer's solution is the initial resuscitation fluid of choice for a hypovolemic child. Because the length of time that a crystalloid fluid remains in the vascular system is so short, a 3:1 ratio of crystalloid fluid to blood lost is used. An initial resuscitative bolus should reflect approximately 25% of the standard circulating volume in the pediatric patient, which is approximately 20 mL/kg. Considering the 3:1 ratio, a bolus of 50 to 60 mL/kg is required to achieve adequate and rapid initial replacement in response to significant volume loss. Specific to trauma care, in any child who does not show at least a minor improvement with the first 20 mL/kg fluid bolus, blood product infusion should begin as soon as possible. The crystalloid bolus may temporarily restore cardiovascular dynamics as it transiently fills and then leaks from the circulatory system. However, until RBC mass is replaced and oxygen transport is restored, the basic process of cellular hypoxia will continue unchecked.

Injured children usually present in one of three ways—normotensive, hypotensive, or in rapidly decom-

Intraosseous Infusion

Intraosseous infusion can provide an adequate alternative site for volume replacement in injured children. This is an effective route for infusion of medication and has been documented as an equally effective means to provide high-volume fluid resuscitation.

The easiest site for intraosseous infusion is the anterior tibia just below the tibial tuberosity. After preparing the skin antiseptically and securing the leg adequately, a site is chosen on the anterior portion of the tibia, 1 to 2 cm distal and medial to the tibial tuberosity. Specially manufactured intraosseous infusion needles are optimal for the procedure, but spinal or bone marrow needles may also be used. Spinal needles that are 18- to 20-gauge work well because they have a trocar to prevent the needle from being obstructed as it passes through the bony cortex into the marrow. Any 14- to 20-gauge needle can be used in an emergency. The needle is placed at a 90-degree angle to the bone and advanced firmly through the cortex into the marrow. Evidence that the needle is adequately within the marrow includes the following:

1. A soft "pop" and lack of resistance after the needle has passed through the cortex
2. Aspiration of bone marrow into the needle
3. Free flow of fluid into the marrow without evidence of subcutaneous infiltration

Intraosseous infusion should be considered during the initial minutes of resuscitation if percutaneous venous cannulation has been unsuccessful. Because the flow rate is limited, the intraosseous route alone will seldom be sufficient.

pensated shock. Few demonstrate evidence of blood loss and hypotension. With the high incidence of potential brain injury, volume replacement must balance restoration of adequate circulating volume against fluid overload with its potentially detrimental effect on evolving cerebral edema.

Children who present in hypovolemic shock and respond to large amounts (50 to 60 mL/kg in 20 mL/kg boluses) of crystalloid resuscitation need blood replacement as soon as possible. As a result of the crystalloid bolus, these patients frequently regain adequate cardiac output. However, the resulting circulating volume has minimal oxygen-carrying capacity. Continuing hypoxia induces a cellular shift to anaerobic metabolism. These children should be resuscitated aggressively and transported without delay to be transfused with RBCs. Only under these circumstances will they have a chance of surviving their hemorrhagic injury.

Disability

Traumatic brain injury (TBI) continues to be the most common cause of death in the pediatric population. Of the fatalities included in the first 40,000 patients in the NPTR, 89% had a CNS injury as either the primary or secondary contributor to mortality. Although many of the most severe injuries are treatable only by prevention, initial resuscitative measures may at least lessen the serious consequences of the child's injury. Again, adequate oxygenation, ventilation, and circulation are the primary considerations. The outcome of children sustaining severe TBI is typically better than in adults; however, the outcome of children younger than 3 years of age is worse than that of older children.

Initial assessment of the LOC is a rapid and reliable prognostic exercise. Regardless of the outcome of the neurologic evaluation on the first examination, any child who sustains potential brain injury may be susceptible to cerebral edema and hypoperfusion. This can even result from trauma that appears minor. Any child who presents with even a transitory loss of consciousness should be assumed to have sustained a significant level of mechanical trauma to the brain stem and reticular activating system.

Even if the LOC returns to normal, the patient should be observed carefully to rule out the possibility of evolving secondary dysfunction as a result of cerebral edema or a space-occupying lesion in the form of a subdural or epidural hematoma. Because brain trauma is frequently the most severe and life-threatening injury, the probability of an injured child requiring an immediate computed tomography (CT) scan for assessment of the CNS is high. Therefore a baseline GCS score should be assessed and repeated during transport. Supplemental oxygen should be administered, and if possible, pulse oximetry should be monitored. Although vomiting is common after a concussion, persistent vomiting is of concern and requires further evaluation.

Like hypoxia, hypovolemia may dramatically worsen the original injury. External hemorrhage must be controlled and the patient's extremities immobilized to limit internal blood loss associated with fractures. An attempt should be made to keep these children in a euvolemic state with intravenous volume resuscitation. On rare occasions, infants may become hypovolemic as a result of intracranial bleeding because of open cranial sutures and fontanelles. In addition, a child with an open fontanelle may better tolerate an expanding intracranial hematoma.

Because the intracranial mass may not present symptoms until rapid decompensation occurs, an infant with a bulging fontanelle should be considered to have a more severe brain injury.

Children with a GCS score of 8 or less may benefit from intubation. However, prolonged attempts at securing an endotracheal airway should not delay transport to an appropriate facility, as long as adequate oxygenation and ventilation with a BVM device can be accomplished.

A child with signs and symptoms of increased intracranial pressure (ICP) (intracranial hypertension), such as a sluggishly reactive or nonreactive pupil, hypertension, bradycardia, and motor deficits, hyperventilation may transiently lower ICP. This is easily achieved in the sensory-depressed or comatose child by initial airway control, ventilation with a bag-valve device via either mask or endotracheal tube, and supplemental high-concentration oxygen. End-tidal CO_2 monitoring can guide management, with the target range being 25 to 30 mm Hg. If capnography is not available, a ventilation rate of 30 breaths/min for children and 35 breaths/min for infants should be used.

During prolonged transports, small doses of mannitol (0.5 to 1 g/kg body weight) may benefit children with evidence of intracranial hypertension; however, use of this medication may result in hypovolemia with insufficient volume resuscitation. Seizures may occur soon after the brain injury; however, recurrent seizure activity is worrisome and may require treatment with intravenous boluses of diazepam (0.1 to 0.2 mg/kg/dose). Diazepam should be used with extreme caution because of the potential side effects of ventilatory depression and hypotension.

Spinal Trauma

The indication for spinal immobilization in a pediatric patient is based on the mechanism of injury and physical findings; the presence of other injuries that suggest violent or sudden movement of the head, neck, or torso; or the presence of specific signs of spine injury, such as deformity, pain, or neurologic deficit. As with adult patients, the correct prehospital management of a suspected unstable spine is manual stabilization; use of a properly fitting cervical collar; and immobilization of the patient to a rigid device so that the head, neck, torso, pelvis, and legs are maintained in a neutral inline position. This should be achieved without inhibiting the patient's ventilation, ability to open the mouth, or any other required resuscitation. The threshold for performing spinal immobilization is often lower in children because of their inability to communicate or otherwise participate in their own assessment (see Indications for Spinal Immobilization algorithm, p. 238).

When most small children are placed on a rigid surface, the relatively larger size of the child's head posterior to the spinal column will result in moving of the head into a flexed position. Padding should be placed under the patient's torso to elevate it enough to allow the head to be in a neutral position. The padding should be continuous and flat from the shoulders to the pelvis and extend to the lateral margins of the torso to ensure that the thoracic, lumbar, and sacral spine are on a flat, continuous, stable platform without movement. Padding should also be placed between the lateral sides of the child and the edges of the board to ensure that no lateral movement occurs when the board is moved or if the patient and board need to be rotated to the side to avoid aspiration of vomitus.

Various new pediatric immobilization devices are becoming available. The prehospital care provider must practice and be familiar with the required adjustments when immobilizing a child with adult-sized equipment. If a vest-type device is used on a child, the prehospital care provider should ensure adequate immobilization and no deleterious side effects. The prehospital care provider should also be familiar with the techniques of immobilizing a young child in a car safety seat.

Thoracic Injuries

As mentioned previously, the extremely resilient rib cage of a child with its incomplete calcification reduces the energy transferred through the thoracic cage to the intrathoracic organs. As a result, a child may have significant organ injury, disruption of vascular anatomy, or simple contusions without even the slightest degree of skeletal abnormality on external examination.

A high index of suspicion is the key to identifying these injuries. Every child who sustains trauma to the chest and torso should be carefully monitored for signs of ventilatory difficulty and shock. Even if no distress is present, the child should be transported without delay to a suitable facility for radiographic chest examination and careful evaluation of cardiopulmonary and ventilatory function. Radiologic evidence of pulmonary contusion has been found in children who, other than having a history of blunt torso trauma, are completely asymptomatic. Pulse oximetry may help identify these problems.

Being aware of this potential problem requires continuous careful monitoring of a child's fluid status to en-

sure prevention of gross intravenous fluid overload. Unlike adults, rib fractures in children are associated with a high risk of death. Even if they are an isolated injury, the presence of one or more fractured ribs is an indication of multisystem trauma, even in the absence of other apparent signs.

The possibility of a cardiac contusion should also be considered in children who sustain blunt thoracic trauma. When transporting a child who has sustained a high-impact blunt thoracic injury, the patient's cardiac rhythm should be monitored once he or she is en route to a medical facility.

The key items in managing thoracic trauma involve careful attention to ventilation and timely transport to an appropriate facility.

Abdominal Injuries

Because of the large size of the torso relative to the extremities in children, abdominal injuries are a common problem. As discussed previously, the presence of blunt trauma to the abdomen; an unstable pelvis; posttraumatic abdominal distention, rigidity, or tenderness; or otherwise unexplained levels of shock can be associated with possible intraabdominal hemorrhage.

The key elements in management of abdominal injuries include fluid resuscitation, supplemental high-concentration oxygen, and rapid transport to an appropriate facility with continued careful monitoring en route.

Extremity Trauma

In comparison to the adult skeleton, a child's skeleton is actively growing and consists of a large proportion of cartilaginous tissue and metabolically active growth plates. The collateral ligaments that hold the skeleton together are frequently stronger and better able to withstand mechanical disruption than the bones to which they are attached. As a result, children with skeletal trauma frequently sustain major deforming forces before developing fractures or disruptions of their bony skeleton.

Primary joint disruption from injury other than penetrating injury is uncommon in comparison with disruption of the diaphyseal or epiphyseal segments of bone. Fractures that involve the growth plate should be carefully identified and managed in a manner that will not only ensure adequate healing but also prevent subsequent displacement or deformity as the child grows. The association of vascular injuries with orthopedic injuries in children should always be considered, and the distal pulse should be evaluated carefully.

In pediatric patients with an isolated extremity injury, even a seemingly minor skeletal injury may require hospital treatment. Because the potential for unrecognized growth plate injury or vascular disruption may result in subsequent impaired limb growth and deformity, such injuries require careful examination and evaluation. Often the provider can rule out the presence of a potentially deforming injury only by radiologic study or, when the slightest suggestion of a decrease in distal perfusion exists, by arteriography.

In the child with more than just isolated extremity injuries, the prehospital care provider must focus on the essentials and not be distracted from potentially life-threatening injuries by the apparent gross deformity sometimes associated with extremity injury. Uncontrolled hemorrhage represents the sole life-threatening condition associated with extremity trauma. In multisystem pediatric and adult trauma patients alike, the initiation of transport to an appropriate facility without delay after completion of the primary survey, resuscitation, and rapid packaging remains paramount in reducing mortality.

Transport

Because timely arrival at an appropriate facility may be the key element in the patient's survival, triage is an important consideration of management.

The tragedy of preventable pediatric traumatic death has been documented in multiple studies reported over the past three decades. As many as 40% of pediatric trauma deaths could be classified as preventable. These statistics have been one of the primary motivations for the development of regionalized pediatric trauma centers where continuous high-quality, sophisticated care can be provided.

In some areas, both pediatric trauma centers and adult trauma centers exist. If the patient experiences only a small delay in transport, the pediatric multisystem trauma patient may benefit from the initial resuscitation capability and definitive care available at a facility specialized in treating traumatized children. However, for many locations the nearest specialized pediatric trauma center is hours away. In such places, the seriously traumatized child should be transported to the nearest adult trauma center. In areas where no specialized pediatric trauma center is nearby, personnel working in adult trauma centers are experienced in the resuscitation and treatment of both adult and pediatric trauma patients. In areas where neither are read-

ily close, the seriously injured child should be transported to the nearest appropriate hospital (for trauma victims) according to local protocols. Aeromedical transport should be considered if appropriate to get a pediatric patient to a pediatric trauma center in a timely manner.

Review of over 15,000 records in the NPTR indicates that 25% of children are injured severely enough to require triage to a designated pediatric trauma center. Use of the PTS will help with appropriate triage.

The Battered and Abused Child

Child abuse is a significant cause of childhood injury. Prehospital care providers must consider the possibility of child abuse when circumstances warrant.

In many jurisdictions, prehospital care providers are legally mandated reporters if they identify potential child abuse. Generally, reporters who act in good faith are protected from legal action by the reported party.

The prehospital care provider should suspect abuse if he or she notes any of the following scenarios:

- A discrepancy exists between the history and the degree of physical injury.
- A prolonged interval has passed between the time of the injury and when medical care is actually sought.
- A history of the injury is inconsistent with the developmental level of the child. For example, a history indicating that a newborn rolled off a bed would be suspect because newborns are developmentally unable to roll over.

Certain injury types also suggest abuse, such as the following (Figure 12-4):

- Multiple bruises in varying stages of resolution
- Bizarre injuries such as bites, cigarette burns, or rope marks
- Sharply demarcated burns or scald injuries in unusual areas

Reporting procedures vary, so prehospital care providers should be familiar with the appropriate agencies that handle child abuse cases in their location. The need to report abuse is emphasized by data suggesting that up to 50% of abused children who are released back to their abusers subsequently die of further abuse episodes.

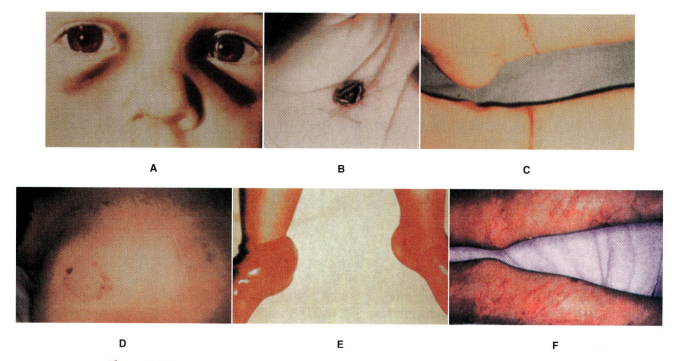

A   B   C

D   E   F

Figure 12-4   Indicators of possible abuse. **A**, "Raccoon eye," or periorbital bruising, a possible indication of anterior fossa skull fracture. **B**, Fresh cigarette burn to palm. **C**, Fresh abrasions of restraint injury. **D**, Human bites. **E**, "Dunking" burns to the feet. **F**, Welts and abrasions to legs as a result of abuse with an electric cord. (*From Sanders M: Mosby's paramedic textbook, ed 2 revised, St Louis, 2001, Mosby.*)

Summary

The initial and continuing prehospital care of the injured child requires application of standard trauma life support principles modified by the unique characteristics of children. Children have the ability to compensate for volume loss longer than adults, but when they exceed their ability to compensate, they deteriorate suddenly and severely. Significant underlying organ and vascular injury can occur without apparent external injury, often with only mild external signs and symptoms. The prehospital care provider should consider children with trauma and the following signs unstable and should transport them without delay to an appropriate facility:

- Difficulty breathing
- Signs of shock or circulatory instability
- Any period of postinjury unconsciousness
- Significant blunt trauma to the thorax
- Fractured ribs
- Significant blunt trauma to the abdomen
- Pelvic fracture

If possible, children with multisystem trauma and a PTS of less than 8 should be transported to a pediatric trauma center.

Scenario Solution

You correctly identify this child as a victim of multisystem trauma who is in shock. Because of the mechanism of injury, you decide that Scott is critically injured. Because of the femur injury combined with the change in mentation, you have to determine the greatest threat to his survivability—the brain injury, the potential volume loss from the femur, or other injuries not yet identified. You correctly identify hypotension and tachycardia, which you assume is related to hypovolemic shock, probably resultant from the femur injury and a possible intraabdominal injury. Initially, Scott's breathing is supported with high-concentration oxygen via a nonrebreather mask. You are prepared to provide more aggressive airway control if his condition deteriorates. If you consider intubation, you may need to consider additional cervical spine protective maneuvers. You may consider rapid sequence induction (RSI) if it is appropriate and you are properly trained.

Because of the nature of the child's injuries, you consult with medical control, who agrees that helicopter transport to a more distant pediatric trauma center is more appropriate than ground transport to a nearby community hospital that has no pediatric critical care, neurosurgical, or orthopedic resources. Brief efforts at peripheral venous access are unsuccessful. You begin crystalloid infusion via an intraosseous line. The patient's mother arrives just as you are transferring care to the helicopter crew.

Review Questions

Answers are provided on p. 414.

1. Pediatric patients are more difficult to communicate with because of which of the following?
   a. They may not have command of language skills relative to the emergency situation
   b. They may be fearful of strangers or persons unknown to them
   c. The prehospital care provider may not be communicating at their developmental level
   d. All the above

2. Which formula is a good method to estimate the systolic blood pressure of a child?
   a. 100 – Age in years
   b. 120 – Age in years
   c. 16+ (Age in years × 10)
   d. 80+ (2 × Age in years)

3. In a child who has 25% to 30% total body surface area burns, what is one of the major secondary considerations in the prehospital setting?
   a. Fluid retention
   b. Hypothermia
   c. Infection
   d. Loss of extremity function

4. What is meant by *adequate ventilation*?
   a. Ventilatory effort
   b. O_2/CO_2 gas exchange
   c. Ventilatory effort and O_2 delivery
   d. Adequate chest rise and effective O_2/CO_2 gas exchange

5. What is the approximate volume loss in the pediatric patient before blood pressure changes are noted?
   a. 25%
   b. 10%
   c. 30%
   d. 5%

6. In the normal child, which general statement is most accurate in comparison with the adult patient?
   a. Blood pressure is higher, heart rate is higher, and ventilatory rate is higher
   b. Blood pressure is lower, heart rate is lower, and ventilatory rate is higher
   c. Blood pressure is lower, heart rate is higher, and ventilatory rate is higher
   d. Blood pressure is lower, heart rate is higher, and ventilatory rate is lower

REFERENCES

American Academy of Pediatrics: *Diagnostic and statistical manual for primary care*, Elk Grove, Ill, 1996, Author.

American College of Surgeons Committee on Trauma: Extremes of age: pediatric trauma. In *Advanced trauma life support for physicians*, Chicago, 2002, American College of Surgeons.

Ball JW, Bindler R: *Pediatric nursing*, ed 2, Norwalk, Conn, 1999, Appleton & Lange.

Brain Trauma Foundation: *Guidelines for prehospital management of traumatic brain injury*, New York, 2000, Author.

Eichelberger MR: *Pediatric trauma: prevention, acute care, and rehabilitation*, St Louis, 1993, Mosby.

Horn LJ, Zasher ND: *Medical rehabilitation of traumatic brain injury*, St Louis, 1996, Mosby.

Marshall LF, Becker DP, Bowers SA et al: The national traumatic coma data bank, *J Neurosurg* 59:276, 1983.

National Center for Injury Prevention and Control, Centers for Disease Control and Prevention: *Fact book for the year 2000: working to prevent and control injury in the United States*. Available at www.cdc.gov/ncipc/cmprfact.htm (accessed 12/17/01).

National Pediatric Trauma Registry: *Facts sheets*. Available at www.nemc.org/rehab/factshee.htm (accessed 12/17/01).

Seidel HS, Ball JW, Daines JE, Benedict GW: *Physical examination*, St Louis, 1999, Mosby.

Sellars CW et al: *Pediatric brain injury: the special case of the very young child*, Houston, 1997, HDI.

Chapter 13

Special Considerations in Trauma of the Elderly

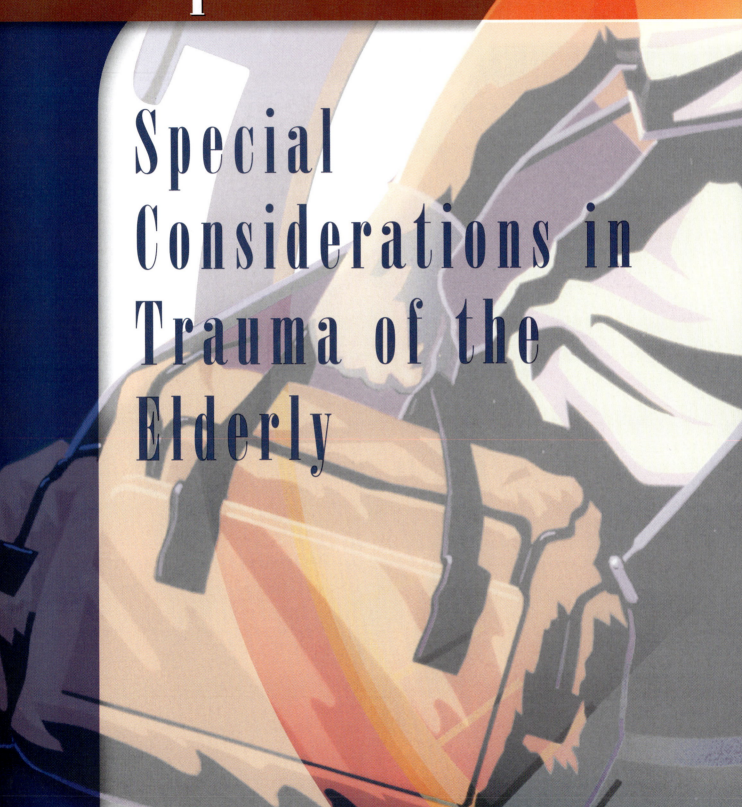

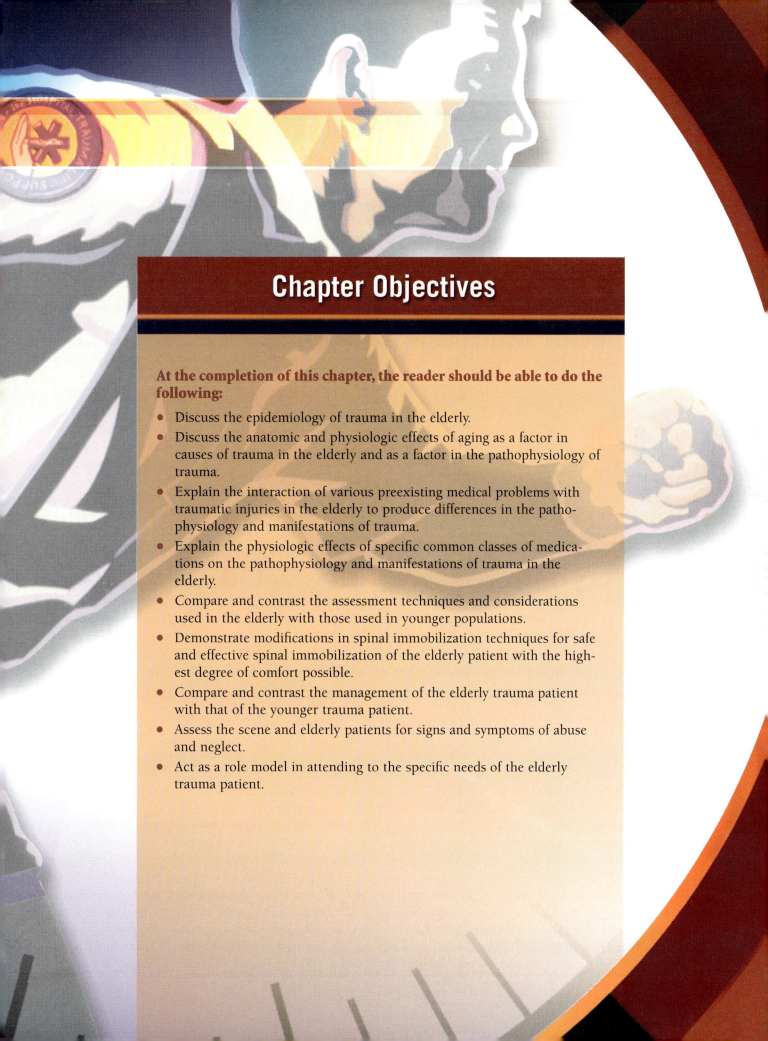

Chapter Objectives

At the completion of this chapter, the reader should be able to do the following:

- Discuss the epidemiology of trauma in the elderly.
- Discuss the anatomic and physiologic effects of aging as a factor in causes of trauma in the elderly and as a factor in the pathophysiology of trauma.
- Explain the interaction of various preexisting medical problems with traumatic injuries in the elderly to produce differences in the pathophysiology and manifestations of trauma.
- Explain the physiologic effects of specific common classes of medications on the pathophysiology and manifestations of trauma in the elderly.
- Compare and contrast the assessment techniques and considerations used in the elderly with those used in younger populations.
- Demonstrate modifications in spinal immobilization techniques for safe and effective spinal immobilization of the elderly patient with the highest degree of comfort possible.
- Compare and contrast the management of the elderly trauma patient with that of the younger trauma patient.
- Assess the scene and elderly patients for signs and symptoms of abuse and neglect.
- Act as a role model in attending to the specific needs of the elderly trauma patient.

Scenario

Sitting outside of your station on a sunny afternoon, you and your crew are startled by a loud crash. Looking toward the noise, you see that a vehicle has struck a tree head-on a block down the street. Your captain calls in the run as you and your partner respond to the scene. Your patient, the driver and sole occupant, is a woman in her mid-seventies who is unresponsive and taking agonal ventilations as you approach. The patient has a laceration on her forehead and a large skin tear on her left forearm that are both bleeding freely. She is wearing a MedicAlert bracelet that indicates that she takes "blood thinners."

Was the vehicle crash the primary event or secondary to a medical event? How does the information that the patient is on anticoagulant therapy affect your level of suspicion for traumatic brain injury and for intraabdominal hemorrhage? How do the patient's age, medical history, and medications interact with the injuries she received to make the pathophysiology and manifestations different from those in younger patients? How will you modify your approach to the management of this patient.

The elderly represent the fastest growing age group in the nation. Gerontologists (medical specialists who study and care for the elderly) divide the term *elderly* into three specific categories:

- Middle age: 50 to 64 years of age
- Late age: 65 to 79 years of age
- Older age: 80 years of age and older

More than 34 million Americans (12% of the U.S. population) are 65 years of age or older, and the size of this group has risen dramatically during the last 100 years. At the same time, fertility rates have dropped, meaning that there will be fewer people under 65 years of age to support the costs of health care and living expenses of those over 65 years of age. By the year 2050, nearly 25% of Americans will be eligible for Medicare, and the population over 85 years of age will grow from 4 million to 19 million.

The elderly present challenges in prehospital care management, second only to those encountered with infants. The sudden illness and trauma in the elderly present a different prehospital care dimension than in younger patients.

Because older persons are more susceptible to critical illness and trauma than the rest of the population, a prehospital care provider needs to consider a wider range of complications in patient assessment and management. Because the elderly access medical care via emergency systems (e.g., 911), rendering care is different than that for patients younger in age. The range of disabilities experienced by the elderly is enormous, and field assessment may take longer than with younger patients. Difficulties in assessment can be expected as a result of sensory deficits in hearing and vision, senility, and physiologic changes.

Advances in medicine and an increasing awareness of healthier lifestyles during the last several decades has resulted in a significant increase in the percentage of the population that is over 65 years of age. Although trauma has its highest frequency in young people and geriatric emergencies are most commonly medical in nature, a growing number of geriatric calls result from or include trauma. Trauma is currently the fifth leading cause of death in the elderly, and trauma deaths in this age group account for 25% of all of the trauma deaths nationwide.

Progress in recent years has not only increased adult life expectancy but has also affected the quality of life and therefore the range of physical activities performed at older ages. As more people live longer and enjoy better health in their older years, more of them travel, drive, and continue active physical pursuits that can result in an associated increase in geriatric trauma. Many who could retire continue to work in spite of a health problem or advancing age.

Recent social changes have increased the number of older people living in independent housing, retirement communities, and other assisted-living opportunities over those in nursing homes or other more guarded and limited environments. This suggests a probable increase in the incidence of simple household trauma, such as falls, in the elderly. The past few years have also seen an increase in geriatric victims of crime in the home and on the streets. Older people are often singled out as "easy marks" and can sustain substantial trauma from crimes of seemingly limited violence—such as purse snatching—when they are struck, are knocked down, or fall.

With the growing awareness of this expanding population at risk, the prehospital care provider must understand the unique needs of an elderly trauma patient. Specifically, prehospital care providers must understand the aging process and the effects of co-existing medical problems on an elderly patient's response to trauma and trauma management. The special considerations outlined in this chapter should be included in the assessment and management of any trauma patient who is 65 years of age or older, physically appears elderly, or is a middle-age adult who has any of the significant medical problems commonly associated with the elderly.

Anatomy and Physiology of Aging

The aging process causes changes in physical structure, body composition, and organ function, and it can create unique problems during prehospital care. The aging process does influence mortality and morbidity rates.

Aging, or senescence, is a natural biologic process and is sometimes referred to as a process of biologic reversal that begins during the years of early adulthood. At this time, organ systems have achieved maturation, and a turning point in physiologic growth has been reached. The body gradually loses its ability to maintain homeostasis (the state of relative constancy of the body's internal environment), and viability declines over a period of years until death occurs.

The fundamental process of aging occurs at the cellular level and is reflected in both anatomic structure and physiologic function. The period of "old age" is generally characterized by frailty, slower mental processes, impairment of psychologic functions, diminished energy, the appearance of chronic and degenerative diseases, and a decline in sensory acuity. Functional abilities are lessened, and the well-known superficial signs and symptoms of older age appear, such as skin wrinkling, changes in hair color and quantity, osteoarthritis, and slowness in reaction time and reflexes (Figure 13-1).

Influence of Chronic Medical Problems

As people age, they experience the normal physiologic changes of aging and can also experience more medical problems. Although some individuals can reach an advanced age without any serious medical problems, statistically an older person is more likely to have one or more significant medical conditions. Usually, proper medical care can control these conditions, avoiding or minimizing exacerbation into repeated acute and often

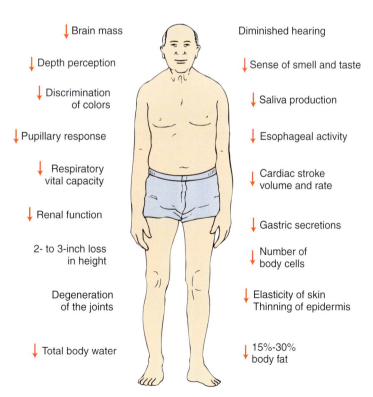

↓ Brain mass

↓ Depth perception

↓ Discrimination of colors

↓ Pupillary response

↓ Respiratory vital capacity

↓ Renal function

2- to 3-inch loss in height

Degeneration of the joints

↓ Total body water

Diminished hearing

↓ Sense of smell and taste

↓ Saliva production

↓ Esophageal activity

↓ Cardiac stroke volume and rate

↓ Gastric secretions

↓ Number of body cells

↓ Elasticity of skin Thinning of epidermis

↓ 15%-30% body fat

Figure 13-1   Changes caused by aging.

life-threatening episodes. Some older individuals have reached advanced age with minimal medical problems, whereas others may live with chronic illnesses and depend on modern medical means. This latter group can deteriorate more rapidly in an emergency situation.

Repeated acute episodes or even the single occurrence of a significant episode can result in chronic residual effects on the body. A patient who has previously had an acute myocardial infarction sustains permanent heart damage. The resultant reduced cardiac capacity continues for the rest of his or her life, affecting the heart and, because of the ensuing chronic decline in circulation, other organs as well.

As a person's age advances, additional medical problems can occur. None are truly isolated because the influence on the body is cumulative. The total influence on the body usually is greater than the sum of each individual effect. As this condition progresses and reduces the quality of the body's vital functions, the individual's ability to withstand the introduction of disease, serious trauma, or even minor trauma is greatly diminished.

Regardless of whether the patient is pediatric, middle-age, or elderly, the priorities, intervention needs, and life-threatening conditions commonly found as a result of serious trauma are the same. Elderly trauma patients die for the same reasons as trauma patients of any age. However, often because of preexisting physical conditions, the elderly can also die from less severe injuries and die sooner than younger patients. Data are available that support the role that preexisting conditions play in the survival of an elderly trauma patient (Table 13-1) and that the more conditions a trauma patient has the higher his or her mortality rate (Table 13-2). Certain conditions are associated with a higher mortality rate because of the way in which they interfere with an elderly patient's ability to respond to trauma (Table 13-3).

Respiratory System

Ventilatory function declines in the elderly partly as a result of the inability of the chest cage to expand and contract and partly from stiffening of the airway. The increased stiffness in the chest wall is associated with a reduction in the ability to expand the chest wall and a stiffening of cartilaginous connections of the ribs. As a result of these changes, the chest cage is less pliable. With declines in the efficiency of the respiratory system, the elderly patient requires more exertion to carry out daily activities. The alveolar surface area decreases with age. The alveolar surface area is estimated to reduce 4% for each decade after 30 years of age. A 70 year old, for example, would have a 16% reduction in his or her alveolar surface area. Any alteration of the already reduced alveolar surface decreases oxygen uptake. Additionally, as the body ages, its ability to saturate hemoglobin with oxygen decreases, leading to lower baseline oxygen saturations as normal and less reserve available.

Impaired cough and gag reflexes along with poor cough strength and diminished esophageal sphincter tone results in an increased risk of aspiration. A reduction in the number of cilia (hair-like processes that

Table 13-1 Percentage of Patients with Preexisting Disease (PED)

Age (yr)	PED (%)
15-24	2.8
25-34	8
35-44	17
45-54	30.8
55-64	44.1
65-74	50
>75	64.9

(Adapted from Milzman DP, Boulanger BR, Rodriguez A et al: Preexisting disease in trauma patients: a predictor of fate independent of age and injury severity score, *J Trauma* 32:236, 1992.)

Table 13-2 Number of Preexisting Diseases (PEDs) and Outcome

Number of PEDs	Survived	Died	Mortality rate (%)
0	6341	211	3.2
1	868	56	6.1
2	197	36	15.5
3 or more	67	22	24.7

(Adapted from Milzman DP, Boulanger BR, Rodriguez A et al: Preexisting disease in trauma patients: a predictor of fate independent of age and injury severity score, *J Trauma* 32:236, 1992.)

propel foreign particles and mucus from the bronchi) predisposes the elderly to problems caused by inhaled particulate matter.

Another factor that affects the respiratory system is a change to the spinal curvature. Curvature changes accompanied by an anteroposterior hump (as seen in osteoporosis patients) often lead to additional ventilatory difficulty (Figure 13-2). Changes that affect the diaphragm can also contribute to ventilatory problems. Stiffening of the rib cage can cause more reliance on diaphragmatic activity to breathe. This increased reliance on the diaphragm makes an older person especially sensitive to changes in intraabdominal pressure. Thus a supine position or an overly filled stomach from a large meal can provoke ventilatory insufficiency. Obesity can also play a part in diaphragm restriction, especially when fat distribution tends to be central.

Ears, Nose, and Throat

Tooth decay, gum disease, and injury to teeth result in the need for various dental prostheses. The brittle nature of capped teeth, fixed bridges, or loose, removable bridges and dentures poses a special problem of possible foreign bodies that can be aspirated and obstruct the airway.

Table 13-3	Prevalence of Preexisting Diseases (PEDs) and Their Mortality Rates			
PED	**Number of patients**	**PED present (%)**	**Total (%)**	**Mortality rate (%)**
Hypertension	597	47.9	7.7	10.2
Pulmonary disease	286	23	3.7	8.4
Cardiac disease	223	17.9	2.9	18.4
Diabetes	198	15.9	2.5	12.1
Obesity	167	13.4	2.1	4.8
Malignancy	80	6.4	1	20
Neurologic disorder	45	3.6	0.6	13.3
Renal disease	40	3.2	0.5	37.5
Hepatic disease	41	3.3	0.5	12.2

(Adapted from Milzman DP, Boulanger BR, Rodriguez A et al: Pre-existing disease in trauma patients: a predictor of fate independent of age and injury severity score, *J Trauma* 32:236, 1992.)

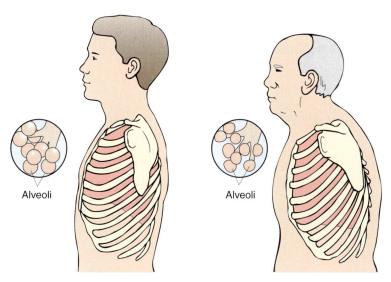

Alveoli

Alveoli

Figure 13-2   Spinal curvature can lead to an anteroposterior hump, which can cause ventilatory difficulties. Reduction in the alveolar surface area can also reduce the amount of oxygen that is exchanged in the lungs.

Changes in the contours of the face result from resorption of the mandible, in part because of absence of teeth (edentulism). The characteristic look is an infolding and shrinking of the mouth. These changes can affect the ability to create an effective seal with a bag-valve-mask (BVM) device and sufficient visualization of the airway during endotracheal intubation. The nose and ears are more elongated than at a younger age because of the continuous growth of cartilage (Figure 13-3).

Cardiovascular System

Diseases of the cardiovascular system are the major cause of death in the elderly. Cardiovascular disease accounts for over 3000 deaths per 100,000 persons over 65 years of age.

Age-related decreases in arterial elasticity lead to increased peripheral vascular resistance. The myocardium and blood vessels rely on their elastic, contractile, and distensible properties to function properly. With aging, these properties decline, and the efficiency of the cardiovascular system to move circulatory fluids around the body decreases. The cardiac output diminishes by approximately 50% from 20 to 80 years of age. As many as 10% of those over 75 years of age will have some degree of overt (asymptomatic) congestive heart failure.

Atherosclerosis is a narrowing of the blood vessels, a condition in which the inner layer of the artery wall thickens while fatty deposits build up within the artery. These deposits, called plaque, protrude above the surface of the inner layer and decrease the diameter of the internal

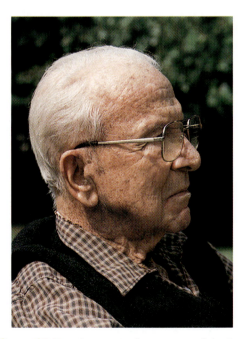

Figure 13-3   Changes in the contour of the face.

channel of the vessel. One result of this narrowing is hypertension, a condition that affects one out of six adults in the United States. The calcification of the arterial wall reduces the ability of the vessels to change size in response to endocrine and central nervous system stimuli. The lowered circulation can adversely affect any of the vital organs and is a common cause of heart disease.

With age, the heart itself shows an increase in fibrous tissue and size (myocardial hypertrophy). Atrophy of the cells of the conduction system result in the increased incidence of cardiac dysrhythmias. In particular, the normal reflexes in the heart that respond to hypotension diminish with age resulting in the inability of elderly patients to appropriately increase their heart rate. Patients with a permanent pacemaker have a fixed heart rate and cardiac output that cannot meet the demands of increased myocardial oxygen consumption that accompanies the stress of trauma.

In the elderly trauma patient, this reduced circulation contributes to cellular hypoxia. The result is cardiac dysrhythmias, acute heart failure, and even sudden death. The ability of the body to compensate for blood loss or other causes of shock is significantly lowered in the elderly due to a diminished inotropic (cardiac contraction) response to catecholamines.

The reduced circulation and circulatory defense responses coupled with increasing cardiac failure produce a significant problem in managing shock in the elderly. Fluid resuscitation needs to be carefully watched because of the reduced compliance of the cardiovascular system and the often "stiff" right ventricle. Care must be taken while treating hypotension and shock so as not to cause volume overloading with aggressive fluid resuscitation.

Nervous System

As individuals age, a decrease occurs in brain weight and in the number of neurons or nerve cells. The weight of the brain reaches its peak (1.4 kg, or 3 lb) at approximately 20 years of age. By 80 years of age the brain loses about 100 grams (about 3½ ounces). The speed with which nerve impulses are conducted along certain nerves also decreases. These decreases result in only small effects on behavior and thinking. Reflexes are slower but not to a significant degree. Compensatory functions can be impaired, particularly in patients with diseases such as Parkinson's disease, resulting in an increased incidence of falls. The peripheral nervous system is also affected by the slowing of nerve impulses, resulting in tremors and an unsteady gait.

General information and vocabulary abilities increase or are maintained, whereas skills requiring mental and muscular activity (psychomotor ability) may decline. The intellectual functions that involve verbal comprehension, arithmetic ability, fluency of ideas, experiential evaluation, and general knowledge tend to increase after 60 years of age in those who continue learning activities. Exceptions are those who develop senile dementia and other disorders like Alzheimer's disease.

The normal biologic aging of the brain is not a predictor for diseases of the brain. However, decreases in the cortical structure of the brain may be involved in mental impairment. As changes occur in the brain, memory can be affected, personality changes, and other reductions in brain function can occur. These changes may involve the need for some form of mental health service. About 10% to 15% of the elderly require professional mental health services. However, when assessing an elderly trauma patient, any impairment in mentation should be assumed to be the result of an acute traumatic insult such as shock, hypoxia, or brain injury.

Sensory Changes

VISION AND HEARING

Overall, approximately 28% of elderly persons have hearing impairment and approximately 13% have visual impairment. Men tend to be more likely to have hearing difficulties, whereas both genders have a similar share of eye-related impairment.

Loss of vision is challenging at any age, and it may be even more problematic for the elderly. The inability to read directions (e.g., on a prescription label) can lead to a disastrous effect. In addition, the elderly experience decreases in visual acuity, ability to differentiate colors, and night vision.

The cells of the lens of the eye are incapable of restoration to their original molecular structure. One of the destructive agents over years of exposure is ultraviolet radiation. Eventually, the lens loses its capability to increase in thickness and curvature. The result is almost universal farsightedness (presbyopia) in persons over 40 years of age, requiring glasses for reading.

As a result of changes to the various structures of the eye, the elderly have more difficulty seeing in dimly lit environments. Decreased tear production leads to dry eyes and itching, burning, and the inability to keep the eyes open for long periods of time.

With age the lens of the eye begins to become cloudy and impenetrable to light. This gradual process results in what is termed a *cataract*, or a milky lens that blocks and distorts light that enters the eye and blurs vision. Some degree of cataract formation is present in 95% of elderly persons. This deterioration of vision increases the risk of a motor vehicle crash (MVC), particularly while driving at night.

A gradual decline in hearing (presbycusis) is also characteristic of aging. Presbycusis is commonly due to loss of conduction of sound into the inner ear and can be assisted to some degree with the use of hearing aids. This hearing loss is most pronounced when the person attempts to discriminate complex sounds, such as when many people are speaking at once or with loud ambient noise present, such as the wailing of sirens.

PAIN PERCEPTION

Because of the aging process and the presence of diseases such as diabetes, the elderly may not perceive pain normally, placing them at increased risk of injury from excesses in heat and cold exposures. Many elderly patients have conditions such as arthritis that result in constant chronic pain. Living with daily pain can cause an increased tolerance to pain. This may result in a patient's failure to identify areas of injury. In evaluating patients, especially those who usually "hurt all over" or who appear to have a high tolerance to pain, the prehospital care provider should locate areas where the pain has increased or where the painful area has enlarged. Whether the pain's characteristics or exacerbating factors have changed since the trauma occurred should also be noted.

Musculoskeletal System

Bone loses mineral as it ages. The loss of bone (osteoporosis) is unequal among the sexes. During young adulthood, bone mass is greater in women than in men. However, bone loss is more rapid in women and accelerates after menopause. With this higher incidence of osteoporosis, older women have a greater probability of fractures, particularly of the neck of the femur (hip).

Older persons are sometimes shorter than they were in young adulthood because of dehydration of the vertebral discs. As the discs flatten, a loss of approximately 2 inches (5 cm) in height occurs between 20 and 70 years of age. Kyphosis (curvature of the spine) in the thoracic region can also contribute to height loss and is commonly caused by osteoporosis (Figure 13-4).

As the bones become more porous and fragile, erosion occurs anteriorly and compression fractures may develop. As the thoracic spine becomes more curved, the head and shoulders appear to be pushed forward (Figure 13-5). If chronic obstructive pulmonary disease (COPD), particularly emphysema, is present, the kyphosis may be more pronounced because of the increased development of the accessory muscles of breathing.

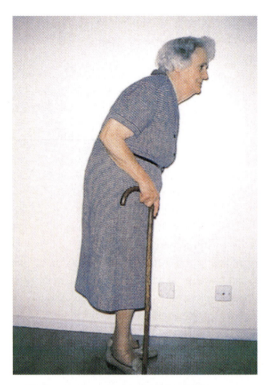

Figure 13-4   Kyphosis, commonly caused by osteoporosis.

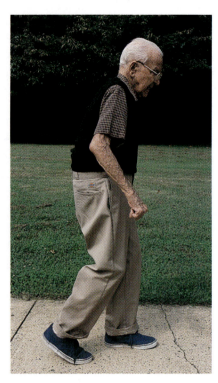

Figure 13-5   Because of the tendency to flex the legs, the arms appear longer.

Osteoarthritis, a form of arthritis in which joints undergo degenerative changes, is characterized by stiffness, deformity, swelling of the joints, and pain. Osteoarthritis usually involves changes in the hands and feet, particularly in the proximal and distal interphalangeal joints, and in the hips and spine (Figure 13-6). The increased tendency to flex the legs makes the arms appear longer even though no change in their anatomic length has actually occurred (see Figure 13-5).

As muscles age, loss of muscle mass occurs, estimated to be 30% between 30 and 80 years of age. Deficits that relate to the musculoskeletal system (e.g., inability to flex the hip or knee adequately with changes in terrain) predispose the elderly to falls. Muscle fatigue in the elderly can cause many problems that affect movement, falls being one of the most frequent. Changes in the body's normal posture are common, and changes of the spine make the curvature become more acute with aging. Some degree of osteoporosis is universal with aging. Because of this progressive bone resorption, the bones become less pliant, more brittle, and more easily broken. The weakening in bone strength coupled with reduced muscle strength caused by less active exercise can result in multiple fractures with only mild or moderate force. As the normal

arthritic process occurs with aging, the range of joint movement becomes more limited.

The entire vertebral column changes with age primarily because of the effects of both osteoporosis and the calcification (osteophysis) of the supporting ligaments. This calcification results in decreased range of motion and narrowing of the spinal canal. The narrowed canal and progressive osteophytic disease put these patients at high risk for spinal cord injury with even minor trauma. The narrowing of the spinal canal is called *spinal stenosis* and increases the likelihood of cord compression without any actual break in the bony cervical spine. The thoracic and lumbar spine degenerate progressively as well, and the combined forces of osteoporosis and posture changes lead to increased falls. The prehospital care provider should maintain a high level of suspicion for spinal injury during patient assessment because over 50% of vertebral compression fractures are asymptomatic.

Skin

As the skin ages, sweat and sebaceous glands are lost. Loss of sweat glands reduces the body's ability to regulate temperature. Loss of sebaceous glands, which produce oil, makes the skin dry and flaky. Production of melanin, the pigment that gives color to skin and hair, declines,

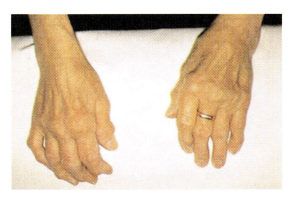

Figure 13-6   Osteoarthritis.

causing an aging pallor. The skin thins and appears translucent primarily because of changes in connective tissue. The thinning and drying of the skin also reduces its resistance to microorganisms, resulting in an increased infection rate with minor trauma. As elasticity is lost, the skin stretches and falls into wrinkles and folds, especially in areas of heavy use, such as those overlying the facial muscles of expression. Loss of fatty tissue can predispose the elderly to hypothermia. This loss of fatty tissue also leads to less padding over bony prominences such as the head, shoulders, spine, buttocks, hips, and heels. Prolonged immobilization without additional padding can result in tissue necrosis and ulceration as well as increased pain and discomfort during treatment and transport.

Renal System

Changes common with aging include reduced levels of filtration by the kidneys and a reduced excretory capacity. These changes should be considered when administering drugs normally cleared by the kidneys. Chronic renal inhibition, commonly found in the elderly, contributes to the lowering of a patient's overall health and ability to withstand trauma.

Immune System

As the immune system ages, its ability to function decreases. A decrease in cell-mediated and humoral responses also results. Coupled with any preexisting nutritional problems common in the elderly, this leads to an increased susceptibility to infection. Sepsis is a common cause of late death after severe or even insignificant trauma in the elderly.

Assessment

Prehospital assessment of the elderly is based on the same method used for all trauma patients. As with all trauma patients, the mechanism of injury should be considered first. This section discusses some special considerations in assessing an elderly trauma patient.

Mechanism of Injury

FALLS

Falls are the leading cause of trauma death and disability in those over 75 years of age. Approximately one third of community-dwelling people over 65 years of age fall each year, increasing to 50% by 80 years of age. Men and women fall with equal frequency, but women are more than twice as likely to sustain a serious injury because of more pronounced weakening of the bones (osteoporosis).

Most falls occur as a result of the inherent nature of aging with the changes in posture and gait. Declining visual acuity from cataracts, glaucoma, and loss of night vision all contribute to the loss of visual clues used by the elderly to navigate safely. Diseases of the central and peripheral nervous systems and the vascular instability of cardiovascular disease further precipitate falls. However, the most important variables contributing to falls in the elderly are physical barriers in their environment, such as slippery floors, stairs, poor-fitting shoes, and poor lighting.

Long bone fractures account for the majority of injuries, with fractures of the hip resulting in the greatest mortality and morbidity rates. The mortality rate from hip fractures is 20% 1 year after the injury and rises to 33% 2 years after the injury. Mortality is most often secondary to pulmonary embolus and the effects of decreased mobility.

VEHICULAR TRAUMA

MVCs are the leading cause of trauma death in the geriatric population between 65 and 74 years of age. An elderly patient is five times more likely to be fatally injured in an MVC than a younger driver, even though excessive speed is rarely a causative factor found in the older age group.

These high fatality rates have been attributed to certain physiologic changes. In particular, the subtle change in memory and judgment in combination with impairment in visual and auditory acuity can result in impaired reaction time.

Alcohol is rarely involved as compared with MVCs in younger persons. Only 6% of fatally injured elderly persons are intoxicated compared with 23% for all other age categories.

Elderly pedestrians represent more than 20% of all pedestrian fatalities. Because of slower walking speeds, the time allowed by traffic signals may be too short for the elderly to safely traverse the crosswalk. This may explain the observation that more than 45% of all elderly pedestrian fatalities occur near a crosswalk.

ASSAULT AND DOMESTIC ABUSE

The elderly are highly vulnerable to crime. Violent assaults have been estimated to account for more than 10% of trauma admissions in the elderly. The need for chronic care because of debilitation may predispose an elderly person to abuse from his or her caregivers.

BURNS

The elderly represent 20% of burn unit admissions with an estimated 1500 fire-related deaths per year. Burn fatalities in the elderly occur from burns of smaller size and severity as compared with other age groups. Fatality rates are seven times those of younger burn victims.

Because of impairments in visual and auditory acuity the elderly may have delayed recognition of house fires. Decreased pain perception can result in more significant burns.

The presence of preexisting medical conditions, such as cardiovascular disease and diabetes, results in poor tolerance to the resuscitative care of burns. Vascular collapse and infection are the most common causes of death from burns.

TRAUMATIC BRAIN INJURY

The brain has undergone a 10% reduction in mass by 70 years of age. The dura mater adheres more closely to the skull, resulting in a loss of some brain volume. One consequence of this is a lower frequency of epidural hemorrhage and a higher frequency of subdural hemorrhage. Because of brain atrophy, a fairly large subdural hemorrhage can exist with minimal clinical findings. The combination of head trauma and hypovolemic shock yields a greater fatality rate.

Airway

Evaluation of the elderly patient begins with assessment of the airway. Changes in mentation may be associated with the tongue blocking the airway. The oral cavity should be examined for foreign bodies, such as dentures, that have become dislodged.

Breathing

Elderly patients who breathe at a rate of less than 10 or greater than 30 breaths/min, similar to any other adult, will not have adequate minute volume and will require positive-pressure assisted ventilations. In most adults a ventilatory rate between 12 and 20 breaths/min is normal and confirms that an adequate minute volume is present. However, in an elderly patient, reduced tidal volume capacity and pulmonary function may result in an inadequate minute volume even at rates of 12 to 20 breaths/min. Breath sounds should be immediately assessed if the ventilatory rate is abnormal.

Circulation

Delayed capillary refilling time is common in the elderly because of less efficient circulation; therefore it is a poor indicator of acute circulatory changes in these patients. Some degree of decreased distal motor, sensory, and circulatory ability in the extremities represents a common normal finding in the elderly.

Some findings can only be interpreted properly by knowing the individual patient's preevent, or "baseline," status. Expected ranges of normal vital signs and other findings usually accepted as standard (normal) are not normal in every individual, and deviation is much more common in the elderly patient. Although the commonly assumed ranges are broad enough to include most individual adult differences, an individual of any age may vary beyond these norms; therefore such variation in elderly patients should be expected. Medication may contribute to these changes. For example, in the average adult, a systolic blood pressure of 120 mm Hg is considered normal and generally unimpressive. However, in the chronically hypertensive patient who normally has a systolic blood pressure of 150 mm Hg, a pressure of 120 mm Hg would be a concern, suggestive of hidden bleeding (or some other mechanism) of such a degree that decompensation has occurred. Likewise, heart rate is a poor indicator of trauma in the elderly because of the effects of medications and the heart's poor response to circulating catecholamines (epinephrine). Quantitative information or signs should not be used in isolation from other findings. However, failing to recognize that such a change occurred or that it is a serious pathologic finding in a particular patient can produce a poor outcome for the patient.

Disability

The prehospital care provider should view all findings together and maintain an increased level of suspicion in the elderly. Wide differences in mentation, memory, and orientation (to the past and present) can exist in the elderly. Significant neurologic trauma should be identified in light of the individual's preinjury, normal status. Unless someone on the scene can describe this status, it should be assumed that the patient has a neurologic injury, hypoxia, or both. The ability to distinguish between a patient's chronic status and acute changes is an essential factor to prevent underreaction or overreaction to the patient's present neurologic status as a key index in evaluating his or her overall condition. However, unconsciousness remains a grave sign in all cases.

The prehospital care provider must carefully select questions to determine the elderly patient's orientation to time and place. People who work 5 days a week with weekends off usually know what day of the week it is. If they do not, it can be assumed that they have some level of disorientation. For those who no longer work a traditional job and who are often surrounded by others who do not, a lack of distinction between days of the week or even months of the year may not indicate disorientation but only of a lack of "calendar" importance in the structure of their lives. Similarly, people who no longer drive pay less attention to roads, town borders, locations, and maps. Although normally oriented, they may not be able to identify their present location. Confusion or the inability to recall events and details long past may be more indicative of how long ago the events occurred rather than how forgetful the individual is. Similarly, the repeated retelling of events long past and seemingly more attention to the far past rather than the immediate past often simply represent a nostalgic lingering on years and events. Such social and psychological compensations should not be considered as signs of senility or a diminished mental capacity.

Expose/Environment

The elderly are more susceptible to ambient environmental changes. They have a decreased ability to respond to changes, decreased heat production, and a decreased ability to rid the body of excessive heat. Thermoregulatory problems are related to an imbalance of electrolytes (e.g., potassium depletion, hypothyroidism, and diabetes mellitus). Other factors include a decreased basal metabolic rate, decreased ability to shiver, arteriosclerosis, and effects of drugs and alcohol. Hyperthermia is affected by cerebrovascular accidents, diuretics, antihistamines, and antiparkinsonian drugs. Hypothermia is affected by decreased metabolism, fat, less efficient peripheral vasoconstriction, and poor nutrition.

Secondary Survey (Focused History/ Physical Examination)

In the assessment of acute illness, the following factors are important to consider after management of urgent life-threatening conditions. More than the average time may be taken in gathering information and taking a history.

- *The body may not respond the same as in younger patients.* Typical findings of serious illness such as

Communication

The prehospital care provider should not approach elderly patients as if they are small children. A common mistake by health care professionals in both the prehospital and emergency department settings is to treat the elderly in this way. Often, well-meaning relatives are so aggressive in reporting the events for an elderly loved one that they take over as the respondent to any inquiries. In such a situation, the fact that the clinical impression and history are from someone other than the patient and may not be correct can easily be overlooked. Not only does this increase the danger of obtaining incomplete or inaccurate information through a third party's impressions and translation, but it also discounts the patient as a mature adult.

Proper adult interaction with the patient is essential in obtaining good information, establishing rapport between the prehospital care provider and the patient, and preserving the dignity to which the patient is entitled. Although additional information from relatives, nursing home personnel, or others can be important, it should not replace the primary information and responses supplied by the patient.

fever, pain, or tenderness may take longer to develop and make it more difficult to evaluate the patient. In addition, many medications will alter the body's response. Often a prehospital care provider will have to depend on history alone.

- *Additional patience may be needed because of the patient's hearing or visual deficits.* Empathy and compassion are essential. A patient's intelligence should not be underestimated merely because communication may be difficult or absent. If the patient has close associates or relatives, they may participate in giving information or may stay nearby to help validate information.

- *Assessment of the elderly requires different questioning tactics.* The patient should be asked for specific versus general information because the elderly tend to respond "yes" to all questions during the assessment process. Asking open-ended questions is a useful tool in evaluating most patients. However, sometimes with the elderly providing specific details from which to choose when dealing with a problem can be helpful. For example, instead of saying "Describe the pain in your hip," ask, "Is the pain in your hip sharp, stabbing, or dull?" or "On a scale of 1 to 10, 10 being the most intense pain, how would you rate the pain?"

- *A significant other may need to be involved.* With the patient's permission, involving the caregiver or spouse may be necessary to gather valid information. Some elderly patients may be reluctant to give information without the assistance of a relative or support person. However, the elderly patient may not want any other person present for many reasons, one of which may be abuse problems. The elderly patient may fear punishment for telling someone, in the presence of the abuser, why he or she has multiple bruise marks. Some problems may embarrass the elderly patient that he or she may not want any family members to know about.
- *Attention should be paid to sensory deficits (hearing, vision, smell, taste, touch, and position).* Given the usual presence of these deficits, maintaining eye contact and speaking more slowly than usual and with suitable volume are important in gathering patient information.
- *Altered comprehension or neurologic disorders are a significant problem for many elderly patients.* These impairments can range from confusion to senile dementia of the type associated with Alzheimer's disease. Not only may these patients have difficulty

in communicating, but they may also be unable to comprehend or help in the assessment. They may be restless and sometimes combative.

- *Firmness, reassurance, and clear, simple (and repeated) questioning may be helpful.* Often a family member or friend can be of assistance.
- *Pay attention to impaired hearing, sight, comprehension, and mobility capabilities.* Eye contact should be made with the patient. The patient may be hearing impaired and depend on watching your lips and other facial movements. Noise, distractions, and interruptions should be minimized. Fluency in speech, an involuntary movement, cranial nerve dysfunction, or difficulty breathing should be noted. Is the patient's movement easy, unsteady, or unbalanced?
- *Shake the patient's hand to feel for grip strength, skin turgor, and body temperature.* The patient should be addressed by his or her last name, unless otherwise told by the patient. Phrases like, "Now, now, you'll be fine" should be avoided. Open-ended questions such as, "Describe the pain in your abdomen, is it . . . ?" should be used, and questions like, "Where does it hurt?" should be avoided.
- *Look for behavioral problems or manifestations that do not fit the scene.* Look at grooming. Are the patient's attire and grooming appropriate for where and how the patient was found? The ease of rising or sitting should be observed.
- *Look at the patient's state of nourishment.* Does the patient appear to be well, thin, or emaciated? Elderly patient's have a decreased thirst response. The kid-

---

Elderly patients present with a host of common complaints. When assessing a geriatric patient, even during a trauma event, knowing what these complaints are can be helpful to the prehospital care provider. The following is a list of some common complaints:

- Alcoholism*
- Constipation or diarrhea
- Dementia*
- Depression*
- Dizziness, vertigo, or syncope
- Dysphagia
- Dyspnea
- Falls
- Fatigue and weakness
- Headache
- Hearing loss*
- Incontinence or inability to void*
- Musculoskeletal stiffness*
- Poor nutrition; loss of appetite
- Sexual dysfunction
- Sleep disorders*
- Visual disorders

*Most frequently repeated complaints.

Medication

Knowledge of a patient's medications can provide key information in determining prehospital care. For example, the use of a beta blocker such as Inderal may account for a patient's bradycardia. In this situation, an increasing tachycardia as a sign of developing shock may not occur. The drug's inhibition of the body's normal sympathetic defense mechanisms can mask the true level of the patient's circulatory deterioration. Such patients can rapidly decompensate, seemingly without warning.

Another common medication in the elderly is warfarin, which is an anticoagulant, or "blood thinner." Any bleeding from trauma will be more brisk and difficult to control when a patient is on an anticoagulant. More importantly, internal bleeding can progress rapidly, leading to shock and death.

neys have a problem in meeting the challenge of injury. The kidney's ability to concentrate urine is decreased, leading to dehydration even before injury. Urine output is a poor measure of perfusion in the elderly. They also have a decreased amount of body fat (15% to 30%) and total body water.

- *Elderly patients have a decrease in skeletal muscle weight, widening and weakening of bones, degeneration of joints, and osteoporosis.* They have an increased probability of fractures with minor injuries and a marked increased risk of fractures to the vertebrae, hip, and ribs.
- *Elderly patients have degeneration of heart muscle cells and fewer pacemaker cells.* The elderly are prone to dysrhythmias as a result of a loss of elasticity of the heart and major arteries. Widespread use of beta and calcium channel blockers and diuretics further complicates this problem. Often after injury, the elderly present with low cardiac output with hypoxia and have no lung injury. Cardiac stroke, volume, and rate decrease as does cardiac reserve, all leading to morbidity and mortality of the elderly trauma patient. An elderly patient with a systolic blood pressure of 120 mm Hg should be considered to be in hypovolemic shock until proven otherwise.
- *An elderly patient's vital capacity is diminished by 50%.* Kyphotic changes in the spine (anteroposterior) result in a ventilation-perfusion mismatch at rest. Hypoxia is much more likely a consequence of shock than it is in younger patients. Elderly patients also have a decreased ability for chest excursions. Lower tidal volumes and lower minute volumes are typical. Reduced capillary oxygen and carbon dioxide exchange are significant. Hypoxemia tends to be progressive.

Management

Airway

The existence of dentures, common in the elderly, may affect airway management. Ordinarily, dentures should be left in place to maintain a better seal around the mouth with a mask. However, partial dentures (plates) may become dislodged during an emergency and occlude or partially block the airway; these should be removed.

Placement of devices to maintain a patent airway, such as a nasopharyngeal airway, can be complicated by severe bleeding if the patient is taking an anticoagulant, such as warfarin or aspirin.

Breathing

The elderly population has a high prevalence of COPD. In the presence of COPD, the ventilatory drive of some patients is not dependent on the level of carbon dioxide in the blood but on diminished blood oxygen levels. However, oxygen should never be withheld from a patient who needs it. The SpO_2 should generally be kept at greater than 95%.

The elderly experience increased stiffness of the chest wall. In addition, reduced chest wall muscle power and stiffening of the cartilage makes the chest cage less flexible. These and other changes are responsible for reductions in lung volumes. The patient may need ventilatory support by assisted ventilations with a BVM device.

Circulation

Hemorrhage in the elderly is controlled somewhat differently than in other patients. The elderly have poor cardiovascular reserve. Vital signs are a poor indicator of shock in the elderly because the patient who is normally hypertensive may be in shock with a systolic blood pressure of 110 mm Hg. Fluid resuscitation should be guided by the index of suspicion for serious bleeding based on the mechanism of injury and an overall appearance of shock.

The use of a pneumatic antishock garment (PASG) may precipitate congestive heart failure and impair ventilation. The decision to place the PASG on an elderly trauma victim requires increased vigilance in observing for associated complications.

Immobilization

Protection of the cervical spine, particularly in trauma patients who have sustained multiple system injury, is an expected standard of care. In the elderly, this standard of care must apply not only in trauma situations but also during acute medical problems in which attempts to maintain airway patency is a priority. Degenerative arthritis of the cervical spine may subject the elderly patient to spinal cord injury from maneuvering the neck, even if the patient has no injury to the spine. Another consideration with improper movement of the cervical spine is the possibility of occlusion of the arteries to the brain, which can result in unconsciousness and even stroke.

When applying a cervical collar to an elderly patient with severe kyphosis, the prehospital care provider must ensure that the collar does not compress the airway or carotid arteries. Less traditional means of immobilization, such as a rolled up towel and head block, can be considered if standard collars are inappropriate.

Padding may need to be placed under the patient's head and between the shoulders when immobilizing the supine elderly patient. Because of the lack of adipose tissue in the frail elderly patient, additional padding will be required when the patient is immobilized to a longboard. The prehospital care provider should look for pressure points where the patient is resting on the board and pad appropriately. When applying the straps to secure the patient, the elderly patient may not be able to fully straighten his or her legs because of decreased range of motion of the hips and knees. This may require the placement of padding under the legs for comfort and security of the patient during transport.

Temperature Control

The elderly patient should be watched closely for hypothermia and hyperthermia during treatment and transportation. Although it is appropriate to expose the patient to facilitate a thorough examination, the elderly are especially prone to heat loss. The effects of various medications may mean that a patient is more prone to overheating; therefore some means of cooling the patient should be considered if the patient is unable to be moved quickly to a controlled environment. Prolonged extrication in the extremes of heat and cold may also place the elderly patient at risk and should be rapidly addressed.

Legal Considerations

Several legal distinctions can become issues when giving care to the elderly. In most of the United States, spouses, siblings, children, spouses of children, and parents have no legal standing in making medical decisions for an adult. Persons with power of attorney or court-appointed conservators may have authority over an individual's financial affairs, but they do not necessarily have control over that individual's personal medical decisions. Even court-appointed custodians or guardians may or may not have the power to make medical decisions, depending on the local laws and on the specific charge of their appointment. The prehospital care provider should only consider such powers to exist when a guardianship of person or a durable power of attorney for health care is specified and clear documentation of such third-party powers is present.

In the midst of a trauma scene, the prehospital care provider may have difficulty making such a fine legal distinction. Because the ambulance was summoned and a "call for help" was made, a prehospital care provider must react on the basis of implied consent in cases of patients who are unconscious or have reduced mental capacity.

Should further clarification be necessary or should anyone attempt prehospital care, the problem should be presented to the police officer in charge at the scene. The law generally provides a protocol for an officer to make a timely decision at the scene, ensuing clarification to occur later at the hospital when time allows. Such events should be documented carefully and completely as a part of the run report.

Abuse and Neglect of the Elderly

Abuse is defined as any action by an elderly person's family member (any relative); associated persons who have daily household contact (housekeeper, roommate); anyone upon whom the elderly are reliant for daily needs of food, clothing, and shelter; or a professional caregiver, who takes advantage of the elderly's person, property, or emotional state.

Reports and complaints of abuse, neglect, and other related problems among the elderly are increasing. The exact extent of elder abuse is not known for several reasons:

- Elder abuse has been largely hidden from society.
- Abuse and neglect in the elderly have varying definitions.
- Elders are uneasy or fearful of reporting the problem to law enforcement agencies or human and social welfare personnel. A typical victim of elder abuse may be a parent who feels ashamed or guilty because he or she raised the abuser. The abused may also feel traumatized by the situation or fear continued reprisal by the abuser.
- Some jurisdictions lack formal reporting mechanisms. Some areas do not even have a statutory provision requiring the reporting of elder abuse.

The physical and emotional signs of abuse, such as rape, beating, or nutritional deprivation, are often overlooked or perhaps are not accurately identified. Older women in particular are not likely to report incidents of sexual assault to law enforcement agencies. Sensory deficits, senility, and other forms of altered mental status (e.g., drug-induced depression) may make it impossible or extremely difficult for the elderly patient to report the maltreatment.

Profile of the Abused

The elderly adult most likely to be abused falls into the following profile:

- Over 65 years of age, especially women over 75 years of age
- Frail
- Multiple chronic medical conditions
- Demented
- Impaired sleep cycle, sleepwalking, or loud shouting during the nighttime
- Incontinent of feces, urine, or both
- Dependent on others for activities of daily living or incapable of independent living

Profile of the Abuser

Because many elderly people live in a family environment and are typically women older than 75 years of age, that environment may provide clues. The abuser is frequently the spouse of the patient or the middle-age daughter-in-law of the patient who is caring for dependent children and dependent parents while perhaps holding full- or part-time employment. Most of these abusers are untrained in the particular care required by the elderly and have little relief time from the constant care demands of their family.

Abuse is not restricted to the home. Other environments like nursing, convalescent, and continuing care centers are sites where the elderly may sustain physical, chemical, or pharmacologic harm. Care providers in these environments may consider the elderly to represent management problems or categorize them as obstinate or undesirable patients. The usual profile of the abuser includes the following signs:

- Existence of household conflict
- Marked fatigue
- Unemployment
- Financial difficulties
- Substance abuse
- Previous history of being abused

Categories of Abuse

Abuse can be categorized in three ways:

1. *Physical abuse.* Physical abuse includes assault, neglect, malnutrition, poor maintenance of the living environment, and poor personal care. The signs of physical abuse or neglect may be obvious, such as the imprint left by an item like a fireplace poker, or subtle, such as malnutrition. The signs of elder abuse are similar to those of child abuse (Figure 13-7).
2. *Psychologic abuse.* Psychologic abuse can take on the forms of neglect, verbal abuse, infantilization, or deprivation of sensory stimulation.

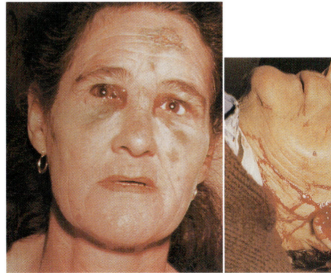

Figure 13-7 Signs of physical abuse of the elderly. **A,** Bruising caused by a punch. This woman agreed to go the hospital only because she was advised to by the police. When about to leave, she mentioned discomfort in her neck. X-ray examination showed a fracture of the body of C6. **B.** Wound of the scalp. The scalp is a common site of elderly abuse that often causes hemorrhagic shock. (*From London PS: A colour atlas of diagnosis after recent injury, London, 1990, Wolfe.*)

3. *Financial abuse.* Financial abuse can include theft of valuables or embezzlement.

Important Points

Many abused patients are terrorized into making false statements for fear of retribution. In the case of elder abuse by family members, fear of removal from the home environment can cause the elderly patient to lie about the origin of the abuse. In other cases of elder abuse, sensory deprivation or dementia may deter adequate explanation. The prehospital care provider should identify abuse and uncover any pathology reported by the patient.

Further trauma may be reduced to a patient by identifying an abusive situation. Reporting a high index of suspicion for abuse can allow for referral and protective services from human, social, and public safety agencies.

Summary

Elderly persons are living healthier, more active, and longer lives than ever before. As a result, trauma has become a significant cause of morbidity and mortality among older adults. Anatomic and physiologic changes associated with aging, chronic disease, and medications can make certain types of trauma more likely, complicate traumatic injuries, and cause a decreased ability to compensate for shock. Many factors in elderly trauma patients can mask early signs of deterioration, increasing the possibility of sudden rapid decompensation without apparent warning. Even simple isolated trauma can progress to an acute systemic condition and produce potentially life-threatening conditions in the elderly. Proactive, timely care is particularly important in the treatment of the elderly trauma patient.

With an elderly trauma patient, more serious injury may have occurred than is indicated by the initial presentation. The injuries and conditions found will have a more profound effect than in a younger patient. By including these considerations, the prehospital care provider will be forewarned, manage the patient in a more anticipatory manner, and provide better, safer care to the older trauma patient.

Scenario Solution

When dealing with trauma in the elderly, you cannot always determine immediately whether the trauma was the primary event or whether it was secondary to a medical event, such as a stroke, myocardial infarction, or syncopal episode. However, you should always consider the possibility that a significant medical event preceded the trauma. The fact that this patient is on anticoagulant therapy and has evidence of impaired blood clotting should alert you that any bleeding from traumatic brain injury or internal injury will be increased as a result. Trauma in the elderly may be exacerbated by the effects of aging, disease, and medications. These factors may also distort the normal findings associated with shock. By the same token, preexisting illness and physiologic changes caused by aging may be aggravated by otherwise less serious trauma, creating a more serious situation in the older trauma patient than the same injury in a younger patient. You should approach the elderly trauma patient with an index of suspicion for injuries whose signs and symptoms may be masked by the effects of aging, disease, or medications and for the possibility of injuries sustained with less significant mechanisms than in younger patients. Of particular concern is modification of cervical spine immobilization because of increased curvature of the spine. Airway management may be more challenging because of changes in facial structure that make achieving a seal with a mask difficult. In addition, for a variety of reasons, the elderly are more prone to aspiration.

Review Questions

Answers are provided on p. 414.

1. Which of the following is an anatomic or physiologic consequence of aging?
   a. Decreased risk of aspiration
   b. Poor retention of newly learned material
   c. Increased risk of wound infection
   d. Increased perception of pain

2. Which of the following BEST describes the most clinically significant effect of osteoporosis and calcification of the spine of the elderly trauma patient in the prehospital setting?
   a. Spinal cord injury may occur with relatively minor trauma to the spine
   b. Reabsorption of bone leads to hypercalcemia
   c. Abnormal lumbar curvature leads to decreased intrathoracic volume
   d. Scoliosis leads to compression of the heart and lungs

3. Which of the following leads to difficulty in investigation of possible abuse or neglect in the elderly?
   a. Attributing signs and symptoms to another cause
   b. Patient's fear of retribution by the abuser
   c. Patient's altered mental status
   d. All of the above

4. The current epidemiologic and demographic trends indicate which of the following?
   a. An increasing proportion of individuals over 65 years of age in the population
   b. A rising incidence of trauma in the elderly
   c. An increased quality of life among the elderly population
   d. All of the above

5. Which of the following is the most important variable contributing to falls in the elderly?
   a. Cataracts
   b. Diseases of the central nervous system
   c. Physical hazards in the environment
   d. Diseases of the cardiovascular system

6. Which of the following factors is NOT associated with an increased risk of abuse or neglect of an elderly patient?
   a. Patient has a sleep disorder
   b. Patient can perform activities of daily living
   c. Caregiver is fatigued
   d. Patient is incontinent

REFERENCES

American College of Surgeons Committee on Trauma: *Advanced trauma life support*, Chicago, 2002, American College of Surgeons.

American Geriatrics Society Foundation for Health in Aging: *2000-2010 decade of health in aging: the challenge: the aging of the U.S. population*, April 20, 2000. Available at www.heathlinaging.org/the challenge.html.

Koyanagi I, Iwasaki Y, Hilda K et al: Acute cervical cord injury without fracture or dislocation of the spinal column, *J Neurosurg* 93(1 suppl):15, 2000.

Milzman DP, Boulanger BR, Rodriquiez A et al: Preexisting disease in trauma patients: a predictor of fate independent of age and injury severity score, *J Trauma* 32:236, 1992.

SUGGESTED READING

DeLisa JA, Gans BM, editors: *Rehabilitation medicine: principles and practices*, ed 2, Philadelphia, 1993, J.B. Lippincott.

Ruskin AP: *Current therapy in psychiatry*, Philadelphia, 1984, W.B. Saunders.

Schwab CW, Shapiro MB, Kauder DR: Geriatric trauma: patterns, care and outcomes. In Mattox KL, Feliciano DV, Moore EE: *Trauma*, ed 4, New York, 1999, McGraw-Hill.

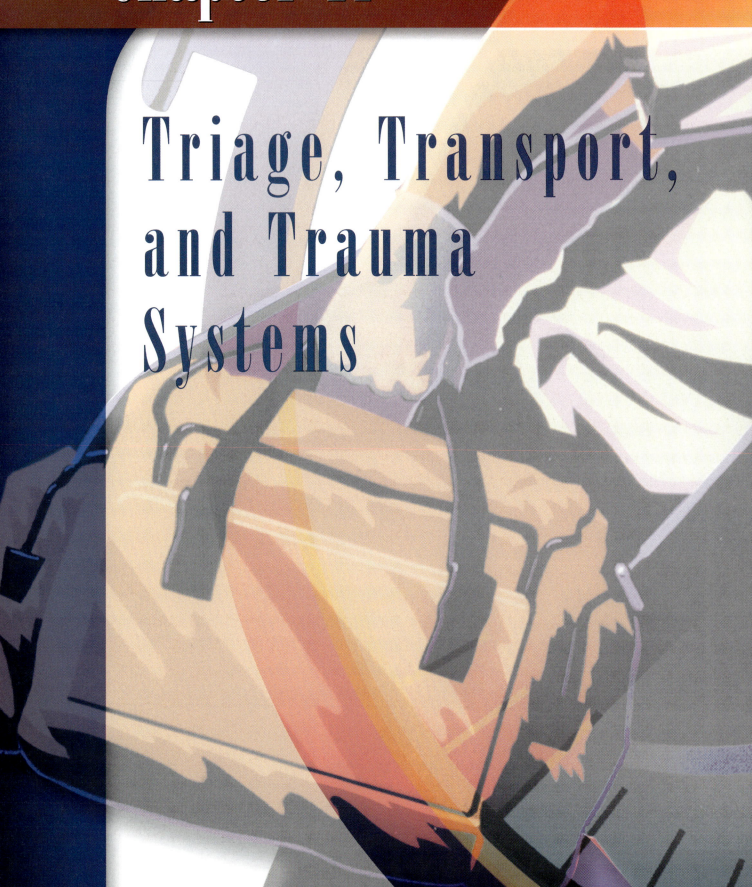

Chapter 14

Triage, Transport, and Trauma Systems

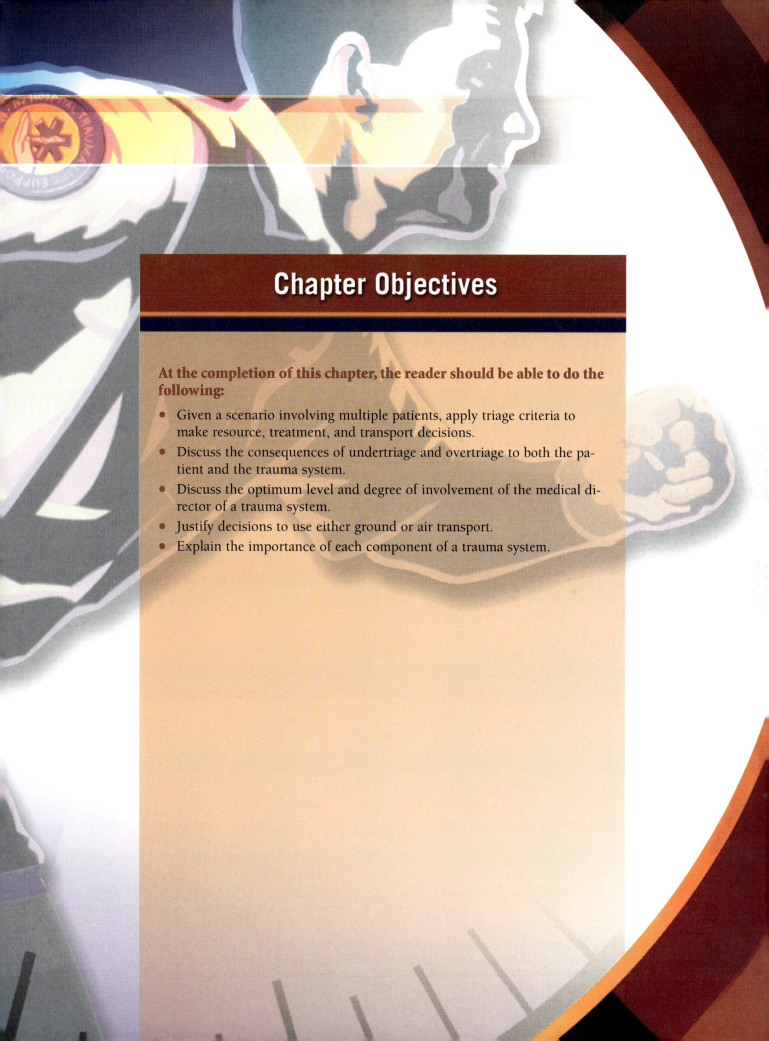

Chapter Objectives

At the completion of this chapter, the reader should be able to do the following:

- Given a scenario involving multiple patients, apply triage criteria to make resource, treatment, and transport decisions.
- Discuss the consequences of undertriage and overtriage to both the patient and the trauma system.
- Discuss the optimum level and degree of involvement of the medical director of a trauma system.
- Justify decisions to use either ground or air transport.
- Explain the importance of each component of a trauma system.

Scenario

Your EMS dispatcher receives a 911 call reporting a multiple motor vehicle crash with seven victims in a rural part of your county. As you travel en route to the scene, you review the assets available to you. Your county system includes a volunteer rescue squad and five ground ambulances. The regional trauma system contains a Level I trauma center that is about 20 minutes away from the scene by ground and two nondesignated hospitals, one of which is 5 minutes from the scene. The Level I trauma center also operates an EMS helicopter.

Upon arrival at the scene, you find that your ambulance is the first to arrive. Two of the victims are out of their vehicles and ambulatory, although they have evidence of injury. One is obviously dead, while the other four are trapped in their vehicles with evidence of significant problems. As you are assessing the scene, the rescue squad and a second ambulance crew arrive.

How do you proceed?

Optimal care of the injured patient throughout the course of his or her injury is required to minimize the death and disability that can occur. Although definitive surgical treatment of injuries rarely occurs in the field, the care that does occur in the field can have a significant influence on the outcome of the patient. Prehospital care providers deliver care in the field in less than optimal conditions to manage the patient, prevent further injury, and deliver the patient to an appropriate medical facility to receive definitive care in the most timely fashion possible. To achieve this requires preplanning and an understanding of the regional trauma system. This chapter discusses some of the issues that should be considered in that preplanning process.

Triage

Triage can refer to several different situations in the prehospital setting. The most common meaning of the term *triage* refers to the need to identify patients with the potential for serious injury to ensure that they are transported to an appropriate trauma center. This form of triage can be difficult because some life-threatening injuries are not immediately obvious in the field. The victims may not demonstrate obvious injury and may be ambulatory at the scene or even refusing transport. Another goal of prehospital care is to minimize scene time, which requires rapid assessment of patients to decide who requires transport rather than attempting to discover all of the injuries that have been sustained. To help make this process more rapid and accurate, triage guidelines should be established beforehand. The most com-

mon triage guidelines are those from the American College of Surgeons Committee on Trauma (Figure 14-1). These guidelines use a four-step process to determine which patients should be taken to a trauma center and, depending upon the structure of the regional trauma system, to which trauma center they should be taken:

1. Physiologic criteria are used to identify unstable patients who should be taken rapidly to the highest level of trauma care available.
2. The anatomy of the injury is considered to identify patients who are physiologically stable but have obvious injuries that will require trauma center care. Patients in both of these categories should be transported to trauma centers with notification to the trauma team that the patient is en route.
3. The mechanism of injury is used to identify patients who are physiologically stable with no obvious injuries yet are at high risk of serious injury as a result of the high energy that is involved in the trauma. Depending on the regional trauma system, these patients should be considered for transport to a trauma center, perhaps after discussion with medical control.
4. Patients with comorbid conditions that may increase their risk should be identified. Transport to a trauma center should be considered after discussion with medical control.

Another important but less common form of triage occurs when the prehospital care provider is dealing with mass casualty incidents (MCIs). This triage involves transporting and treating the injured patients in a

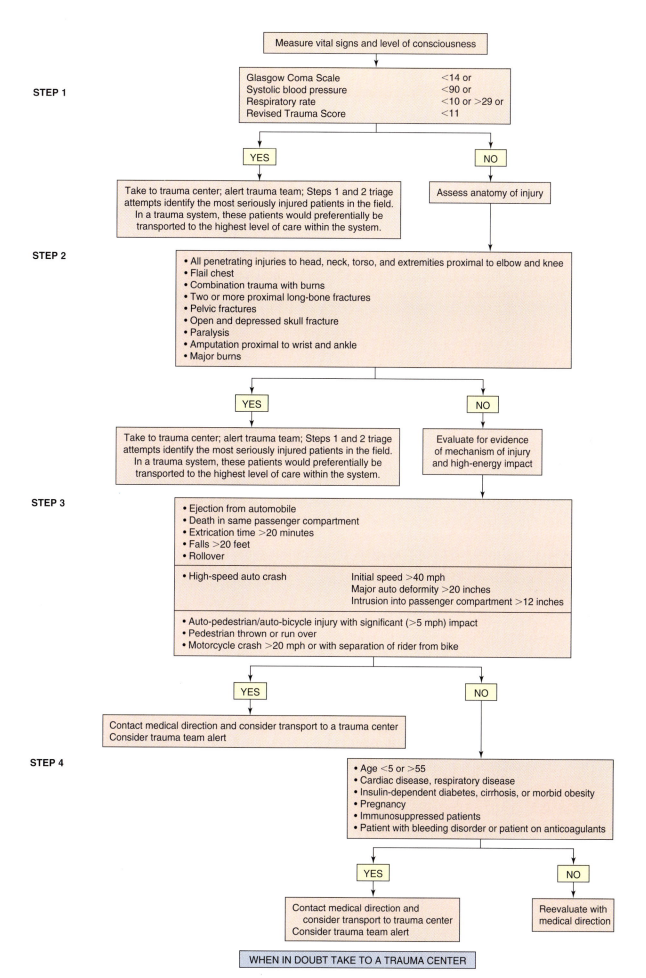

Figure 14-1 Triage decision scheme. (*From American College of Surgeons Committee on Trauma: Resources for optimal care of the injured patient: 1999, Chicago, 1998, American College of Surgeons.*)

way that will result in the best outcome for the most patients. Two situations can arise when dealing with MCIs:

1. Multiple victims will be present, but the number of patients and severity of injuries are such that the resources available in the field and in the regional trauma system can deal with all of them efficiently. In this case, patients should be triaged as described previously—by attempting to identify those with the most immediate life-threatening injuries and ensuring that they receive rapid transport to the highest level of trauma care available.
2. The number and severity of injuries are such that the resources of the trauma care system are overwhelmed. In this case, resources must be deployed in such a way that those patients with the greatest chance of survival are treated in a timely fashion. This situation will generally require the activation of region-wide disaster plans that have been previously designed and practiced and will often require several levels of medical control, including in the field.

Undertriage and Overtriage

The prehospital care provider must consider triage decisions and the state of the regional trauma care system before applying these decisions in the field in order to minimize undertriage and overtriage. *Undertriage* occurs when seriously injured patients are not recognized as such and are mistakenly taken to nontrauma centers. This results in increased morbidity and mortality rates in these patients. Although some undertriage will occur in almost any system, most trauma systems (and the triage scheme outlined previously) have been designed to minimize undertriage, thus minimizing avoidable death and disability. However, this design tends to increase *overtriage*, which occurs when minimally or noninjured patients are taken to trauma centers. Although this generally does not result in significant problems for the patients, it can lead to a strain on the trauma center that has to deal with more patients with its limited resources. This can lead to internal problems triaging multiple patients and increased costs to the center. The goal of a regional trauma system should be to accept an overtriage rate that will not overtax the trauma centers but will result in an acceptably low level of undertriage to minimize unnecessary morbidity and mortality rates in injured patients. The performance improvement programs of the agencies involved should monitor the undertriage rate carefully and reexamine it as conditions in the system change.

Medical Direction

Appropriate triage, as discussed previously, depends on an understanding of the trauma system in which the prehospital care provider is operating and of risk factors and appropriate treatment of various traumatic injury patterns. These issues should be discussed with the medical director before the traumatic event occurs. Prehospital care providers must make assessments and deliver care under the control of a physician. Therefore these discussions should result in written protocols that can direct most prehospital care. Occasionally, a situation will arise that falls outside the norm of events that are covered by the protocols. A trauma system must allow rapid and reliable access to direct online medical direction through either phone or radio discussions with a physician. This system of combined offline and online medical control will allow the most efficient management of most trauma situations using preestablished protocols, while allowing for flexibility and support in unusual situations.

Transport

Survival of severely injured patients depends on rapid transport of the patient to a center that offers immediate definitive surgical treatment of those injuries, not transport by whatever means is available to the nearest hospital. The patient should be transported by the most rapid, safe means, after initial management, to the nearest center that can provide definitive care. Depending on the regional trauma system, this can be carried out in several ways.

Before transport, the patient must access the system to activate the emergency medical service (EMS). In most parts of North America, this can occur via the 911 call system, which provides immediate access to an EMS dispatcher. Globally, a similar activation is available with several different call systems.

Once the prehospital care providers arrive and after they have assessed the scene, immobilization and extrication proceeds. The patient may require procedures that may immediately save his or her life, such as endotracheal intubation and chest decompression. Immobilization of the patient to a long backboard and splinting of extremity injuries will help move the patient and minimize further injury. Intravenous access may be initiated en route to the medical facility. Adequate time should be taken at the scene to allow for safe transport of the patient. However, excessive scene time should be avoided because definitive surgical treatment for most injuries cannot be provided in the field and the patient will risk continued bleeding, shock, and other complications. If the injury occurs within minutes of the trauma center, a load-and-go technique in which the patient is immobilized to a long backboard for easy movement with rapid transport to the trauma center will often provide the best outcome. In a rural area with prolonged transport time to the trauma center, initial transport to a local hospital may be useful to provide advanced resuscitation and stabilization of the patient in preparation for the trip to the trauma center. However, evaluation of the patient at the initial hospital must not delay transport to the trauma center.

In most regional transport systems, two organized transport options are available—ground transport and air transport (helicopter). Both provide the capability to transport and monitor patients.

Ground Transport

For most injured patients, ground transport is the best option, providing rapid response to most scenes. They can carry a large amount of equipment, they have monitoring capability, and the weight of the vehicle is never a problem. Ground tranport vehicles are more economical to operate, and most systems will have many ground transport units with several levels of graduated care available. Especially in urban areas, ground transport vehicles can reach the scene and package and transport the patient to the trauma center more rapidly than a helicopter can get off the ground and find a landing site. The highest risk with ground transport is often the risk of collisions with other vehicles that have not noticed the ambulance running with lights and sirens. Safety for the patient, crew, and bystanders requires a careful approach.

Air Transport

Civilian helicopter transport of the injured began after its usefulness was demonstrated in the Korean and Vietnam wars. Its use in civilian transport, although widespread, has been controversial. Helicopters can provide rapid transport over longer distances or more difficult terrain than ground ambulances. In rural areas, helicopters may allow delivery of advanced life support to areas that are unable to provide it. However, helicopters are more expensive than ground transport vehicles, often have limited access to the scene because of weather and/or terrain, and may provide safety issues for the patient, crew, and bystanders. In many situations, helicopters will not provide more rapid transport because they must be activated (usually after ground transport units are on the scene), takeoff, fly to the scene, and land. The patient must then be loaded for the flight back and unloaded once on the ground. For ground transports of less

than 15 minutes, loading into the ambulance and driving to the trauma center will usually be faster than waiting for a helicopter.

Trauma Systems

This chapter has made several references to decision-making based on the regional trauma system in which the prehospital care provider functions. Therefore the prehospital care provider must understand what the term *trauma system* means and how trauma systems may differ. Discussions on management of the injured used to center on prehospital care and hospital (or trauma center) care as important but separate issues. The trauma system recognizes that outcomes for the injured are improved by developing a system that integrates care throughout the process—beginning in the field, extending to hospitalization, and following through the completion of rehabilitation. This system tries to meet the needs of all injured patients in an area while minimizing the overtriage and undertriage rates. It also includes prevention and public education activities to try to minimize injuries. Organization of a system such as this requires public support and has financial and political implications that cause systems to be developed differently based on the circumstances. A regional trauma system in a major metropolitan area will differ significantly from one in a rural area that covers several states.

A regional trauma system is organized based on the needs of the region and the resources that are available to meet those needs. The American College of Surgeons has established criteria that are frequently used in determining trauma center designation. These criteria may be adapted based on a region's resources:

1. A Level I trauma center should be a regional resource center and is usually based in large population areas.
2. A Level II trauma center provides comprehensive trauma care, either in a population-dense region where it can supplement the Level I trauma center or in less populous areas where it may be the highest level of care available. Both of these centers provide immediate surgical availability and differ mainly in educational and research activities.
3. A Level III trauma center usually has general surgical coverage and the ability to manage many injured patients but should be closely linked to a higher level center for the most severely injured patients.
4. A Level IV trauma center is usually in a rural area with the ability to provide initial stabilization.

The concept of the trauma system has evolved over time. Initially systems were considered only in terms of the trauma centers and the care that they could deliver to the injured patients (exclusive trauma systems). However, evaluation of the current regional trauma system includes not only the trauma centers available in that system but other components as well (Figure 14-2).

Several prehospital companies may operate in a trauma system with varying levels of training and support, especially a system that covers a large area. Dispatch may be handled from several different points, resulting in problems with communication and coordination. Guidelines for the use of aeromedical transport should be in place, and the prehospital care provider should consider them carefully. The ability of nontrauma hospitals to provide initial stabilization and provide care for less severely injured patients should also be considered. Knowledge of all of these regional components before arriving at the scene will allow for improved management of injured patients throughout the system. Discussion of issues that arise between various agencies will help provide better care in the future. Each component of the regional trauma system should have a quality improvement process that examines ways to improve care delivery. The system should also allow all of the components of the regional trauma system to discuss these quality improvement issues together.

Increased integration of all of the components involved in the care of the injured patient will lead to improved outcomes as trauma systems continue to evolve. One area of weakness in most systems continues to be communication between various agencies and documentation of what has been done for the patient and how they

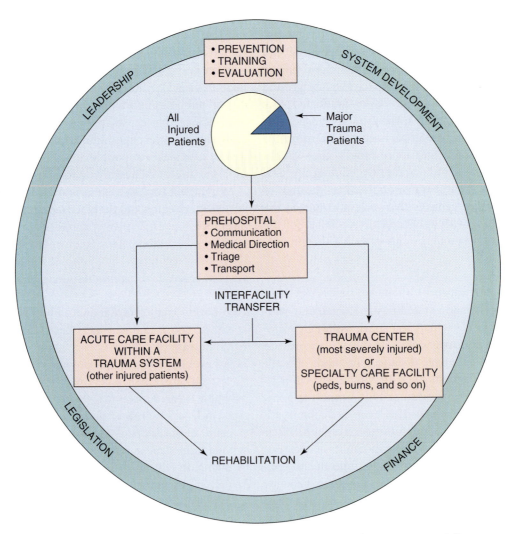

Figure 14-2 Components of an inclusive trauma care system. (*From American College of Surgeons Committee on Trauma: Resources for optimal care of the injured patient: 1999, Chicago, 1998, American College of Surgeons.*)

responded. This means that as patients move through the system, efforts are often duplicated and time is wasted. Continued development of integrated regional systems, combined with the use of new technologies such as telemedicine, should allow more seamless movement of the patient through the system with less duplication and waste of time. This integration, combined with continuous quality improvement, will help prehospital care providers ensure that the right patient gets to the right place at the right time.

Summary

Optimal outcomes for trauma patients depend on organized regional trauma systems. A regional trauma system is preplanned based on the resources of the community. The American College of Surgeons Committee on Trauma (ACS-COT) has led the way in the development of regional trauma systems. Their contribution includes creating criteria for designation of trauma centers and triage guidelines.

The prehospital care provider must have a thorough understanding of the underlying principles and purposes of a trauma system and must be well versed in the specifics of his or her own regional trauma system. All components of the trauma system must operate well to ensure efficient, effective, seamless delivery of emergency medical care. In particular, the prehospital care provider must be familiar with the triage guidelines of his or her system, the resources available in the community, and the trauma designation and capabilities of hospitals in the area. A sound process of decision-making should be based on established criteria to optimally use system resources without unduly stressing the system or jeopardizing patient outcomes.

To maximize the effectiveness of trauma systems, all parties must participate in continuous quality improvement processes to increase system efficiency, remove barriers to system operation, and enhance integration of trauma system components.

Scenario Solution

With seven patients in this incident, the numbers temporarily overwhelm your resources. Therefore you should rapidly assess the patients as you have done to have a better idea of how to direct resources as they arrive. You should leave the fatally injured patient in place and calm down the "walking wounded" temporarily, if their vital signs are acceptable, while resources are concentrated on the more severely injured trapped patients. If enough help arrives, you should consider transporting these "walking wounded" to the nearby hospital so they can be evaluated there, perhaps with a rapid return of the ambulance to the scene. Lifesaving interventions can be done as the remaining patients are extricated. Because extrication is involved and the trauma center is a 20-minute drive away, you should consider mobilizing the helicopter, assuming that a safe landing site is nearby and someone is available to help ensure their safe landing. However, if the extrication is not prolonged or the landing site is not nearby and requires transport of the patient to the helicopter, you should probably transport the patients directly to the trauma center by ground with advanced warning to allow mobilization of the trauma team.

Review Questions

Answers are provided on p. 414.

1. *Triage* refers to which of the following?
   a. The process by which the American College of Surgeons ensures that injured patients bypass local hospitals
   b. The practice of sending all injured patients to trauma centers
   c. The means to prevent overload of trauma resources
   d. The process of ensuring that potentially seriously injured patients receive the appropriate level of care

2. *Triage* problems include which of the following?
   a. Seriously injured patients are not taken to a trauma center
   b. All injured patients are taken to a single trauma center
   c. Undertriage can lead to unnecessary death and disability
   d. All of the above

3. Medical directors of EMS systems:
   a. Have no role in prehospital care
   b. Are responsible for all care delivered
   c. Interfere with rapid care of injured patients
   d. Must be in direct radio communication at all times

4. When transporting injured patients, which of the following is true?
   a. Helicopter transport is always faster and better than ground transport
   b. Load-and-go techniques do not require immobilization
   c. The prehospital care provider should use the most rapid method that is safest for everyone involved
   d. The prehospital care provider should always take the patients directly to trauma centers

5. Regional trauma systems have which of the following characteristics?
   a. Are all designed in the same way
   b. Have no role for consideration of nontrauma centers
   c. Are not important in rural areas
   d. Are affected by local politics and financial considerations

REFERENCES

American College of Surgeons Committee on Trauma: *Resources for optimal care of the injured patient: 1999*, Chicago, 1998, American College of Surgeons.

Callahan M: Emergency medical services base station function and design: on-line medical control, *Prehosp Emerg Care* July-September, 1989.

Clawson JJ, Forbuss R, Hauert SA, and other members of the Emergency Medical Response Task Force: Use of warning lights and siren in emergency medical vehicle response and patient transport, *Prehosp Emerg Care* April-June, 1994.

National Association of Emergency Medical Service Physicians: Air medical dispatch: guidelines for trauma scene response, *Prehosp Emerg Care* 7(1):75, 1992.

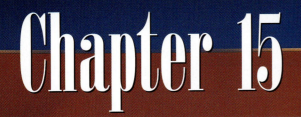

Chapter 15

Golden Principles of Prehospital Trauma Care

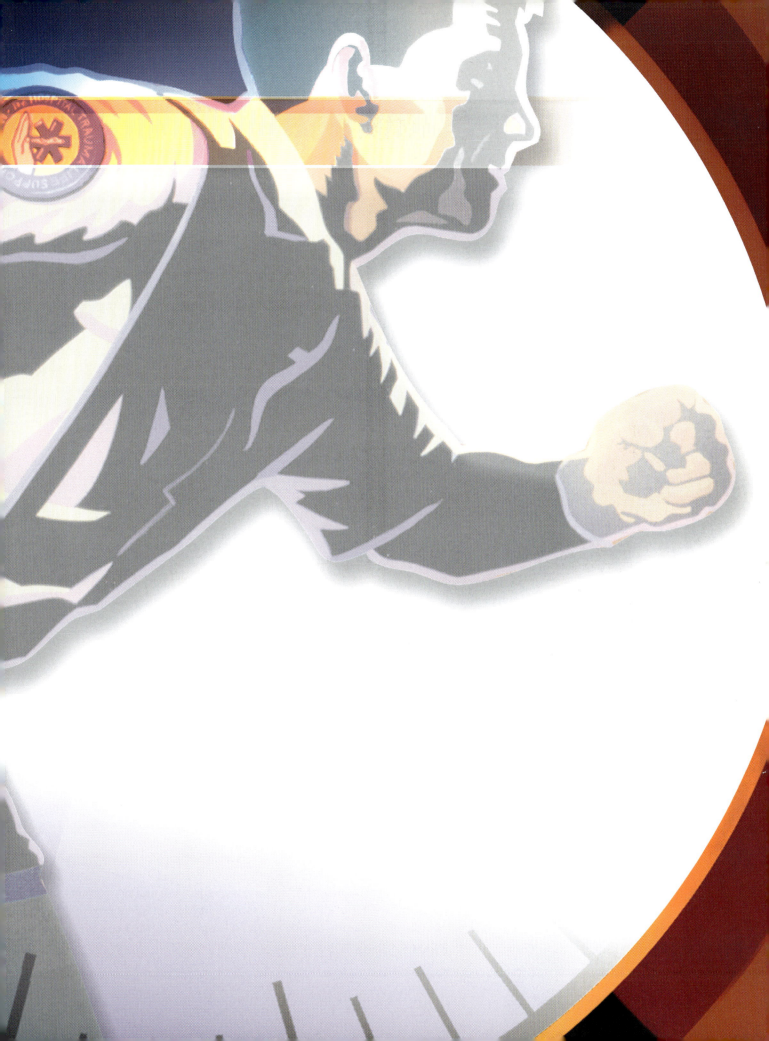

In the late 1960s, R Adams Cowley, M.D., conceptualized the notion of a crucial time period during which it was important to begin definitive patient care for a critically injured trauma patient. In an interview he said, "There is a 'golden hour' between life and death. If you are critically injured, you have less than 60 minutes to survive. You might not die right then: it may be 3 days or 2 week later—but something has happened in your body that is irreparable."

Is there a basis for this concept? The answer is definitely "yes." However, an important realization is that a patient does not always have the luxury of a "Golden Hour." A patient with a penetrating wound of the heart may have only a few minutes to reach definitive care before the shock caused by the injury becomes irreversible. At the other end of the spectrum is a patient with slow, ongoing internal hemorrhage from an isolated femur fracture. Such a patient may have several hours to reach definitive care and resuscitation. Because the "Golden *Hour*" is not a strict 60-minute time frame and varies from patient to patient based on the injuries, the more appropriate term is the "Golden *Period*." If a critically injured patient is able to obtain definitive care, namely hemorrhage control and resuscitation, within his or her Golden Period, then the chance of survival is greatly improved.

No call, scene, or patient is the same. Each requires flexibility of the team to act and react to situations as they develop. The management of prehospital trauma must reflect these contingencies. The goal, however, has not changed: gain access to the patient, identify and treat life-threatening injuries, package and transport to the closest appropriate facility in the least amount of time. The majority of the techniques and principles discussed are not new, and most are taught in an initial education program. This text is different in several ways.

1. It provides current evidence-based practices of management of the trauma patient.
2. It provides a systematic approach for establishing priorities of patient care for trauma patients who have sustained injury to multiple body systems.
3. It provides an organizational scheme for interventions.

The Prehospital Trauma Life Support (PHTLS) program teaches that the prehospital care provider can make correct judgments leading toward a good outcome only if the prehospital care provider is provided with a good base of knowledge. The foundation of the PHTLS program is that patient care should be judgment driven, not protocol driven, hence the medical detail provided in this course. This chapter addresses the key aspects of prehospital trauma care and "brings it all together."

Why Patients Die

As discussed in Chapter 6, the metabolic processes of the human body are driven by energy just like any other machine. Just as machines, the human body generates its own energy but must have fuel to do this. Fuel for the body is oxygen and glucose. The body can store glucose as complex carbohydrates (glycogen) and fat to use at a later time. However, oxygen cannot be stored. It must be constantly supplied to the cells of the body. Atmospheric air, containing oxygen, is drawn into the lungs by the action of the diaphragm and intercostal muscles. Oxygen then diffuses across the alveolar and capillary walls, where it binds to the hemoglobin in the red blood cells and is transported to the body's tissues by the circulatory system. There, in the presence of oxygen, the cells of the tissues "burn" glucose though a complex series of metabolic processes (glycolysis, Krebs cycle, and electron transport) to produce the energy needed for all body functions. This energy is stored as adenosine triphosphate (ATP). Without enough energy (ATP), essential metabolic activities fail to function normally and organs begin to fail. Shock is viewed as a failure of energy production in the body. The sensitivity of the cells to oxygen deprivation varies from organ to organ. The cells within an organ can be fatally damaged yet continue to function for a period of time. This delayed death of cells, leading to organ failure, was what Dr. Cowley referred to in his statement quoted in the opening paragraph. A discussion of the complications of prolonged shock can be found in Chapter 6.

The condition described by Dr. Cowley—*shock*—resulted in death if a patient was not treated promptly. His definition included getting the patient to the operating room for control of internal hemorrhage. The American College of Surgeons Committee on Trauma has used this concept of a Golden Hour to emphasize the importance of getting a patient to a facility where expert trauma care is immediately available.

The Golden Period represents a time period during which shock is worsening, but this condition is almost always *reversible* if proper care is received. Failure to initiate appropriate interventions aimed at improving oxygenation and controlling hemorrhage allows shock to progress, becoming *irreversible*. For trauma patients to have the best chance of survival, interventions should start in the field with prehospital care providers and then continue in the emergency department, the operating

When the heart is deprived of oxygen, the myocardial cells cannot produce enough energy to pump blood to the other tissues. For example, a patient has lost a significant number of red blood cells and blood volume from a gunshot wound to the aorta. The heart continues to beat for several minutes before failing. Refilling the vascular system, after the heart has been without oxygen for several minutes, will not restore the function of the injured cells of the heart. This process is called *irreversible shock*. The specific condition in the heart is known as *pulseless electrical activity* (PEA). Cellular function is still present; however, it is not sufficient to pump blood to the body's cells. The patient has an ECG rhythm but not enough contractile power to force blood out of the heart to the rest of the body.

Another example of this same process but with a less severe outcome is congestive heart failure. Many of the cells of the heart have been damaged by ischemia secondary to coronary artery disease, but some are not. The damage is not complete, so enough functioning cells are left for the pumping process to continue.

Although ischemia, as seen in severe shock, may damage virtually all tissues, the damage to the organs does not become apparent at the same time. In the lungs, acute respiratory distress syndrome (ARDS) often develops within 48 hours after an ischemic insult, whereas acute renal failure and hepatic failure typically occur several days later. Although all body tissues are affected by insufficient oxygen, some tissues are more sensitive to ischemia. For example, a patient who has sustained a traumatic brain injury may develop cerebral edema (swelling) that results in permanent brain damage. Although the brain cells cease to function and die, the rest of the body may survive for years.

room, and the intensive care unit. Trauma is a "team sport." The patient "wins" when all members of the trauma team—from those in the field to those in the trauma center—work together to care for an individual patient.

The Golden Principles of Prehospital Trauma Care

The preceding chapters discuss the assessment and management of patients who have sustained injury to specific body systems. Although this text presents the body systems individually, most severely injured patients have injury to more than one body system, hence the name multisystem trauma patient (also known as polytrauma). A prehospital care provider must effectively recognize and prioritize the treatment of patients with multiple injuries. The following represent the Golden Principles of Prehospital Trauma Care:

1. Ensure the Safety of the Prehospital Care Providers and the Patient.

Prehospital care providers must ensure that scene safety remains their highest priority. This includes not only the safety of the patient, but their own safety as well. Based on information provided by dispatch, potential threats can often be surmised before arrival at the scene. For a motor vehicle crash, threats may include traffic, hazardous materials, fires, and downed power lines; for a shooting victim, one should be aware that the perpetrator may still remain in the area. When violent crime is involved, law enforcement personnel should first enter the scene and secure the area. A prehospital care provider who takes needless risk may also become a victim—in doing so he or she is no longer of help to the original trauma patient. Except in the most unusual circumstances, only those with proper training should attempt rescues.

Another fundamental aspect of safety involves the use of standard precautions. Blood and other body fluids can transmit infections, such as HIV and hepatitis viruses. Protective gear should always be worn, especially when caring for trauma patients where blood is present.

The safety of the patient and possible hazardous situations should also be identified. Even if a patient involved in a motor vehicle crash has no life-threatening conditions identified in the primary survey, rapid extrication is appropriate if threats to patient safety are noted, such as a significant potential for fire or a precarious vehicle position.

2. Assess the Scene Situation to Determine the Need for Additional Resources.

During the response to the scene and immediately upon arrival, a quick size-up is performed to determine the need for additional or specialized resources. Examples include additional EMS units to accommodate the number of patients, fire suppression equipment, special rescue teams, power company personnel, medical helicopters, or physicians to aid in the triage of a large number of patients. The need for these resources should be anticipated and requested as soon as possible.

3. Recognize the Kinematics that Produced the Injuries.

Chapter 2 provides the reader with a foundation of how energy can translate into injury to the trauma patient. As the scene and the patient are approached, the kinematics of the situation can be noted. Understanding the principles of kinematics leads to better patient assessment. Knowledge of specific injury patterns aids in predicting injuries and knowing where to look. Consideration of the kinematics should not delay the initiation of patient assessment and care but can be included in the global scene assessment and questions asked of the patient and bystanders. The kinematics may also play a key role in determining the destination facility for a given trauma patient (see Chapter 14). The key aspects of the kinematics noted at the scene

---

Box 15-1

Critical Trauma Patient—Scene Time of 10 Minutes or Less

Presence of any of the following life-threatening conditions:
- Inadequate or threatened airway
- Impaired ventilation as demonstrated by the following:
  - Abnormally fast or slow ventilatory rate
  - Hypoxia (Spo$_2$ <95% even with supplemental oxygen)
  - Dyspnea
  - Open pneumothorax or flail chest
  - Suspected pneumothorax
- Significant external hemorrhage or suspected internal hemorrhage
- Shock, even if compensated
- Abnormal neurologic status
  - GCS score ≤13
  - Seizure activity
  - Sensory or motor deficit
- Penetrating trauma to the head, neck, or torso, or proximal to the elbow and knee in the extremities
- Amputation or near amputation proximal to the fingers or toes
- Any trauma in the presence of the following:
  - History of serious medical conditions (e.g., coronary artery disease, chronic obstructive pulmonary disease, bleeding disorder)
  - Age >55 years
  - Hypothermia
  - Burns
  - Pregnancy

---

should also be relayed to the physicians at the receiving facility.

4. Use the Primary Survey Approach to Identify Life-Threatening Conditions.

The central concept in the PHTLS program is the emphasis on the primary survey adopted from the Advanced Trauma Life Support Program for Physicians, taught by the American College of Surgeons Committee on Trauma. This brief survey allows vital functions to be rapidly assessed and life-threatening conditions to be identified through systematic evaluation of Airway, Breathing, Circulation, Disability, and Expose/Environment (Box 15-1). On initial approach of the scene and as field care is provided, the prehospital care provider receives input from several senses (sight, hearing, smell, touch) that must be sorted, placed in a priority scheme of life- or limb-threatening injuries, and used to develop a plan for correct management.

The primary survey involves a "treat as you go" philosophy. As life-threatening problems are identified, care is initiated at the earliest possible time. Although taught in a stepwise fashion, many aspects of the primary survey can be performed simultaneously. During transport, the primary survey should be reassessed at reasonable intervals so that the effectiveness of the interventions can be evaluated and new concerns addressed.

In children, pregnant patients, and the elderly, injuries should be considered to be more serious than their outward appearance, have a more profound systemic influence, and have a greater potential for producing rapid decompensation. In pregnant patients, there are at least two patients to care for—the mother and the fetus—both of which may have sustained injury. Compensatory mechanisms differ from younger adults and may not reveal abnormalities until the patient is profoundly compromised.

The primary survey also provides a framework to establish management priorities when faced with numerous patients. For example, at a multiple casualty incident, those patients with serious problems identified with their airway, ventilation, or perfusion are managed and transported before those patients with only altered levels of consciousness.

5. Provide Appropriate Airway Management while Maintaining Cervical Spine Stabilization.

Management of the airway remains the highest priority in the management of critically injured patients. This should be accomplished while maintaining the head and neck in a neutral inline position. The "essential skills" of airway management should be performed with ease: manual clearing of the airway, manual maneuvers to open the airway (trauma jaw thrust and trauma chin lift), suctioning, and the use of oropharyngeal and naso-pharyngeal airways.

For those properly trained, endotracheal intubation is the "gold standard" technique for controlling an airway. Endotracheal intubation should be considered for all trauma patients who are unable to protect their airway, including those who have a Glasgow Coma Scale (GCS) score of 8 or less, require high concentrations of oxygen to maintain an SpO_2 greater than 95%, or require assisted ventilations because of a decreased ventilatory rate or decreased minute volume. Intubation may also be considered for those patients with potential threats to their airway, such as an expanding hematoma in the neck or findings consistent with airway or pulmonary burns. After performing endotracheal intubation, a combination of clinical assessments and adjunct devices should be used, if practical, to confirm that the tube has been properly placed. After moving an intubated patient, tube placement should always be confirmed.

When intubation is indicated but cannot be performed, there are several back-up options (see Airway Management Algorithm, p. 99). Ventilation can be attempted using the essential skills alone, or ventilation can be attempted with a dual lumen airway or a laryngeal mask airway. If adequate ventilation can be achieved, additional attempts at intubation by using either retrograde or digital techniques may be considered. If ventilation cannot be accomplished, percutaneous transtracheal ventilation is an acceptable option.

The decision to attempt intubation involves weighing the potential risks and benefits of intubation along with the distance to the closest appropriate facility. Although performing intubation in the field seems to make sense, there is no conclusive evidence that endotracheal intubation results in lower morbidity or mortality rates in the trauma patient. *In some circumstances, such as the close proximity of an appropriate receiving facility, the most prudent decision may be to focus on the essential skills of airway management and rapidly transport the patient to that facility.*

6. Support Ventilation and Deliver Oxygen to Maintain an SpO_2 Greater than 95%.

Assessment and management of ventilation is another key aspect in the management of the critically injured patient. The normal ventilatory rate in the adult patient is 12 to 20 ventilations per minute. A rate slower than this often significantly interferes with the body's ability to oxygenate the red blood cells passing though the pulmonary capillaries and remove the CO_2 produced by the tissues. These bradypneic patients require assisted or total ventilatory support with a bag-valve-mask (BVM) connected to supplemental oxygen (FiO_2 >0.85). When patients are tachypneic (adult rate >20 breaths/min), their minute ventilation (tidal volume multiplied by their ventilatory rate) should be estimated. When faced with a patient who has a significant decrease in his or her minute volume (rapid, shallow ventilations), ventilations should be assisted with a BVM connected to supplemental oxygen (FiO_2 >0.85). If available, end-tidal CO_2 monitoring ($ETCO_2$) can prove useful to ensure sufficient ventilatory support. A sudden decrease in the $ETCO_2$ may indicate dislodgment of the endotracheal tube or a sudden decrease in perfusion (profound hypotension or cardiopulmonary arrest).

Supplemental oxygen is administered to any trauma patient with obvious or suspected life-threatening conditions. If available, pulse oximetry can be used to titrate the oxygen administration to keep the SpO_2 greater than 95%. If concern exists about the accuracy of a pulse oximetry reading or if this technology is not available, oxygen can be administered via a non-rebreathing mask to the spontaneously breathing patient and a BVM connected to supplemental oxygen (FiO_2 >0.85) for those patients receiving assisted or total ventilatory support.

7. Control Any Significant External Hemorrhage.

In the trauma patient, significant external hemorrhage is a finding that requires immediate attention. Extremity injuries and scalp wounds, such as lacerations and partial avulsions, may be associated with life-threatening blood loss. Most external hemorrhage is readily controlled by the application of direct pressure at the bleeding site, or if resources are limited, by the use of a pressure dressing created with gauze 4 × 4 pads and an elastic bandage. If direct pressure fails to control external hemorrhage from an extremity, other options include elevation (provided that there are no suspected fractures or dislocations) and pressure applied to pressure points. Tourniquets should be applied only as a last resort to control exsanguinating hemorrhage.

When faced with a patient in obvious shock from external hemorrhage, measures aimed at resuscitation (such as the administration of intravenous fluids) should be avoided before adequately controlling the bleeding.

Attempted resuscitation will never be successful in the face of ongoing external hemorrhage.

8. Provide Basic Shock Therapy, Including Restoring and Maintaining Normal Body Temperature and Appropriately Splinting Musculoskeletal Injuries.

At the end of the primary survey, the patient's body is exposed in order to quickly scan for additional life-threatening injuries. Once this is completed, the patient should be re-covered because hypothermia can be fatal to a critically injured trauma patient. The patient in shock is already handicapped by a marked decrease in energy production resulting from widespread inadequate tissue perfusion. If the patient's body temperature is not maintained, severe hypothermia can ensue. Hypothermia drastically impairs the ability of the body's blood clotting system to achieve hemostasis. Blood coagulates (clots) as the result of a complex series of enzymatic reactions that leads to the formation of a fibrin matrix that traps red blood cells and stems bleeding. These enzymes function in a very narrow temperature range. A drop in body temperature below 95° F (35° C) may significantly contribute to the development of a coagulopathy (decreased ability for blood clotting to occur). Therefore it is important to maintain and restore body heat through the use of blankets and a warmed environment inside the ambulance.

When a fracture of a long bone occurs, surrounding muscle and connective tissue is often torn. This tissue damage, along with bleeding from the ends of the broken bones, can result in significant internal hemorrhage. This blood loss can range from about 500 mL with a humerus fracture up to 1 to 2 L with a single femur fracture. Rough handling of a fractured extremity can worsen the tissue damage and aggravate bleeding. For this reason, as well as for pain management, fractured extremities are splinted.

With a critically injured trauma patient, there is no time to splint each individual fracture. Instead, immobilizing the patient to a long backboard will splint virtually all fractures in an anatomic position and diminish internal hemorrhage. The one possible exception to this is a midshaft fracture of the femur. Because of the spasm of the very strong muscles in the thigh, the muscles contract, causing the bone ends to override one another, thereby damaging additional tissue. These types of fractures are best managed by use of a traction splint if time allows its application during transport. For the vast majority of trauma calls where no life-threatening conditions are identified in the primary survey, each suspected extremity injury can be appropriately splinted.

9. Consider the Use of the Pneumatic Antishock Garment for Patients with Decompensated Shock (SBP <90 mm Hg) and Suspected Pelvic, Intraperitoneal, or Retroperitoneal Hemorrhage, and in Patients with Profound Hypotension (SBP <60 mm Hg).

When a trauma patient in *decompensated* shock has suspected pelvic, intraperitoneal, or retroperitoneal hemorrhage, application and inflation of the pneumatic antishock garment (PASG) may decrease and even tamponade serious internal bleeding. Some research data indicate that trauma patients with profound hypotension (systolic blood pressure <60 mm Hg) might also benefit from the use of the PASG. Trauma patients with a significant mechanism of injury may be log-rolled into the PASG. The device is then inflated if hypotension occurs, especially if transport times are prolonged (i.e., >15-20 minutes). The PASG is probably ineffective when used solely as a splint for the lower extremity. It is contraindicated when there is penetrating trauma to the thorax, evisceration of abdominal organs, impaled objects in the abdomen, or pregnancy, and in traumatic cardiopulmonary arrest.

10. Maintain Manual Spinal Stabilization until the Patient Is Immobilized on a Long Backboard.

When contact with a trauma patient is made, manual stabilization of the cervical spine should be provided and maintained until the patient is either (a) immobilized on a long backboard, or (b) deemed not to meet indications for spinal immobilization (see Indications for Spinal Immobilization Algorithm, p. 238). Satisfactory spinal immobilization involves immobilization from the head to the pelvis. Immobilization should not interfere with the patient's ability to open his or her mouth nor impair ventilatory function.

For the victim of penetrating trauma, spinal immobilization is performed if the patient has a neurologic complaint or if a motor or sensory deficit is noted on physical examination. In the setting of blunt trauma, spinal immobilization is indicated if the patient has an altered level of consciousness (GCS score of <15); a neurologic complaint; or spinal tenderness, an anatomic abnormality, or motor or sensory deficit identified on physical examination. If the patient has sustained a concerning mechanism of injury, spinal immobilization is indicated if the patient has evidence of alcohol or drug intoxication, a significant distracting injury, or an inability to communicate because of an age or language barrier.

11. For Critically Injured Trauma Patients, Initiate Transport to the Closest Appropriate Facility within 10 Minutes of Arrival on Scene.

Numerous studies have demonstrated that delays in transporting trauma patients to appropriate receiving facilities lead to increases in mortality rates. Although prehospital care providers have become proficient at endotracheal intubation, ventilatory support, and administration of intravenous fluid therapy, most critically injured trauma patients are in hemorrhagic shock and are in need of two things that cannot be provided in the prehospital setting—blood and control of internal hemorrhage. Because human blood is a perishable product, it is impractical for administration in the field under most circumstances. Crystalloid solution restores intravascular volume but does not replace the oxygen-carrying capacity of the lost red blood cells. Although some blood substitutes have shown promising results in early clinical trials, none is nearing approval for use in the field setting. Similarly, control of internal hemorrhage almost always requires emergent surgical intervention best performed in an operating room. Resuscitation can never be achieved in the face of ongoing internal hemorrhage. Therefore the goal of a prehospital care provider should be to spend as little time on scene as possible.

This concern for limiting scene time should not be construed as a "scoop and run" mentality where no attempts are made to address key problems before initiating transport. Instead, the PHTLS program advocates a philosophy of "limited scene intervention," focusing on a rapid assessment aimed at identifying threats to life and performing interventions that are believed to improve outcome. Examples include airway and ventilatory management, control of external hemorrhage, and spinal immobilization. Precious time should not be wasted on procedures that can be instituted en route to the receiving facility. Patients who are critically injured (see Box 15-1) should be transported within 10 minutes of the arrival of EMS on the scene—the Platinum 10 Minutes of the Golden Period. Reasonable exceptions to the Platinum 10 Minutes include situations that require extensive extrication or time needed to secure an unsafe scene, such as law enforcement ensuring that the perpetrator is no longer present.

The closest hospital may not be the most appropriate receiving facility for many trauma patients. Those patients who meet certain physiologic, anatomic, or mechanism of injury criteria benefit from being taken to a trauma center—a facility that has special expertise and resources for managing trauma (see Chapter 14). Each community, through a consensus of surgeons, emergency physicians, and prehospital care providers, must decide where these types of trauma patients should be transported. These decisions should be incorporated into protocols that designate the best destination facility—the closest appropriate facility. In some situations, it is appropriate to bypass nontrauma centers to reach a trauma center. Even if this produces a moderate increase in the transportation time, the overall time to definitive care will be shorter. Ideally, in the urban setting, a critically injured patient arrives at a trauma center within 25 to 30 minutes of being injured. The hospital also must work equally efficiently to continue resuscitation and if necessary get the patient quickly to the operating room (all within the Golden Period) to control hemorrhage.

12. Initiate Warmed, Intravenous Fluid Replacement En Route to the Receiving Facility.

Initiation of transport of a critically injured trauma patient should never be delayed simply to insert intravenous catheters and administer fluid therapy. Although crystalloid solutions do restore lost blood volume and improve perfusion, they do not transport oxygen. Additionally, restoring normal blood pressure may result in additional hemorrhage from damaged blood vessels that have clotted off. While en route to the receiving facility, two large-bore IV catheters can be inserted and an infusion of warmed (102° F [39° C]) crystalloid solution, preferably lactated Ringer's solution, can be started. Warmed solution is given to aid in the prevention of hypothermia. For adult patients in Class II, III, or IV hemorrhagic shock, an initial bolus of 1 to 2 L of crystalloid solution is given. Intravenous fluid therapy is then titrated to maintain a mean blood pressure of 60 to 65 mm Hg (systolic blood pressure of 80 to 90 mm Hg). Intravenous lines and fluid therapy may be initiated during extrication or while awaiting the arrival of an air medical helicopter. These situations do not result in a delay in transport to initiate volume resuscitation. Basic providers should consider a rendezvous with an advanced life support service (by air or ground units) when faced with lengthy transportation time.

13. Ascertain the Patient's Medical History and Perform a Secondary Survey When Life-Threatening Problems Have Been Satisfactorily Managed or Have Been Ruled Out.

If life-threatening conditions are found in the primary survey, key interventions should be performed and the patient prepared for transport within the Platinum 10 Minutes. Conversely, if life-threatening conditions are not identified, a secondary survey is performed. The secondary survey is a systematic, head-to-toe physical examination that serves to identify all injuries. At this time an AMPLE history (Allergies, Medications, Past medical history, Last meal and Events preceding the injury) is also obtained. For critically injured trauma patients, a secondary survey is performed if time permits and once life-threatening conditions have been appropriately managed. In some situations where the patient is located in close proximity to an appropriate receiving facility, a secondary survey may never be completed. This approach ensures that the prehospital care provider's attention is focused on the most serious problems—those that may result in death if not properly managed—and not on lower-priority injuries. The patient should be reassessed frequently because patients who initially present without non–life-threatening injuries may subsequently develop them.

14. Above All, Do No Further Harm.

The medical principle that states "Above all, do no further harm" dates back to the ancient Greek physician Hippocrates. Applied to the prehospital care of the trauma patient, this principle can take many forms: developing a back-up plan for airway management before initiating rapid sequence intubation, protecting a patient from flying debris during extrication from a damaged vehicle, or controlling significant external hemorrhage before initiating volume resuscitation. Recent experience has shown that prehospital care providers can safely perform many of the life-saving skills that can

be delivered in a trauma center. However, with that said, the issue is not, "What *can* providers do for critically injured trauma patients?" but rather, "What *should* providers do for critically injured trauma patients?"

When caring for a critically injured patient, the provider must ask himself or herself if their actions at the scene and during transport will reasonably benefit the patient. If the answer to this question is either "no" or "uncertain," then those actions should be withheld and emphasis placed on getting the trauma patient to the closest appropriate facility. From arrival on the scene, interventions should be limited to those that prevent or treat physiologic deterioration. Trauma care must follow a given set of priorities that establish an efficient and effective plan of action, based on available time frames and any dangers present at the scene, if the patient is to survive. Appropriate intervention and stabilization should be integrated and coordinated between the field, the emergency department, and the operating room. Every provider at every level of care and at every stage of treatment must be in harmony with the rest of the team.

One study, discussed in the Introduction of this text, demonstrated that critically injured trauma patients arriving at one trauma center had a worse outcome when transported by EMS rather than private vehicle. A significant factor that probably accounts for the increased mortality rate is the actions by well-intentioned prehospital care providers who failed to understand that trauma is a *surgical* disease—most critically injured patients require immediate surgery to save their lives. Anything that delays operative intervention translates into more hemorrhage, more shock, and ultimately death.

Of course, even with the best-planned and executed resuscitation, not all trauma patients can be saved. However, with attention focused on the reasons for early traumatic death, a much larger percentage of patients may survive and there may be a lower residual morbidity rate than without the benefit of correct and expedient field management. *The fundamental principles taught in PHTLS—rapid assessment, key field interventions, and rapid transport to the closest appropriate facility—have been shown to improve outcomes in critically injured trauma patients.*

Summary

The following are the Golden Principles of Prehospital Trauma Care:

1. Ensure the safety of the prehospital care providers and the patient.
2. Assess the scene situation to determine the need for additional resources.
3. Recognize the kinematics that produced the injuries.
4. Use the primary survey approach to identify life-threatening conditions.
5. Provide appropriate airway management while maintaining cervical spine stabilization.
6. Support ventilation and deliver oxygen to maintain an SpO_2 greater than 95%.
7. Control any significant external hemorrhage.
8. Provide basic shock therapy, including restoring and maintaining normal body temperature and appropriately splinting musculoskeletal injuries.
9. Consider the use of the pneumatic antishock garment for patients with decompensated shock (SBP <90 mm Hg) and suspected pelvic, intraperitoneal, or retroperitoneal hemorrhage, and in patients with profound hypotension (SBP <60 mm Hg).
10. Maintain manual spinal stabilization until the patient is immobilized on a long backboard.
11. For critically injured trauma patients, initiate transport to the closest appropriate facility within 10 minutes of arrival on scene.
12. Initiate warmed, intravenous fluid replacement en route to the receiving facility.
13. Ascertain the patient's medical history and perform a secondary survey when life-threatening conditions have been satisfactorily managed or have been ruled out.
14. Above all, do no further harm.

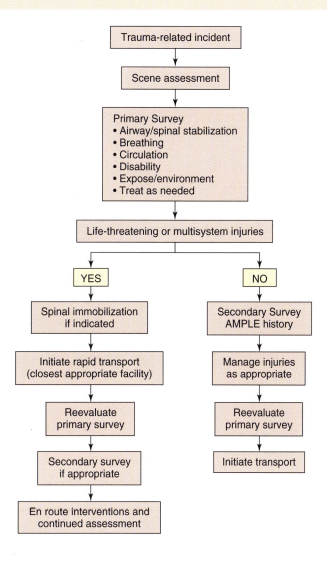

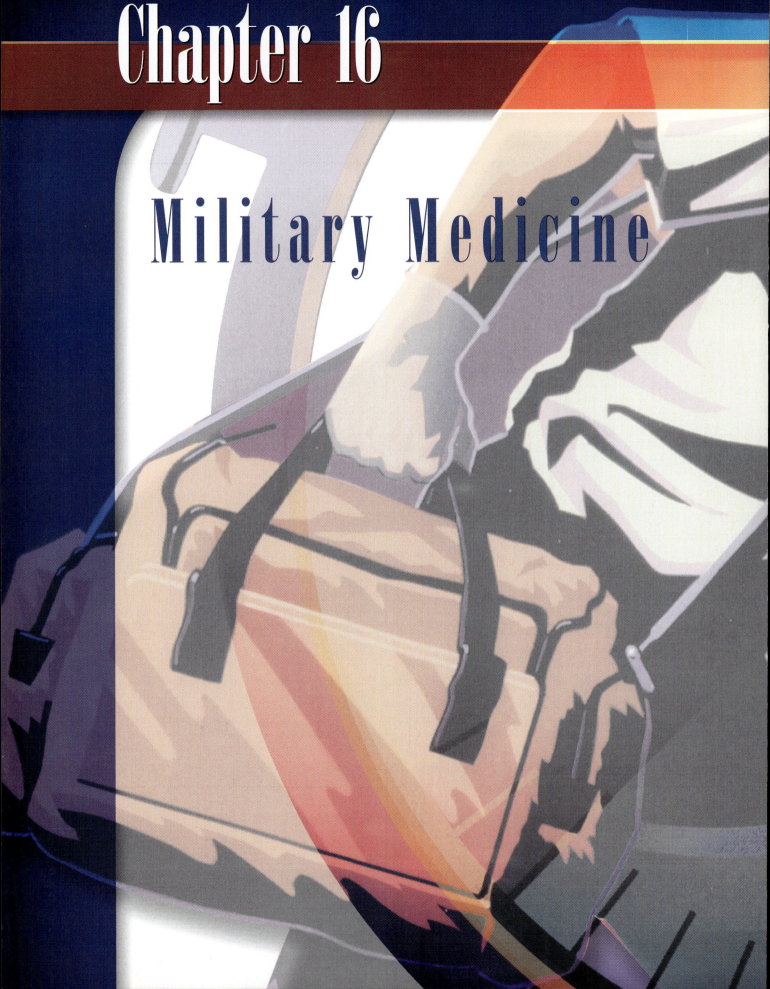

Chapter 16

Military Medicine

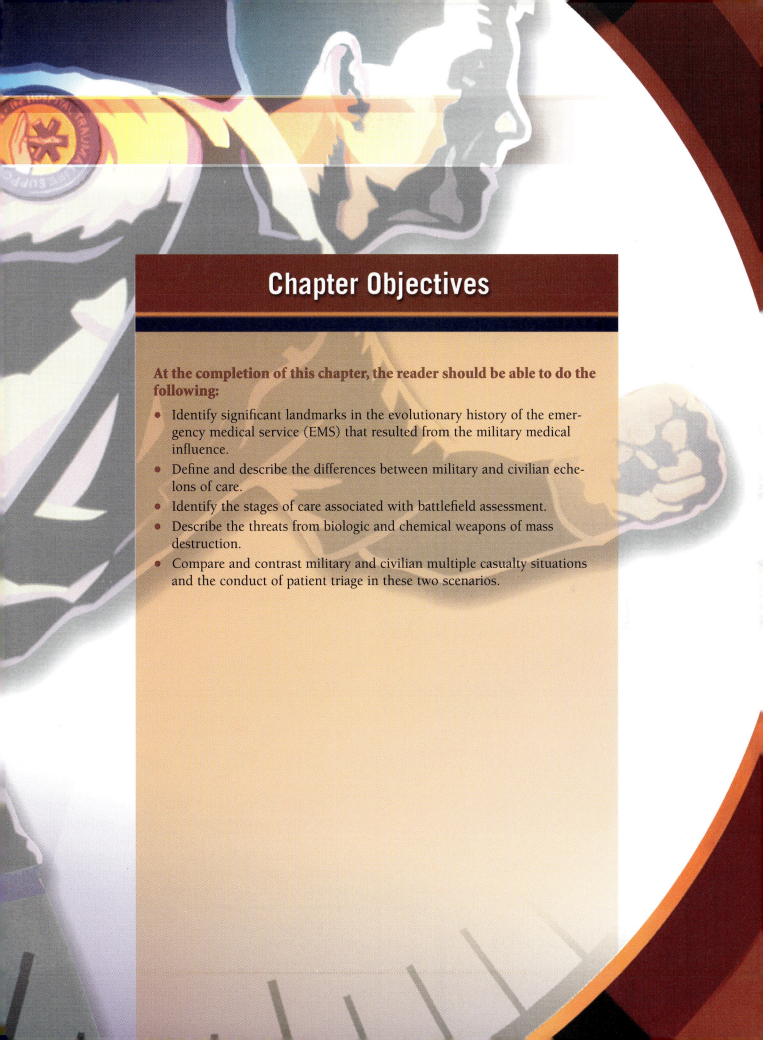

Chapter Objectives

At the completion of this chapter, the reader should be able to do the following:

- Identify significant landmarks in the evolutionary history of the emergency medical service (EMS) that resulted from the military medical influence.
- Define and describe the differences between military and civilian echelons of care.
- Identify the stages of care associated with battlefield assessment.
- Describe the threats from biologic and chemical weapons of mass destruction.
- Compare and contrast military and civilian multiple casualty situations and the conduct of patient triage in these two scenarios.

Scenario

A 24-person Special Operations Forces (SOF) team is ordered to raid a cocaine laboratory in South America. The cocaine laboratory is located in a dense jungle area protected by an estimated hostile strength of 15 men with automatic weapons. The raid will be accomplished by use of a riverine craft approximately 6 kilometers from the target. As the patrol reaches the target area, a booby trap injures the point man (no pulse or ventilations) and the patrol leader (massive trauma to the leg with femoral arterial bleeding). You experience heavy incoming direct and indirect fire as the laboratory security force responds to the explosive blast. The planned extraction of the SOF team is by boat, 1 kilometer from the target area.

As the medic accompanying the SOF team, how would you triage the patients regarding treatment and order of evacuation? What additional information would help you make medical management decisions at this point? Do you recognize any barriers to proper patient management at the scene? How can you work around these barriers? Outline the steps you would take to manage these patients.

Prehospital Trauma Life Support (PHTLS) had its birth on the battlefields of Europe and during the American Civil War. Exigencies of war have driven the evolution of military medical care throughout history with innovations in equipment, principles of care, and training founded on the need to improve combat survivability. Lessons learned in war were applied on the home front as returning medics and corpsmen adapted them to address increasing levels of industrial-based trauma in the civilian sector. The civilian emergency medical services (EMS) system would develop from this, maintaining many of the original concepts such as scene safety (avoid becoming a casualty, avoid incurring additional casualties), primary survey (manage life-threatening injuries, avoid additional injuries), and transport (evacuate the casualty as quickly and safely as possible to definitive care).

Despite similarities, significant differences have historically existed between civilian PHTLS and military requirements on the battlefield (Table 16-1). However, the gap between battlefield trauma management and civilian PHTLS is diminishing as the threat of terrorist attacks grows worldwide. Conventional explosive devices and weapons of mass destruction (chemical, biologic, and nuclear) make the civilian population vulnerable to multiple casualty situations traditionally faced only by those in combat.

Most combat-related deaths occur near the site of injury before the casualty reaches an established medical treatment facility (MTF). Highly trained nonphysicians provide health care on or near the front lines, and patients are transported to various levels of MTFs for further care. These combat medics have a scope of practice beyond that of their civilian counterparts. Basic first aid is the starting point, but modifications and ingenuity are expected and acceptable when applying basic protocols in a hostile situation. The restrictive environment of the battlefield significantly influences patient care decisions. Mission accomplishment may have a higher priority than immediate evacuation, an apparent conflict with generally accepted patient care standards. Immediate evacuation may not even be an option, and long-term

Table 16-1 Differences Between Civilian and Military PHTLS

Civilian	Military
Patients are usually limited in number, and medical resources are not overwhelmed.	A large number of injuries can quickly overwhelm available resources.
Patients are located in secure areas.	Patients are located in nonsecure areas.
Access to supplies and advice is available.	Supplies are limited, and the provider is isolated.
The prehospital phase is generally short.	The prehospital phase is often extended.
Evacuation times to definitive care are generally short.	Evacuations may be delayed.

supportive care may be required. Once more, lessons learned in combat can be extended into civilian practice.

Military and civilian health care agencies are increasingly involved in cooperative efforts to provide relief operations during natural or man-made disasters such as hurricanes, floods, earthquakes, chemical spills, or nuclear power plant incidents. Civil-military interoperability has become critical, and the two communities can learn from and complement each other as they continue to fine tune their skills. Familiarity with this chapter will help civilian providers and their military counterparts.

Military Medics and Emergence of Prehospital Care

Military and civilian prehospital care providers share a common heritage of unparalleled commitment to service at great personal risk and sacrifice. The civilian EMS system can be traced to developments and innovations within the military.

Military Medicine—The Early Years

Armies have not always provided medical care during combat. Wounded soldiers, through most of history, relied on themselves or the compassion of fellow soldiers for care. Those on the losing side often faced death at the hands of their victors. Officers sometimes pooled resources and hired a surgeon to accompany them into war, but the common soldier rarely counted on such a luxury. One notable exception was the Holy Roman Empire, which established a military health care system with hospitals (valetudinaria) at their permanent frontier posts, providing institutionalized care for their deployed soldiers. However, when the Empire fell, the idea of an army being responsible for the health of its soldiers was lost for centuries.

Battlefield care reemerged in the first modern nation-states of Europe as the armies of postrevolutionary France organized a system of prehospital care that included a corps of litter bearers (bracardiers) to remove the wounded from the field and the flying ambulance, or ambulance volante, of Baron Dominique Jean Larrey to transport surgeons forward and patients to the rear. These concepts of clearing the battlefield and rapidly transporting patients to field hospitals were expanded greatly during the American Civil War.

The early phases of the American Civil War clearly illustrated that neither army was adequately prepared for handling battlefield casualties. At the first Battle of Manassas (Bull Run), wounded soldiers were left on the battlefield for as long as 5 days. The American people reacted with horror and disgust, leading to the reform of the U.S. Army's medical department. Charles Tripler, medical director of the Army of the Potomac, suggested that some soldiers be trained in the use of litters, and daily litter drills were instituted in 1861. Jonathan Letterman replaced Tripler and established an ambulance corps under the command of a medical officer. Enlisted personnel drilled on evacuation standards, and the senior noncommissioned officer with each ambulance train was examined on his knowledge of bandaging and dressings. This system was extended to all Union armies, by law, for the duration of the war.

Lessons learned during the American Civil War had a great influence on civilian care, and many postwar developments were direct outgrowths of wartime experiences. Dr. Edward B. Dalton served as a volunteer medical officer in the Army of the Potomac, worked with the ambulance system, and fully understood the value of prehospital care and dedicated transport. When later appointed sanitary superintendent for New York City, he suggested the establishment, in 1869, of a military-like ambulance system based in city hospitals for handling trauma cases. Each ambulance was to carry ". . . a box beneath the driver's seat, containing a quart flask of brandy, two tourniquets, a half dozen bandages, a half dozen small sponges, some splint material, pieces of old blanket for padding, strips of various lengths with buckles, and a 2 ounce vial of persulfate of iron." A young doctor accompanied each ambulance; the idea of a dedicated paraprofessional corps that could provide medical services was not part of the initial U.S. civilian ambulance system. Several European systems, such as those from the British Order of St. John, were staffed with volunteers trained to provide a certain extent of prehospital care.

During the expansion of the American West, military surgeons were faced with a choice of accompanying isolated patrols or providing medical care at the base post for soldiers who stayed behind or who were retrieved from combat. Many surgeons resorted to training enlisted personnel to accompany the patrols and provide initial medical coverage. This extension of medical coverage by paraprofessionals continues today.

The Paraprofessional in Forward Care

When the battleship Maine was destroyed in Havana Harbor in 1898, the United States mobilized for war against Spain. Hospital corpsmen played a vital role and led volunteer surgeons, like Nicholas Senn, to report, "The fate of the wounded rest in the hands of the one who applies the first dressing." The absolute need for prehospital care by trained personnel in the military was universally recognized by World War I. Twentieth-century advances in science and technology enhanced the medics' ability to deliver that care.

Medics and corpsmen leaving the service took their skills into civilian positions. Many went to work for fire and police departments or for mortuaries at a time when undertakers often had the only vehicles in which a patient could be transported. They began to work with ambulance services, providing various levels of first aid care. Organized teaching of first aid began to grow under the auspices of the American Red Cross, the Boy Scouts of America, and other groups, reflecting a growing awareness of the value of prehospital care.

The Modern Prehospital Care Provider

The conflict in Vietnam expanded in the 1960s, and the evening news graphically revealed the vital role played by the combat medic in saving lives. They were at the site of the injury, initiated first aid measures, and participated in rapid patient evacuations back to prestationed trauma hospitals. A transformation occurred in the concept of civilian prehospital care in 1965. A concern arose over mass trauma as part of highway safety and civil defense, and the National Academy of Sciences (NAS) published its *Accidental Death and Disability: The Neglected Disease of Modern Society*. This paper pointed out that over half of U.S. ambulance services were provided by morticians; that most of these, as well as most municipal-based ambulances, were geared toward a "collect and run mentality"; and that no care was provided before or during transport. Supplies were virtually nonexistent, and generally accepted standards for competency or training of ambulance personnel did not exist.

The findings of this paper led to the Highway Safety Act of 1966, requiring states to develop EMS programs. This was the first comprehensive effort in the United States to establish a professional, standardized, prehospital EMS. Military manuals were used to compile training programs for prehospital care providers. The National Registry of EMTs was established in 1970, and certification ensured a recognizable civilian profession.

Many early prehospital care providers were influenced by their military experience, where their scope of practice was much wider than civilian agencies allowed. In 1970 the NAS recommended that ambulance attendants develop advanced medical training programs.

Standard advanced provider training and certification criteria were established in 1977. By 1979, 45 states were participating in paramedic training and all 50 had authorized use of advanced providers in their EMS systems.

Military Medical Evacuation and Today's Lifeflight

The use of helicopters was introduced into civilian EMS programs in 1970 when the NAS recommended an evaluation program using Department of Defense helicopters in conjunction with civilian authorities. Five demonstration areas were established for the Military Assistance to Safety and Traffic (MAST) program. Helicopter evacuation was so successful that, despite costs, 22 additional areas were soon added. The Commission of Emergency Medical Services, the American Medical Association, and the Department of Transportation published air ambulance guidelines in 1981. Civilian EMS had achieved mature independence.

Military Health Services Support Organization

Echelons (Levels) of Care

Field medical assets of the United States military are organized into five increasingly sophisticated echelons of care. Each echelon builds upon the capabilities of the previous level and adds additional services. Echelons extend from the point of wounding, illness, or injury (usually at the lowest level) and provide a continuum of care. Military medical doctrine is evolving from a fixed facility concept to a more fluid system to improve the survivability of wounded soldiers. Advanced capabilities are being moved further forward in the echelons with the idea of balancing maximal care with required mobility.

ECHELON OF CARE I

Echelon I is care at the unit level, accomplished by individual soldiers or a trained medical corpsman. All military personnel are taught basic first aid upon entry into the service. The United States Army augments this capability with its Combat Lifesaver Program, which instructs nonmedical personnel in skills beyond basic first aid. Echelon I also includes mobile aid stations, staffed by medical technicians, one physician and one physician's assistant, that move with the units they support. They function out of small tents or vehicles, such as armored personnel carriers, when in a mechanized unit. Care at this level includes restoration of the airway by surgical procedure, administration of intravenous fluids and antibiotics, and stabilization of wounds and fractures. The goal of medical management at the echelon I level is to return the patient to duty or to stabilize the patient for evacuation to the next appropriate level of care.

ECHELON OF CARE II

Echelon II involves a team of physicians, physician's assistants, nurses, and medical technicians capable of basic resuscitation, stabilization, and surgery along with x-ray examination, pharmacy, and temporary holding facilities. Many echelon II facilities have limited laboratories, and this is the first level of care that has transfusion capabilities (group O liquid packed red blood cells [RBCs]). Surgery procedures are limited to emergency procedures to prevent death or loss of limb or body function.

Like echelon I facilities, echelon II units must be small and mobile. The size is determined by the predicted number and types of casualties during an operation based on previous experience and analysis of the enemy threat. An example of an echelon II unit is the United States Air Force ten-bed facility. It has 51 personnel assigned in support of ten holding beds and one operating room, with enough supplies to perform 50 major surgical cases. Ground or air evacuation is available to transfer the patients to more capable treatment facilities if required.

ECHELON OF CARE III

Echelon III facilities have capabilities normally found in fixed medical treatment facilities and are located in environments with a lower enemy threat. The goal of echelon III is restoration of functional health and includes resuscitation, initial or delayed wound surgery, and postoperative treatment. More extensive services such as laboratory, x-ray examination, and pharmacy are available with a full range of blood products. Care proceeds with greater preparation and deliberation.

ECHELON OF CARE IV

Echelon IV further expands on the capabilities of the echelon III facility by providing definitive therapy within the theater of operations for patients who can be returned to duty within the time set by the theater evacuation policy. The theater evacuation policy (the amount of time a casualty can remain in the theater) depends on enemy threat, the type of mission, the size of the force, air frame availability, and bed occupancy and availability. If the patient cannot be returned to duty within the spec-

ified time, evacuation is required, usually to the continental United States (CONUS). Definitive care in an echelon IV facility is normally provided by a fleet hospital ship, a general hospital, or an overseas MTF.

ECHELON OF CARE V

Convalescent, restorative, and rehabilitative care are provided at echelon V. This care is provided by military hospitals, Department of Veterans Affairs (VA) hospitals, or civilian hospitals located in the United States.

COMPARISON OF MILITARY AND CIVILIAN SYSTEMS OF CARE

The military system of echeloned medical care can be compared with the civilian trauma system spread out across the theater of operations. If the integrated trauma system used in the civilian community is broken down into parts, it closely matches the military system. Echelon I is comparable with care rendered by paramedics and civilian critical care helicopter units. Echelon II facilities are comparable with the resuscitation areas in Level I trauma centers. Echelons III and IV provide the restorative surgery and medical care provided in acute and intermediate trauma center wards. Echelon V units provide the rehabilitative and support services that are offered in the follow-up phase of care in truly integrated trauma systems.

ECHELON COORDINATION

Military echelon system units are small and geographically separated; superb coordination is required to make the system work. Central control of patient movement within and out of the theater is critical and relies on good communications, the visibility of casualty flow through all the medical facilities in the theater (to minimize overload of any one facility), and the availability and control of evacuation assets. Proper triage techniques minimize the stress on any one level by ensuring that workloads are appropriate for the degrees of specialization, level of care, and resources. Stable patients, even with serious wounds, may bypass intermediate echelons and be sent directly to definitive care if the transport time is short.

Prehospital Care in the Tactical Environment

General Considerations

Throughout their careers, military medical personnel may be called upon to treat trauma victims in two types of situations—in combat and in routine life on or off military installations. For noncombat situations, such as motor vehicle crashes, training incidents on the base, falls at home, and civilian acts of violence, the PHTLS guidelines described elsewhere in this manual apply. These guidelines should be followed and the appropriate EMS system activated. This chapter deals specifically with military combat trauma. The recommendations herein apply solely to the tactical prehospital setting.

Ninety percent of combat wound fatalities die on the battlefield before reaching a medical treatment facility.[1] This fact of war emphasizes the need for continued improvement in combat prehospital care. Trauma care training for military corpsmen and medics has been based primarily on the principles taught in the Advanced Trauma Life Support (ATLS) course.[2] ATLS provides a standardized approach to the management of trauma that has proved very successful when used in the setting of a hospital emergency department. The value of at least some aspects of ATLS in the *prehospital* setting, however, has been questioned, even in the civilian sector.[3-23] Military authors have voiced additional concerns about the applicability of ATLS in the combat setting.[24-31] Mitigating factors such as darkness, hostile fire, resource limitations, prolonged evacuation times, unique battlefield casualty transportation issues, command and tactical decisions affecting healthcare, hostile environments, and provider experience levels pose constraints different from the hospital emergency department. These differences are profound and must be carefully reviewed when trauma management strategies are modified for combat application.

For example, Zajtchuk, Jenkins, Bellamy, and their colleagues recommended combat casualty care guidelines for U.S. Army combat medics prior to the Gulf War that differed somewhat from ATLS guidelines.[25] Butler's "Tactical Combat Casualty Care in Special Operations" paper in 1996 provided a comprehensive review of prehospital care in the Special Operations tactical setting along with a set of recommended Tactical Combat Casualty Care (TCCC) guidelines for use by Special Operations corpsmen, medics, and pararescuemen (PJs).[31] These TCCC guidelines were published in the fourth edition of the PHTLS: *Basic and Advanced Prehospital Trauma Life Support*.[32] Additionally, civilian medical organizations like the Wilderness Medical Society have published their own recommendations for the care of trauma patients in environments of interest to their members.[33] The ATLS course and its principles are well accepted as the standard of care once the patient reaches the Emergency Department of an MTF. Difficulties arise,

however, as civilian ATLS principles are extrapolated onto the battlefield setting. This chapter addresses those difficulties in light of the requirement to best achieve all *three* goals of TCCC: (1) treat the casualty, (2) prevent additional casualties, and (3) complete the mission.

Committee on Tactical Combat Casualty Care

Like all medical management strategies, the TCCC guidelines require periodic review and updating. Establishing a standing multiservice Committee on Tactical Combat Casualty Care (COTCCC) was first stated as a requirement by the Commander of the Naval Special Warfare Command.[34] This Committee was founded in 2002 by the U.S. Special Operations Command, and continued support of this effort has been approved by the Navy Bureau of Medicine and Surgery (BUMED). The committee comprises a triservice group of trauma specialists, operational medical officers, and combat medical personnel. It will continue to monitor developments in the field of TCCC and propose changes to the guidelines as appropriate. The updated TCCC guidelines in Boxes 16-1 to 16-3 and the explanatory text in this chapter are the results of the efforts of the COTCCC during workshops held in 2002.

Box 16-1

Basic TCCC Management Plan Care Under Fire

1. Expect casualty to stay engaged as a combatant if appropriate.
2. Return fire as directed or required.
3. Try to keep yourself from being shot.
4. Try to keep the casualty from sustaining additional wounds.
5. Airway management is generally best deferred until the Tactical Field Care phase.
6. Stop any life-threatening external hemorrhage:
   - Use a tourniquet for extremity hemorrhage
   - For nonextremity wounds, apply pressure and/or a HemCon dressing
7. Communicate with the patient if possible.
   - Offer reassurance and encouragement
   - Explain first aid actions

Box 16-2

Basic TCCC Management Plan Tactical Field Care

1. Casualties with an altered mental status should be disarmed immediately.
2. *Airway management*
   a. Unconscious casualty without airway obstruction:
      - Chin-lift or jaw-thrust maneuver
      - Nasopharyngeal airway
      - Place casualty in recovery position
   b. Casualty with airway obstruction or impending airway obstruction
      - Chin-lift or jaw-thrust maneuver
      - Nasopharyngeal airway
      - Place casualty in recovery position
      - Surgical cricothyroidotomy (with lidocaine if conscious) if above measures unsuccessful
3. *Breathing*
   - Consider tension pneumothorax and decompress with needle thoracostomy if casualty has torso trauma and respiratory distress
   - Sucking chest wounds should be treated by applying a Vaseline gauze during expiration, covering it with tape or a field dressing, placing the casualty in the sitting position, and monitoring for development of a tension pneumothorax
4. *Bleeding*
   - Assess for unrecognized hemorrhage and control all sources of bleeding
   - Assess for discontinuation of tourniquets after application of hemostatic dressing (HemCon) or a pressure dressing
5. *IV*
   - Start an 18-gauge IV or saline lock, if indicated
   - If resuscitation is required and IV access is not obtainable, use the intraosseous route
6. *Fluid resuscitation*
   - Assess for hemorrhagic shock; altered mental status in the absence of head injury and weak or absent peripheral pulses are the best field indicators of shock.
     a. If not in shock:
        - No IV fluids necessary
        - PO fluids permissible if conscious

   b. If in shock:
      - Hextend 500 mL IV bolus
      - Repeat once after 30 minutes if still in shock
      - No more than 1000 mL of Hextend
   - Continued efforts to resuscitate must be weighed against logistical and tactical considerations and the risk of incurring further casualties
   - If a casualty with TBI is unconscious and has no peripheral pulse, resuscitate to restore the radial pulse
7. *Inspect and dress known wounds*
8. *Check for additional wounds*
9. *Analgesia as necessary*
   a. Able to fight:
      - Rofecoxib 50 mg PO qd
      - Acetaminophen 1000 mg PO q6h
   b. Unable to fight:
      - Morphine 5 mg IV/IO
      - Reassess in 10 minutes
      - Repeat dose q10min as necessary to control severe pain
      - Monitor for respiratory depression
      - Promethazine 25 mg IV/IO/IM q4h
10. *Splint fractures and recheck pulse*
11. *Antibiotics: recommended for all open combat wounds*
    - Gatifloxacin 400 mg PO qd
    - If unable to take PO (shock, unconscious, or penetrating torso injuries), cefotetan 2 g IV (slow push over 3-5 minutes) or IM q12h
12. *Communicate with the patient if possible*
    - Encourage, reassure
    - Explain care
13. *Cardiopulmonary resuscitation*
    - Resuscitation on the battlefield for victims of blast or penetrating trauma who have no pulse, no ventilations, and no other signs of life will not be successful and should not be attempted.

Box 16-3

Basic TCCC Management Plan Combat Casualty Evacuation (CASEVAC) Care

1. *Airway management*
   a. Unconscious casualty without airway obstruction:
      - Chin-lift or jaw-thrust maneuver
      - Nasopharyngeal airway
      - Place casualty in recovery position
   b. Casualty with airway obstruction or impending airway obstruction:
      - Chin-lift or jaw-thrust maneuver
      - Nasopharyngeal airway
      - Place casualty in recovery position *or*
        Laryngeal mask airway/ILMA *or*
        Combitube *or*
        Endotracheal intubation *or*
        Surgical cricothyroidotomy (with lidocaine if conscious)
   c. Spinal immobilization is not necessary for casualties with penetrating trauma
2. *Breathing*
   - Consider tension pneumothorax and decompress with needle thoracostomy if casualty has torso trauma and respiratory distress
   - Consider chest tube insertion if no improvement and/or long transport anticipated
   - Most combat casualties do not require oxygen, but administration of oxygen may be of benefit for the following types of casualties:
        Low oxygen saturation by pulse oximetry
        Injuries associated with impaired oxygenation
        Unconscious patient
        TBI patients (maintain oxygen saturation >90)
   - Sucking chest wounds should be treated with a Vaseline gauze applied during expiration, covering it with tape or a field dressing, placing the casualty in the sitting position, and monitoring for the development of a tension pneumothorax
3. *Bleeding*
   - Reassess for unrecognized hemorrhage and control all sources of bleeding
   - Assess for discontinuation of tourniquets after application of hemostatic dressing (HemCon) or a pressure dressing
4. *IV*
   - Reassess need for IV access
   - If indicated, start an 18-gauge IV or saline lock

- If resuscitation is required and IV access is not obtainable, use intraosseous route
5. *Fluid resuscitation*
   - Reassess for hemorrhagic shock—altered mental status (in the absence of brain injury) and/or abnormal vital signs
   a. If not in shock:
      - IV fluids not necessary
      - PO fluids permissible if conscious
   b. If in shock:
      - Hextend 500 mL IV bolus
      - Repeat after 30 minutes if still in shock
      - Continue resuscitation with PRBC, Hextend, or LR as indicated
        If a casualty with TBI is unconscious and has no peripheral pulse, resuscitate as necessary to maintain a systolic blood pressure of 90 mm Hg or above
6. *Monitoring*
   Institute electronic monitoring of pulse oximetry and vital signs if indicated
7. *Inspect and dress wound if not already done*
8. *Check for additional wounds*
9. *Analgesia as necessary*
   a. Able to fight:
      - Rofecoxib 50 mg PO qd
      - Acetaminophen 1000 mg PO q6h
   b. Unable to fight:
      - Morphine 5 mg IV/IO
      - Reassess in 10 minutes
      - Repeat dose q10min as necessary to control severe pain
      - Monitor for respiratory depression
      - Promethazine 25 mg IV/IO/IM q4h
10. *Reassess fractures and recheck pulses*
11. *Antibiotics: recommended for all open combat wounds*
    - Gatifloxacin 400 mg PO qd
    - If unable to take PO (shock, unconscious, or penetrating torso injuries), cefotetan 2 g IV (slow push over 3-5 minutes) or IM q12h
12. Pneumatic antishock garment (PASG) may be useful for stabilizing pelvic fractures and controlling pelvic and abdominal bleeding. Their application and extended use must be carefully monitored. They are contraindicated for casualties with thoracic and brain injuries.

Stages of Care in TCCC

Casualty management during combat missions can be divided into three distinct phases.[31] This approach recognizes a particularly important principle—performing the correct intervention at the correct time in the continuum of field care. A medically correct intervention performed at the wrong time in combat may lead to further casualties.

1. *Care Under Fire* refers to care rendered at the scene of the injury while both the medic and the casualty are under effective hostile fire. The risk of additional injuries being sustained at any moment is extremely high for both casualty and rescuer. Available medical equipment is limited to that carried by each operator and the medic.
2. *Tactical Field Care* is the care rendered once the casualty and his unit are no longer under effective hostile fire. It also applies to situations in which an injury has occurred on a mission but hostile fire has not been encountered. Medical equipment is still limited to that carried into the field by mission personnel. Time prior to extraction may range from a few minutes to many hours.
3. *Combat Casualty Evacuation Care* (CASEVAC) is the care rendered while the casualty is being evacuated by an aircraft, ground vehicle, or boat for transportation to a higher echelon of care. Any additional personnel and medical equipment prestaged in these assets will be available during this phase. The term "CASEVAC" should be used to describe this phase since the Air Force reserves "MEDEVAC" to describe a noncombat medical transport.

Basic TCCC Management Plan

An updated basic management plan for each of the three phases of TCCC is presented in Boxes 16-1 to 16-3. This plan is a generic sequence of steps that serves as a starting point from which development of tailored, scenario-based management plans may begin. A detailed rationale for each step outlined in the basic management plan was presented in the fourth edition of this publication.[32] Modifications to the TCCC guidelines by the COTCCC are discussed below. As before, treatment principles in the ATLS course have been followed except where specific tactical considerations require a departure.

Care Under Fire

Very limited medical care should be attempted while the casualty and his unit are under effective hostile fire, as reflected in Box 16-1. Suppression of hostile fire and moving the casualty to a safe position are major considerations at this point. Significant delays for a detailed examination or consummate treatment of all injuries are ill advised while one is under effective enemy fire. Casualties who have sustained injuries that are not life threatening and that do not preclude further participation in the fight should continue to assist the unit in suppressing hostile fire and in any other way possible to achieve mission success. It may also be critical for the combat medic or corpsman to help suppress hostile fire before attempting to provide care. This can be especially true in small unit operations where friendly firepower is limited and every man's weapon may be needed to prevail. If hostile fire is not effectively suppressed, it may be necessary to move the casualty to cover. Casualties whose wounds do not prevent them from moving themselves to cover should do so to avoid exposing the medic or other aid givers to unnecessary hazard. Management of an impaired airway is temporarily deferred until the patient is safe, thereby minimizing the risk to the rescuer and avoiding the difficulty of managing the airway while dragging the casualty. Further discussion of casualty movement is presented in Box 16-4.

The temporary use of a tourniquet to manage life-threatening extremity hemorrhage is recommended. This principle is supported by the wealth of Vietnam conflict combat casualty data indicating that exsanguinations from extremity injuries represented the number one cause of preventable battlefield deaths.[35] Direct pressure and compression dressings are less desirable than tourniquets in this setting because their application at the site of injury may result in delays getting the casualty and the rescuer to cover, and they may provide poorer control of hemorrhage while the casualty is being moved. Mabry et al reported on the lives saved in Mogadishu in 1993 by properly applied tourniquets.[36] In recent experience by the Israeli Defense Force (IDF), the use of tourniquets in combat settings confirmed that they are effective and safe even when their use is prompted by tactical rather than clinical indications. There were very few and minimal complications resulting from their use.[37]

The standard "web belt through the buckle" tourniquet issued by the military for many years has not been well received by the combat medic community. Combat medics have often carried makeshift tourniquets composed of an encircling soft bandage tightened by a makeshift windlass. Some commercially available tourniquets were tested in a study sponsored by the U.S. Special Operations Command and found to be unsatisfactory.[38] Several newly designed tourniquets are now being

Box 16-4

Movement of Casualties

CARE UNDER FIRE

Usually, the best first step in saving a casualty is to control the tactical situation. If possible, casualties should move to cover without assistance so as not to expose a rescuer to unnecessary risk. If a casualty is unable to move and is unresponsive, he is likely beyond help, and risking the lives of rescuers is not warranted. If a casualty is responsive and unable to move, then a rescue plan should be developed.

1. Determine the potential risk to the rescuers, keeping in mind that **rescuers should not move into a zeroed-in position.** Did the casualty trip a booby trap or mine? Where is fire coming from? Is it direct or indirect (rifle, machine gun, grenade, mortar, etc.)? Are there electrical, fire, chemical, water, mechanical, or other environmental hazards?
2. Consider assets. What can rescuers provide in the way of covering fire, screening, shielding, and rescue-applicable equipment?
3. Make sure all understand their role in the rescue and which movement technique is to be used (drag, carry, rope, stretcher, etc.). If possible, let the casualty know what the plan is so that he can assist as much as possible by rolling to a certain position, attaching a drag line to web gear, identifying hazards, etc.

The fastest method for moving a casualty is dragging along the long axis of the body by two rescuers. This drag can be used in buildings, shallow water, snow, and down stairs. It can be accomplished with the rescuers standing or crawling. The use of the casualty's web gear, tactical vest, a drag line, poncho, cloth-ing, or improvised harness makes this method easier. However, holding the casualty under the arms is all that is necessary. A one-rescuer drag can be used for short distances, but it is more difficult for the rescuer, is slower, and is less controlled. The great disadvantage of dragging is that the casualty is in contact with the ground, and this can cause additional injury in rough terrain. The firefighter's carry can be used, but it may expose too much of the rescuer and the casualty to hostile fire. Otherwise, it can be used over rough terrrain with potentially less injury to the casualty from contact with the ground.

TACTICAL FIELD CARE

Once the tactical situation is controlled or the casualty has been moved to cover, further movement should be easier. The casualty can be disarmed and mission-essential gear distributed to other team members. Here again, the firefighter's carry can be used for short distances, but it is very exhausting for both the casualty and the rescuer. If the casualty is conscious, a saddleback carry can be used. It is less stable and more difficult for the rescuer, however. The two-person carry is accomplished by having the casualty sit on a rifle, board, pack frame, or other object, which is then carried by a rescuer on either side. If the casualty can hold on to the rescuers, then each rescuer will have one arm free to fire a weapon or move obstacles. If the casualty cannot hold on, then the rescuers can take turns holding the casualty. The two-person fore-and-aft carry can be used in narrow areas, but it does not allow either rescuer a free hand. For longer distances, a conventional or improvised litter should be used. Either the Sked or Stokes basket make better litters for rough terrain, building interiors, or areas where the litter must be raised or lowered more than 3 meters. These litters can be dragged by two rescuers if necessary, rather than carried by four. The folding litter or a body bag are the next best options, but they have little or no support for the casualty's spine and are difficult to drag by two rescuers. The Army litter

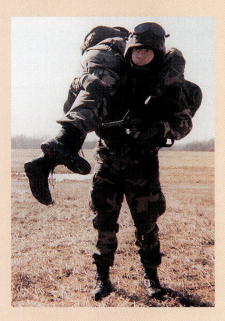

Firefighter's carry.

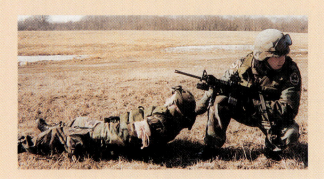

One-person drag.

has no good way to restrain the casualty and is difficult to use over rough terrain. An improvised litter can be made from a poncho, poncho liner, blanket, field jackets, doors, or any other materials that may be available. If the casualty is a victim of blunt trauma and spinal injury is suspected, then rigid support may be better than nonrigid. A cervical collar can be improvised from a SAM splint or other material and applied to the casualty before moving. When moving casualties long distances, tourniquets, dressings, splints, and IV lines should be checked periodically to assure they are intact. Casualties should be protected as much as possible from the elements (sun, rain, wind, cold, snow, blowing sand, insects) during transport and observed for signs of hypothermia, dehydration, and heat illness.

CASEVAC CARE

Conventional litters should be available during this phase. The casualty should be made as comfortable as possible and kept warm and dry. If an improvised litter is used, it should be padded and field expedient material replaced with conventional splints, tourniquets, dressings, etc. as soon as feasible. If decontamination is needed, it should be carried out prior to evacuation, if tactically feasible.

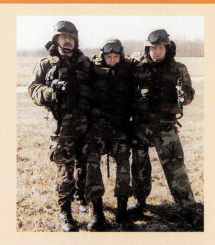

Two-person rifle carry.

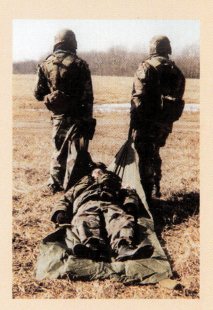

Poncho drag.

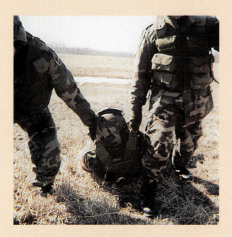

Two-person drag.

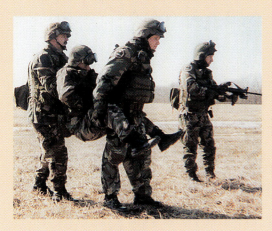

Two-person fore-and-aft carry.

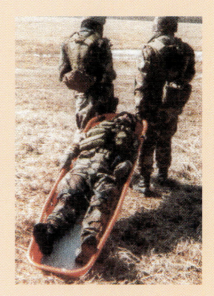

Stokes basket.

field tested by the U.S. Army, including a double-buckle tourniquet, designed for ease of self-application with one hand in the event of a traumatic amputation of a hand or arm, and a ratchet design. Whatever tourniquet is selected must be both effective in controlling arterial bleeding and quickly applied under field conditions.

If the site of the bleeding is accessible without surgical incision, first responders can also achieve hemostasis in some cases of nonextremity hemorrhage using hemostatic agents in conjunction with direct pressure. A number of external agents have been approved by the U.S. Food and Drug Administration (FDA) for this indication and have recently been evaluated in a standardized fashion in tactically relevant animal models. The Rapid Deployment Hemostat® (RDH) bandage is a proprietary formulation of poly-N-acetyl glucosamine that has not proved as efficacious as other options in trials at the U.S. Army Institute of Surgical Research (USAISR).[39] TraumaDex is a starch polymer that has been shown to reduce bleeding in some trauma models, but it has not been proved at this time to equal the other options in severe bleeding models.[40] QuickClot is an FDA-approved powder of proprietary formulation. This agent was introduced by the Marine Corps in mid-2002, the first combat test and evaluation of an active hemostatic agent by the U.S. Armed Forces. QuickClot has been found effective in severe bleeding models,[41] but when not meticulously applied, it can produce an exothermic reaction with temperatures up to 90° C. The heat produced under this circumstance could potentially cause pain and collateral tissue damage.[41] To minimize the risk posed by this exothermic potential, excess blood and fluid must first be removed from the application site. The powder format may prove difficult to apply properly on the battlefield, especially at night.

In November 2002, another active hemostatic agent, the HemCon® dressing, was approved by the FDA for external use. The HemCon dressing is another proprietary formulation of poly-N-acetyl glucosamine that has proved effective in a severe bleeding model in trials at the USAISR.[43] Recombinant factor VIIa is another hemorrhage control agent currently under evaluation in a multicenter trial. It has anecdotally proved efficacious in cessation of bleeding in trauma patients with severe bleeding and acquired coagulopathies.[44] It is currently not recommended for field use, but it may ultimately prove valuable in forward surgical units for some patients.

Further evaluation and development will yield more information on currently approved external hemostatic agents, and intense research in the area of other agents that can control hemorrhage in the field is underway.

New agents are likely to be available soon. Efficacy will be demonstrated in severe hemorrhage models and in the durability, ease of use, cost, tactical relevance, and shelf life of the product. As of this writing, there is currently no direct data to demonstrate that either QuickClot or the HemCon dressing is more effective at achieving hemostasis. However, because of its safety and ease of application, the HemCon dressing represents the best current option for external hemostasis on the battlefield in casualties whose bleeding sites are not amenable to the use of a tourniquet.

A casualty may exsanguinate before any medical help arrives,[45] so the importance of achieving rapid, definitive control of life-threatening hemorrhage on the battlefield cannot be overemphasized. Furthermore, standard field dressings and direct pressure may not work reliably to control exanguinating extremity hemorrhage.[45] Therefore, every combatant should carry both a tourniquet and a hemostatic dressing as part of the personal gear loadout and should be trained in their use.

There is no requirement to immobilize the spine before moving a casualty out of a firefight if he has sustained only penetrating trauma. Arishita, Vayer, and Bellamy examined the value of cervical spine immobilization in penetrating neck injuries in Vietnam. They determined that only 1.4% of patients with penetrating neck injuries might have benefited from cervical immobilization.[24] Hostile fire poses a much more significant threat in this setting, to both casualty and rescuer, than spinal cord injury from failure to immobilize the cervical spine.[24] For casualties with significant blunt trauma in the Care Under Fire phase, the risk of spinal cord injury remains a major consideration.[36] In this circumstance, the risk of cord injury from neck movement must be weighed against the risk of additional hostile fire injuries while immobilizing the cervical spine.

Combat is a frightening experience, and being wounded, especially seriously, can generate tremendous anxiety and fear. Engaging a casualty with reassurance is therapeutically beneficial, and communication is just as important in patient care on the battlefield as it is in the MTF.

Tactical Field Care

Recommended guidelines for this phase of care are shown in Box 16-2.

In the combat setting, there are four primary reasons for an individual to exhibit an altered state of consciousness: traumatic brain injury, pain, shock, and analgesic medications. An armed combatant with an altered state of consciousness poses a serious threat of injury to others in the unit should he employ his weapons inappropriately. Anyone noted to have an altered state of consciousness should be disarmed immediately, including secondary weapons and explosive devices.[46]

Unconscious casualties should have their airways opened with the chin-lift or jaw-thrust maneuvers. If spontaneous ventilations are present and there is no respiratory distress, further airway management is best achieved with a nasopharyngeal airway. It is more easily tolerated than an oropharyngeal airway if the patient suddenly regains consciousness,[2] and it is probably less likely to be dislodged during transport.[31] These casualties should be placed in the semiprone recovery position (Figure 16-1) to prevent aspiration of blood, mucus, or vomitus.

Should an airway obstruction develop or persist despite the use of a nasopharyngeal airway, a more definitive airway will be required. The ability of experienced paramedical personnel to perform endotracheal intubation has been well documented.[6,47-56] Most studies reported use of cadaver training, operating room intubations, supervised initial intubations, or a combination of these methods in teaching the skill. They also stressed the importance of continued practice to maintain proficiency. This technique may be prohibitively difficult in the tactical environment, however, for a number of reasons[31]: (1) there have been no studies examining the ability of well-trained but relatively inexperienced military medics to accomplish endotracheal intubation on the battlefield; (2) many corpsmen and medics have never performed an intubation on a live patient or even a cadaver; (3) standard endotracheal intubation techniques entail the use of a tactically compromising white light in the laryngoscope; (4) endotracheal intubation can be extremely difficult in a casualty with maxillofacial injuries[25]; and (5) esophageal intubations are probably much less recognizable on the battlefield.

Endotracheal intubation may be difficult to accomplish even in the hands of more experienced paramedical personnel under less austere conditions.[57] One study, which examined first-time intubationists trained with mannequin intubations alone, noted an initial success rate of only 42% in the ideal confines of the operating room with paralyzed patients.[54] Another study examined basic EMTs who had been trained in intubation and found that only 53 of 103 patients were successfully intubated.[58] Even in civilian settings with experienced paramedical personnel, another report documented that in 27 of 108 prehospital intubations, the tube was misplaced upon arrival in the Emergency Department.[59] Some reports of successful intubation by military combat

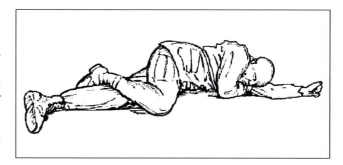

Figure 16-1   Semiprone recovery position.

medical personnel use mannequin intubation by just-trained corpsmen as an outcome measure,[60] which may not be an accurate indicator of success under actual battlefield conditions. The usefulness of this procedure was further questioned in a study in which prehospital endotracheal intubation was not found to improve outcome in patients with severe head injuries.[61]

Significant airway obstruction in the combat setting is likely to be the result of penetrating wounds of the face or neck in which blood or disrupted anatomy precludes good visualization of the vocal cords. Cricothyroidotomy is therefore preferable to intubation in these cases, if the combat corpsman or medic has been trained in this procedure.[25,31] Cricothyroidotomy has been reported safe and effective in trauma victims,[62] but it is not without complications.[63,64] Even so, it is felt to provide the best chance for successful airway management in this setting. Furthermore, it can be performed under local anesthesia with lidocaine in an awake patient.

Thermal or toxic gas injuries are important considerations in certain tactical situations. Airway edema is aggravated by fluid administration, and this may lead to acute upper airway obstruction. Airway burns should be suspected if fire occurs within a confined space, the patient has cervicofacial burns, singeing of the nasal hairs, carbonaceous sputum or complaints of sore throat, hoarseness, or wheezing. Cricothyroidotomy is the airway of choice in the Tactical Field Care Phase for these casualties.

A presumptive diagnosis of tension pneumothorax should be made when significant respiratory distress develops in the setting of torso trauma. The diagnosis of tension pneumothorax on the battlefield should not rely on such typical clinical signs as decreased breath sounds, tracheal deviation, or hyperresonance to percussion because these signs may not always be present.[65] Even if they are present, they may be exceedingly difficult to appreciate on the battlefield. A patient with penetrating chest trauma will generally have some degree of hemo/pneumothorax as a result of the primary wound. The additional trauma caused by a needle thoracostomy would not be expected to significantly worsen his condition should he not actually have a tension pneumothorax.[56]

Paramedics are authorized to perform needle thoracentesis in some civilian emergency medical services.[51,56] Combat corpsmen and medics should also be proficient in this technique. Chest tubes are not recommended in this phase of care for the following reasons: (1) they are not needed to provide initial treatment for a tension pneumothorax, (2) they are more difficult and time-consuming for relatively inexperienced medical personnel, especially in the austere battlefield environment, (3) chest tube insertion is probably more likely to cause additional tissue damage and subsequent infection than needle thoracostomy, and (4) no documentation of benefit from battlefield tube thoracostomy by paramedical personnel was found in the literature.[31] Tube thoracostomy is generally not part of the paramedic's scope of care in civilian EMS settings,[51,56] and no studies were found that address the use of this procedure by corpsmen and medics in combat settings.

Needle thoracentesis with a 14-gauge needle was found to rapidly relieve elevated intrapleural pressure in a swine model of traumatic tension pneumothorax.[66] The therapeutic effect was sustained for 4 hours, and this procedure was found to be equivalent to tube thoracostomy with a 32F chest tube for the observation period.[66] The ease and speed of performance and the decreased likelihood of complications make needle thoracentesis the procedure of choice for relieving tension pneumothorax on the battlefield. Cannula length is an important consideration here,[67] since the pectoral muscles must be penetrated, and in young soldiers, they can be very thick. Even though it may be difficult to appreciate in field settings, if there is no rush of air when the needle is inserted, then either it did not go in far enough or there was no tension pneumothorax there. Medics of the 75th Ranger Regiment currently pack 10-gauge 3-inch needle/catheters for this procedure (personal communication, SFC Rob Miller). Any patient who has undergone needle thoracentesis for relief of tension pneumothorax must be continually reassessed. Catheters used for this purpose are subject to occlusion by clotting and kinking.

An open pneumothorax (sucking chest wound) may result from large defects in the chest wall and may interfere with ventilation. These wounds are treated by applying a vaseline gauze during expiration, covering the gauze with tape or a field dressing, placing the casualty in the sitting position, and monitoring for the possible development of a tension pneumothorax.

Tourniquets applied during the Care Under Fire phase should be replaced with direct pressure and/or HemCon dressings when the tactical situation allows, with care to assure continued hemostasis.

Although ATLS teaches starting two large bore (14- or 16-gauge) intravenous catheters for fluid resuscitation in trauma cases,[2] the 18-gauge catheter is preferred in the field setting because of the ease of cannulation.[31] Crystalloid and colloid solutions can be administered rapidly through an 18-gauge catheter, and blood products requiring the larger cannulae are not given in the field.[68,69] Blood products may be administered in the CASEVAC phase or later at an MTF, but field-placed IV cannulae will normally be replaced there anyway because of the risk of contamination.

Despite its ubiquity, the benefit of prehospital fluid resuscitation in trauma patients has not been established.* The ATLS course proposes initial fluid resuscitation with 2 liters of a crystalloid. Other options are no fluid resuscitation until hemorrhage is definitively controlled or limited (hypotensive) resuscitation to achieve a perfusing systolic blood pressure of about 70 mm Hg. Additionally, there has been controversy over the fluid to be used. Choices have included crystalloid, colloid, synthetic colloid, blood products, and the new hemoglobin solutions. The beneficial effect from crystalloid and colloid fluid resuscitation in hemorrhagic shock has been demonstrated largely in animal models where the volume of hemorrhage is controlled experimentally and resuscitation is initiated after the hemorrhage has been stopped.[21,22] Multiple studies using uncontrolled hemorrhagic shock models have found that aggressive fluid resuscitation before surgical repair of a vascular injury is associated with either no improvement in survival or increased mortality when compared to no resuscitation or hypotensive resuscitation.† This lack of benefit is presumably due to interference with vasoconstriction, as the body attempts to adjust to the loss of blood, and interference with hemostasis at the bleeding site. Two studies were found in which aggressive fluid resuscitation improved the outcome of uncontrolled hemorrhagic shock.[74,75] Both of these studies used rat tail amputation models, which may not correlate well with uncontrolled hemorrhage on the battlefield from intrathoracic and intraabdominal injuries. Some studies have noted that

---

*References 3, 6-8, 10-12, 14, 16, 19, 21, 25, 71.
†References 9, 10, 15, 17-21, 72, 73.

fluid resuscitation proved to be of benefit only after previously uncontrolled hemorrhage was stopped.[76-78]

Three studies were found that address this issue in humans. One large study of 6,855 trauma patients found that although hypotension was associated with a significantly higher mortality rate, the administration of prehospital IV fluids did not reduce this mortality.[14] A retrospective analysis of patients with ruptured abdominal aortic aneurysms showed a survival rate of 30% for patients who were treated with aggressive preoperative colloid fluid replacement in contrast to a 77% survival rate for patients in whom fluid resuscitation was withheld until the time of operative repair.[79] The author strongly recommended that aggressive fluid resuscitation be withheld until the time of surgery in these patients. Bickell and colleagues published a large prospective trial examining this issue in 598 victims of penetrating torso trauma.[4,13] They found that aggressive prehospital fluid resuscitation of hypotensive patients with penetrating wounds of the chest and abdomen was associated with a higher mortality than seen in those for whom aggressive volume replacement was withheld until the time of surgical repair. Further analysis of this data found that this difference was most significant in those patients with wounds of the chest, with abdominal wounds showing little difference in survival between early and delayed fluid resuscitation.[80] Although confirmation of these findings in other randomized, prospective human studies has not yet been obtained, no human studies were found that demonstrated any benefit from fluid replacement in patients with ongoing hemorrhage. Continuing hemorrhage must be suspected in battlefield casualties with penetrating abdominal or thoracic injury until surgical repair is effected.

Hespan (6% hetastarch) was recommended in the 1996 TCCC paper as better alternative for fluid resuscitation in the Tactical Field Care phase than lactated Ringer's (LR) solution.[31] LR is a crystalloid, which means that the primary osmotically active particle is sodium. Since the sodium ion distributes throughout the entire extracellular fluid compartment, LR moves rapidly from the intravascular space to the extravascular space. This shift has significant implications for fluid resuscitation. For example, if a trauma patient is infused with 1000 mL of LR, only 200 mL of that volume will remain in the intravascular space 1 hour later.[81-83] This is not a problem in the civilian setting, since the average time for transport of the patient to the hospital in an ambulance is less than 15 minutes,[13,14] after which surgical control of hemorrhage can be rapidly achieved. In the military setting, however, where several hours may elapse before a casu-

alty arrives at an MTF, effective volume resuscitation may be difficult to sustain with LR.

In contrast, the large hetastarch molecule is retained in the intravascular space and there is no loss of fluid into the interstitium. Hetastarch osmotically promotes fluid influx into the vascular space from the interstitium such that an infusion of 500 mL of hetastarch results in an intravascular volume expansion of almost 800 mL,[83] and this effect is sustained for 8 hours or longer.[84] Although concerns have been voiced about coagulopathies and changes in immune function associated with the use of hetastarch,[23,85-88] these effects are not seen with infusions of less than 1500 mL.[86-90] Several papers have found hetastarch to be a safe and effective alternative to LR in resuscitating patients with controlled hemorrhagic shock.[91,92] Hetastarch is also believed to be an acceptable alternative to LR for intraoperative fluid replacement.[93]

The 1993 Ben Taub study found that aggressive prehospital fluid resuscitation of hemorrhagic shock resulting from penetrating trauma to the chest or abdomen produced a greater mortality than KVO fluids only.[4] This resulted in a recommendation in the original TCCC paper to withhold aggressive fluid resuscitation from individuals with penetrating torso trauma.[31] At the 1998 Special Operations workshop on Urban Warfare casualties, however, there was a clear consensus among the panelists that should a casualty with uncontrolled hemorrhage have mental status changes or become unconscious (correlating to a systolic blood pressure of 50 mm Hg or less), he should be given enough fluid to resuscitate him to the point where his mentation improves (correlating to a systolic blood pressure of 70 mm Hg or above). Panel members stressed the importance of not trying to aggressively administer IV fluids with the goal of achieving "normal" blood pressure in casualties with penetrating truncal injuries.[46]

The consensus conferences held in 2001 and 2002 under the sponsorship of the Office of Naval Research and other agencies promoted the concepts of minimal fluid resuscitation in the setting of uncontrolled hemorrhage and the use of alternative fluids that yield logistical advantages of lighter weight and smaller volume in the ruck sack.[94] The report from the Institute of Medicine in 1999 titled "Fluid resuscitation; state of the science for treating Combat Casualties and Civilian injuries" recommended that 7.5% hypertonic saline (HTS) be initially used for fluid resuscitation. The rationale for this recommendation was that lactated Ringer's has been shown to have detrimental immunologic effects and that further research was needed to find the optimal resuscitation fluid.[95-112] HTS was recommended since it has been used in numerous clinical trials with minimal consequences, and in patients with traumatic brain injury, it may have potential benefits. HTS has also been shown to be immunosuppressive, which may cause the complications (such as ARDS) often seen after massive resuscitation. However, the main reason for the recommendations of HTS was its logistical advantage. The problem with the use of 7.5% HTS is that it is not currently manufactured or available. Therefore, in the consensus conferences in 2001 and 2002, the recommendation was that a colloid solution such as hetastarch be used until HTS is more readily available. It is also unclear if the resuscitative effect of a single infusion of HTS lasts as long as that of a comparable infusion of a colloid solution. This point deserves further investigation.

A technique of minimal fluid resuscitation in the field in casualties with uncontrolled hemorrhage was promoted in a recent paper by Holcomb.[113] Whereas the 1996 TCCC guidelines called for Special Operations medics to give 1000 mL of Hespan to all casualties meeting the requirement for resuscitation, Holcomb proposed that all casualties in shock (defined by absent peripheral pulses or altered mental status in the absence of brain injury) be given a 500 mL bolus of Hextend. If no improvement is noted in 30 minutes, the bolus is repeated once. This modification has several advantages:

1. Logistics: not all casualties will require 1000 mL of hetastarch, thus saving fluid and time for other casualties.
2. Rebleeding; titration of fluids based on a monitored physiologic response may avoid the problem of excessive blood pressure elevation and fatal rebleeding from previously clotted sites.
3. Training; basing the fluid therapy on the premise of responders vs. nonresponders follows the lead of the ACS Committee on Trauma in the ATLS course and allows for a single approach to patients with both controlled and uncontrolled hemorrhage.

Interestingly, this recommendation for "hypotensive" resuscitation is a rebirth of similar principles employed in World War II by Beecher.[114]

Although hetastarch has a theoretical advantage over crystalloids for resuscitating combat casualties on the battlefield because of its sustained intravascular presence, there is little convincing clinical evidence in trauma patients that any one crystalloid or colloid works better than others. However, a multifold reduction in medical equipment weight is achieved by substitution of hetastarch solution for LR.[31] This is clearly of logistical

benefit to military medics, enabling them to carry the smallest volume and weight of resuscitation fluid consistent with effective practice.[113,115]

The Hextend formulation of hetastarch has not been widely used as a front-line resuscitation fluid, thus clear evidence of its superiority is lacking. However, hetastarch solutions mixed in saline (Hespan) increase blood loss compared to the identical hetastarch mixed in a balanced electrolyte solution, a lactate buffer, and physiologic levels of glucose (Hextend).[116] A protective influence of Hextend against multiple organ injury after hepatoenteric ischemia-reperfusion has been reported. The effect has been attributed to a potential antioxidant effect of the hetastarch molecule.[117] For the near future, hypertonic saline dextran is not available, so Hextend is the recommended resuscitation fluid for the Tactical Field Care phase. The 500 mL boluses recommended should be administered as rapidly as possible using manual pressure on the IV bag or inflatable IV bag cuffs.

The most significant concern with the proposed battlefield resuscitation algorithm is that it cannot be rigorously evaluated in clinical trials. It is based on a combination of historical information, recent animal studies, civilian and military trauma experience, and expert opinion. The realities of war prevent prospective randomized blinded resuscitation studies on the battlefield, so now, as in the past, insightful recommendations from those knowledgeable in trauma physiology and experienced in trauma care must provide the basis for military medical doctrine.[114,118,119] Further modification will be warranted as ongoing research and development efforts yield new and relevant information. This issue was extensively discussed during the combat fluid resuscitation conferences,[94] with unanimous agreement that this approach is sound. Optimally, future analysis will also include review of injury data prospectively collected in a military trauma registry.

It may be difficult to establish intravenous access in casualties in shock. A sternal intraosseous (IO) device offers an alternative route for administering fluids and medications in this situation.[120,121] This allows the medic to avoid more difficult and invasive techniques like central venous cannulation or saphenous cutdown. IO access is far easier to obtain in the dark and requires minimal aseptic technique.

An additional change from the previous recommendations entails the administration of oral fluids to casualties with penetrating trauma. This recommendation is based on observations from trauma surgeons attached to forward-deployed MTFs, noting that many casualties are kept NPO for prolonged periods in anticipation of eventual surgery. With transportation delays superimposed on the dehydration often present in combat operations before wounding, these casualties come to surgery markedly dehydrated. This may adversely affect their chance of survival, and the observed risk of emesis and aspiration is remarkably low. Under the new guidelines, therefore, oral fluids are recommended for all casualties with a normal state of consciousness, including those with penetrating torso trauma.

The last recommended change to the fluid resuscitation guidelines is a modified fluid regimen for an individual with traumatic brain injury (TBI) and shock. In this individual, decreased state of consciousness may be due to either the TBI or hemorrhagic shock from associated injuries. Hypotension in the presence of brain injury has been found to be associated with a significant increase in mortality.[122] Because of the need to ensure adequate cerebral perfusion pressure, this casualty should receive IV or IO fluids until he has a palpable radial pulse, commensurate with a systolic blood pressure of at least 80 mm Hg.

The optimal resuscitation fluid for use by combat medics remains an open question and is currently a topic of great interest in military medical research. Studies planned in the near future at the USAISR and other laboratories will evaluate hetastarch solutions, crystalloids, 5% hypertonic saline, and hemoglobin-based oxygen carrying solutions in combat-appropriate trauma models. Animal models used in studies performed to address fluid resuscitation issues on the battlefield should include a significant delay to surgical repair to simulate the prolonged evacuation times combat operations often entail. Care should be taken in attempting to extrapolate the results of resuscitation fluid studies in the civilian sector to the battlefield, since average prehospital time in urban areas is usually very short. However, civilian studies may provide all the available human trauma data. Additionally, resuscitation studies must address both controlled and uncontrolled hemorrhagic shock since the preoperative clinical objectives may be different.

It is common for intravenous lines started in the field to become dislodged during casualty transport. One system for securing IV lines that has proved useful in TCCC is inserting an 18-gauge, 1¼ inch catheter along with a saline lock. The saline lock is then secured with Tegoderm over the site. Fluids and medications are then given by inserting a second 18-gauge, 1¼ inch needle and catheter through the lock and then withdrawing the needle. The catheter is left in place and secured with a circumferential Velcro wrap (Linebacker) to prevent it from being dislodged (personal communication, SFC Rob Miller, 75th Ranger Regiment).

As in civilian settings, the type of analgesic given in TCCC depends on the severity of the casualty's pain. Beecher noted in his WWII survey that many men were fairly unruffled by seemingly horrific wounds sustained in battle, though the same wounds in a civilian setting would be expected to produce agonizing pain.[123] If the wounds are not significantly painful, no analgesia is indicated. For mild to moderate pain, 50 mg of rofecoxib (orally each day) and 1000 mg of acetaminophen (orally every 6 hours) are given with the goal of preserving normal sensorium and allowing the casualty to continue as a combatant. Rofecoxib (Vioxx) is a cyclo-oxygenase-2 (Cox-2) inhibitor and does not cause the platelet dysfunction seen with nonselective NSAIDs.[124,125] It also provides a more favorable side effect profile than seen with other Cox-2 inhibitors. It does not exhibit the same hypersensitivity responses in sulfa-sensitive individuals that have been reported with valdecoxib (Bextra)[126] and celecoxib (Celebrex),[127] and it carries no such contraindication. It is important to realize that platelet dysfunction is an important consideration even for individuals with relatively minor wounds until they have been evacuated to a medical treatment facility or their operating base. The first wounds sustained by a casualty in combat may not, unfortunately, be the last.

If the casualty's wounds require more potent analgesia (bony injuries and burns are typically the most painful), it should be achieved with morphine, preferably administered intravenously.[31] Intravenous administration allows for much more rapid onset and more accurate titration of narcotic dose than the intramuscular route. An initial dose of 5 mg is given and repeated at 10-minute intervals until adequate analgesia is achieved. It is common for individuals who have received high doses of morphine to experience nausea and vomiting, so promethazine 25 mg should be given to prevent this side effect.

Infection is an important late cause of morbidity and mortality in battlefield wounds. Cefoxitin was previously proposed because of its excellent spectrum of action, low incidence of side effects, and low cost.[31] Several significant changes in the antibiotics used in TCCC have recently been proposed by O'Connor and Butler.[128]

The logistical burden of reconstituting and injecting parenteral medications makes the use of oral antibiotics an attractive alternative when possible. In some cases (penetrating abdominal trauma, unconsciousness, shock), oral antibiotics are clearly not an option. In patients without contraindications, however, oral antibiotic prophylaxis is feasible. The USSO-COM-sponsored workshop on Tactical Management of Urban Warfare Casualties held in Tampa in December, 1998, focused on the Battle of Mogadishu and identified a number of potential improvements in the battlefield care of combat casualties.[46] Participants in this workshop noted that an orally administered antibiotic would have several advantages. Giving antibiotics to a wounded teammate would require no more than having him swallow a tablet with a gulp of water from a canteen, and it would eliminate the need for mixing and parenteral administration. With a long-acting oral antibiotic, SOF combat medics could easily carry an adequate supply of antibiotics to cover the entire unit for several days.

Penicillins are not a good choice in this setting because they cause too many severe allergic reactions, require too frequent dosing, and are not active against most gram-negative organisms. The fluoroquinolones, on the other hand, have an excellent spectrum of antibacterial action. Ciprofloxacin has good coverage against *Pseudomonas* species but little activity against anaerobes.[129,130] Levofloxacin has more action against gram-positive organisms than ciprofloxacin but is less effective against *Pseudomonas* and is not reliably effective against anaerobes. Levofloxacin does have some activity against *Pseudomonas* and is indicated for urinary tract infections caused by this organism.[131] Trovafloxacin is effective against gram-positive, gram-negative, and anaerobic organisms.[129] Moxifloxacin and gatifloxacin are fourth-generation fluoroquinolones that have an enhanced spectrum of activity. Trovafloxacin, gatifloxacin, and moxifloxacin yield low minimum inhibitory concentrations against most groups of anaerobes.[130,132] One study found that moxifloxacin's activity against *Clostridium* and *Bacteroides* species was in the same range as metronidazole and superior to that of clindamycin.[133] Another study found that "in general, moxifloxacin was the most potent fluoroquinolone for gram-positive bacteria while ciprofloxacin, moxifloxacin, gatifloxacin, and levofloxacin demonstrated equivalent potency against gram negative bacteria."[134] A third study found that moxifloxacin was almost as active as trovafloxacin, as active as gatifloxacin, and more active than levofloxacin and ciprofloxacin against the anaerobes tested, including *Clostridium* species.[135] Blood levels of the fluoroquinolones achieved with oral dosing are similar to those achieved with IV dosing, so oral administration does not significantly reduce the bioavailability of these agents.

Use of a fourth-generation fluoroquinolone has an additional benefit for use in Special Operations. Since these operations often entail immersion in seawater or fresh water, infections with pathogens found in these environments must be considered as well. Wounds contaminated with seawater are susceptible to infections with *Vibrio* species, gram-negative rods that can result in an overwhelming gram-negative sepsis with 50% mortality.[138] Contamination of wounds with fresh water may result in infections with *Aeromonas* species, also a gram-negative rod.[136] The excellent gram-negative coverage of fourth-generation fluoroquinolones makes them a good choice in these circumstances.

In addition to the advantage of oral administration, the fluoroquinolones require less frequent dosing. Both moxifloxacin and gatifloxacin are given as a single daily 400 mg dose. Imagine a SOF unit with three seriously wounded individuals who cannot be extracted for 48 hours. To maintain antibiotic coverage with cefoxitin for all three casualties would require 24 doses—a quantity that Special Operations medics are not likely to carry. In contrast, 6 tablets of one of the fluoroquinolones would suffice for the same period.

The fluoroquinolones also have an excellent safety profile. A review in the October 1999 *Mayo Clinic Proceedings* states that they are tolerated as well or better than any other class of antibacterial agents.[129] The best-known toxic effect of the fluoroquinolones has been the severe hepatotoxicity seen with trovafloxacin use, but this was seen in only 140 patients out of 2.5 million prescriptions and was usually seen after long-term (more than 28 days) use of the medication. Another disadvantage of trovafloxacin is that its absorption is delayed by morphine, which may be used in combat casualties.[129] Gastrointestinal upset is seen in about 5% of patients treated with fluoroquinolones, and mild allergic reactions (rash, urticaria, and photosensitivity) are seen in 1% to 2% of patients. Mild CNS symptoms (headache and dizziness) are also encountered in 5% to 10% of patients treated with the fluoroquinolones.[129]

One of the considerations in a medication chosen for use by ground troops in the field is its ability to maintain its activity in hot and cold environments. The recommended storage temperature for gatifloxacin is 77° F, with 59° F to 86° F listed as the acceptable temperature range. If true, this would limit the drug's usefulness to ground combat troops. Correspondence on this issue with the manufacturer, Bristol-Myers Squibb, has indicated that gatifloxacin tablets have excellent stability at higher temperatures, with documented maintenance of efficacy for 6 months at 104° F and 3 months at 122° F (personal correspondence, Brett Schenk and Steve Sharpe, Bristol-Myers Squibb).

Gatifloxacin is a good choice for single-agent therapy based on its excellent spectrum of coverage, good safety profile, and once-a-day dosing. Moxifloxacin would be an acceptable second choice. A third choice might be levofloxacin, but since levofloxacin has only limited activity against anaerobes, another drug must be added to achieve coverage against these organisms. The most active drugs for the treatment of anaerobic infections are clindamycin and metronidazole.[137] Relatively few anaerobes are resistant to clindamycin, and few, if any, are resistant to metronidazole.[137] Metronidazole has the advantage of having a less severe side effect profile than clindamycin.

Based on the discussion above, either moxifloxacin or gatifloxacin would be a good choice for an oral antibiotic for use on the battlefield. A cost comparison of these two agents performed by the Naval Hospital Pensacola pharmacy in August of 2002 found that the cost to the U.S. government for a single dose of moxifloxacin was $5.09 while a single dose of gatifloxacin was only $1.86. This cost comparison is based on DOD-wide pricing schedules (personal communication, LT Roger Bunch and LCDR Tony Capano). Based on the much lower cost of gatifloxacin with other factors being approximately equal, gatifloxacin emerges as the best choice for an oral antibiotic.

The use of oral antibiotics is not advisable in some casualties. An unconscious casualty is not able to take the medication. An individual in shock will have a reduced mesenteric blood flow that might interfere with absorption of an oral agent. Casualties with penetrating abdominal trauma may have a mechanical disruption of the gastrointestinal tract that would impede absorption of an oral antibiotic. Effective antibiotic prophylaxis is especially important in this group of patients. A large group of patients (338) with penetrating trauma to the abdomen was reported by Dellinger et al.[138] Even in this civilian trauma center setting, 24% of patients developed wound infections and nine individuals died as a result.

Use of cefotetan as an alternative to cefoxitin as a battlefield antibiotic was first proposed by O'Connor.[139] Cefotetan is a similar medication with the same broad spectrum of action but with a longer half-life that allows every-12-hour dosing. Both cefoxitin and cefotetan were recommended by Osmon as prophylactic agents for adults undergoing colorectal surgery[140] and by Conte for trauma victims with a ruptured viscus.[141]

Luchette et al published a meta-analysis of antibiotic prophylaxis in penetrating trauma in 2000.[142] The more successful regimens included cefoxitin, gentamycin with clindamycin, tobramycin with clindamycin, cefotetan, cefamandole, aztreonam, and gentamycin alone. Nichols and colleagues compared cefoxitin to a gentamycin/clindamycin combination in penetrating abdominal trauma and found them to be equivalent.[143] Jones

and colleagues compared cefoxitin, cefamandole, and a tobramycin/clindamycin combination in patients with penetrating colon trauma.[144] They concluded that both cefoxitin and the tobramycin/clindamycin combination were superior to cefamandole. In 1992, Fabian compared cefoxitin to cefotetan directly. His study of 515 patients found no difference in efficacy between the two agents.[145]

While cefoxitin and cefotetan appear to be equal in efficacy, the longer half-life and comparable cost make cefotetan a better choice. Cefoxitin remains a viable alternative and a good second choice.

Cardiopulmonary resuscitation of a battlefield casualty who has sustained blast or penetrating trauma is not appropriate.[31,146] Prehospital resuscitation of trauma patients in cardiac arrest has been fraught with futility even in urban settings where the victim is close to trauma centers. For example, Branney and colleagues reported a 2% survival rate (14 of 708) among patients receiving emergency department thoracotomy who arrived at the emergency department with absent vital signs.[147] In a more recent study, Rosemurgy, Norris, et al reported no survivors out of 138 trauma patients who sustained a prehospital cardiac arrest in whom resuscitation was attempted.[148] The authors recommended that resuscitation of trauma victims in cardiopulmonary arrest not be attempted even in the civilian prehospital setting, primarily because of the large economic cost entailed in these uniformly unsuccessful attempts. In the tactical combat setting, the cost of attempting to resuscitate patients with inevitably fatal wounds will be measured in additional lives lost as combat medical personnel are exposed to hostile fire during resuscitation efforts and care is withheld from casualties with potentially survivable wounds. Successful completion of the unit's mission may also be unnecessarily jeopardized by these efforts. Only in the case of nontraumatic disorders such as hypothermia, near drowning, or electrocution should cardiopulmonary resuscitation be performed in the tactical prehospital setting.

CASEVAC Care

The use of a CASEVAC asset to evacuate the wounded from the battlefield presents the opportunity to bring in additional medical equipment and personnel to treat the casualties. This opportunity led to the recommendation to establish designated Combat Casualty Transportation Teams for Special Operations forces.[31] This additional medical expertise and equipment will allow for the expanded diagnostic and therapeutic measures outlined in Box 16-3 for the CASEVAC phase of care.

Care in this phase more closely approximates ATLS guidelines. The opportunity to carry additional equipment and a (possibly) more favorable environment in which to work make a more varied selection of airway management interventions possible. Endotracheal intubation, the laryngeal mask airway,[149] the intubating laryngeal mask airway,[150] and the esophageal-tracheal combitube[151] are all potentially feasible alternatives in this phase if the nasopharyngeal airway is insufficient to manage the airway. Schwartz and his colleagues reported success in performing endotracheal intubation with the aid of night vision goggles.[152] Surgical cricothyroidotomy remains a valuable option if needed.[153]

Several improvements in fluid resuscitation may be possible in the CASEVAC phase. Electronic monitoring, if available, may yield a better understanding of the casualty's status. Casualties with traumatic brain injuries should be maintained with a systolic blood pressure of 90 mm Hg or higher in this phase. Asanguinous fluids restore blood volume but do not replace oxygen-carrying capacity. When logistically feasible, O-positive or O-negative packed red blood cells should be available in this phase for use when indicated and under appropriate protocols. Rhesus factor compatibility is an issue only in females with reproductive capability. Both the British Special Air Service (personal communication, Dr. John Naevin, former 22nd SAS Regimental Surgeon) and the IDF[154] have used packed red blood cells (PRBCs) successfully in casualty transport platforms. Israeli medical personnel store the PRBCs in a special field refrigerator that maintains a temperature between 33° F (1° C) and 39° F (6° C), and they expand them with 250 mL of saline solution before administration.[154] Use of PRBCs in the field has had an excellent safety record in the IDF.[154]

The potential for casualties to develop hypothermia and a secondary coagulopathy makes adequate warming an important function in preparation for and during CASEVAC.[155] Concomitant use of the Thermal Angel device, the Rescue Wrap, and gel heaters has been employed in combat operations in both fixed-wing and rotary aircraft. This combination has proved able to increase a casualty's temperature in ambient temperatures below freezing (personal communication, TSgt Steve Cum).

The proposal for Combat Casualty Transportation Teams and the additional care that they provide should be evaluated by the conventional forces for applicability in their units.

Scenario-Based Training

Despite the effort that has gone into developing a combat-appropriate trauma management plan, the bottom line remains that no single plan will suffice for all situations. This realization led to the concept of scenario-

based management plans.[31] Representative scenarios are presented in Boxes 16-5 through 16-12. The medical and tactical issues to be addressed in most of these scenarios have been addressed previously.[156,157] Figures 16-3 and 16-4 are from action in Mogadishu on 3 October 1993. This engagement resulted in the greatest number of US casualties in a single firefight since Vietnam (18 dead, 73 wounded). In addition, there was a delay of 15 hours

Box 16-5

Urban Warfare Scenario—Fast Rope Casualty

- 16-person Ranger team—security element for building assault
- 70-foot fast rope insertion
- One person misses rope and falls
- Unconscious
- Bleeding from mouth and ears
- Taking fire from all directions from hostile crowds
- Anticipated extraction by ground convoy in 30 minutes

Box 16-6

Urban Warfare Scenario—Helicopter Hit by RPG Round

- Hostile and well-armed (AK-47s, RPG) enemy in urban environment
- Building assault to capture members of a hostile clan
- In Blackhawk helicopter trying to cover helo crash site
- Flying at 300 foot altitude
- Left door gunner with six-barrel M-134 minigun (4000 rpm)
- Hit in hand by ground fire
- Another crew member takes over mini-gun
- RPG round impacts under right door gunner
- Windshields blown out
- Smoke filling aircraft
- Right minigun not functioning
- Left minigun without a gunner and firing uncontrolled
- Pilot—transiently unconscious, now becoming alert
- Co-pilot—unconscious, lying forward on helo's controls
- Crew member
    Leg blown off
    Lying in puddle of his own blood
    Femoral bleeding

before the first wounded were evacuated to a Combat Support Hospital. Scenarios like these, based on actual past events, help to raise the level of interest in ensuing discussions.

Boxes 16-7 through 16-9 deal with a parachute insertion and subsequent land warfare phase, with injuries of different magnitudes sustained on landing. The medical care of these casualties is relatively straightforward, but they require difficult tactical decisions of the mission commander.

Boxes 16-10 through 16-12 deal with casualty scenarios that occur during diving operations. This is a very important aspect of the training for SEAL and Marine Reconnaissance mission commanders because the underwater environment has such a large impact on casualty management and because this area is not addressed in civilian medical literature.

As one examines these scenarios, it becomes apparent that the appropriate care for a casualty may vary based on how critical the mission is, the anticipated time to evacuation, and the environment in which the casualty occurs. Any management plan for a combat casualty discussed in the planning phase should be considered advisory rather than directive in nature, since only infrequently will an actual casualty situation unfold exactly as anticipated. It is obviously not possible to plan for every casualty scenario, but review of several casualty scenarios most appropriate for an impending operation is a valuable exercise in the planning process.

Box 16-7

Tib/Fib Fracture on Parachute Insertion

- 12-person SF team
- Interdiction operation for weapons convoy
- Night parachute jump from a C-130
- 4-mile patrol over rocky terrain to the objective
- Planned helicopter extract near target
- One jumper sustains an open fracture of his left tibia and fibula on landing

---

Box 16-8

Multiple Trauma from Parachute Collapse

- 16-person SF team
- Interdiction operation on a weapons convoy
- Night static line jump from C-130
- 4-mile patrol over rocky terrain to objective
- Planned helicopter extraction near target
- One jumper has canopy collapse 40 feet above the drop zone
    - Open facial fractures with blood and teeth in the oropharynx
    - Bilateral ankle fractures
    - Open angulated fracture of the left femur

Box 16-9

Fatality from Parachute Malfunction

- 16-person SF team
- Interdiction operation on a weapons convoy
- Night static line jump from C-130
- 4-mile patrol over rocky terrain to objective
- Planned helicopter extraction near target
- One jumper has streamer, obviously dead on DZ

Box 16-10

Underwater Explosion on Ship Attack

- Ship attack
- Launch from PC 12 miles out
- One hour transit in two Zodiacs
- Seven SEAL swim pairs
- Zodiacs approach to within 1 mile from harbor
- Turtleback half mile, then purge and go on bag
- Charge dropped in water by hostile forces at target ship
- Swim buddy unconscious

Box 16-11

CNS Oxygen Toxicity during Ship Attack

- Launch from PC 12 miles out
- One hour transit in two Zodiacs
- Seven SEAL swim pairs
- Zodiacs approach to within 1 mile from harbor
- 78° F water—wet suits
- Turtleback half mile, then go on bag
- Very clear, still night—transit depth 25 feet
- Diver notes that buddy is disoriented and confused, with arm twitching

TCCC Skills List

Individuals other than medics may be called upon to provide medical care on the battlefield. Each combatant should be able to perform life-saving interventions, such as the application of a tourniquet, and simple tasks, such as self-administration of oral antibiotics and analgesics. This is the goal of an Army program called "Combat Lifesaver" in which nonmedics receive basic medical training in specified life-saving skills. A list of each type of potential first responder and the skills that each should possess is provided in Table 16-2.

Tactical Medicine for Small Unit Mission Commanders

Although the TCCC protocol is gaining increasing acceptance throughout the U.S. Department of Defense and allied military forces,[158-165] this protocol by itself is not adequate training for the management of combat trauma in the tactical environment. Since casualty scenarios in small-unit operations entail tactical problems as well as medical ones, the appropriate management plan for a particular casualty must be developed with an appreciation for the entire tactical situation.[31] This approach has been developed through a series of workshops carried out by SOF medical personnel in association with appropriate medical specialty groups such as the Undersea and Hyperbaric Medical Society, the Wilderness Medical Society, and the Special Operations Medical Association.[46,156,157]

The most recent of these workshops, which addressed the Tactical Management of Urban Warfare Casualties in

Table 16-2   Tactical Combat Casualty Care Skills List

Skill	Individual operator	Combat lifesaver	Medic
Overview of Tactical Medicine Training	X	X	X
Hemostasis			
Apply tourniquet	X	X	X
Apply direct pressure	X	X	X
Apply HemCon dressing	X	X	X
Apply PASG			X
Casualty Transport Techniques	X	X	X
Airway			
Chin-lift/jaw-thrust maneuver	X	X	X
Nasopharyngeal airway	X	X	X
Cricothyroidotomy			X
ILMA			X
Endotracheal intubation			X
Combitube			X
Breathing			
Needle thoracostomy		X	X
Treat open pneumothorax	X	X	X
Chest tube			X
Administer oxygen			X
Intravenous access/therapy			
Assess for shock	X	X	X
Start an IV/saline lock		X	X
Obtain intraosseous access			X
IV fluid resuscitation		X	X
IV analgesia			X
IV antibiotics			X
Administer PRBCs			X
Intramuscular therapy			
IM morphine	X	X	X
IM antibiotics			X
Oral antibiotics	X	X	X
Oral analgesia	X	X	X
Fracture management			
Splinting	X	X	X
Traction splinting		X	X
Electronic monitoring			X

Special Operations, noted that several of the casualty scenarios studied from the Mogadishu action in 1993[166] had very important tactical implications for the mission commanders.[46] The unconscious fast-rope fall victim in Box 16-5 resulted in a decision by the mission commander to split the forces in his ground convoy, detaching three of the 12 vehicles to take the casualty back to base immediately, leaving the remaining nine to extract the rest of the troops. The helicopter crash described in Figure 16-4 resulted in the pilot's body being trapped in the wreck. Several discrete elements from the target building sustained multiple casualties as they moved toward the crash site to assist. The casualties eventually outnumbered those who were able to maneuver, forcing the elements to remain stationary and preventing them from consolidating their forces. When a rescue convoy finally reached the embattled troops at the crash site, there was a delay of approximately 3 hours while the force worked feverishly to free the trapped body. Several hundred troops and over 25 vehicles were vulnerable to counterattack during this period. These scenarios made it obvious to members of the workshop panel that training only combat medics in tactical medicine is not enough.

McRaven has compiled accounts of a number of special operations that may be used for scenario development.[167] If tactical medicine involves complex decisions about both tactics and medicine, then we must train the tactical decision makers—the mission commanders—as well as combat medical personnel in this area.[46] A customized course in Tactical Medicine for SEAL and Ranger Mission Commanders has been developed and incorporated into the training for mission commanders in those units. The Tactical Medicine course provides a rationale for why mission commanders need training in this area. While it is true that the combat medic takes care of the casualty, the mission commander runs the mission, and *what's best for the casualty and what's best for the mission may be in direct conflict.* The question is often not just whether or not the mission can be completed successfully without the wounded individual(s); the issue may well be that continuing the mission will adversely affect the outcome for the casualty. If the mission is to be successfully accomplished, the mission commander may have to make some very difficult decisions about the care and movement of casualties. Additional reasons to train mission commanders in tactical medicine include:

1. The importance of having the commander know that the care provided in TCCC may be substantially different than the care provided for the same injury in a noncombat setting.
2. The unit may be employed in such a way that there is no corpsman, medic, or PJ immediately available to the injured individual
3. The corpsman, medic, or PJ may be the first team member shot

Although the use of helmets and body armor are not feasible for every combat operation, the Mogadishu experience documents the efficacy of individual protective clothing in preventing potentially lethal injuries.[36] Tactical Medicine training should emphasize the benefits of these devices where operationally feasible.

Weapons of Mass Destruction

Weapons of mass destruction (WMD) include nuclear devices, biologic agents, and chemical substances. Historically, WMD have been considered as a single class of weapons, but they differ significantly in their use, presentation, and concepts of casualty management. Nuclear weapons may be encountered in the civilian sector as radiation accidents or spills. The technology required to use a nuclear weapon is still substantial in comparison with that required for chemical or biologic agents. A significantly increased threat exists that terrorist groups or hostile nations may use chemical and/or biologic weapons against the United States. These weapons are readily available to determined parties. Each type of weapon is discussed along with its general management principles.

Nuclear Weapons

Thermal burns and a variety of traumas complicated by differing degrees of radiologic contamination are the most likely injuries to be encountered in survivors of a nuclear blast. Multiple delayed effects may be anticipated, but early treatment will deal with relatively standard trauma management. Decontamination should be conducted as soon as possible but should not delay lifesaving treatment. A radiologic spill or incident may occur with or without associated trauma. A simple acronym—SWIMS—will suffice for most incidents: *S*top the spill, *W*arn others, *I*solate the area, *M*inimize contamination, and *S*ecure ventilation if in an enclosed building. Many civil defense agencies are well versed in the management of nuclear events, and further information can be obtained through these sources.

Biologic Warfare Agents

Biologic weapons are among the most insidious and dangerous ever devised by humankind. They have been characterized as the poor person's atomic bomb, a cheaper and less sophisticated alternative to chemical, nuclear, or conventional weapons. Biologic agents can be produced at low cost and in a covert manner, and they can be spread easily using readily available equipment. They are capable of producing a large number of casualties, and the first sign of an attack may be days after the actual event when symptoms of a disease begin to appear. Biologic warfare agents (BWAs) fall into four broad categories:

1. *True biologic agents* are living microorganisms (pathogens) that have the ability to cause disease in humans and/or animals and can cause plant destruction. These include viruses, bacteria, fungi, and rickettsiae.
2. *Biologic vectors* are insect vectors that have been purposefully infected with a pathogen in an attempt to propagate the spread of a disease. Various insect vectors exist within nature, usually endemic to a specific region, and often act as intermediate breeding grounds for local pathogens. Mosquitoes act in this way for the spread of malaria, and infected fleas do the same for plague.
3. *Toxins* of biologic origin, strictly speaking, are chemicals, but they are generally classified as BWAs because of their production within living things. Examples include botulinum and cholera toxins.
4. *Bioregulators* are chemicals that occur naturally, in small amounts within the body, to regulate such functions as heart rate and blood pressure; they may be synthetically derived to achieve the same purposes. In altered concentrations, these agents may lead to various adverse actions, such as paralysis, loss of consciousness, or death. Given their specificity for use against the human system, they are included as BWAs.

The primary means of exposure to most of these agents is via the respiratory tract. The gastrointestinal tract is the second major route of exposure for many infectious agents and toxins, normally through the ingestion of contaminated food or water supplies.

Weight for weight, BWAs are inherently more toxic than either chemical or conventional weapons, have a much higher specificity for their intended targets than chemical weapons, and effectively disseminated, provide the largest area coverage of any type of weapon. However, once they are disseminated, BWAs tend to degrade quickly.

Two primary methods of dissemination of BWAs exist, both of which depend on weather conditions for maximum effectiveness. The first is from a point source weapon such as a bomb or stationary aerosol generator, which disseminates the agent from a single location. The second is a line source weapon that disseminates the agent from a moving platform, such as a spray tank mounted on a vehicle (truck or aircraft). Line source weapons can disperse large amounts of an agent over much wider areas than point source weapons and are significantly more effective.

FACTORS AFFECTING DISSEMINATION OF BIOLOGIC WARFARE AGENTS

Atmospheric conditions can dramatically alter the dispersal and subsequent effectiveness of BWAs. High winds tend to disperse BWAs over a wider area and dilute their concentrations. Unstable winds, especially those with gusty, unpredictable patterns, will provide a less uniform spread. Sunlight, particularly the ultraviolet portion, tends to break down toxic agents and kill pathogens through rapid drying. Rain tends to wash an agent out of the air and clear surfaces.

Terrain is equally important in the dispersal patterns and subsequent effectiveness of BWAs. Flat, unobstructed territory or an open expanse of water allows for maximum potential distribution. Urban settings or hilly, rugged terrain prevents even distribution, increases vertical dilution, and tends to reduce effective concentrations over a distance.

Early detection allows personnel to take protective cover in time to prevent exposure. However, limitations in technology make this extremely difficult to achieve. BWA detectors are in development but are currently of questionable reliability.

Personnel entering a targeted area may lack effective protection, become casualties themselves, and spread the disease further. Delayed effects make it difficult to even discern when and where the attack was conducted. An outbreak of disease may cause significant death or illness yet still mimic a naturally occurring epidemic.

Should biologic agents be of concern, three points should be remembered:

1. Avoid contamination if possible.
2. Decontamination should be conducted, if possible, to eliminate or reduce the hazard from exposed personnel and equipment. Decontamination often involves caustic materials and bleaches to neutralize

the agent and thus may damage equipment. The secondary infectious hazard is minimal, and treatment may proceed even in the absence of full decontamination.

3. Maintain a high index of suspicion. Look for unusual diseases or patterns of disease if a biologic incident was possible. Seek treatment early if you develop symptoms after responding to a call. Prompt and effective medical treatment is necessary to counteract the effects of the agents and minimize casualties. Treatment is effective in the majority of commonly used agents, but in some cases, by the time symptoms appear, it may be too late to treat effectively; in other cases, no effective treatment exists.

CHARACTERISTICS OF BIOLOGIC WARFARE AGENTS

General characteristics that determine the usefulness of BWAs include the following:

1. *Infectivity.* This involves the ability of an agent to reliably infect a person or animal exposed to it.
2. *Virulence.* This characteristic relates the agent's ability to incapacitate or kill an intended target once exposure and infection have occurred.
3. *Incubation period.* The incubation period is the lag between the time when infection occurs and the time when symptoms of the disease become apparent. BWAs rarely cause instant casualties; with the exception of certain toxins, BWAs tend to have effects only after their incubation period.
4. *Stability.* Most biologic agents are unstable when compared with chemical agents. Stability is the ability to maintain virulence and other characteristics over time and under varying ecologic conditions.
5. *Environmental persistence.* Persistence is closely related to stability and is the ability of an organism to survive in the environment long enough to have the desired effect.
6. *Resistance.* This is the ability of an agent to withstand normal medical countermeasures.
7. *Protection.* This is the ability of an attacker to protect his or her troops with a vaccine or other protective measure not available to the opponent.
8. *Controllability.* This is the ability to predict, with some measure of assuredness, the extent and nature of the BWA's effects given a specific set of employment parameters.
9. *Producibility.* The most likely agents used by developing countries are cheap, are easy to produce, and can be readily obtained on the global market. Only

about 30 pathogens have been considered as likely BWAs out of the several hundred known to affect humans and animals.

ANTHRAX

Anthrax is often discussed as the prototypical BWA. *Bacillus anthracis*, the causative organism for anthrax, occurs naturally in horses, cattle, and sheep. Anthrax is highly toxic and stable in an aerosolized form. Once released, exposure can occur through inhalation, ingestion, or wounds in the skin. An inhalation dose of less than one microgram can be fatal in days. The normal incubation period is 3 to 5 days but may be as little as 24 hours with a larger exposure.

Cutaneous anthrax has a mortality rate approaching 20% if left untreated but less than 1% after treatment. However, inhalation anthrax approaches a much higher mortality rate. Treatment of suspected cases must begin before the onset of symptoms or it is likely to be ineffective. Even with treatment, survivors may be incapacitated for months and require retreatment because of relapses. Protection against an anthrax attack currently includes the use of personal protective gear and a mask if the attack is detected in time. However, current detection methods may be unreliable if warning of an attack is early enough to prevent exposure, and detectors are not routinely deployed with at-risk units. An anthrax vaccine is available.

Chemical Warfare Agents

Chemical agents fall into five main categories: nerve agents, vesicants, cyanide, lung agents, and riot control agents. Although the potential for terrorist activity exists, these agents may be encountered during cleanup of lands where old chemical munitions were stored or during hazardous materials (HAZMAT) incidents involving spills of organophosphate insecticides or other industrial chemicals such as phosgene or cyanide. Chemical agents are primarily liquids that produce contact hazards but are even more dangerous as they vaporize. They may be persistent (staying on the ground for more than 24 hours) or nonpersistent (evaporating within 24 hours). In liquid form, these agents are heavier than water and may be covered by puddles. In vapor form, they are heavier than air and tend to collect in low spots. As with biologic agents, the primary considerations are contamination avoidance, decontamination, and movement of decontaminated patients from a contaminated to a clean area. In many circumstances, patients should be treated on site and moved after appropriate decontamination is achieved. Failure to do this may result in widespread contamination and increased casualties. Responders to a chemical incident must protect themselves by use of appropriate suits and masks or they will risk becoming casualties as well.

NERVE AGENTS

Nerve agents cause involuntary skeletal muscle activity and excessive secretion from lachrymal, nasal, salivary, and sweat glands into the airways and gastrointestinal tract. Constriction of muscles within the airway produces bronchoconstriction similar to that seen in asthma; in the gastrointestinal tract it leads to cramps, vomiting, and diarrhea. The single most effective treatment for exposure to nerve agents is atropine. Atropine will reduce secretions and reduce activity in smooth muscle but has little effect on excess activity of skeletal muscles. Nerve agents penetrate normal clothing and skin to be absorbed into the body. Clinical effects will depend on the route and amount of agent exposure.

VESICANTS

Vesicants are substances that cause burning of the skin with redness and blistering. These agents are liquids but produce damage in the vapor form as well. Damage begins to occur almost immediately on contact with the skin, and the best management is early and thorough decontamination of the affected areas. Clinical effects may be delayed for several hours and increase in severity over several days; death usually occurs as a result of damage to the respiratory tract. Early responders may not see significant lesions because the effects are often delayed.

CYANIDE

Cyanide is a common industrial chemical that has been used as a poison for centuries. It is found in cigarette smoke and in some types of foods. Cyanide inhibits the ability of cells to use oxygen and causes death by cellular hypoxemia. Although large doses produce rapid death, smaller doses may be effectively treated with rapid administration of the antidotes, support of circulation as necessary, and administration of oxygen.

LUNG AGENTS

Lung agents are a class of compounds that cause pulmonary edema. The most important of these is phosgene, a common industrial compound. Teflon, when it burns, may give off perfluoroisobutylene, another agent in this class. Generally, these agents produce damage to the alveolar-capillary membrane with onset of symptoms between 2 and 24 hours depending on the

level of exposure. Patients should be observed for a 24-hour period and triaged based on the severity of symptoms that develop.

RIOT CONTROL AGENTS

Riot control agents (RCAs) are in common use by law enforcement agencies but are not usually of great concern to first responders. Medical treatment is not generally indicated after exposure because the effects are self-limiting; however, some rare complications are worthy of note:

- Persons with reactive airway disease may develop prolonged bronchospasm after exposure to RCAs. Standard treatment for a severe asthmatic attack may be required.
- Moderate to severe conjunctivitis has been reported after exposure that occasionally requires treatment by an ophthalmologist.
- A delayed-onset contact dermatitis may develop that may require follow-up medical care.

DECONTAMINATION

Decontamination is vital in any chemical incident and has two main goals:

1. *To minimize injury to the casualty.* This must be done within minutes after exposure to be effective. The best and most effective decontamination is that performed within the first minute after exposure to a liquid chemical agent. If decontamination is delayed 15 to 60 minutes, it may do little to assist the casualty. If the agent was a nerve agent, the casualty may be dead. The best and often quickest decontamination is physical removal of the agent. Any clothing that has been contaminated should be removed, and the skin should be cleaned of any residual. Large amounts of water under pressure or a scraper-type object may be effective. Substances that will chemically destroy or detoxify the agent are commonly used for decontamination. Sodium hypochlorite is a primary agent. Undiluted bleach followed by washing may be effective, and specially prepared decontamination kits are available.

2. *To prevent contamination of rescue personnel, EMS personnel, transport units, and the receiving medical facility.* Before a casualty is decontaminated, all personnel in contact with the casualty must wear appropriate protective equipment. A significant risk exists of contaminating vehicles and medical facilities from a chemical casualty. A strict decontamination area must be established with a clean area on one side and

the contaminated area on the other. Any person who is symptomatic or asymptomatic, casualty, or medical care provider who goes from a contaminated area to a clean uncontaminated area, such as a medical treatment area, must be decontaminated. Casualties or medical personnel who have not undergone decontamination procedures may contaminate the entire air system of a hospital by spreading a vapor agent.

Specific protective equipment to investigate includes the following:

- Personal equipment
  - Masks, the M40 or older M17A2, and suits
  - Self-contained breathing apparatus (SCBA) approved for civilian use
  - Standard chemical clothing is available to civilian emergency agencies through the Defense Logistics Agency
  - Civilian responders should have the responder suit
- Detection equipment
  - Chemical detection kits
- Medical items
  - Mark I nerve agent antidote kit: decontaminable litter made of monofilament polypropylene fabric, which allows drainage of liquids, does not absorb chemical agents, and is easily decontaminated for reuse
  - Fiberglass long backboards—nonpermeable and easily decontaminated

Triage

The most important concept in the successful management of multiple casualties is triage. Triage is the sorting of casualties into treatment categories by a designated officer. Categories are determined based on the severity of injury and likelihood of recovery, given limited treatment resources. Resources consist of time, personnel, and equipment. The objective is to provide survival for as many patients as possible. The triage officer's responsibility is to sort the casualties; he or she does not treat patients and is often alone without equipment. In an ideal situation, a senior experienced trauma or general surgeon should conduct triage because these individuals are most qualified to make the necessary life and death decisions. In practice, many other personnel may be forced to do triage based on circumstances. Patients are triaged and retriaged at each level of care, and treatment categories may change based on availability of resources. Two types of triage deserve special mention—field and hospital triage.

Field Triage

Field triage occurs near the site of injury. This can be the battlefield in wartime or the site of a disaster in peacetime. The triage officer may be a physician but will more likely be a corpsman. The broad categories of patients in the field include (1) those who are about to die (the agonal), (2) those who are more scared than wounded, and (3) all others. Little can be done for the agonal, and the minimally injured should be removed from the scene and returned to duty as soon as possible. Those with more serious injuries need to be treated initially and moved to an MTF as quickly as possible. Two categories are designated based on injury severity and threat to integrity of airway, breathing, and circulation (primary survey). These include the traditional "immediate" and "urgent" categories. This determination is based on the premise that little can be accomplished at the scene in terms of reversing instability and that outcome will be determined at the MTF.

Hospital Triage

Hospital triage is considerably more precise than field triage. The triage officer is the surgeon who is most experienced in trauma care. He or she only sorts patients and rarely treats them. Three categories constitute the simplest, most used method of triage:

1. The "walking wounded" are patients whose injuries would heal with little or no therapy. They constitute approximately 65% of the patients seen. They are moved to a separate area of the MTF where their injuries are treated by a physician and a nurse if staffing permits.
2. The "expectant" are patients who will probably die no matter what treatment is performed and would tie up significant resources in the process. They are moved to a separate area of the MTF and made as comfortable as possible. They number fewer than 10% of the casualties and are attended by only a single nurse.
3. The "priority" are patients for whom a meaningful survival can be achieved by immediate or prompt intervention and treatment. They number about 25% of the patient load.

Despite obvious differences, military (battlefield) triage and civilian (disaster) triage adhere to those basic levels of casualty sorting. The next section provides a comparison of casualty management after the terrorist bombing of the U.S. Marine Corps facility in Beirut, Lebanon, in 1983 and the terrorist bombing of the A.P. Murrah Federal Building in Oklahoma City in 1995.

Comparison of Civilian versus Military Casualty Management

The Beirut bomb resulted in 346 casualties among whom 234 (68%) died immediately. The battalion aid station, located on the fourth floor of the building, was destroyed, and the medical officer and numerous corpsmen were killed, resulting in a lack of initial medical capability at the scene. Of the 112 survivors, 7 subsequently died (6%) and 6 of these succumbed in association with a delay in treatment secondary to entrapment within the building. Most of the survivors (64%) were flown by helicopter off shore to the USS Iwo Jima where they were triaged. Twenty-four casualties were flown from the scene to Europe and Cypress after the arrival of U.S. and British Air Ambulance Units. Fifteen survivors with minor injuries remained on shore and all survived. Eight casualties were taken to local Lebanese hospitals where one died.

The Oklahoma City bomb caused 759 casualties among whom 167 (22%) died immediately. Of the 83 (11%) survivors who were hospitalized, 1 died. The remaining 509 casualties were treated as outpatients. The field triage officer in this disaster was an emergency medicine resident from the nearby University Hospital.

Extenuating Factors Related to Battlefield Triage

Triage in the combat zone is stressed by obvious extenuating circumstances. The ongoing conflict poses risks to the integrity of the MTF and those components integral to patient transport and evacuation. Casualty care is problematic but may be remarkably efficient despite the difficulties.

Resource limitations are present in both battlefield and domestic occurrences. Contingency planning can minimize shortfalls in both scenarios, and protocols should be established for each. A major treatment facility, whether it be a combat casualty support hospital or a Level I trauma center, must have a disaster plan. It should be published, updated routinely, and periodically rehearsed.

Environmental Concerns with Triage

Environmental concerns in disaster management include casualty and medical personnel protection against heat, cold, wind, rain, dust, flood, and storm. Sources of water and electricity may be jeopardized, communications disrupted, and transportation rendered impossible. Contingency planning is essential, and these issues should be addressed in standard disaster plans. Exposure to nuclear, biologic, or chemical agents has become of increased concern in recent years.

Triage is best done at a distance from the actual scene of a terrorist act. An initial blast may be followed by a second, larger detonation designed to maim and kill those responding to the first.

Summary

The emergence of prehospital care is deeply rooted in military tradition, dating as far back as the sixteenth century. The modern prehospital care provider is simply an evolution of the bracardier of revolutionary France. The Vietnam conflict was responsible for quantum leaps in what we now regard as prehospital care. With ever-changing conditions in the geopolitical picture, future advancements in EMS can already be predicted by what we now see in the Department of Defense.

Echelons (levels) of care improve the survivability of wounded soldiers by moving more advanced capabilities further forward in the echelon system. The military-derived system of echelons of care is the civilian counterpart spread across a theater of operation.

Prehospital care in the tactical environment requires specialized training for physicians, corpsmen, and medics. Because of the complicating effects of battlefield conditions (e.g., darkness, enemy fire, and equipment limitations), scene safety is not always feasible. Care under fire calls for an occasional variance from what we consider normal protocol because of these unique circumstances. Before any combat operation or mission can be undertaken, special attention must be directed at a basic medical care plan.

Weapons of mass destruction are the most insidious and dangerous threat devised by humankind. Early detection and decontamination are the most important priorities in countering biologic or chemical warfare agents. Concurrent injuries should be treated as in a conventional setting.

The most important concept in successful management of multiple casualties, whether in the battlefield or on the home front during peacetime, is triage. Triage in the combat zone is stressed by extenuating circumstances.

Scenario Solution

The point man who sustained the injuries resulting in no pulse or ventilations would be placed in the "expectant" category. No time or equipment would be used in a resuscitation attempt. The point man will be extracted with the team. The patrol leader with the femoral hemorrhage would be placed in the "immediate" category.

Can the patient be stabilized well enough to be extracted with the team as planned? If not, what is the Combat Casualty Evacuation (CASEVAC) care plan? How soon can CASEVAC arrive at the patrol's present location? Does. the CASEVAC aircraft have the necessary equipment to extract the patients from the patrol's present location (e.g., jungle penetrator, Stokes litter)?

Incoming direct and indirect fire make it necessary for the patrol to either suppress hostile fire using fire support (e.g., artillery, naval gunfire, close air support) or break contact and move out of their present position immediately. Transport of the patient is a priority, and more definitive care may be delayed until the patrol is in a suitable location.

The patrol leader will receive a pressure dressing or a tourniquet placement until the medic or corpsman can remove him from hostile fire. Later, during movement or at the extraction site, the patient will receive a more definitive dressing and advanced lifesaving procedures, including 3:1 volume replacement with lactated Ringer's solution and a full primary and secondary survey to identify any other conditions that may have previously gone unrecognized.

Review Questions

Answers are provided on p. 414.

1. The first comprehensive effort in America to upgrade or establish prehospital care was required by states because of which of the following?
   a. National Academy of Sciences recommendation in 1970
   b. Commission of Public Charities and Corrections of New York City in 1869
   c. Highway Safety Act of 1966
   d. Commission of EMS or DOT in 1981

2. Which echelon of care is characterized by its mobility and staffing of medical technicians, one physician, and one physician's assistant?
   a. Echelon I
   b. Echelon II
   c. Echelon III
   d. Echelon IV

3. Which stage of care applies to a situation in which care of an injury is provided while on a mission with no hostile fire?
   a. Combat Casualty Evacuation Care
   b. Care Under Fire
   c. Tactical Field Care
   d. Battlefield Care

4. Which chemical warfare agent is distinguished with signs of involuntary skeletal muscle activity, bronchoconstriction, cramps, vomiting, diarrhea, and excessive secretion from lachrymal, nasal, salivary, and sweat glands into the airways and gastrointestinal tract?
   a. Cyanide
   b. Lung agents
   c. Nerve agents
   d. Vesicants

5. Field triage will most likely be performed by whom?
   a. Surgeon (with the most experience)
   b. Nurse
   c. Physician's assistant
   d. Corpsman

REFERENCES

1. Bellamy RF: The causes of death in conventional land warfare: implications for combat casualty care research, *Mil Med* 149:55, 1984.

2. Alexander RH, Proctor HJ: *Advanced Trauma Life Support 1993 Student Manual*, Chicago, 1993, American College of Surgeons.

3. Krausz MM: Controversies in shock research: hypertonic resuscitation—pros and cons, *Shock* 3:69, 1995.

4. Bickell WH, Wall MJ, Pepe PE, et al: Immediate versus delayed fluid resuscitation for hypotensive patients with penetrating torso injuries. *N Engl J Med* 331:1105, 1994.

5. Honigman B, Rohwder K, Moore EE, et al: Prehospital advanced trauma life support for penetrating cardiac wounds, *Ann Emerg Med* 19:145, 1990.

6. Smith JP, Bodai BI: The urban paramedic's scope of practice, *JAMA* 253:544, 1985.

7. Smith JP, Bodai BI, Hill AS, et al: Prehospital stabilization of critically injured patients: a failed concept, *J Trauma* 25:65, 1985.

8. Dronen SC, Stern S, Baldursson J, et al: Improved outcome with early blood administration in a near-fatal model of porcine hemorrhagic shock, *Am J Emerg Med* 10:533, 1992.

9. Stern SA, Dronen SC, Birrer P, et al: Effect of blood pressure on hemorrhage volume and survival in a near-fatal hemorrhage model incorporating a vascular injury, *Ann Emerg Med* 22:155-163, 1993.

10. Chudnofsky CR, Dronen SC, Syverud SA, et al: Early versus late fluid resuscitation: lack of effect in porcine hemorrhagic shock, *Ann Emerg Med* 18:122, 1989.

11. Bickell WH: Are victims of injury sometimes victimized by attempts at fluid resuscitation? *Ann Emerg Med* 22:225, 1993.

12. Chudnofsky CR, Dronen SC, Syverud SA, et al: Intravenous fluid therapy in the prehospital management of hemorrhagic shock: improved outcome with hypertonic saline/6% dextran 70 in a swine model, *Am J Emerg Med* 7:357, 1989.

13. Martin RR, Bickell WH, Pepe PE, et al: Prospective evaluation of preoperative fluid resuscitation in hypotensive patients with penetrating truncal injury: a preliminary report, *J Trauma* 33:354, 1992.

14. Kaweski SM, Sise MJ, Virgilio RW: The effect of prehospital fluids on survival in trauma patients, *J Trauma* 30:1215, 1990.

15. Gross D, Landau EH, Klin B, et al: Treatment of uncontrolled hemorrhagic shock with hypertonic saline solution, *Surg Gynecal Obstet* 170:106, 1990.

16. Deakin CD, Hicks IR: AB or ABC: prehospital fluid management in major trauma, *J Accid Emerg Med* 11:154, 1994.

17. Bickell WH, Bruttig SP, Millnamow GA, et al: Use of hypertonic saline/dextran versus lactated ringer's solution as a resuscitation fluid after uncontrolled aortic hemorrhage in anesthetized swine, *Ann Emerg Med* 21:1077, 1992.

18. Dontigny L: Small-volume resuscitation, *CJS* 35:31, 1992.

19. Krausz MM, Bar-Ziv M, Rabinovici R, et al: "Scoop and run" or stabilize hemorrhagic shock with normal saline or small-volume hypertonic saline? *J Trauma* 33:6, 1992.

20. Gross D, Landau EH, Assalia A, et al: Is hypertonic saline resuscitation safe in uncontrolled hemorrhagic shock? *J Trauma* 28:751, 1988.

21. Kowalenko J, Stern S, Dronen S, et al: Improved outcome with hypotensive resuscitation of uncontrolled hemorrhagic shock in a swine model, *J Trauma* 33:349, 1992.

22. Krausz MM, Klemm O, Amstislavsky T, et al: The effect of heat load and dehydration on hypertonic saline solution treatment on uncontrolled hemorrhagic shock, *J Trauma* 38:747, 1995.

23. Napolitano LM: Resuscitation following trauma and hemorrhagic shock: is hydroxyethyl starch safe? *Crit Care Med* 23:795, 1995.

24. Arishita GI, Vayer JS, Bellamy RF: Cervical spine immobilization of penetrating neck wounds in a hostile environment, *J Trauma* 29:332, 1989.

25. Zajtchuk R, Jenkins DP, Bellamy RF, et al, editors: *Combat casualty care guidelines for Operation Desert Storm*, Washington, DC, 1991, Office of the Army Surgeon General Publication.

26. Bellamy RF: How shall we train for combat casualty care? *Mil Med* 152:617, 1987.

27. Baker MS: Advanced Trauma Life Support: is it adequate stand-alone training for military medicine? *Mil Med* 159:587, 1994.

28. Wiedeman JE, Jennings SA: Applying ATLS to the Gulf War, *Mil Med* 158:121, 1993.

29. Heiskell LE, Carmona RH: Tactical emergency medical services: an emerging subspecialty of Emergency Medicine, *Ann Emerg Med* 23:778, 1994.

30. Ekblad GS: Training medics for the combat environment of tomorrow, *Mil Med* 155:232, 1990.

31. Butler FK, Hagmann J, Butler EG: Tactical combat casualty care in special operations, *Mil Med* 161(Supplement): 1, 1996.

32. McSwain N, editor: Military medicine. *Prehospital Trauma Life Support*, ed 4, St Louis, 1999, Mosby, pp 316-331.

33. *Practice guidelines for wilderness medical emergencies*. Indianapolis, 1995, Wilderness Medical Society.

34. Commander, Naval Special Warfare Command letter of 29 May 1997.

35. Maughon JS: An inquiry into the nature of wounds resulting in killed in action in Vietnam, *Mil Med* 135:8, 1970.

36. Mabry RL, Holcomb JB, Baker A, et al: US Army Rangers in Somalia: an analysis of combat casualties on an urban battlefield, *J Trauma* 49:515, 2000.

37. Lakstein D, Blumenfeld A, Sokolov T, et al: Tourniquets for hemorrhage control in the battlefield—a four year accumulated experience, accepted for publication, *J Trauma*.

38. Calkins MD, Snow C, Costello M, Bentley TB: Evaluation of possible battlefield tourniquet systems for the far-forward setting. *Mil Med* 165:379, 2000.

39. Sondean JL, Pusateri AE, Coppes VG, et al: Comparison of ten different hemostatic dressings in an aortic injury. Accepted for publication, *J Trauma*.

40. Alam HB, Gemma B, Miller D, et al: Comparative analysis of hemostatic agents in a swine model of lethal extremity injury, accepted for publication, *J Trauma*.

41. Pusateri AE, Wright J: United States Army Institute of Surgical Research, unpublished data.

42. Reference deleted in proof.

43. Pusateri AE, McCarthy SJ, Gregory KW, et al. Effect of a Chitosan-based hemostatic dressing on blood loss and survival in a model of severe venous hemorrhage and hepatic injury in swine, accepted for publication, *J Trauma*.

44. Martinowitz U, Kenet G, Segal E, et al: Recombinant activated factor VII for adjunctive hemorrhage control in trauma, *J Trauma* 51:431, 2001.

45. Carey ME: Analysis of wounds incurred by U.S. Army Seventh Corps personnel treated in corps hospitals during Operation Desert Storm, February 20 to March 10, 1991, *J Trauma* 40: S165, 1996.

46. Butler FK, Hagmann JH, et al: Tactical management of urban warfare casualties in special operations, *Mil Med* 165 (4, supp: 1-48), 2000.

47. Sladen A: Emergency endotracheal intubation: who can—who should? *Chest* 75:535, 1979.

48. Stewart RD, Paris PM, Winter PM, et al: Field endotracheal intubation by paramedical personnel: success rates and complications, *Chest* 85:341, 1984.

49. Jacobs LM, Berrizbeitia LD, Bennet B, et al: Endotracheal intubation in the prehospital phase of emergency medical care, *JAMA* 250:2175, 1983.

50. Pointer JE: Clinical characteristics of paramedics' performance of endotracheal intubation, *J Emerg Med* 6:505, 1988.

51. Lavery RF, Doran J, Tortella, BJ, et al: A survey of advanced life support practices in the United States, *Prehosp Disaster Med* 7:144, 1992.

52. DeLeo BC: Endotracheal intubation by rescue squad personnel, *Heart Lung* 6:851, 1977.

53. Stratton SJ, Kane G, Gunter CS, et al: Prospective study of manikin-only versus manikin and human subject endotracheal intubation training of paramedics, *Ann Emerg Med* 20:1314, 1991.

54. Trooskin SZ, Rabinowitz S, Eldridge C, et al: Teaching endotracheal intubation using animals and cadavers, *Prehosp Disaster Med* 7:179, 1992.

55. Stewart RD, Paris PM, Pelton GH, et al: Effect of varied training techniques on field endotracheal intubation success rates, *Ann Emerg Med* 13:1032, 1984.

56. Cameron PA, Flett K, Kaan E, et al: Helicopter retrieval of primary trauma patients by a paramedic helicopter service, *Aust NZ J Surg* 63:790, 1993.

57. Reinhart DJ, Simmons G: Comparison of placement of the laryngeal mask airway with endotracheal tube by paramedics and respiratory therapists, *Ann Emerg Med* 24:260, 1994.

58. Sayre MR, Sakles JC, Mistler AF, et al: Field trial of endotracheal intubations by basic EMTs, *Ann Emerg Med* 31:228, 1998.

59. Katz SH, Falk JL: Misplaced endotracheal tubes by paramedics in an urban emergency medical services system, *Ann Emerg Med* 37:32, 2001.

60. Calkins MD, Robinson TD: Combat trauma airway management: endotracheal intubation versus laryngeal mask airway versus combitube use by SEAL and reconnaissance combat corpsmen, *J Trauma* 46:927, 1999.

61. Murray JA, Demetriades D, Berne TV, et al: Prehospital intubation in patients with severe head injury, *J Trauma* 49:1065, 2000.

62. Salvino CK, Dries D, Gamelli R, et al: Emergency cricothyroidotomy in trauma victims, *J Trauma* 34:503, 1993.

63. McGill J, Clinton JE, Ruiz E: Cricothyroidotomy in the emergency department, *Ann Emerg Med* 11:361, 1982.

64. Erlandson MJ, Clinton JE, Ruiz E, et al: Cricothyroidotomy in the emergency department revisited, *J Emerg Med* 7:115, 1989.

65. Mines D: Needle thoracostomy fails to detect a fatal tension pneumothorax, *Ann Emerg Med* 22:863, 1993.

66. Holcomb JB, Pusateri AE, Kerr SM, et al: Initial efficacy and function of needle thoracentesis versus tube thoracostomy in a swine model of traumatic tension pneumothorax, accepted for publication, *J Trauma*.

67. Britten S, Palmer SH, Snow TM: Needle thoracocentesis in tension pneumothorax: insufficient cannula length and potential failure, *Injury* 27(10):758, 1996.

68. Aeder MI, Crowe JP, Rhodes RS, et al: Technical limitations in the rapid infusion of intravenous fluids, *Ann Emerg Med* 14:307, 1985.

69. Hoelzer MF: Recent advances in intravenous therapy, *Emerg Med Clin North Am* 4:487, 1986.

70. Lawrence DW, Lauro AJ: Complications from IV therapy: results from field-started and emergency department-started IV's compared, *Ann Emerg Med* 17:314, 1988.

71. Kramer GC, Perron PR, Lindsey DC, et al: Small volume resuscitation with hypertonic saline dextran solution, *Surgery* 100:239, 1986.

72. Shaftan GW, Chiu C, Dennis C, et al: Fundamentals of physiological control of arterial hemorrhage, *Surgery* 58:851, 1965.

73. Milles G, Koucky CJ, Zacheis HG: Experimental uncontrolled arterial hemorrhage, *Surgery* 60:434, 1966.

74. Krausz MM, Horne Y, Gross D: The combined effect of small-volume hypertonic saline and normal saline in uncontrolled hemorrhagic shock, *Surg Gynecol Obstet* 174:363, 1992.

75. Sindlinger JF, Soucy DM, Greene SP, et al: The effects of isotonic saline volume resuscitation in uncontrolled hemorrhage, *Surg Gynecol Obstet* 177:545, 1993.

76. Landau EH, Gross D, Assalia A, et al: Treatment of uncontrolled hemorrhagic shock by hypertonic saline and external counterpressure, *Ann Emerg Med* 18:1039, 1989.

77. Rabinovici R, Krausz MM, Feurstein G: Control of bleeding is essential for a successful treatment of hemorrhagic shock with 7.5 percent NaCl solution, *Surg Gynecol Obstet* 173:98, 1991.

78. Landau EH, Gross D, Assalia A, et al: Hypertonic saline infusion in hemorrhagic shock treated by military anti-shock trousers (MAST) in awake sheep, *Crit Care Med* 21:1554, 1993.

79. Crawford ES: Ruptured abdominal aortic aneurysm: an editorial, *J Vasc Surg* 13:348, 1991.

80. Wall M: AAST presentation, 1994.

81. Rainey TG, Read CA: The pharmacology of colloids and crystalloids. In Baltimore CB, editor: *The pharmacologic approach to the critically ill patient,* Baltimore, 1988, Williams & Wilkens, pp 219-240.

82. Carey JS, Scharschmidt BF, Culliford AL, et al: Hemodynamic effectiveness of colloid and electrolyte solutions for replacement of simulated blood loss, *Surg Gynecol Obstet* 131:679, 1970.

83. Marino PL: Colloid and crystalloid resuscitation. In *The ICU Book,* Malvern PA, 1991, Lea & Febiger, pp 205-216.

84. Mortelmans Y, Merckx E, van Nerom C, et al: Effect of an equal volume replacement with 500 cc 6% hydroxyethyl starch on the blood and plasma volume of healthy volunteers, *Eur J Anesth.* 12:259, 1995.

85. Lucas CE, Denis R, Ledgerwood AM, et al: The effects of Hespan on serum and lymphatic albumin, globulin, and coagulant protein, *Ann Surg* 207:416, 1988.

86. Sanfelippo MJ, Suberviola PD, Geimer NF: Development of a von Willebrand-like syndrome after prolonged use of hydroxyethyl starch, *Am J Clin Pathol* 88:653, 1987.

87. Strauss RG: Review of the effects of hydroxyethyl starch on the blood coagulation system, *Transfusion* 21:299, 1981.

88. Dalrymple-Hay MB, Aitchison R, Collins P, et al: Hydroxyethyl starch-induced acquired von Willebrand's disease, *Clin Lab Haematol* 14:209, 1992.

89. Macintyre E, Mackie IJ, Ho D, et al: The haemostatic effects of hydroxyethyl starch (HES) used as a volume expander, *Intensive Care Med* 11:300, 1985.

90. Via D, Kaufman C, Anderson D, et al: Effect of hydroxyethyl starch on coagulopathy in a swine model of hemorrhagic shock resuscitation, *J Trauma* 50:1076, 2002.

91. Falk JL, O'Brien JF, Kerr R: Fluid resuscitation in traumatic hemorrhagic shock, *Crit Care Clin* 8(2):323, 1992.

92. Shatney CH, Krishnapradad D, Militello PR, et al: Efficacy of hetastarch in the resuscitation of patients with multisystem trauma and shock, *Arch Surg* 118:804, 1983.

93. Ratner LE, Smith GW: Intraoperative fluid management, *Surg Clin North Am* 73:229, 1993.

94. Champion HR: The Combat Fluid Resuscitation Conferences, accepted for publication, *J Trauma*.

95. Rhee P, Koustova E, Alam HB: Searching for the optimal resuscitation method: recommendations for the initial fluid resuscitation of combat casualties, accepted for publication, *J Trauma*.

96. Rhee P, Burris D, Kaufmann C, et al: Lactated ringer's resuscitation causes neutrophil activation after hemorrhagic shock, *J Trauma* 44:313, 1998.

97. Burris D, Rhee P, Kaufmann C, et al: Controlled resuscitation in uncontrolled hemorrhagic shock, *J Trauma* 46:216, 1998.

98. Deb S, Martin B, Sun L, et al: Lactated ringer's resuscitation in hemorrhagic shock rats induces immediate apoptosis, *J Trauma* 46:582, 1999.

99. Sun L, Ruff P, Austin B, et al: Early upregulation of ICAM-1 and VCAM-1 expression in rats with hemorrhagic shock and resuscitation, *Shock* 11:416, 1999.

100. Rhee P, Wang D, Ruff P, et al: Human neutrophil activation and increased adhesion by various resuscitation fluids, *Crit Care Med* 28:74, 2000.

101. Alam HB, Sun L, Deb S, et al: Increase in E and P selectin expression is immediate and depends on the fluid used for resuscitation in rats, 5th International Congress on Trauma, Shock, Inflammation and Sepsis, 2000, pp 331-335.

102. Alam HB, Austin B, Koustova E, Rhee P: Ketone Ringer's solution attenuates resuscitation induced apoptosis in rat lungs following hemorrhagic shock, 5th International Congress on Trauma, Shock, Inflammation and Sepsis, 2000, pp 63-66.

103. Deb S, Sun L, Martin B, et al: Resuscitation with Hetastarch and lactated Ringer's induces early apoptosis in the lung through the Bax protein following hemorrhagic shock, *J Trauma* 49:47, 2000.

104. Rhee P, Morris J, Durham R, et al: Ascending dose, parallel group, double-blind, placebo-controlled, dose finding study of rhu MAB CD18 in patients with traumatic hemorrhagic shock, *J Trauma* 49:611, 2000.

105. Alam HB, Austin B, Koustova E, Rhee P: Resuscitation induced pulmonary apoptosis and intracellular adhesion molecule-1 expression are attenuated by the use of ketone Ringer's solution in rats, *Surg Forum* LI:181, 2000.

106. Alam HB, Sun L, Ruff P, et al: E- and P-selectin expression depends on the resuscitation fluid used in hemorrhaged rats, *J Surg Res* 94:145, 2000.

107. Alam HB, Austin B, Koustova E, Rhee P: Resuscitation induced pulmonary apoptosis and intracellular adhesion molecule-1 expression are attenuated by the use of ketone Ringer's solution in rats, *J Am Coll Surg* 193(3):255, 2001.

108. Lieberthal W, Fuhro R, Alam H, et al: Comparison of a 50% exchange-transfusion with albumin, hetastarch, and modified hemoglobin solutions, *Shock* 7:61-69, 2002.

109. Gushchin V, Stegalkina S, Alam HB, et al: Cytokine expression profiling in human leukocytes after exposure to hypertonic and isotonic fluids, *J Trauma* 52:867, 2002.

110. Koustova E, Stanton K, Gushchin V, et al: Effects of lactated Ringer's solutions on human leukocytes, *J Trauma* 52:872, 2002.

111. Alam HB, Stegalkina S, Rhee P, Koustova E: cDNA array analysis of gene expression following hemorrhagic shock and resuscitation in rats, *Resuscitation* 54(2):189, 2002.

112. Alam H, Koustova E, Stanton K, et al: Differential effects of various resuscitation fluids on neutrophil activation following hemorrhagic shock in swine, submitted to *Shock*.

113. Holcomb JB: Fluid resuscitation in modern combat casualty care: lessons learned from Somalia, accepted for publication, *J Trauma*.

114. Beecher HK: The management of traumatic shock. In Beecher HK, editor: *Resuscitation and anesthesia for wounded men*, Springfield, IL, 1949, Banerstone House, pp 123-127.

115. Pearce FJ, Lyons WS: Logistics of parenteral fluids in battlefield resuscitation, *Mil Med* 164:653, 1999.

116. Gan TJ, Bennett-Guerrero E, Phillips-Bute B, et al: Hextend, a physiologically balanced plasma expander for large volume use in major surgery: a randomized phase III clinical trial, Hextend Study Group, *Anesth Analg* 88(5):992, 1999.

117. Nielsen VG, Tan S, Brix AE, et al: Hextend (hetastarch solution) decreases multiple organ injury and xanthine oxidase release after hepatoenteric ischemia-reperfusion in rabbits, *Crit Care Med* 25:1565, 1997.

118. Debakey ME: *Surgery in World War II: Vol II. General Surgery,* Washington, Dc, 1956, US Government Printing Office.

119. Churchill ED: *Surgeon to Soldiers.* Philadelphia, 1972, JB Lippincott.

120. Dubrick MA, Holcomb JB: A review of intraosseous vascular access: current status and military application, *Mil Med* 165:552, 2000.

121. Calkins MD, Fitzgerald G, Bentley TB, Burris D: Intraosseous infusion devices: a comparison for potential use in Special Operations, *J Trauma* 48:1068, 2000.

122. Manley G, Knudson MM, Morabito D, et al: Hypotension, hypoxia, and head injury, *Arch Surg* 136:1118, 2001.

123. Beecher HK: Pain in men wounded in battle, *Ann Surg* 123:96, 1946.

124. Buttar N, Wang K: The "aspirin" of the new millennium: cyclooxygenase-2 inhibitors. *Mayo Clin Proc* 75:1027, 2000.

125. McCrory C, Lindahl SGE: Cyclooxygenase inhibition for postoperative analgesia, *Anesth Analg* 95:169, 2002.

126. FDA: Pharmacia update Bextra label with new warnings. *FDA Talk Paper,* T02-43, Nov. 15, 2002.

127. *Physicians Drug Reference,* ed 56, 2002, Product information: Celebrex®; Contraindications. 2780-84.

128. O'Connor K, Butler FK: Antibiotics in tactical combat casualty care 2002, accepted for publication, *Mil Med.*

129. Walker RC: The fluoroquinolones, *Mayo Clin Proc* 74:1030, 1999.

130. Appelbaum PC: Quinolone activity against anaerobes, *Drugs* 58(Suppl 2):60, 1999.

131. *Mosby's GenRx,* ed 11, 2001; quoted on MD Consult website.

132. Hoellman DB, Kelly LM, Jacobs MR, Appelbaum PC: Comparative antianaerobic activity of BMS 284756, *Antimicrob Agents Chemother* 45:589, 2001.

133. Seciale A, Musumeci R, Blandino G, et al: Minimal inhibitory concentrations and time-kill determination of moxifloxacin against aerobic and anaerobic isolates, *Int J Antimicrob Agents* 19:111, 2002.

134. Mather R, Karenchak LM, Romanowski EG, Kowalski RP: Fourth generation fluoroquinolones: new weapons in the arsenal of ophthalmic antibiotics, *Am J Ophthalmol* 133:463, 2002.

135. Ackerman G, Schaumann R, Pless B, et al: Comparative activity of moxifloxacin in vitro against obligately anaerobic bacteria, *Eur J Clin Microbiol Infect Dis* 19:228, 2000.

136. Auerbach PS, Halstead B: Injuries from non-venomous aquatic animals. In Auerbach PS, editor: *Wilderness medicine,* ed 4, St Louis, 2001, Mosby, pp 1418-1449.

137. Brooks GF, Butel JS, Morse SA: Infections caused by anaerobic bacteria. In *Medical microbiology,* New York, 2001, Lange Medical Books, pp 268-269.

138. Dellinger EP, Oreskovich MR, Wertz MJ: Risk of infection following laparotomy for penetrating abdominal injury, *Arch Surg* 119:20, 1984.

139. O'Connor K: War wound prophylaxis, Special Operations Medical Association Presentation, December, 2000.

140. Osmon DR: Antimicrobial prophylaxis in adults, *Mayo Clinic Proc* 75:98, 2000.

141. Conte JE: Manual of antibiotics and infectious diseases, ed 8, Baltimore, 1995, Williams & Wilkins.

142. Luchette FA, Borzotta AP, Croce MA, et al: Practice management guidelines for prophylactic antibiotic use in penetrating abdominal trauma: the EAST practice management guidelines work group, *J Trauma* 48:508, 2000.

143. Nichols RL, Smith JW, Klein DB, et al: Risk of infection after penetrating abdominal trauma, *N Engl J Med* 311:1065, 1984.

144. Jones RC, Thal ER, Johnson NA, Gollihar LN: Evaluation of antibiotic therapy following penetrating abdominal trauma, *Ann Surg* 201:576, 1985.

145. Fabian TC, Croce MA, Payne LW, et al: Duration of antibiotic therapy for penetrating abdominal trauma: a prospective trial, *Surgery* 112:788, 1992.

146. Battistella FD, Nugent W, Owings JT, Anderson JT: Field triage of the pulseless trauma patient, *Arch Surg* 134:742, 1999.

147. Branney SW, Moore EE, Feldhaus KM, et al: Critical analysis of two decades of experience with postinjury emergency department thoracotomy in a regional trauma center, *J Trauma* 45:87, 1988.

148. Rosemurgy AS, Norris PA, Olson SM, et al: Prehospital cardiac arrest: the cost of futility, *J Trauma* 35:468, 1993.

149. Martin SE, Ochsner G, Jarman RH, et al: Use of the laryngeal mask airway in air transport when intubation fails, *J Trauma* 47:352, 1999.

150. Joo HS, Kapoor S, Rose DK, Naik VN: The intubating mask airway after induction of general anesthesia versus awake fiberoptic intubation in patients with difficult airways, *Anesth Analg* 92:1342, 2001.

151. Blostein PA, Koestner AJ, Hoak S: Failed rapid sequence intubation in trauma patients: esophageal tracheal combitube is a useful adjunct, *J Trauma* 44:534, 1998.

152. Schwartz RB, Gillis WL, Miles RJ: Orotracheal intubation in darkness using night vision goggles, *Mil Med* 166:984, 2001.

153. Fortune JB, Judkins DG, Scanzaroli D, et al: Efficacy of prehospital surgical cricothyrotomy in trauma patients, *J Trauma* 42: 832, 1997.

154. Barkana Y, Stein M, Maor R, et al: Prehospital blood transfusion in prolonged evacuation, *J Trauma* 46:176, 1999.

155. Holcomb JB, Pusateri A, Harris RA, et al: Dry fibrin sealant dressings reduce blood loss, resuscitation volume, and improve survival in hypothermic coagulopathic swine with Grade V liver injuries, *J Trauma* 47:233, 1999.

156. Butler FK, Smith DJ, editors: *Tactical management of diving casualties in special operations,* Bethesda, 1998, Undersea and Hyperbaric Medical Society Workshop Report.

157. Butler FK, Zafren K, editors: Tactical management of wilderness casualties in special operations, *Wilderness Environ Med* 9:62, 1998.

158. Richards TR: Commander, Naval Special Warfare Command letter 1500 Ser 04/0341, 9 April 1997.

159. Allen RC, McAtee JM: Pararescue medications and procedures manual, *Air Force Special Operations Command Publication,* January 1999.

160. Krausz MM: Resuscitation strategies in the Israeli Army, presentation to the Institute of Medicine Committee on Fluid Resuscitation for Combat Casualties, 17 September 1998.

161. Pappas CG: The Ranger medic *Mil Med* 166(5):394, 2001.

162. Malish RG: The preparation of a Special Forces company for pilot recovery, *Mil Med* 164:881, 1999.

163. De Lorenzo RA: Medic for the millennium: the U.S. Army 91W health care specialist, *Mil Med* 166(8):685, 2001.

164. Naevin J, Dunn RLR: The Combat Trauma Life Support Course: resource-constrained first responder trauma care for special forces medics, *Mil Med* 167:566, 2002.

165. Butler FK: Tactical medicine training for SEAL mission commanders, *Mil Med* 166(7):625, 2001.

166. Bowden M: Blackhawk down, New York, 1999, Atlantic Monthly Press.

167. McRaven W: Spec Ops—Case studies in Special Operations warfare: theory and practice. Novato, CA, 1995, Presidio Press.

Acknowledgments

The authors express their appreciation to the many individuals, both military and civilian, who have assisted with this project. Special thanks are also extended to the Special Operations corpsmen, PJs, and medics who will risk their lives in future conflicts while using these guidelines to save their wounded teammates.

Thanks also to the Naval Operational Medical Institute that conducted this research effort, the U.S. Special Operations Command Biomedical Initiatives Steering Committee for its sponsorship of the COTCCC in 2002/2003, and the Navy Bureau of Medicine and Surgery for its planned future sponsorship of this effort.

THE COMMITTEE ON TACTICAL COMBAT CASUALTY CARE: 2002 U.S. SPECIAL OPERATIONS COMMAND/U.S. NAVY BUREAU OF MEDICINE AND SURGERY

Chairman–CAPT Stephen Giebner
COL Robert Allen
COL Frank Anders
CAPT Steve Anderson
COL James Bagian
COL Ron Bellamy
1LT Bart Bullock
CAPT Frank Butler
Dr. Howard Champion
TSGT George Cum
CAPT Roger Edwards
LTC Stephen Flaherty
CDR Scott Flinn
MAJ John Gandy
CDR Jeff Timby
HMCM Gary Welt

CAPT Larry Garsha
COL John Holcomb
Dr. David Hoyt
LTC Donald Jenkins
COL Jay Johannigman
MSG John Kennedy
CPT Robert Mabry
Dr. Norman McSwain
SFC Robert Miller
MAJ Kevin O'Connor
CAPT Edward Otten
LTC Tyler Putnam
CDR Peter Rhee
CAPT Larry Roberts
Executive Assistants:
  LT David Anderson,
  Ms. Shannon Addison

Appendix

Patient Care Beyond the Golden Period

A common assumption is that delayed transportation applies only to rural regions; however, this is not always the case. Transportation can also be prolonged in an urban service (e.g., bad weather, heavy traffic, etc.). In many instances the patient does not arrive at the hospital within the Golden Period. Some of the situations are specific to extrication and some are specific to transportation, but most involve both. Transport may not be delayed for hours, but if a prehospital crew has a 45-minute extrication time and are delayed en route to the medical facility, delivery of a patient may take over an hour. No one is immune to delays in transport.

Prolonged Extrication

Prolonged extrication can refer to a period of time from 10 minutes up until the patient is actually extricated. Situations include extrication from a vehicle, out of a hotel room, out of a tall building, out of a sports stadium, or out of a house around which the house itself or stairs inside the house are difficult to maneuver. For example, it may take a long time to extricate a patient with a fractured hip who is wedged between the tub and the toilet. Spine precautions should be taken with the patient while maneuvering him or her down three flights of stairs. Extricating a patient from a hotel room when the hotel does not have a service elevator and the only elevator is 5 feet by 5 feet can also prove difficult. A standard long backboard and stretcher do not fit within this space. More than two people may be required to extricate a patient, and the crew may have to wait for backup. A wooden long backboard can break while CPR is being performed. All of these instances can delay extrication and a patient's arrival at the receiving facility.

The primary concern when caring for any patient is to "do no further harm." Thus keeping the patient safe on an extrication scene is of utmost importance. Regardless of the number of people on the scene, the patient is the most important person and must be kept safe in the middle of the machinery, generators, noise, and personnel. The patient should be covered with blankets to prevent shards of glass and metal from causing further injury. Extra straps and tape should be used to secure the patient to the extrication device to ensure that the patient will not move or fall out of the device. The safest and easiest extrication device for each individual patient should be chosen; what may be the best for one patient may not be the best for another. Multiple extrication baskets, boards, and chairs are available on the market. A provider should use the one most familiar, easiest to use, and safest to accommodate the patient.

On an extrication scene with so many people, advice, and machinery, it is easy to forget why the teams are at the scene. A patient or patients who have been involved in horrible and frightening experience are at the center of every situation. *Do not forget about the patient.* The patient should be told when a loud noise will occur or if movement may be felt. One person on the extrication team should only talk to and inform the patient about what is going on in the environment. This is a good time to elicit the patient's history and complete as much of the primary and secondary surveys as possible.

Prolonged Transportation

Prolonged transportation is defined as transportation from the scene to the closest appropriate facility that takes longer than 10 to 15 minutes. Transportation time can be much longer, taking 45 minutes to 1 hour before arriving at an emergency department; occasionally transport times can take 2 to 3 hours. In the Australian Outback, initial transport times can be up to 48 hours; this is an extreme example, but it does occur. The prehospital care provider may be able to rendezvous with an advanced life support unit or helicopter en route and transfer patient care; the responding unit may never see the receiving facility. Delayed transportation includes a host of problems, some of which are discussed in the following section.

Managing Prolonged Patient Care

For whatever reason that transportation is delayed or prolonged, the principles of patient care remain the same. The medical priorities do not change.

Any prehospital care provider can observe that a patient is in shock when his or her blood pressure is at

50 mm Hg. However, an astute provider observes that the patient is going to go into shock when he or she gets tachypneic. The body accumulates carbon dioxide with decreased energy production. Chemoreceptors interpret this and send a signal to increase the ventilatory rate. During prolonged transport, it is important to prevent a descending cascade of events from occurring through early intervention. Prolonged transport is more stressful and requires the provider to think more, concentrate more, and pay more attention to subtle signs.

During a prolonged transport situation, there is an opportunity to conduct the primary and secondary surveys in detail and repeat the primary survey to reevaluate the patient. For that reason, the steps in management of a prolonged transport are the same as the steps in the initial primary survey with emphasis on those things most likely to occur in a prolonged transport situation.

AIRWAY

Brain Injury. The Advanced Trauma Life Support (ATLS®) standard for intubating a patient is a Glasgow Coma Scale (GCS) score of 8 or less. However, this does not mean that the patient with a GCS score of 10 is not going to have a GCS score of 8 in 15 minutes and require intubation. A mental status with a change in the GCS score from 12 to 11 to 10 should alert a prehospital care provider that the patient is deteriorating. The most likely reason for deterioration with a brain injury is brain swelling, which is a result of hypoxia. Hypoxia, produced by incomplete or inadequate ventilation or decreased perfusion, makes a brain injury worse (see Chapter 8).

The response to a deteriorating mental status is aggressive ventilation and oxygenation. Based on the Fick Principle, the most important step is to ensure that the red blood cells (RBCs) are adequately oxygenated in the lungs. The second step is to ensure that adequate perfusion exists to deliver these RBCs to the brain.

Difficult Intubation. Intubation is not normally a difficult skill in controlled circumstances. Accomplishment of intubation requires practice, knowledge of anatomy, and visualization of the vocal cords. The most important part of intubation is visualization of the endotracheal tube passing through the vocal cords, which can be incredibly difficult in some situations. Each intubation is unique; therefore the PHTLS program teaches how to intubate a patient using several different techniques. In trauma, intubation has only two rules:

1. Maintain cervical spine stabilization, if indicated.
2. Visualize the tube passing through the vocal cords.

After intubation, the position of the tube should be checked by use of both clinical assessments and adjunctive devices (see Chapter 4). These checks should be repeated after the tube is secured, each time the patient is moved, every 5 minutes during transport, and anytime there is concern that things "just don't look right."

BREATHING

A patient with significant blunt trauma to the chest may have, in addition to any fractured ribs apparent on physical examination, an associated pulmonary contusion or pneumothorax.

A pulmonary contusion is a bruised segment of the lung. Pulmonary contusion results from blood clogging the alveoli or an injury that produces edema in the wall between the alveolus and the capillary. The associated decrease in oxygenation that can occur can be managed en route to the receiving facility. This is achieved by increasing the end-expiratory pressure after ventilation. An in-depth analysis of the physiology is beyond the scope of the PHTLS course; however, understanding and being able to use positive end-expiratory pressure (PEEP) in prolonged transport is important.

A simple pneumothorax under continuous positive-pressure ventilation can easily convert into a tension pneumothorax that requires decompression. Therefore on prolonged transports when a patient does require ventilatory support, breath sounds on each side of the lungs should be listened to frequently. If breath sounds decrease on one side and ventilatory compliance decreases, a tension pneumothorax may be present and the steps of decompression should be initiated.

Prolonged transports also require an oxygen concentration as close to 100% (FiO_2 of 1.0) as possible throughout. If a patient requires prolonged ventilation, a mechanical ventilator in the ambulance optimizes the ventilation of a patient en route.

CIRCULATION

As noted in Chapter 3, circulation is divided into two components:

1. Stopping of ongoing hemorrhage
2. Oxygen delivery via the RBCs to the tissue (perfusion)

Ongoing hemorrhage is a major concern during prolonged transport. External hemorrhage can usually be visualized and controlled by use of pressure dressings. Because internal hemorrhage is deep to the skin, it cannot be visualized and direct pressure cannot be applied to it. Assessment of ongoing hemorrhage should be gauged by the body's response, including tachypnea, tachycardia, falling blood pressure, and distention. Distention can be swelling of the abdominal cavity or swelling of the part involved with hemorrhage, such as the thigh.

Temporary management of internal hemorrhage during prolonged transport can involve indirect pressure, such as with an air splint on an extremity or with a pneumatic antishock garment (PASG) on the abdomen.

For prolonged transport, the patient's ventilatory rate, pulse rate, and blood pressure should be assessed. However, to completely assess perfusion, urinary output should also be measured and monitored and insertion of a urinary catheter may be necessary. Decreased perfusion of oxygenated blood should be managed by fluid replacement using a crystalloid solution (preferably lactated Ringer's) and blood if available. A deteriorating patient with ongoing hemorrhage is an indication to rendezvous with a helicopter for more rapid transport to a trauma center.

Hemorrhage control may be one of the most difficult aspects of prolonged transportation. The best place to control bleeding is the operating room (OR). If that option is not available, the prehospital care provider should use direct pressure, elevation, and pressure points. For lower-extremity bleeding, a PASG can provide direct pressure. Manual holding of direct pressure can tie up one provider, preventing him or her from performing other skills. However, gross hemorrhage is a life-threatening injury that must be managed in the primary survey. The number of IV sites and the amount of IV fluid that has been given do not matter if it is escaping through a wound that has not clotted.

Difficult IV Access and Choice of IV Fluids. IV access can be difficult to initiate and typically is most challenging when the IV is needed the most. In trauma, the rules for IV access are as follows:

- Choose the closest available vein to the heart (use the arm and not the leg if both are accessible).
- Use the largest-bore catheter that the vein can accommodate (a 14-gauge catheter is large enough to deliver fluids quickly).
- Keep the catheter pointed toward the heart (do not initiate an IV pointing distal to the extremity). If the external jugular is the vein chosen to initiate the IV, point the IV toward the heart, not the head.
- If possible, access two IV sites, preferably bilaterally and not both in one extremity.

Lactated Ringer's solution contains calcium as one of the electrolytes in the fluid, whereas normal saline does not. Inside a bag of donated blood is a substance that impedes the clotting cascade so the blood does not clot. If blood and lactated Ringer's solution that contains calcium are administered through the same line, the clotting cascade will be initiated and blood will clot in the tubing. For this reason, only normal saline can be infused with blood at the same IV site.

The IV fluid of choice in trauma is lactated Ringer's solution unless blood will also be hung; in this case, normal saline should be used. If two IV sites are used, one should be used to initiate blood and normal saline and the other to continue administration of lactated Ringer's solution.

DISABILITY

Assessment of a patient's neurologic status to identify deterioration is important. Continuously monitoring vital signs and other components of the primary survey while en route is also important. Assessment of vital signs at least every 5 minutes is imperative.

EXPOSE/ENVIRONMENT

A patient's energy production may be compromised by ongoing hemorrhage and the beginning of shock; therefore the patient's body temperature should be preserved as much as possible. The patient should be kept warm by giving warm IV fluids, keeping the patient compartment warm, keeping the patient covered with blankets, and using heaters. IV bags can be placed over a vent in the ambulance for a few minutes with the heater of the unit on to raise the temperature in the bag before initiating fluid. Extremities with the IV sites should be kept warm by covering them with a blanket.

SPECIAL CONSIDERATIONS

Pressure Ulcers. Pressure ulcers are not normally associated with prehospital care; however, on extended trips, with the patient lying supine on a long backboard in the same position for a long period of time, pressure wounds are an issue. Pressure ulcers develop as a result of unrelieved pressure to a specific area or region of the body, usually the sacrum. Incontinent patients are at a greater risk of developing these pressure sores. If a patient is properly immobilized, he or she should not be able to shift his or her weight to relieve the pressure. Also, an ambulance is not built for comfort. Because the unit is large and top heavy, the ride is usually bumpy. If the EMS crew knows that the patient will be secured to a long-board with an extended transport time in the back of a bumpy unit, they should take precautions, such as padding the patient's bony prominences as much as possible without compromising spinal immobilization. As little as 2 hours with constantly applied pressure can lead to oxygen deprivation to an area, and the resulting accumulation of metabolic by-products can produce irreversible tissue damage. Padding can decrease the likelihood of this condition.

Pain Management. Pain management on extended transports is important. An EMS system should develop local protocols to address this issue. A patient in pain will have an elevated heart rate and blood pressure. In this situation, the patient's pain should be treated in addition to the injuries; however, some pain medication will cause vasodilatation, so this action may not be desirable. Patients who are in compensated hypovolemic shock are much more susceptible to hypotension from the administration of intravenous narcotics.

Extremity Injuries. Extremities can be placed in strange positions after trauma and can by themselves pose problems with extrication. Extremities can be lodged in machinery, such as a grinder, axle, or escalator. Extremities can also be trapped under or within items such as stairs, trains, vehicles, motorcycles, or chains. Entrapped extremities that must be extricated introduce a different realm of trauma and thought process. Extremities that are trapped (versus extremities that are trapped and amputated or trapped and shredded) are usually without a blood supply and thus oxygen supply. Therefore no matter what kind of metabolism the rest of the body is using (aerobic versus anaerobic), that extremity is using anaerobic metabolism because of the lack of oxygen. For example, one of the main complications of a fractured femur is compartment syndrome. Compartment syndrome is a complication that may become apparent during prolonged transport. This syndrome can develop within 6 hours of injury and can cut off circulation distal to the fracture.

Compartment Syndrome. Compartment syndrome occurs when a structure in an enclosed space is deprived of blood supply because the vessels have been compressed to the point where they cannot supply adequate oxygen to prevent anaerobic metabolism. Any space-occupying mass in a closed compartment in the extremity, such as a large hematoma, reduces the amount of space that can be occupied by other things. The most common result is a reduction in the size of the arteries, capillaries, and veins. This reduction of blood flow reduces the amount of oxygen delivered to the cells, produces ischemia, and leads to anaerobic metabolism. This causes the cells to swell, which further increases the pressure inside the space and further reduces blood flow. The ischemia and anaerobic metabolism worsen, which leads to more swelling and more pressure. At some point in this process the cells begin to die. This condition is cyclic, and if it is not recognized and corrected, it can be an emergent situation. Compartment syndrome also compromises the tissue distal to the injury because the distal tissue does not receive the nutrients it requires.

Any injury to an extremity has the potential to cause compartment syndrome. Signs and symptoms of compartment syndrome include the following:

- Pain greater than expected that typically increases by passive stretching of the involved muscles
- Decreased sensation or functional loss of the nerves distal to the injury
- Tense swelling of the involved area.

The most important signs for the prehospital care provider to assess are the six P's—*pain*, *pulselessness*, *paralysis*, *paresthesia*, *pallor*, and *puffiness*. Since nerves are the most sensitive part of the body, one of the first signs of compartment syndrome is paresthesia of the web space. The web space is the space between the thumb and the first finger and the space between the first and second toes. If a patient has no feeling in this space, compartment syndrome should be suspected. Weakness or paralysis of involved muscles and loss of pulses in the affected extremity are late signs of compartment syndrome.

Compartment syndrome can be definitively managed only in the hospital. In the field it should be managed like a fracture. The position in which the patient was found and the presence or absence of pulses, movement, sensation, and color should be reported to the receiving facility and properly documented on the run report.

Myoglobinuria. Patients who have extremities trapped often have crush injuries. One of the complications of a patient with this type of injury is myoglobinuria, which is defined as myoglobin from muscle tissue that is excreted in the urine. This complication would not be relevant to the prehospital provider except in the case of prolonged transportation. Myoglobinuria results from a loss of arterial blood flow, therefore loss of oxygen to the distal extremity, and therefore ischemia and death of skeletal muscle cells. When skeletal muscle cells die, they lyse (rupture), releasing potassium and myoglobin.

Myoglobin is a large molecule that gives muscle its reddish color. Because of the anaerobic metabolism, lactic acids are being produced and are also released from the cell when it lyses. Although these conditions are not a risk factor during the entrapment period, once the extremity is no longer trapped, blood and oxygen are allowed to return to it, allowing by-products to circulate to the rest of the body. Lactic acid production leads to the body becoming acidotic, and the myoglobin release can lead to renal failure. Myoglobin is a large molecule; as it circulates through the body it can block the filtering system of the kidneys, producing acute renal failure.

Myoglobinuria can develop within 6 hours of injury. Treatments to prevent these conditions include increased IV fluids to perfuse the kidneys and administration of sodium bicarbonate to neutralize the acidosis. One sign of myoglobinuria is dark red or crimson-colored urine with a decreased urine output.

Other Considerations. Another condition of which the prehospital care provider should be aware during prolonged transport is the development of fat emboli. A crush injury that fractures bone can lead to fat droplets leaking out of the fracture site and entering the circulation. These droplets can potentially lodge in the pulmonary system. Signs include chest pain, shortness of breath, and a decreased oxygen saturation.

If an extremity appears as though it is almost completely severed from the body but is still trapped, a physician may be able to come to the scene and perform an amputation. Contacting medical control and painting a realistic picture of the scene and the amount of time it may take to extricate a patient may make this a viable option. Another option, if ordered by medical control, may be to bring packed RBCs to the scene to start replacing blood products. In general, blood must be used and completely infused within 4 hours of leaving the blood bank; therefore initiation of blood products should not be delayed once they have arrived at the scene.

Answer Key

Chapter 1

1. a
2. c
3. d
4. a
5. d
6. d

Chapter 2

1. c
2. a
3. b
4. b
5. d
6. a
7. c
8. a
9. d
10. d

Chapter 3

1. c
2. d
3. d
4. a
5. c
6. d
7. a
8. d
9. a

Chapter 4

1. c
2. d
3. a
4. a
5. b

6. a
7. b

Chapter 5

1. a
2. c
3. d
4. a
5. d
6. a
7. c
8. c
9. b
10. a

Chapter 6

1. b
2. c
3. d
4. c
5. c
6. a
7. b
8. a
9. a
10. d

Chapter 7

1. b
2. d
3. a
4. d
5. a

Chapter 8

1. a
2. d

3. d
4. b
5. d
6. a
7. a
8. c

Chapter 9

1. b
2. d
3. a
4. d
5. c

Chapter 10

1. c
2. b
3. e
4. d
5. d

Chapter 11

1. a
2. c
3. a
4. b
5. c
6. a
7. d
8. a
9. b

Chapter 12

1. d
2. d
3. b
4. b

5. a
6. c

Chapter 13

1. c
2. a
3. d
4. d
5. c
6. b

Chapter 14

1. d
2. d
3. b
4. c
5. d

Chapter 16

1. c
2. a
3. c
4. c
5. d

Glossary

accelerated motion A sudden surge or increase in motion, e.g., from the transferring of motion in a rear-impact collision; occurs as a slower moving or stationary object is struck from behind.

acetabulum The cup-shaped hip socket on the lateral surface of the pelvis that holds the head of the femur.

acidosis Accumulation of acids and decreased pH of the blood.

adolescent A child with the body size and physical development normally found in children between 13 and 16 years of age. An arbitrary grouping of older children based on the similar physical characteristics common to these near-adult ages.

acute respiratory distress syndrome (ARDS) Respiratory insufficiency as a result of damage to the lining of the capillaries in the lung, leading to the leakage of fluid into the interstitial spaces and alveoli.

acute tubular necrosis (ATN) Acute damage to the renal tubules, usually due to ischemia associated with shock.

adult A person (generally 16 years of age or older) whose body has reached maturity and has finished its progression through the phases of pediatric growth and development.

aerobic metabolism Oxygen-based metabolism that is the body's principal combustion process.

afterload The pressure against which the left ventricle must pump out (eject) blood with each beat.

air bags Bags that automatically inflate in front of the driver or passenger upon collision to cushion the impact. The bags absorb the energy slowly by increasing the body's stopping distance. These bags are only designed to cushion forward motion on the initial impact.

alveoli Where the respiratory system meets the circulatory system and gas exchange occurs.

Alzheimer's disease A form of brain disease commonly associated with premature senile dementia.

amnesia A loss of memory.

amputation A severed part or a part that is pathologically or surgically totally separated (removed) from the rest of the body.

anaerobic metabolism Metabolism not using oxygen.

anatomical splinting "Splinting" the body on a long backboard, in a supine position and securing the patient to the board.

angina (angina pectoris) A cramping, crushing midsternal chest pain caused by myocardial anoxia. It often radiates to either arm, most commonly the left, and is associated with a feeling of suffocation and impending death.

anisocoria Inequality of pupil size.

anterior cord syndrome A result of bony fragments or pressure on spinal arteries.

anterocaudad Forward and toward the feet.

anterograde amnesia Amnesia for events occurring after the precipitating trauma; inability to form new memories.

anticoagulant A substance or drug that prevents or delays coagulation or the forming of blood clots.

antihypertensive A drug that reduces high blood pressure (hypertension). Some drugs that increase urine production (diuretics) lower the blood pressure by decreasing blood fluid volume.

aortic tear Complete or partial tear of one or more layers of tissue of the aorta.

apnea An absence of spontaneous breathing.

arachnoid mater (arachnoid membrane) Spiderweb-like transparent membrane between the dura mater and the pia mater. The middle of the three meningeal membranes surrounding the brain.

ARDS See *acute respiratory distress syndrome*.

ataxic breathing Erratic breathing with no rhythm. Commonly associated with head injury and increased intracranial pressure.

atelectasis Collapse of alveoli or part of the lung.

atherosclerosis A narrowing of the blood vessels, a condition in which the inner layer of the artery wall thickens while fatty deposits build up within the artery.

atlas First cervical vertebra (C1); the skull perches upon it.

avulsion The ripping or tearing away of a part; a flap or partially separated tissue or part.

axis Second cervical vertebra (C2); its shape allows for the wide possible range of rotation of the head. Also, an imaginary line that passes through the center of the body.

bag-valve-mask (BVM) device Mechanical resuscitation device consisting of a self-inflating bag made of plastic or rubber and several one-way valves. Squeezing the bag results in positive-pressure ventilation through a mask or endotracheal tube. May be used with or without supplementary oxygen.

baroreceptor   A sensory nerve ending that is stimulated by changes in pressure. Baroreceptors are found in the walls of the atria of the heart, vena cava, aortic arch, and carotid sinus.

basilar skull fracture   Fracture to the floor of the cranium.

Battle's sign   Discoloration posterior and slightly inferior to the outer ears due to bleeding into the subcutaneous tissue caused by an occipital basilar skull fracture.

blunt trauma   Nonpenetrating trauma caused when there is a temporary cavity in the body caused by a rapidly moving object with a small frontal projection concentrating its energy in one area.

body surface area (BSA)   Outer surface of the body covered by the skin. Percentage of the body's total surface area represented by any body part. Used as one factor in determining size of a burn.

bradycardia   Pulse rate less than 60 beats per minute.

brain stem   The stemlike part of the brain that connects the cerebral hemispheres with the spinal cord.

bronchioles   The smaller divisions of the bronchial tubes.

Broselow Resuscitation Tape   A commercially available system for estimating pediatric medication dosing and equipment sizing based on patient length.

Brown-Séquard syndrome   Caused by penetrating injury and involves hemitransection of the spinal cord involving only one side of the cord.

capillaries   The smallest blood vessels. Minute blood vessels that are only one cell wide, allowing for diffusion and osmosis through the capillary walls.

capnography (end-tidal carbon dioxide)   A monitoring device that measures the partial pressure of carbon dioxide in a sample of gas. It can correlate very closely to the arterial partial pressure of carbon dioxide ($PaCO_2$).

cardiac output   The volume of blood pumped by the heart at each contraction (reported in liters per minute).

cardioaccelerator center   The brain center that activates the sympathetic response that increases the rate of the heart.

cardiogenic shock   Shock that results from failure of the heart's pumping activity; causes can be categorized as either intrinsic, a result of direct damage to the heart itself, or extrinsic, related to a problem outside the heart.

cardioinhibitory center   A part of the medulla that slows or inhibits the heart's activity.

cardiovascular   Referring to the combination of the heart and blood vessels.

cataract   Milky lens that blocks and distorts light entering the eye and blurs vision.

catecholamines   Group of chemicals produced by the body that work as important nerve transmitters. The main catecholamines made by the body are dopamine, epinephrine (also called adrenaline), and norepinephrine. They are part of the body's sympathetic defense mechanism used in preparing the body to act.

caudad   Toward the tail (coccyx).

cavitation   Forcing tissues of the body out of their normal position; to cause a temporary or permanent cavity (e.g., when the body is struck by a bullet, the acceleration of particles of tissue away from the missile produces an area of injury where the large temporary cavity occurs).

central cord syndrome   Usually occurs with hyperextension of the cervical area.

central neurogenic hyperventilation   Pathologic rapid and shallow ventilatory pattern associated with head injury and increased intracranial pressure.

cephalad   Toward the head (away from the tail).

cerebellum   A portion of the brain that lies dorsal to the medulla oblongata and is concerned with coordination of movement.

cerebral perfusion pressure   The difference between the mean arterial pressure (MAP) and the intracranial pressure (ICP).

cerebrospinal fluid (CSF)   A fluid found in the subarachnoid space and dural sheath; acts as a shock absorber, protecting the brain and spinal cord from jarring impact.

cerebrum   The largest part of the brain; responsible for the control of specific intellectual, sensory, and motor functions.

cervical flexion   Rotating the head forward or downward, causing bending of the neck.

cervical spine   The neck area of the spinal column containing seven vertebrae (C1–C7).

chemical burn   Burn that occurs when skin comes into contact with various caustic agents.

chemoreceptor cells   Cells that stimulate nerve impulses by reacting to chemical stimuli. Certain chemoreceptor cells control the ventilatory rate.

chemoreceptor   A sensory nerve ending that is stimulated by and reacts to certain chemical stimuli; located outside of the central nervous system. Chemoreceptors are found in the large arteries of the thorax and neck, the taste buds, and the olfactory cells of the nose.

Cheyne-Stokes breathing   Pathologic ventilatory pattern with periods of shallow, slow breathing increasing to rapid, deep breathing and then returning to shallow, slow breathing followed by a short apneic period. Commonly associated with traumatic brain injury and increased intracranial pressure.

chin lift   A way to open the airway of a patient with suspected cervical spine compromise. Adaptation of chin lift airway maneuver that includes manual immobilization of the head in a neutral in-line position.

cilia   Hair-like processes that propel foreign particles and mucus from the bronchi.

closed fracture   A fracture of a bone in which the skin is not interrupted.

coccygeal spine   The most caudad part of the spinal column; contains the three to five vertebrae that form the coccyx.

Colles' fracture   Fracture of the wrist. If the victim falls forward onto outstretched hands to break a fall, this may result in a silver fork deformity.

compartment syndrome   The ischemia and compromised circulation that can occur from vascular injury. The cellular edema produces increased pressure in a closed facial or bony compartment.

compensated shock   Inadequate peripheral perfusion as evidenced by signs of decreased organ perfusion but with normal blood pressure.

complete cord transection   All spinal tracts are interrupted, and all cord functions distal the site are lost.

complication   An added difficulty that occurs secondary to an injury, disease, or treatment. Also, disease or incident superimposed upon another without being specifically related yet affecting or modifying the prognosis of the original disease.

compression injuries   Injuries caused by severe crushing and squeezing forces; may occur to the external structure of the body or to the internal organs.

compression   Type of force involved in impacts resulting in a tissue, organ, or other body part being squeezed between two or more objects or body parts.

concussion   A diagnosis made when an injured patient shows an alteration in neurologic function, most commonly a loss of consciousness, and no intracranial abnormality is identified by computed tomography (CT) scan.

conduction   The transfer of heat between two objects in direct contact with each other.

consensual reflex   The reflexive constriction of one pupil when a strong light is introduced into the other eye. A lack of consensual reflex is considered a positive sign of brain injury or eye injury.

contracoup injury   An injury to parts of the brain located on the side opposite that of the primary injury.

contraindication   Any sign, symptom, clinical impression, condition, or circumstance indicating that a given treatment or course of treatment is inappropriate and therefore outside of accepted medical practice. Relative contraindication is usually considered as a contraindication but under special circumstances may be overruled by a physician as an accepted medical practice on a case-by-case basis.

contralateral   On the opposite side.

contusion   A bruise or bruising.

convection   The heating of water or air in contact with a body, removing that air (such as wind) or water, and then having to heat the new air or water that replaces what left.

cord compression   Pressure on the spinal cord caused by swelling, which may result in tissue ischemia and in some cases may require decompression to prevent a permanent loss of function.

cord concussion   Results from the temporary disruption of the spinal cord functions distal to the injury.

cord contusion   Bruising or bleeding into the spinal cord's tissue, which may also result in a temporary loss of cord functions distal to the injury.

cord laceration   Occurs when spinal cord tissue is torn or cut.

coup injury   An injury to the brain located on the same side as the point of impact.

cranial vault   The skull or cranium.

crepitus   Crackling sound made by bone ends grating together.

cyanosis   Blue coloring of skin, mucous membranes, or nail beds indicating unoxygenated hemoglobin and a lack of adequate oxygen levels in the blood; usually secondary to inadequate ventilation or decreased perfusion.

decerebrate posturing   Characteristic posture present in an individual with decerebrate rigidity. When a painful stimulus is introduced, the extremities are stiff and extended and the head is retracted. One of the forms of pathologic posturing (response) commonly associated with increased intracranial pressure.

decorticate posturing   A characteristic pathologic posture of a patient with increased intracranial pressure; when a painful stimulus is introduced, the patient is rigidly still with the back and lower extremities extended while the arms are flexed and fists clenched.

definitive care   Care that resolves the patient's illness or injury after a definitive diagnosis has been established. Clear and final care that is without question what the particular patient needs for his or her individual problem.

density   The number of particles in each given area of tissue.

dermis   Layer of skin just under the epidermis made up of a framework of connective tissues containing blood vessels, nerve endings, sebaceous glands, and sweat glands.

diaphragmatic rupture (diaphragmatic herniation)   A tearing or cutting of the diaphragm so that the abdominal and thoracic cavities are no longer separated, allowing abdominal contents to enter the thoracic cavity. Usually a result of increased intraabdominal pressure producing a tear in the diaphragm.

diaphyseal   Part of or affecting the shaft of a long bone.

diastole   Ventricular relaxation (ventricular filling).

diastolic blood pressure   The resting pressure between ventricular contractions measured in millimeters of mercury (mm Hg).

diffusion   The movement of solutes (substances dissolved in water) across a membrane.

distributive shock   Shock that occurs when the vascular container enlarges without a proportional increase in fluid volume.

Don Juan syndrome   The pattern that often occurs when victims fall or jump from a height and land on their feet. Bilateral calcaneus (heel bone) fractures are often associated with this syndrome. After the feet land and stop moving, the body is forced into flexion as the weight of the still-moving head, torso, and pelvis come to bear. This can cause compression fractures of the spinal column in the thoracic and lumbar areas.

down-and-under pathway   When a vehicle ceases its forward motion, the occupant usually continues to travel downward into the seat and forward into the dashboard or steering column.

dura mater   The outer membrane covering the spinal cord and brain; the outer of the three meningeal layers. Literally means "tough mother."

dural sheath   A fibrous membrane that covers the brain and continues down to the second sacral vertebra.

dysarthria   Difficulty speaking.

dysrhythmia (cardiac)   Abnormal, disordered, or disturbed rhythm of the heart.

ecchymosis   A bluish or purple irregularly formed spot or area resulting from a hemorrhagic area below the skin.

edema   A local or generalized condition in which some of the body tissues contain an excessive amount of fluid; generally includes swelling of the tissue.

edentulism   The absence of teeth.

electrolytes   Substances that separate into charged ions when dissolved in solution.

endotracheal intubation   Insertion of a large tube into the trachea for direct ventilation from outside of the body. The most desirable way of achieving definitive control of the airway in trauma patients.

epidermis   The outermost layer of the skin, which is made up entirely of epithelial cells with no blood vessels.

epidural hematoma   Arterial bleeding that collects between the skull and dura mater.

epidural space   Potential space between the dura mater surrounding the brain and the cranium. Contains the meningeal arteries.

epiphyseal   The end of the long bone.

escharotomy   A removal of sloughed tissue formed on the skin and underlying tissue of severely burned areas.

eucapnia   Normal blood carbon dioxide level.

evaporation   Change from liquid to vapor.

event phase   The phase that begins at the time of impact between one moving object and a second object. The occurrence of an incident.

evisceration   When a section of the intestine or other abdominal organ is displaced through an open wound and protrudes externally outside the abdominal cavity.

exsanguination   Total loss of blood volume, producing death.

external respiration   The transfer of oxygen molecules from the atmosphere to the blood.

fight-or-flight response   A defense response that the sympathetic nervous system produces that simultaneously causes the heart to beat faster and stronger, constricts the arteries to raise blood pressure, and increases the ventilatory rate.

Fio$_2$ Fraction of oxygen in inspired air stated as a decimal. An Fio$_2$ of 0.85 means that 85 hundredths or 85% of the inspired air is oxygen.

flail chest   A chest with an unstable segment produced by multiple ribs fractured in two or more places or including a fractured sternum.

flexion   A bending movement around a joint that decreases the angle between the bones at the joint. In the cervical region it is a forward bending motion of the head, bringing the chin nearer to the sternum.

foot-pounds of force   A measure of mechanical force brought to bear. Force equals mass times deceleration or acceleration.

foramen magnum   The opening at the base of the skull.

foramina   Small opening.

fracture   A broken bone. A simple fracture is closed without a tear or opening in the skin. An open fracture is one where the initial injury or bone end has produced an open wound at or near the fracture site. A comminuted fracture has one or more free-floating segments of disconnected bone.

frostbite   The actual freezing of body tissue as a result of exposure to freezing or below-freezing temperatures.

full-thickness (third-degree) burns   Burn to the epidermis, dermis, and subcutaneous tissue (possibly deeper). Skin may look charred or leathery and may be bleeding.

G force (gravitational force) Actual force of acceleration or deceleration or of centrifugal force.

gastric ventilation Air undesirably forced down the esophagus and into the stomach rather than into the lungs.

geriatric Dealing with aging and the diagnosis and treatment of injuries and diseases affecting the elderly.

Glasgow Coma Scale A scale for evaluating and quantifying level of consciousness or unconsciousness by determining the best responses to standardized stimuli of which the patient is capable.

global overview The simultaneous 15- to 30-second overview of the patient's condition. The global overview focuses on the patient's immediate ventilatory, circulatory, and neurologic status.

Golden Period The period of time a patient has to reach definitive care to achieve the best possible outcome.

heat cramps Acute painful spasms of the voluntary muscles after hard physical work in a hot environment, especially when not acclimated to the temperature.

heat exhaustion Results from excessive fluid and electrolyte loss through sweating and lack of adequate fluid replacement when the patient is exposed to high environmental temperatures for a sustained period of time, usually several days.

heat stress index The combination of ambient temperature and relative humidity.

heat stroke An acute and dangerous reaction to heat exposure characterized by high body temperature.

hematocrit A measure of the packed cell volume of red blood cells in the total blood volume.

hemianesthesia Loss of sensation on one side of the body.

hemiparesis Weakness limited to one side of the body.

hemiplegia Paralysis on one side of the body.

hemoglobin The molecule found in red blood cells that carry oxygen.

hemopericardium Blood accumulation inside the pericardial space that can lead to pericardial tamponade.

hemorrhage Bleeding. Also, a loss of a large amount of blood in a short period of time, either outside or inside the body.

hemothorax Blood in the pleural space.

homeostasis A constant, stable internal environment. Balance necessary for healthy life processes.

hypercarbia Increased level of carbon dioxide in the body.

hyperchloremia Increase in the blood chloride level.

hyperextension Extreme or abnormal extension. A position of maximum extension. Hyperextension of the neck is produced when the head is extended posterior to a neutral position and can result in a fracture or dislocation of the vertebrae or in spinal cord damage in patients with an unstable spine.

hyperflexion Extreme or abnormal flexion. A position of maximum flexion. Increased flexion of the neck can result in a fracture or dislocation of the vertebrae or in spinal cord damage in patients with an unstable spine.

hyperkalemia Increased blood potassium.

hypertension Having a blood pressure greater than the upper limits of the normal range. Generally considered to exist if the patient's systolic pressure is greater than 150 mm Hg.

hypertensive crisis A sudden severe increase in blood pressure exceeding 200/120 mm Hg.

hyperthermia Body temperature much higher than normal range.

hypertonic Osmotic pressure greater than serum or plasma.

hypoglycemia Decreased blood glucose.

hypoperfusion Inadequate perfusion (bathing) of cells with properly oxygenated blood.

hypopharynx The lower portion of the pharynx that opens into the larynx anteriorly and the esophagus posteriorly.

hypotension Blood pressure below normal acceptable range.

hypothenar eminence Fleshy part of the palm along the ulnar margin.

hypothermia Subnormal core body temperature below normal range, usually between 78° and 90° F (26° and 32° C).

hypotonic A solution of lower osmotic pressure than another. Also, having a lower osmotic pressure than normal serum or plasma.

hypovolemia Inadequate (below normal range) fluid blood volume.

hypovolemic shock Shock caused by loss of blood.

hypoxia (hypoxemia) Deficiency of oxygen. Inadequate available oxygen. Lack of adequate oxygenation of the lungs due to inadequate minute volume (air exchange in the lungs) or a decreased concentration of oxygen in the inspired air. Cellular hypoxia is inadequate oxygen available to the cells.

immune system A related group of responses of various body organs that protects the body from disease organisms, other foreign bodies, and cancers. The main components of the immune response system are the bone marrow, thymus, lymphoid tissues, spleen, and liver.

incisura (tentorial incisura) Opening in the tentorium cerebelli at the junction of the midbrain and the cerebrum. The brain stem is inferior to the incisura.

incomplete cord transection Transection of the spinal cord in which some tracts and motor/sensory functions remain intact.

infant A child between 7 weeks and 1 year of age.

injury A harmful event that arises from the release of specific forms of physical energy or barriers to normal flow of energy.

internal respiration The movement or diffusion of oxygen molecules from the red blood cells into the tissue cells.

interstitial fluid The extracellular fluid located between the cell wall and the capillary wall.

intervertebral disc Cartilage-like discs that lie between the body of each vertebra and act as shock absorbers.

intervertebral foramina A notch through which nerves pass in the inferior lateral side of the vertebra.

intracellular fluid Fluid within the cells.

intracranial hypertension Increased intracranial pressure.

intraosseous Within the bone substance.

intubation Passing a tube into a body aperture. Endotracheal intubation is the insertion of a breathing tube through the mouth or nose into the trachea to provide an airway for oxygen or an anesthetic gas.

ipsilateral On the same side.

ischemia Local and temporary deficiency of blood supply due to obstruction of circulation to a body part or tissue.

ischemic sensitivity The sensitivity of the cells of a tissue to the lack of oxygen and usefulness of anaerobic metabolism before cell death occurs.

jaw thrust A maneuver that enables the airway of a trauma patient to be opened while the head and cervical spine are manually maintained in a neutral inline position.

jugular vein distention (JVD) Backup of pressure on the right side of the heart resulting in venous pooling and neck vein distention (engorgement) due to decreased filling of the left heart and reduced left heart output.

kinematics The process of looking at the mechanism of injury of an incident to determine what injuries are likely to have resulted from the forces and motion and changes in motion involved. The science of motion.

kinetic energy (KE) Energy available from movement. Function of the weight of an item and its speed. KE = one-half of the mass times the velocity squared.

kyphosis A forward, humplike curvature of the spine commonly associated with the aging process. Kyphosis may be caused by aging, rickets, or tuberculosis of the spine.

laws of motion Scientific laws relating to motion. Newton's first law of motion: A body at rest will remain at rest and a body in motion will remain in motion unless acted upon by some outside force.

ligament A band of tough, fibrous tissue connecting bone to bone.

ligamentum arteriosum A remnant of fetal circulation and point of fixation at the arch of the aorta.

logroll A way to turn a person with a possible spine injury from one side to the other or completely over while manually protecting the spine from excessive, dangerous movement. Used to place patients with a suspected unstable spine onto a longboard.

lucid interval Period of normal mental functioning between periods of disorientation, unconsciousness, or mental illness.

lumbar spine Part of the spinal column found at the lower back inferior to the thoracic spine, containing the five lumbar vertebrae (L1–L5).

mass (multiple) casualty incident (MCI) An incident (such as a plane crash, building collapse, or fire) that produces a large number of victims from one mechanism, at one place and at the same time.

mass The victim's weight.

mean arterial pressure The average pressure in the vascular system, estimated by adding one-third of the pulse pressure to the diastolic pressure.

mechanical energy Form of energy dealing with movement.

mediastinum The middle of the thoracic cavity containing the heart, great vessels, trachea, mainstem bronchi, and esophagus.

medulla (medulla oblongata) Part of the brain stem. The medulla is the primary regulatory center of autonomic control of the cardiovascular system.

meninges Three membranes that cover the brain tissue and the spinal cord.

metabolic acidosis Acidosis resulting from increase in acids other than carbonic acid.

metabolism The sum of all physical and chemical changes that take place within an organism; all energy and material transformations that occur within living cells.

minute volume The amount of air exchanged each minute; calculated by multiplying the volume of each breath (tidal volume) by the number of breaths per minute (rate).

myocardial contusion A bruising of the heart or the heart muscle.

myocardium The middle and thickest layer of the heart wall; composed of cardiac muscle.

nares (singular: naris) The openings in the nose that allow passage of the air from the outside to the throat. The anterior nares are the nostrils. The posterior nares are a pair of openings in the back of the nasal cavity where it connects with the upper throat.

nasopharyngeal airway An airway that is placed in the nostril and follows the floor of the nasal cavity directly posterior to the nasopharynx. This airway is commonly tolerated by patients with a gag reflex.

nasopharynx The upper portion of the airway, situated above the soft palate.

neural arches Two curved sides of the vertebrae.

neurogenic shock Shock that occurs when a cervical spine injury damages the spinal cord above where the nerves of the sympathetic nervous system exit.

newborn A child from birth to 6 weeks of age.

nonpatent airway An obstructed airway.

nonrebreather reservoir mask (NRB) An oxygen mask with a reservoir bag and nonrebreather valves that allow the exiting of exhaled air. It delivers high oxygen concentrations of between 85% and 100% to the patient when attached to a high-liter-flow oxygen source.

obtundation A sensory dullness.

occipital condyles The two rounded knuckle-like bumps at the end of the occipital bone at the back of the head.

oculomotor nerve The third cranial nerve; controls pupillary constriction.

odontoid process The toothlike protrusion on the upper surface of the second vertebra (axis) around which the first cervical vertebra (atlas) turns, allowing the head to rotate through approximately 180 degrees.

offline medical direction Written protocols that can direct most prehospital care.

oncotic pressure Pressure that determines the amount of fluid within the vascular space.

online medical direction Medical direction that allows the prehospital care provider to discuss patient care over the radio or phone while in the field.

open fracture A fracture of a bone in which the skin is broken.

open pneumothorax (sucking chest wound) A penetrating wound to the chest causes the chest wall to be opened, producing a preferential pathway for air moving from the outside environment into the thorax.

oropharyngeal airway An airway that, when placed in the oropharynx superior to the tongue, holds the tongue forward to assist in maintaining an open airway. It is only used in patients with no gag reflex.

oropharynx The central portion of the pharynx lying between the soft palate and the upper portion of the epiglottis.

osmosis The movement of water (or other solvent) across a membrane from an area that is hypotonic to an area that is hypertonic.

osteoporosis A loss of normal bone density with thinning of bone tissue and the growth of small holes in the bone. The disorder may cause pain (especially in the lower back), frequent broken bones, loss of body height, and various poorly formed parts of the body. Commonly a part of the normal aging process.

overtriage The problem of minimally or noninjured patients being taken to trauma centers.

oxygen consumption The volume of oxygen consumed by the body in 1 minute.

palpation Process of examining by application of the hands or fingers to the external surface of the body to detect evidence of disease, abnormalities, or underlying injury.

paradoxical motion The motion caused by the combination of the lower pressure in the chest and the higher atmospheric pressure outside the chest that causes a flail segment to move inward, rather than outward, during inspiration.

paradoxical pulse Condition in which the patient's systolic blood pressure drops more than 10 to 15 mm Hg during each inspiration, usually due to the effect of increased intrathoracic pressure.

paraanesthesia Loss of sensation in the lower extremities.

paraplegia Paralysis of the lower extremities.

parasympathetic acute stress reaction Slows bodily functions and may result in syncope.

parasympathetic nervous system The division of the nervous system that maintains normal body functions.

paresis Undue localized weakness or partial (less than total) paralysis related in some cases to nerve inflammation or injury.

parietal pleura A thin membrane that lines the inner side of the thoracic cavity.

Parkland formula Formula for fluid replacement of the burned patient.

partial-thickness (second-degree) burns Burns to both the epidermis and dermis. Skin presents with reddened areas; blisters; or open, weeping wounds.

patent airway An open unobstructed airway of sufficient size to allow for normal volumes of air exchange.

pathophysiology The study of how normal physiologic processes are altered by disease or injury.

PEARRL Pupils equal and round, reactive to light. The term used when checking the patient's eyes to determine if they are round, appear normal, and appropriately react to light by constricting, or whether they are abnormal and unresponsive. Generally the presence of consensual reflex is included in this examination term.

pediatric trauma score (PTS) A clinical scoring system based on clinical information that has been known to be predictive of severity of injury and can be used for triage decision making.

pediatric Dealing with children; dealing with injuries and diseases affecting children (birth to 16 years of age).

penetrating trauma   Trauma when an object penetrates the skin. Generally produces both permanent and temporary cavities.

percutaneous transtracheal ventilation (PTV)   A procedure where a 16-gauge or larger needle through which the patient is ventilated is inserted directly into the lumen of the trachea through the cricothyroid membrane or directly through the tracheal wall.

perfusion   Fluid passing through an organ or a part of the body. Also, the surrounding and bathing of a tissue or cell with blood or fluid parts of the blood.

pericardial space   A potential space existing between the heart muscle (myocardium) and the pericardium.

pericardial tamponade   Compression of the heart by blood collecting in the pericardial sac, which surrounds the heart muscle (myocardium); also sometimes called cardiac tamponade.

pericardiocentesis   A procedure to remove accumulated blood inside the pericardial space.

pericardium   A tough, fibrous, flexible but inelastic membrane that surrounds the heart.

peristalsis   The propulsive, muscular movements of the intestines.

peritoneal space   Space in the anterior abdominal cavity that contains the bowel, spleen, liver, stomach, and gallbladder. The peritoneal space is lined with the peritoneum.

peritoneum   Lining of the abdominal cavity.

peritonitis   Inflammation of the peritoneum.

phantom pain   The experience of sensation in the missing part or limb after amputation.

pharynx   The throat; a tubelike structure that is a passage for both the breathing and digestive tracts. Oropharynx: area of the pharynx posterior to the mouth; nasopharynx: area of the pharynx beyond the posterior nares of the nose.

pia mater   A thin vascular membrane closely adhering to the brain and spinal cord and proximal portions of the nerves. The innermost of the three meningeal membranes that cover the brain.

pleura   A thin membrane that lines the inner side of the thoracic cavity and the lungs. The part that lines the thoracic cavity is called the parietal pleura; the fold covering the lung is called the visceral pleura.

pleural fluid   Fluid that creates surface tension between the two pleural membranes and causes them to cling together.

pneumatic antishock garment (PASG)   A garment designed to put pressure on the lower portion of the body and prevent pooling of blood in the abdomen and pelvis. Also called military or medical antishock trousers (MAST).

pneumothorax   Injury that produces air in the pleural space; commonly associated with a collapsed lung. A pneumothorax can be open with an opening through the chest wall to the outside or closed resulting from blunt trauma or a spontaneous collapse.

postevent phase   This phase begins as soon as the energy from the crash is absorbed and the patient is traumatized. The phase of prehospital care that includes response time, "golden period," and critique of a call.

preevent phase   This phase includes all of the events that precede the incident (e.g., ingestion of drugs and alcohol) and conditions that predate the incident (e.g., acute or pre-existing medical conditions). This phase includes injury prevention and preparedness.

preload   The volume and pressure of the blood coming into the heart from the systemic circulatory system (venous return). The process outside of the heart in the vena cava.

premature ventricular contraction   A premature, irregular, extra contraction of the ventricles due to an ectopic stimulus, causing a contraction rather than the normal stimuli from the normal pacing node. Second most common abnormal rhythm of the heart.

presbycusis   Gradual decline in hearing.

presbyopia   Farsightedness.

preschooler   A child with the body size and physical development normally found in children between 2 and 6 years of age. An arbitrary grouping of children based on the similar physical characteristics common to these ages.

priapism   Occurs when the penis remains erect, usually for a long period. It may be caused by a urinary stone or an injury to the lower spinal column.

primary brain injury   Direct trauma to the brain and associated vascular injuries.

primary injuries of blasts   Injuries that are caused by the pressure wave of the blast (e.g., pulmonary bleeding, pneumothorax, perforation of the gastrointestinal tract).

primary survey   The initial assessment of airway, breathing, circulation, disability, and environment/expose to identify and manage any life-threatening injuries.

psychogenic shock   A temporary neurogenic shock as a result of psychological stress (fainting).

pulmonary contusion   A bruising of the lungs. This can be secondary to blunt or penetrating trauma.

pulmonary diffusion   Movement of oxygen from the alveoli across the alveolar capillary membrane and into the red blood cells or the plasma.

pulmonary function   Controlled patent airway, ventilation, diffusion, and perfusion, resulting in arterial blood that contains adequate oxygen for aerobic metabolism and a proper level of carbon dioxide to maintain tissue acid-base balance.

pulse oximeter A machine that provides measurement of arterial oxyhemoglobin saturation. It is determined by measuring the absorption ratio of red and infrared light passed through the tissue.

pulse pressure The increase in pressure (surge) that is created as each new bolus of blood leaves the left ventricle. Also, the difference between the systolic and diastolic blood pressures (systolic pressure minus diastolic pressure equals pulse pressure).

quadriplegia Paralysis of all four extremities.

raccoon eyes (periorbital ecchymosis) Very distinct ecchymotic area around each eye, limited by the orbital margins.

radiation The direct transfer of energy from a warm object to a cooler one by infrared radiation.

rapid deceleration mechanism A series of three collisions that occur when a vehicle suddenly ceases forward motion. Collision of (1) the vehicle, (2) the occupant inside the vehicle, and (3) the occupant's internal organs.

rapid sequence intubation A method of patient preparation for intubation that includes pharmacologic adjuncts for sedation and muscle relaxation.

residual volume Air that remains trapped in the alveoli and bronchi that cannot be forcibly exhaled.

respiration The total ventilatory and circulatory steps involved in the exchange of oxygen and carbon dioxide between the outside atmosphere and the cells of the body. Sometimes in medicine limited to meaning breathing and the steps in ventilation.

respiratory tract The pathway for air movement between the outside air and the alveoli; includes the nasal cavity, oral cavity, pharynx, larynx, trachea, bronchi, and lungs.

response time From the time an incident occurs until arrival of emergency medical services on scene.

retrograde amnesia Loss of memory for events and situations just preceding the time (immediate preinsult period) of the patient's injury or illness. Also, loss of memory for past events.

retroperitoneal space Space in the posterior abdominal cavity that contains the kidneys, ureters, bladder, reproductive organs, inferior vena cava, abdominal aorta, pancreas, a portion of the duodenum, colon, and rectum.

revised trauma score A method for scoring and quantifying the severity of trauma in pediatric patients.

rotational impact When one vehicle strikes the front or rear side of another, causing it to rotate away from the point of impact. Also, when one corner of the vehicle strikes an immovable object or one moving slower or

in the opposite direction of the vehicle, resulting in it rotating.

rule of nines A topographic breakdown (mostly of 9% and 18% portions) of the body in order to estimate the amount of body surface covered by burns.

sacral spine Part of the spinal column below the lumbar spine containing the five sacral vertebrae (S1–S5), which are connected by immovable joints to form the sacrum. The sacrum is the weight-bearing base of the spinal column and is also a part of the pelvic girdle.

safety Evaluation of all possible dangers and ensuring that no unreasonable threats or risks still exist.

SAR Search and rescue.

scalp The outermost covering of the head.

scene Environment to be evaluated in which injury occurred. In a motor vehicle crash this includes evaluation of the number of vehicles, the forces that acted upon each, and the degree and type of damage to each.

school-age child A child with the body size and physical development normally found in children between about 6 and 12 years of age. An arbitrary grouping of children based upon the similar physical characteristics common to these ages.

secondary survey Head-to-toe evaluation of the trauma patient. This assessment is only done after the primary survey is complete and there are no immediate life-threatening problems; usually done en route in urgent patients.

secondary brain injury An extension of the magnitude of the primary brain injury by factors that result in a larger, more permanent neurologic deficit.

secondary injuries of blasts Injuries that occur when the victim is struck by flying glass, falling mortar, or other debris from the blast.

semipermeable membrane Membrane that will allow fluids (solvents) but not the dissolved substance to pass through it.

senescence The process of aging.

sensory examination A gross examination of sensory capability and response to determine the presence or absence of loss of sensation in each of the four extremities.

sepsis Infection.

septic shock Shock resulting from locally active hormones, due to widespread systemic infection, causing damage to the walls of blood vessels, producing both peripheral vasodilation and a leakage of fluid from the capillaries into the interstitial space.

shear Change-of-speed force resulting in a cutting or tearing of body parts.

shock A widespread lack of tissue perfusion with oxygenated red blood cells that leads to anaerobic metabolism and decreased energy production.

sinoatrial node   Node at junction of superior vena cava with right cardiac atrium; regarded as the pacing or starting point of the heartbeat. In healthy patients, pacing from this node causes atrial contraction, is slowed, and then results in producing ensuing contraction of the ventricles.

situation   Events, relationships, and roles of those parties who, with the patient, were involved in a call. The situation (e.g., domestic dispute, single vehicle crash without an apparent reason, elderly person living alone, a shooting) is important in scene assessment.

skull (cranium)   Several bones that fuse into a single structure during childhood.

sniffing position   A slightly superior anterior position of the midface.

spinal shock   A term that refers to an injury to the spinal cord that results in a temporary loss of sensory and motor function.

spinal stenosis   Narrowing of the spinal canal.

spinous process   Tail-like structure on the posterior region of the vertebrae.

sprain   An injury in which ligaments are stretched or even partially torn.

strain   A soft tissue injury or muscle spasm that occurs around a joint anywhere in the musculature.

stroke volume   The volume of blood pumped out by each contraction (stroke) of the left ventricle.

subarachnoid hemorrhage   Bleeding into the cerebrospinal–fluid—filled space.

subarachnoid space   Space between the pia mater proper and arachnoid membrane; contains cerebrospinal fluid and meningeal veins. The sub arachnoid space is a common site of subdural hematomas.

subcutaneous layer   Layer of skin just under the dermis that is a combination of elastic and fibrous tissue as well as fat deposits.

subdural hematoma   A collection of blood between the dura mater and the arachnoid membrane.

superficial (first-degree) burns   Burns to the epidermis only; red, inflamed, and painful skin.

supine hypotension syndrome   Decrease in blood pressure caused by compression of the vena cava by the uterus.

surgical cricothyrotomy   A procedure to open a patient's airway that should be considered a "last resort." It is a procedure that is accomplished by cutting a slit into the cricoid cartilage in the neck to open the airway into the trachea.

sympathetic acute stress reaction   The "fight-or-flight" response in which bodily functions increase and pain masking occurs.

sympathetic nervous system   Division of the nervous system that produces the fight-or-flight response.

synovial fluid   Fluid found inside joints.

systemic vascular resistance   The amount of resistance to the flow of blood through the vessels. It increases as the vessel constricts. Any change in lumen diameter or vessel elasticity can influence the amount of resistance.

systole   Ventricular contraction.

systolic blood pressure   Peak blood pressure produced by the force of the contraction (systole) of the ventricles of the heart.

tachycardia   Abnormally fast rate of heartbeats; defined as a rate over 100 beats per minute in an adult.

tachypnea   Increased breathing rate.

tendon   A band of tough, inelastic, fibrous tissue that connects a muscle to bone.

tension pneumothorax   Condition when the air pressure in the pleural space exceeds the outside atmospheric pressure and cannot escape. The affected side becomes hyperinflated, compressing the lung on the involved side and shifting the mediastinum to partially collapse the other lung. A tension pneumothorax is usually progressive and is an imminently life-threatening condition.

tentorial herniation   Normally the cerebrum (brain) is supratentorial. When part of the brain is pushed down through the incisura as a result of increased intracranial pressure, tentorial herniation occurs.

tentorium cerebelli (tentorium)   An infolding of the dura that forms a covering over the cerebellum. The tentorium is a part of the floor of the upper skull just below the brain (cerebrum).

tertiary injuries of blasts   The third group of injuries sustained in a sequence (or pattern) of injury-producing events, such as explosions. Injuries that occur when the victim becomes a missile and is thrown against some object. These injuries are similar to those sustained in ejections from vehicles, in falls from significant heights, or when the victim is thrown against an object by the force wave resulting from an explosion. Tertiary injuries are usually obvious injuries.

thoracic spine   The part of the spinal column between the cervical spine (superiorly) and the lumbar spine (inferiorly) containing the 12 thoracic vertebrae (T1–T12). The 12 pairs of ribs connect to the thoracic vertebrae.

thorax (thoracic cavity)   Hollow cylinder supported by 12 pairs of ribs that articulate posteriorly with the thoracic spine and 10 pairs that articulate anteriorly with the sternum. The 2 lowest pairs are only fastened posteriorly (to the vertebrae) and are called floating ribs. The thoracic cavity is defined and separated inferiorly by the diaphragm.

tidal volume Normal volume of air exchanged with each ventilation. About 500 mL of air is exchanged between the lungs and the atmosphere with each breath in a healthy adult at rest.

toddler A child with the body size and physical development normally found in children between about 1 and 2 years of age.

tonsil-tip catheter Rigid suction catheter designed for rapid removal of large amounts of fluid, vomitus, blood, and debris from the mouth and pharynx to avoid aspiration.

total lung capacity The total volume of air in the lungs after a forced inhalation.

toxemia Distribution throughout the body of poisonous products of bacteria (toxins) growing in a focal or local site.

trauma chin lift This maneuver is ideally used to relieve a variety of anatomic airway obstructions in patients who are breathing spontaneously. It is accomplished by grasping the chin and lower incisors and then lifting to pull the mandible forward.

trauma jaw thrust This maneuver allows an open airway with little or no movement of the head and cervical spine. The mandible is thrust forward by placing the thumbs on each zygomatic arch and placing the index and long fingers under the mandible and at the same angle, thrusting the mandible forward.

traumatic aneurysm An abnormal dilation, bursting, or tearing of a major blood vessel (usually an artery) caused by or related to an injury.

traumatic asphyxia Blunt and crushing injuries to the chest and abdomen with marked increase of intravascular pressure, producing rupture of the capillaries.

Trendelenburg position Simultaneous lowering of the patient's head while elevating the patient's legs. Usually done by raising the foot end of a flat bed or longboard higher than the head end. In this position (with the abdomen higher than the thorax) the weight of the abdominal contents presses on the diaphragm, producing some ventilatory difficulty. A modified Trendelenburg position with the head and torso horizontal and only the legs elevated will minimize ventilatory problems.

triage French word meaning "to sort"; a process in which a group of patients is sorted according to their priority of need for care. When only several patients are involved, triage involves alternating from patient to patient, meeting all of the patients' highest priority needs first, then moving to lower priority items. In a mass casualty incident with a large number of patients involved, triage is done by determining both urgency and potential for survival.

tumble End-over-end motion. Bullets commonly tumble when resistance is met by the leading edge of the missile.

undertriage The problem that arises when seriously injured patients are not recognized as such and are mistakenly taken to nontrauma centers.

up-and-over pathway The body's forward motion carries it up and over the steering wheel; the chest or abdomen commonly impacts the steering wheel and the head strikes the windshield. In the semisitting position common in passenger vehicles, once the down-and-under motion has ended as the knees are stopped by the dashboard, the body then continues in an up-and-over movement. In some trucks, where the driver is sitting fully upright with his feet stopped by the pedals, the up-and-over movement may occur initially.

vagal Dealing with stimulation of the vagus (tenth cranial) nerve. The parasympathetic system's response that slows the heart rate and reduces the force of contractions, keeping the body within workable limits. This response can normally override the sympathetic nervous system's chemical release, keeping the heart rate in an acceptable range. Accidental vagal stimulation, however, can result in producing an undesirable bradycardia, further reducing the patient's cardiac output and circulation.

vagus nerve The tenth cranial nerve; when stimulated, slows the heart rate regardless of levels of catecholamines. It contains motor and sensory functions and a wider distribution than any of the other cranial nerves.

velocity Quickness of motion. Speed, as in the speed of a moving mass.

ventilation Movement of air into and out of the lungs through the normal breathing process. The mechanical process by which air moves from the atmosphere outside the body through the mouth, nose, pharynx, trachea, bronchi, and bronchioles, and into and out of the alveoli. To ventilate a patient is to provide positive-pressure inspirations with a ventilating device, such as a bag-valve-mask device, and then alternately allowing time for passive exhalation to occur; used in patients who are apneic or who cannot provide adequate ventilation for themselves.

vertebra Any of the 33 bony segments of the spinal column.

vertebral body Area of the vertebrae that bears most of the weight of the spine.

vertebral foramina Opening in the vertebral body.

visceral pleura A thin membrane that covers the outer surface of each lung.

whistle-stop catheter (whistle-tip catheter) A soft catheter used for suctioning the nasal passage, deep oropharynx, or endotracheal tube; allows for controlled intermittent suction. Its name is derived from the opening (whistle-stop) found in the side of the proximal end of the catheter. Suction is not produced at the distal tip until this hole or port is covered with one of the operator's fingers, producing a closed system to the opening at the distal tip.

zygomatic arches   The bones that form the superior area of the cheeks of the face. Laterally, superior to the molars, these extend more anteriorly than the maxilla, giving the individual some of his or her unique facial structure; commonly called the cheekbones.

Index

Page numbers followed by *f* indicate figures; *t,* tables; *b,* boxes.

Geriatric trauma—cont'd
  mechanism of injury, 343-344
  secondary survey, 345-347
  legal considerations of, 348
  management of, 347-348
Glasgow Coma Scale (GCS), 72-73, 73f, 213, 213t, 323
Golden hour, 4, 65
Golden Period, 366-367
Grand mal seizures, 218
Groin straps for sitting mobilization, 260-261
Ground transport, 359
Gunshot to chest wall, 146f
Gunshot wound scenario, 396b

H
Haddon, William J., 16
Haddon matrix, 16, 17f
Hampton, Oscar, 5
Havana Harbor, 377
Hazardous materials (HAZMAT), 399
Head
  examination of, 79
  immobilization of, 244
  inline position of, maintenance of, 243-244
  manual inline stabilization of, 241
  weight of, 231
Head injuries
  from blunt trauma, 36-37, 36f, 38f, 47, 47f
  from penetrating trauma, 56-57
Head trauma, 206-223
  anatomy of, 206-207
  assessment of, 212-214
  management of, 217-218
  pathophysiology of, 208-212
  physiology of, 208
  specific conditions, 214-216
  transportation of, 218-219
Hearing and aging, 341
Heart, 164-165
  blood pumping through, 164f-165f
  trapped between sternum and thoracic wall, 150f
Heart muscle, damage to, 175
Heart rates
  during pregnancy, 180, 200
  of athletes, 180
Heart valves, disruption of, 176
Heat. See Thermal trauma.
Heat cramps, 303-304
Heat exhaustion, 303
Heat index, 305b
Heat-related conditions and injuries, 294-305
  burns, 294-303
  systemic, 303-305
Heat stress index, 304
Heat stroke, 304-305
Height, range for children, 319t
Helicopter hit by RPG round scenario, 394b
Helicopters, 359
  evacuation with, 378
Helmet removal in spine management, 268-270
Hematologic failure, 176-177

Hematomas, 215-217
HemCon dressing, 386
Hemoglobin-based oxygen carriers, 186
Hemopericardium, 151
Hemopneumothorax, 150
Hemorrhage, 178, 277
  assessment of, 280-281
  in pediatric trauma, 318
  management of, 70-71, 284
    during shock, 182
    external, 369-370
    on battlefield, 386
    retroperitoneal, 184
Hemorrhagic shock, 172-173
  classification of, 173t
  pneumatic antishock garment for, 184
Hemothorax, 150, 150f
Hemostasis, 386
Hepatic failure, 177
Hespan. See Hetastarch (Hespan).
Hetastarch (Hespan), 186, 389-390
Highway Safety Act of 1966, 378
Hip fractures, 343
Holy Roman Empire, military health care system, 377
Home injuries, statistics related to, 12b
Hospital triage, 401
Hospitals in Holy Roman Empire, 377
Humerus fractures, blood loss with, 370
Hydrofluoric acid, 301
Hydrogen fluoride, 301
Hypercapnia, cause of in head trauma, 210
Hypercarbia, 138
Hyperextension, 234
  prevention of, 242f
Hyperflexion, 234
Hyperglycemia, cause of in brain injury, 210
Hyperrotation, 234
Hypertension, intracranial, 209, 211-212
Hyperthermia, primary, 307
Hypertonic crystalloid solutions, 186
Hypertonic saline, 186, 389-390
Hypocapnia, cause of in head trauma, 210
Hypoglycemia, cause of in brain injury, 210
Hypopharynx, 94
Hypotension, cause of in brain injury, 210
Hypothalamus, shell of, 293
Hypothermia, 307-310
  assessment of, 309
  definition of, 307
  in elderly, 343
  management of, 309-310
  severity of, 307-308
Hypoventilation, 95
Hypovolemia in pediatric trauma, 328
Hypovolemic shock, 172-174
  assessment of, 179t
Hypoxia, 179-180, 340
  cause of in head trauma, 209-210
  endotracheal intubation for, 296
  in pediatric trauma, 317-318
  with gag reflex, rapid sequence intubation for, 296